T0200206

THE WASHINGTON MANUAL™
OF EMERGENCY MEDICINE

THE WASHINGTON MANUAL™
OF EMERGENCY MEDICINE

Mark D. Levine, MD, FACEP
Associate Professor, Division of Emergency Medicine
Course Director, Medical Student Education
Washington University School of Medicine
Assistant Medical Director, St. Louis Fire Department
St. Louis, Missouri

W. Scott Gilmore, MD, EMT-P, FACEP, FAEMS
Assistant Professor, Division of Emergency Medicine
Washington University School of Medicine
Attending Physician SSM Health St. Mary's Hospital
Medical Director, St. Louis Fire Department
St. Louis, Missouri

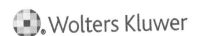. Wolters Kluwer

Philadelphia • Baltimore • New York • London
Buenos Aires • Hong Kong • Sydney • Tokyo

Acquisitions Editor: Sharon Zinner
Development Editor: Ashley Fischer
Editorial Coordinator: Alexis Pozonsky
Marketing Manager: Rachel Mante Leung
Production Project Manager: Linda Van Pelt
Design Coordinator: Holly Reid McLaughlin
Manufacturing Coordinator: Beth Welsh
Prepress Vendor: SPi Global

Library of Congress Cataloging-in-Publication Data
Names: Levine, Mark D., MD editor. | Gilmore, William S. (William Scott), editor. | Washington University (Saint Louis, Mo.). School of Medicine. Division of Emergency Medicine, issuing body.
Title: The Washington manual of emergency medicine / [edited by] Mark D. Levine, William S. Gilmore.
Other titles: Manual of emergency medicine
Description: First edition. | Philadelphia : Wolters Kluwer, [2018] | Includes bibliographical references and index.
Identifiers: LCCN 2017029417 | ISBN 9781496379252
Subjects: | MESH: Emergency Service, Hospital | Emergency Medicine–methods | Emergencies
Classification: LCC RC86.7 | NLM WX 215 | DDC 616.02/5–dc23 LC record available at https://lccn.loc.gov/2017029417

We dedicate this manual to all of our teachers and mentors, including our prehospital providers, nurses, and nursing staff, and to all of those who continue to support and teach us along the way.

Preface

We have the honor and privilege of creating the first edition of the *Washington Manual of Emergency Medicine*. The Washington Manual series is known world over as a high quality resource for students and residents alike, and we are thrilled to join this esteemed publication series.

We would like to thank the residents and faculty who took time out of their busy schedules to write and review the chapters. Special appreciation goes out to Dr. Brent Ruoff, who provided the scheduling and support to allow us to undertake this endeavor. We cannot express enough gratitude to Andrea Ramirez who had the daunting job of keeping all of the paperwork in order. Thanks also to Dr. Tom DeFer, who guided the publishers in our direction. And to our families, without whose support we could never have achieved what we have today, our love and gratitude goes without saying.

Mark D. Levine, MD, FACEP
W. Scott Gilmore, MD, EMT-P, FACEP, FAEMS

Contributors

Enyo Ablordeppey, MD, MPH
Assistant Professor
Director of Critical Care Ultrasound
  Training Program
Washington University School of Medicine
St. Louis, Missouri

Aldo Andino, MD
Resident
Division of Emergency Medicine
Washington University School of Medicine
Barnes-Jewish Hospital and St. Louis
  Children's Hospital
St. Louis, Missouri

Chandra Aubin, MD
Associate Professor
Division of Emergency Medicine
Washington University School of Medicine
St. Louis, Missouri

Kevin Baumgartner, MD
Resident
Division of Emergency Medicine
Washington University School of Medicine
Barnes-Jewish Hospital and St. Louis
  Children's Hospital
St. Louis, Missouri

Rebecca Bavolek, MD
Associate Clinical Professor
Department of Emergency Medicine
David Geffen School of Medicine at UCLA
  Ronald Reagan UCLA Medical Center
Los Angeles, California

Vincent Boston, MD
Resident
Division of Emergency Medicine
Washington University School of Medicine
Barnes-Jewish Hospital and St. Louis
  Children's Hospital
St. Louis, Missouri

Joseph Brancheck, MD
Resident
Department of Internal Medicine
Washington University School of Medicine
St. Louis, Missouri

Christopher Brooks, MD, FACEP
Associate Professor
Division of Emergency Medicine
Washington University School of Medicine
St. Louis, Missouri

Blake Bruton, RN, MD
Resident
Washington University School of Medicine
Barnes-Jewish Hospital and St. Louis
  Children's Hospital
St. Louis, Missouri

Robert Bucelli, MD, PhD
Assistant Professor
Department of Neurology
Washington University School of Medicine
St. Louis, Missouri

Matthew Burford, MD
Clinical Fellow
Department of Neurology
Washington University School of Medicine
St. Louis, Missouri

Bob Cambridge, DO, MPH
Attending Physician
R. Adams Cowley Shock Trauma Center
Batimore, Maryland

Christopher R. Carpenter, MD, MSc
Associate Professor
Division of Emergency Medicine
Washington University School of Medicine
St. Louis, Missouri

Douglas Char, MD, MA
Professor
Washington University School of Medicine
St. Louis, Missouri

Stephanie Charshafian, MD
Chief Resident
Division of Emergency Medicine
Washington University School of
  Medicine
Barnes-Jewish Hospital and St. Louis
  Children's Hospital
St. Louis, Missouri

Rahul Chhana, MD
Resident
Department of Medicine
Washington University School of Medicine
St. Louis, Missouri

Kelly Counts, APRN, ACNP-BC, FNP-C
NP/PA Lead–Emergency Services
Washington University School of Medicine
St. Louis, Missouri

Christina Creel-Bulos, RN-BSN, MD
Resident
Division of Emergency Medicine
Washington University School of Medicine
Barnes-Jewish Hospital and St. Louis Children's Hospital
St. Louis, Missouri

Kevin M. Cullison, MD
Instructor
Division of Emergency Medicine
Washington University School of Medicine
St. Louis, Missouri

Tracy Cushing, FNP-BC, ANP-BC, NP-C
Nurse Practitioner
Division of Emergency Medicine
Washington University School of Medicine
Barnes-Jewish Hospital
St. Louis, Missouri

Julianne S. Dean, DO
Fellow
Anesthesia Critical Care, BCEM
Department of Anesthesia
Washington University School of Medicine
Barnes-Jewish Hospital
St. Louis, Missouri

Tanya Devnani, MD
Resident
Division of Medicine
Washington University School of Medicine
St. Louis, Missouri

Maia Dorsett, MD, PhD
Clinical Fellow, Emergency Medical Services
Division of Emergency Medicine
Washington University School of Medicine
St. Louis, Missouri

William Dribben, MD
Assistant Professor
Division of Emergency Medicine
Washington University School of Medicine
St. Louis, Missouri

S. Eliza Dunn, MD
Assistant Professor
Division of Emergency Medicine
Washington University School of Medicine
Washington University Medical Sciences Outreach Lead
Monsanto Company
St. Louis, Missouri

Kurt Eifling, MD
Resident
Division of Emergency Medicine
Washington University School of Medicine
Barnes-Jewish Hospital and St. Louis Children's Hospital
St. Louis, Missouri

Carol Faulk, MD
Resident
Department of Internal Medicine
Washington University School of Medicine
Barnes Jewish Hospital
St. Louis, Missouri

Caitlin Fuqua, MD
Resident
Division of Emergency Medicine
Washington University School of Medicine
Barnes Jewish Hospital and St. Louis Children's Hospital
St. Louis, Missouri

Gary M. Gaddis, MD, PhD
Professor
Division of Emergency Medicine
Washington University School of Medicine
St. Louis, Missouri

W. Scott Gilmore, MD, EMT-P, FACEP, FAEMS
Assistant Professor
Division of Emergency Medicine
Washington University School of Medicine
Attending Physician
SSM Health St. Mary's Hospital
Medical Director
St. Louis Fire Department
St. Louis, Missouri

P. Gabriel Miranda Gomez, MD
Resident
Division of Emergency Medicine
Washington University School of Medicine
Barnes-Jewish Hospital and St. Louis
   Children's Hospital
St. Louis, Missouri

Daniel S. Greenstein, MD
Resident
Division of Emergency Medicine
Washington University School of
   Medicine
Barnes-Jewish Hospital and St. Louis
   Children's Hospital
St. Louis, Missouri

Matthew Greer, MD
Critical Care Fellow
Department of Medicine
Washington University School of
   Medicine
Barnes-Jewish Hospital
St. Louis, Missouri

Martin H. Gregory, MD
Resident
Department of Medicine
Washington University School of
   Medicine
St. Louis, Missouri

Maureen Gross, MD
Clinical Fellow
Sports Medicine
Department of Orthopedics
Washington University School of
   Medicine
St. Louis, Missouri

Emily Harkins, MD MPH
Resident
Division of Emergency Medicine
Washington University School of Medicine
Barnes-Jewish Hospital and St. Louis
   Children's Hospital
St. Louis, Missouri

Stephen Hasak, MD, MPH
Clinical Fellow
Division of Gastroenterology
Department of Medicine
Washington University School of Medicine
Barnes-Jewish Hospital
St. Louis, Missouri

Laura Heitsch, MD
Assistant Professor
Division of Emergency Medicine and
   Department of Neurology
Washington University School of Medicine
St. Louis, Missouri

SueLin M. Hilbert, MD, MPH, FACEP
Assistant Professor
Division of Emergency Medicine
Washington University School of Medicine
St. Louis, Missouri

Christopher Holthaus, MD
Assistant Professor
Division of Emergency Medicine
Washington University School of Medicine
St. Louis, Missouri

Lucy Hung Humberg, JD, MD
Chief Resident
Division of Emergency Medicine
Washington University School of Medicine
Barnes-Jewish Hospital and St. Louis
   Children's Hospital
St. Louis, Missouri

Stacey House, MD, PhD
Assistant Professor Director of Research in
   Emergency Medicine
Division of Emergency Medicine
Washington University School of Medicine
St. Louis, Missouri

Randall A. Howell, DO
Assistant Professor
Division of Emergency Medicine
Washington University School of
  Medicine
St. Louis, Missouri

Steven Hung, MD
Chief Resident
Division of Emergency Medicine
Washington University School of
  Medicine
Barnes-Jewish Hospital and St. Louis
  Children's Hospital
St. Louis, Missouri

Louis Jamtgaard, MD
Attending Physician
Department of Emergency Medicine
Mosaic Life Care
St. Joseph, Missouri

Reuben D. Johnson, MD
Assistant Professor
Division of Emergency Medicine
Washington University School of
  Medicine
St. Louis, Missouri

Randy Jotte, MD
Associate Professor
Division of Emergency Medicine
Washington University School of
  Medicine
St. Louis, Missouri

Deborah Shipley Kane, MD
Assistant Professor
Ultrasound Fellowship Director
Division of Emergency Medicine
Washington University School of
  Medicine
St. Louis, Missouri

Peter Kang, MD
Resident Physician
Department of Neurology
Washington University School of
  Medicine
Barnes-Jewish Hospital
St. Louis, Missouri

Jacob Keeperman, MD, FACEP,
FAEMS
Assistant Professor
Division of Critical Care Medicine
Assistant Professor
Division of Emergency Medicine
Washington University School of
  Medicine
St. Louis, Missouri

Grant Kleiber, MD
Assistant Professor
Department of Surgery, Division
  of Plastic and Reconstructive Surgery
Washington University School of Medicine
St. Louis, Missouri

Daniel C. Kolinsky, MD
Resident
Division of Emergency Medicine
Washington University School of Medicine
Barnes-Jewish Hospital and St. Louis
  Children's Hospital
St. Louis, Missouri

Christopher Lawrence, MD
Chief Resident
Division of Emergency Medicine
Washington University School of
  Medicine
Barnes-Jewish Hospital and St. Louis
  Children's Hospital
St. Louis, Missouri

Mark D. Levine, MD, FACEP
Associate Professor
Division of Emergency Medicine
Course Director
Medical Student Education
Washington University School of
  Medicine
Assistant Medical Director
St. Louis Fire Department
St. Louis, Missouri

Lawrence Lewis, MD
Professor
Division of Emergency Medicine
Washington University School of Medicine
St. Louis, Missouri

Stephen Y. Liang, MD, MPHS
Assistant Professor
Divisions of Emergency Medicine and
  Infectious Diseases
Washington University School of
  Medicine
St. Louis, Missouri

Chien-Jung Lin, MD, PhD
Fellow, Cardiovascular Division
Department of Medicine
Washington University School of Medicine
Barnes-Jewish Hospital
St. Louis, Missouri

David B. Liss, MD
Clinical Fellow
Medical Toxicology
Division of Emergency Medicine
Washington University School of
  Medicine
St. Louis, Missouri

Matthew C. Loftspring, MD, PhD
Resident
Department of Neurology
Washington University School of Medicine
Barnes-Jewish Hospital
St. Louis, Missouri

Lydia Luangruangrong, MD
Attending Physician
Kaiser Permanente
San Leandro/Freemont
Department of Emergency Medicine
San Francisco, California

Al Lulla, MD
Resident
Division of Emergency Medicine
Washington University School of Medicine
St. Louis, Missouri

Aurora Lybeck, MD
Clinical Instructor
Medical College of Wisconsin
Milwaukee, Wisconsin

Sara Manning, MD
Attending Physician
University of Maryland Medical Center
Baltimore, Maryland

Jordan Maryfield, MD
Resident
Department of Internal Medicine
Washington University School of Medicine
Barnes-Jewish Hospital
St. Louis, Missouri

Nicole Messenger, MD
Resident
Division of Emergency Medicine
Washington University School of Medicine
Barnes-Jewish Hospital and St. Louis
  Children's Hospital
St. Louis, Missouri

Christopher P. Miller, MD
Resident Physician
Division of Emergency Medicine
Washington University School of
  Medicine
Barnes-Jewish Hospital and St. Louis
  Children's Hospital
St. Louis, Missouri

Sahar Morkos El Hayek, MD
Resident
Division of Emergency Medicine
Washington University School of
  Medicine
Barnes-Jewish Hospital and St. Louis
  Children's Hospital
St. Louis, Missouri

Daniel K. Mullady, MD, FASGE
Associate Professor
Director
Interventional Endoscopy
Division of Gastroenterology
Department of Medicine
Washington University School of
  Medicine
St. Louis, Missouri

Sonya Naganathan, MD
Resident
Division of Emergency Medicine
Washington University School of
  Medicine
Barnes-Jewish Hospital and St. Louis
  Children's Hospital
St. Louis, Missouri

Joan Noelker, MD
Instructor
Division of Emergency Medicine
Washington University School of Medicine
St. Louis, Missouri

Alicia Oberle, MD
Clinical Fellow
Ultrasound
Division of Emergency Medicine
Washington University School of Medicine
Barnes-Jewish Hospital
St. Louis, Missouri

Lauren O'Grady, MD
Chief Resident
Division of Emergency Medicine
Washington University School of Medicine
Barnes-Jewish Hospital and St. Louis
  Children's Hospital
St. Louis, Missouri

David Page, MD
Fellow, Critical Care
Department of Medicine
Division of Pulmonary and Critical Care
  Medicine
Washington University School of
  Medicine
St. Louis, Missouri

Peter Panagos, MD, FACEP, FAHA
Associate Professor
Division of Emergency Medicine and
  Department of Neurology
Washington University School of
  Medicine
St. Louis, Missouri

Anna Arroyo Plasencia, MD, SFHM
Assistant Professor
Department of Medicine
Michigan Medicine
University of Michigan
Ann Arbor, Michigan

Robert Poirier, MD, MBA
Assistant Professor
Division of Emergency Medicine
Washington University School of Medicine
St. Louis, Missouri

Gregory M. Polites, MD, FACEP
Associate Professor
Division of Emergency Medicine
Washington University School of Medicine
St. Louis, Missouri

Louis H. Poppler, MD, MSCI
Resident
Division of Plastic and Reconstructive
  Surgery
Washington University School of Medicine
St. Louis, Missouri

Amanda Poskin, ANP
Department of Internal Medicine
Division of Pulmonary Medicine
Washington University School of Medicine
St. Louis, Missouri

Niall Prendergast, MD
Resident
Department of Internal Medicine
Washington University School of Medicine
Barnes-Jewish Hospital
St. Louis, Missouri

Gregory Ratti, MD
Instructor
Department of Hospital Medicine
Washington University School of Medicine
St. Louis, Missouri

Nicholas Renz, MD
Instructor
Division of Emergency Medicine
Washington University School of Medicine
St. Louis, Missouri

Carla Robinson-Rainey, ACNP-BC
Staff
Division of Emergency Medicine
Washington University School of Medicine
Barnes-Jewish Hospital
St. Louis, Missouri

Laura Ruble, MS, MD
Resident Physician
Division of Emergency Medicine
Washington University School of Medicine
Barnes-Jewish Hospital and St. Louis
  Children's Hospital
St. Louis, Missouri

Evan Schwarz, MD, FACEP, FACMT
Assistant Professor
Medical Toxicology Section Chief
Division of Emergency Medicine
Washington University School of
  Medicine
St. Louis, Missouri

David Seltzer, MD
Assistant Professor
Division of Emergency Medicine
Washington University School of Medicine
St. Louis, Missouri

Jeffrey Siegler, MD, EMT-P, EMT-T
Instructor
Division of Emergency Medicine
Washington University School of
  Medicine
St. Louis, Missouri

Elizabeth Silbermann, MD
Resident
Department of Neurology
Washington University School of Medicine
St. Louis, Missouri

Clark Samuel Smith, MD
Clinical Fellow
Emergency Medical Services
Denver Health Medical Center
Denver, Colorado

A. Benjamin Srivastava, MD
Resident
Department of Psychiatry
Washington University School of Medicine
Barnes-Jewish Hospital
St. Louis, Missouri

Daniel Theodoro, MD
Assistant Professor
Division of Emergency Medicine
Washington University School of Medicine
St. Louis, Missouri

Jason Wagner, MD
Assistant Professor
Division of Emergency Medicine
Washington University School of Medicine
St. Louis, Missouri

Xiaowen Wang, MD
Resident
Department of Medicine
Washington University School of Medicine
Barnes-Jewish Hospital
St. Louis, Missouri

Michael Weaver, MD
Chief Resident
Clinical Instructor
Department of Internal Medicine
Washington University School of Medicine
Barnes-Jewish Hospital
St. Louis, Missouri

Aimee Wendelsdorf, MD
Clinical Fellow
Critical Care
Department of Anesthesia
Washington University School of Medicine
Barnes-Jewish Hospital
St. Louis, Missouri

Brian T. Wessman, MD, FACEP, FCCM
Associate Professor
Department of Anesthesiology
Divisions of Critical Care Medicine and
  Emergency Medicine
Washington University School of Medicine
St. Louis, Missouri

Michael Willman, MD
Chief Resident
Division of Emergency Medicine
Washington University School of Medicine
Barnes-Jewish Hospital and St. Louis
  Children's Hospital
St. Louis, Missouri

Nathan Woltman, MD
Assistant Professor
Department of Emergency Medicine
Johns Hopkins School of Medicine
Baltimore, Maryland

Diana Zhong, MD
Resident
Department of Medicine
Washington University School of Medicine
Barnes-Jewish Hospital
St. Louis, Missouri

Contents

Environmental Emergencies

Gastrointestinal Emergencies

Psychiatric Emergencies

Renal and GU Emergencies

Pulmonary Emergencies

Toxicology

Traumatic Emergencies

Procedures

Operational Aspects of Emergency Medicine

1 Cardiovascular Emergencies: Acute Coronary Syndrome

Xiaowen Wang and Stacey House

GENERAL PRINCIPLES

Definition

- Acute coronary syndrome (ACS) encompasses a spectrum of illnesses from ST elevation myocardial infarction (STEMI), non-ST elevation myocardial infarction (NSTEMI) to unstable angina (UA).
- STEMI: myocardial ischemia with persistent ST elevation on electrocardiogram (ECG) and release of biomarkers that indicate myocardial necrosis.
  - ST elevation is seen at the J point in at least two contiguous leads, ≥2 mm (men) or ≥1.5 mm (women) in leads V2–V3, and/or ≥1 mm in other contiguous chest or limb leads. New left bundle-branch block (LBBB) is considered as an STEMI equivalent.
  - In early phases of STEMI, before ST elevation develops, T-wave changes may be observed.
- NSTEMI: myocardial ischemia without ST elevation and with positive myocardial biomarkers.
- UA: patients with ACS but no ST elevation on ECG and no positive myocardial biomarkers that suggest myocardial damage.

Epidemiology/Etiology

- Chest pain accounts for 9% (or 5.5 million) of noninjurious ED visits annually.
- In the United States, ~1.1 million patents are admitted annually to hospitals with NSTEMI/UA and ~300,000 patients with STEMI.

Pathophysiology

- NSTEMI/UA usually happens a with sudden imbalance between oxygen consumption and demand of the myocardium. This could be due to obstruction of coronary arteries but also could be due to vasospasm (Prinzmetal angina), myocardial injury due to nonischemic causes, or increased oxygen demand without coronary obstruction.
- In STEMI, obstruction is usually due to sudden plaque rupture and thrombotic occlusion of coronary arteries.

DIAGNOSIS

- STEMI or new LBBB with signs and symptoms of an acute ischemic event is an indication for immediate reperfusion therapy.

Clinical Presentation

History

- For NSTEMI and UA, the patient commonly presents with pressure-type chest pain, usually described as "heavy," "squeezing," or "crushing." Pain can radiate to the arms and less commonly to the abdomen, back, jaw, and neck.

- Chest pain can be accompanied by diaphoresis, weakness, light-headedness, dizziness, nausea, vomiting, or anxiety.
- Pain usually lasts more than 10 minutes. For chest pain associated with STEMI, it can last more than 30 minutes.
- Females, older patients (>75 years of age), patients with diabetes, renal insufficiency, or dementia may have atypical anginal symptoms.
- Atypical presentations, such as stabbing/pleural pain, indigestion, epigastric pain, fatigue, or weakness can also represent ACS even in the absence of chest pain.

Physical Examination
- Heart sounds may have an S4, a paradoxical splitting of S2, or new mitral regurgitation murmurs.
- The patient may have signs of heart failure or other vascular disease.

Differential Diagnosis
- Cardiovascular: aortic dissection, pericarditis, aortic aneurysm
- Pulmonary: pulmonary embolism, pleuritis, pneumonia, pneumothorax
- Gastrointestinal: esophageal spasm, gastroesophageal reflux disease (GERD), pancreatitis, peptic ulcer, hepatobiliary disease
- Musculoskeletal: costochondritis, cervical radiculopathy
- Skin: herpes zoster
- Hematologic: sickle cell crisis/acute chest

Diagnostic Criteria and Testing
- Risk stratification: patients with TIMI score of 0 and negative high-sensitivity troponin after 2 hours of presentation can be ruled out for ACS using accelerated diagnostic protocols. Patients with TIMI score ≥ 3 should be considered for therapies such as low molecular weight heparin (Table 1.1).

Laboratories
- Troponin: serial troponin I or T levels should be measured at presentation and 3–6 hours after symptom onset. In a patient with initial normal serial troponin levels, additional troponin levels should be obtained beyond 6 hours if there is high clinical suspicion or if the patient has abnormal ECGs.
  - With high-sensitivity troponin assays, patients with chronic elevations in troponin levels will be identified; thus, the serial changes of troponin levels are important. Patients with renal failure and some patients with heart failure are more likely to have chronic elevations of troponin.

TABLE 1.1	TIMI Risk Score (1 Point for Each)

1. Age > 65 y
2. Known coronary artery disease (CAD) (stenosis >50%)
3. 2+ episodes of chest pain in 24 h
4. ST segment or T-wave changes
5. Elevated cardiac biomarkers
6. Acetylsalicylic acid in the last 7 d
7. 3+ CAD risk factors

Data from Antman EM, Cohen M, Bernink PJ, et al. The TIMI risk score for unstable angina/non-ST elevation MI: a method for prognostication and therapeutic decision making. *J Am Med Assoc* 2000;284:835–42.

- Creatine kinase myocardial isoenzyme (CK-MB): with contemporary troponin assays, CK-MB is not useful for diagnosis of ACS. However, CK-MB is useful to estimate MI size and to screen for new ischemia in the case of a chronically elevated or decreasing troponin.

Electrocardiography
- A 12-lead ECG should be performed within 10 minutes of patient's arrival.
- For NSTEMI and UA, ECG may show ST depression, T-wave inversions, or transient ST elevation. ECG can also be normal in 1–6% of patients, especially with occlusions in left circumflex and right coronary artery.
- STEMI: ST elevation is seen at the J point in at least two contiguous leads, ≥2 mm (men) or ≥1.5 mm (women) in leads V2–V3, and/or ≥1 mm in other contiguous chest or limb leads. New LBBB is considered as an STEMI equivalent.

Scarbossa criteria – criteria to evaluate an acute infarction in the presence of a preexisting LBBB. The criteria are given a point scale of 0-5 and three or more points is highly specific (with lower sensitivity) for an acute MI

- ST segment elevation of 1 mm or more that is in the same direction (concordant) as the QRS complex in any lead – 5 points.
- ST segment depression of 1 mm or more in any lead from V1 to V3 – 3 points.
- ST segment elevation of 5 mm or more that is discordant with the QRS complex – 2 points.
- The ECG can be initially normal or nondiagnostic. If this is the case, the ECG should be repeated at 15–30 intervals during the first hour, especially if symptoms recur.

Imaging
- There is no radiographic study that is specific for diagnosing ACS.
- Echocardiogram: can help to identify any wall motion abnormalities.

Diagnostic Procedures
- Coronary CT angiography: in patients who are low risk, coronary CT angiography can be more cost-effective and achieve more rapid diagnosis than stress myocardial perfusion imaging.
- Stress test: for patients with possible ACS but normal ECG and serial cardiac markers, it is reasonable to have the patient undergo stress testing (treadmill ECG, stress echocardiography, or stress myocardial perfusion imaging) before discharge or within 72 hours after discharge.

TREATMENT

Medications
- Aspirin 325 mg should be administered.
- Nitrates can reduce LV preload and increase blood flow to coronary arteries. They should be avoided in patients with hypotension, marked tachycardia or bradycardia, RV infarction, or phosphodiesterase −5 inhibitor use within 24–48 hours.
- Beta-blockers can be initiated in the first 24 hours in STEMI patients who do not have contraindications (heart failure, low output state, cardiogenic shock, PR > 0.24 seconds, second- or third-degree heart block, active asthma/reactive airway disease).
- Angiotensin-converting enzyme (ACE) inhibitors and angiotensin receptor blockers (ARBs) should be initiated within 24 hours in STEMI patients with heart failure, anterior infarction, or EF ≤ 0.4 unless contraindicated. ARBs should be given to patients who are intolerant of ACE inhibitors.

- Morphine has potential beneficial effects by providing analgesic and anxiolytic effects, causing venodilation and modest reduction in heart rate. However, there are observational studies that have demonstrated increased adverse events in patients with ACS and acute decompensated heart failure.
- Anticogulants
  - Clopidogrel: initial loading dose of 300–600 mg is recommended.
  - Prasugrel: initial loading dose of 60 mg.
  - Ticagrelor: initial loading dose of 180 mg.
  - Enoxaparin: 1 mg/kg subcutaneous every 12 hours or 12 mg/kg subcutaneous daily for patients with creatinine clearance < 30 mL/min.
  - Bivalirudin: 0.1 mg/kg loading dose followed by 0.25 mg/kg per hour.
  - Fondaparinux: 2.5 mg subcutaneous daily.
  - Unfractionated heparin: loading dose of 60 IU/kg (maximum of 4000 IU) with initial infusion of 12 IU/kg/h (maximum of 1000 IU/h), adjusted per hospital protocol.
  - Argatroban: used in patients with heparin-induced thrombocytopenia, with initial dose of 2 mcg/kg/min.

Other Nonpharmacologic Therapies

- Percutaneous coronary intervention (PCI)
  - STEMI:
    - **PCI-capable hospital:** if patient is initially seen at a PCI-capable hospital, patient should be sent to the cath lab for primary PCI. The time between first medical contact (FMC) and balloon time should be within 90 minutes.
    - **Non–PCI-capable hospital:** the patient should be transferred to PCI-capable facility if the FMC to balloon time is expected to be <120 minutes. If FMC to balloon time is expected to be over 120 minutes, patients should be given fibrinolytic agent within 30 minutes of arrival, assuming no contraindications for fibrinolytic therapy.
      - The patient should still be urgently transferred to PCI-capable facility if the patient develops evidence of failed reperfusion or reocclusion.
      - After thrombolysis, patients should still be transferred within 3–24 hours for angiography and revascularization as part of an invasive strategy.
    - For a patient with STEMI and cardiogenic shock or acute severe heart failure, primary PCI should still be performed.
  - NSTEMI/UA: a patient who has failed medical therapy, has objective evidence of ischemia, or is very high risk should undergo early invasive testing (within 24 hours).

SPECIAL CONSIDERATIONS

Disposition

- For a low risk patient (TIMI score of 0, normal ECG, normal high-sensitivity troponin at 0 and 2 hours), a 2-hour accelerated diagnostic protocol can be used if the patient has appropriate outpatient follow-up. The HEART score[4] (Table 1.2) predicts adverse cardiac events, and low-risk patients with a score 0–3 have <2% risk of major adverse events at 6 weeks out from incident. It is reasonable to discharge the patient with daily aspirin, short-acting nitroglycerin, with instructions of activity levels and appropriate outpatient follow-up for further testing.
  - For a patient with possible ACS but normal serial ECGs and cardiac troponins should undergo a stress test before discharge or within 72 hours of discharge.
  - For a patient with NSTEMI/UA and patients with recurrent symptoms, positive troponin, or ischemic ECG changes, admission is warranted.

TABLE 1.2	HEART Score[4] for Chest Pain Patients	
		Score
History	Highly suspicious	2
	Moderately suspicious	1
	Slightly suspicious	0
ECG	Significant ST depression	2
	Nonspecific repolarization disturbance	1
	Normal	0
Age	≤65 y	2
	45–65 y	1
	<45 y	0
Risk factors	≥3 risk factors or history of atherosclerotic disease	2
	1 or 2 risk factors	1
	No risk factors known	0
Troponin	>2× normal limit	2
	1–2× normal limit	1
	≤normal limit	0
		Total

0–3: 2.5% risk of adverse cardiac event. Patients can be discharged with follow-up.
4–6: 20.3% risk of adverse cardiac event. Patients should be admitted to the hospital for trending of troponin and provocative testing.
≥7: 72.7% risk of adverse cardiac event, suggesting early invasive measures with these patients and close coordination with inpatient cardiology.
From Six AJ, Backus BE, Kelder JC. Chest pain in the emergency room: value of the HEART score. *Neth Heart J* 2008;16(6):191–6, with permission.

- Patients with STEMI, continuing angina, hemodynamic instability, persistently uncontrolled arrhythmias, or large MI should be admitted to coronary care unit and for reperfusion therapy.

SUGGESTED READINGS

Amsterdam EA, Wenger NK, Brindis RG, et al. 2014 AHA/ACC guideline for the management of patients with non-ST-elevation acute coronary syndromes: a report of the American College of Cardiology/American Heart Association Task Force on Practice Guidelines. *Circulation* 2014;130:e344–426.

O'Gara PT, Kushner FG, Ascheim DD, et al. 2013 ACCF/AHA guideline for the management of ST-elevation myocardial infarction: a report of the American College of Cardiology Foundation/American Heart Association Task Force on Practice Guidelines. *J Am Coll Cardiol* 2013;61:e78–140.

Pitts SR, Niska RW, Xu J, Burt CW. *National Hospital Ambulatory Medical Care Survey: 2006 Emergency Department Summary. National Health Statistics Reports; No. 7.* Hyattsville, MD: National Center for Health Statistics, 2008.

Six AJ, Backus BE, Kelder JC. Chest pain in the emergency room: value of the HEART score. *Neth Heart J* 2008;16(6):191–6.

Sgarbossa EB, Pinski SL, Barbagelata A, et al. Electrocardiographic diagnosis of evolving acute myocardial infarction in the presence of left bundle-branch block. GUSTO-1 (Global Utilization of Streptokinase and Tissue Plasminogen Activator for Occluded Coronary Arteries) Investigators. *N Engl J Med* 1996;334:481.

Tabas JA, Rodriguez RM, Seligman HK, Goldschlager NF. Electrocardiographic criteria for detecting acute myocardial infarction in patients with left bundle branch block: a meta-analysis. *Ann Emerg Med* 2008;52:329.

Cardiovascular Emergencies: Approach to ECGs and Arrhythmias

Clark Samuel Smith and Rebecca Bavolek

Electrical Conduction of the Heart

NORMAL CARDIAC CONDUCTION CYCLE

- Normal conduction begins at SA node, which has an intrinsic rate of 60–100 bpm.
- Impulses travel through the internodal tracts in the left and right atria to the AV node.
- The AV node has a 0.04-second delay in transmission to ventricles to allow time for adequate ventricular filling.
- The AV node is surrounded by junctional pacemaker cells with an intrinsic rate of 40–60 bpm
- Electrical impulse continues down the bundle of His and divides into branches.
- Impulse terminates in Purkinje fibers, which are a fast-conduction network of fibers located beneath the endocardium.
  - Purkinje fibers have an intrinsic pacemaker rate of 20–40 bpm.

The ECG is a graphic representation of the electrical activity generated by the heart. It is recorded from 10 different contact points called leads. Three of the leads are created as a result of vector addition.

- Six precordial (anterior to lateral chest) leads   V1–V6
- Three limb leads (left arm, right arm, left leg)   I, II, III
- Three augmented leads, created by adding vectors of the limb leads   aVR, aVL, and aVF

Leads

- Six unipolar leads are placed along the left chest to obtain the horizontal view of the heart.
- Limb leads are placed on the extremities to obtain vectors of the heart.
- Impulses moving toward a lead yield a positive deflection, while impulses moving away from a lead yield a negative deflection on the tracing.

ECG Grid System

- Horizontal axis—time
  - Each small box = 0.04 seconds
- Vertical axis—voltage
  - Each small box = 0.1 mV

Systematic Approach to Reading ECGs

- Rate
  - Count the number of P waves in a 6-second interval (30 large boxes) and multiply times 10.

- Find a QRS complex that falls on a heavy line and then assign numbers in a sequence to subsequent heavy lines—300, 150, 100, 75, 60, and 50. Whichever number is closest to the next P wave is the approximate bpm.
- Rhythm
  - Check to see if every P wave has a QRS complex following and if each QRS has a preceding P wave (sinus rhythm).
  - Check to see if spaces between each complex in the strip are equal.
    - Rhythms with slight variations (~0.04 seconds) between complexes are regular.
    - If irregular, is there a pattern to the irregularity?
- Axis—determined by evaluating the direction of QRS complex in lead I and aVF
- P wave—represents atrial depolarization
  - Should precede each QRS complex.
  - Normally rounded and upright.
  - Duration normally 0.06–0.12 seconds, amplitude is normally 2–3 mm.
  - Notched or large P waves may indicate atrial enlargement or hypertrophy.
  - Inverted P waves may indicate that the impulse is not originating in SA node.
  - Varying P waves may indicate that several different areas within the atria are generating the impulse.
- PR interval—represents the time the impulse takes to traverse the atria through the AV node, bundle of His, and down the left/right bundles
  - Measured from beginning of P wave to the beginning of QRS complex.
  - Normally 0.12–0.2 seconds in duration.
  - Prolonged PR interval may indicate conduction delay.
  - Shortened PR interval may indicate an alternate conduction pathway or "accessory pathway."
- QRS complex—represents depolarization of the ventricles
  - Should follow the PR interval.
  - Height and deflection depend on the lead being assessed.
  - Duration—measured from beginning of the Q wave to the end of the S wave.
  - Prolonged interval may indicate ventricular conduction problems.
  - Deep Q waves (>25% of R-wave height) are an indication of prior infarction.
  - Missing QRS may indicate conduction deficits.
- ST segment
  - Measured from the end of QRS complex to the beginning of the T wave.
  - Elevated or depressed ST segments may indicate myocardial infarction or ischemia (or pericarditis in some cases).
- T wave—represents ventricular repolarization
  - Follows the ST segment.
  - Normally rounded with a height of about 0.5 mm in chest leads but up to 10 mm in precordial leads.
  - Generally, direction of deflection should be the same as the deflection of the QRS complex.
  - Peaked or tented T waves may indicate hyperkalemia.
  - Inverted T waves may indicate myocardial ischemia.
- QT interval—measures time needed for ventricular depolarization and repolarization
  - Measured from beginning of QRS complex to the end of the T wave.
  - Duration varies by age and sex, and heart rate should not be longer than ½ of RR interval (the QT interval, corrected for heart rate [QTc] = QT/square root of RR interval).

○ Prolongation of QT interval may be congenital or related to medications.
○ Shortened QT interval may be drug toxicities or electrolyte abnormalities.
- J point
  ○ Is the junction between the termination of the QRS complex and the beginning of the ST segment.
  ○ Elevation or depression of the J point is seen with the various causes of ST segment abnormality.
  ○ Notching of the J point is seen with benign early repolarization.
  ○ A positive deflection at the J point is termed an Osborn wave and is characteristically seen with hypothermia.

ECG INTERPRETATION

Normal Sinus Rhythm
- Normal sinus rhythm (NSR) 1:1 relationship of P wave to QRS complex
- Rate: 60–100 bpm

Premature Atrial Contraction (PAC)
- Pathophysiology: extra beats that originate outside the sinus node of the atria
  ○ Ectopic P waves appear earlier than the next expected sinus beat and may or may not be conducted through to the AV node.
- Benign but may represent electrolyte abnormality or medication side effect.
- Treatment: based on severity of underlying abnormality

Sinus Tachycardia
- Pathophysiology: exactly like sinus rhythm with a faster rate
- Rate: Ventricular rate 100–160
- Treatment: correct the underlying cause

Sinus Bradycardia
- Pathophysiology: sinus rhythm with slower rate
- Rate: ventricular rate < 60
- Treatment:
  ○ Atropine—does not work for transplanted hearts
  ○ Transcutaneous or transvenous pacing
  ○ Vasopressor—epinephrine
  ○ Glucagon/HCO_3—for beta-blocker toxicity

Paroxysmal Supraventricular Tachycardia (PSVT)
- Pathophysiology: P waves are abnormal and may not be visible due to an ectopic atrial pacemaker or re-entry system that bypasses the AV node to depolarize ventricle.
- Rate: 120–200 bpm, regular, and narrow QRS complexes
- Treatment:
  ○ Stable patient: vagal maneuvers first followed by medical cardioversion through AV node blockade
    ▪ Other techniques—Valsalva and carotid massage (contraindicated in pts >60 years, history of CVA, or bruit on exam)
  ○ Unstable patient: synchronized cardioversion (120–200 J biphasic, 200 J monophasic)

- Adenosine—usually dosed as 6 mg push and then if not successful, two successive 12 mg IV pushes
- Calcium channel blockers or beta-blockers

Atrial Flutter (AF)
- Pathophysiology: rapid atrial rhythm with a typical sawtooth pattern on ECG.
- Only select impulses will be transmitted so there is usually a block.
- Rate: atrial rate at ~300 bpm
- Treatment: see atrial fibrillation.

Atrial Fibrillation (AFib)
- Pathophysiology: irregularly irregular rhythm (no visible P waves or PR interval). The atrium sends out hundreds of electrical impulses (300–600) but no actual contraction, so QRS are narrow leading to an uncontrolled ventricular response rate of 120–200 bpm.
- Rate: irregularly irregular 120–200 bpm
- Treatment: in patients that have been in a-fib for >48 hours (or unknown length of time), rate control instead of rhythm control is recommended because of the chance of clot formation and propagation. Anticoagulation should be started prior to rate or rhythm control.
  - Unstable patient: synchronized cardioversion (120–200 J biphasic, 200 J monophasic)
  - Stable patient with rapid ventricular response (a-fib w/RVR)
    - Rate control through AV nodal blockage: calcium channel blockers and beta-blockers

Multifocal Atrial Tachycardia
- Pathophysiology: three different morphologies of P waves all in one lead with a rhythm that is irregularly irregular. The PP, PR, and RR intervals all vary within one lead.
- Treatment: rate and symptom control with calcium channel blockers, magnesium, and beta-blockers.
- Digoxin and cardioversion are usually ineffective for multifocal atrial tachycardia (MAT).

Premature Ventricular Contractions
- Pathophysiology
  - Appear as abnormal QRS complexes during another rhythm.
  - Originate in the ventricular myocardium (slow) ectopic foci.
  - Isolated premature ventricular contractions (PVCs) is benign and usually not felt.
  - Frequent PVCs may degenerate into unstable rhythms (ventricular tachycardia or ventricular fibrillation).
    - Bigeminy—Every 2nd beat is a PVC.
    - Trigeminy—Every 3rd beat is a PVC.
- Five ECG Characteristics of PVCs
  - Occur earlier than next expected QRS
  - Wide QRS complex (>0.12 seconds)
  - Abnormal morphology
  - Absence of preceding P wave
  - ST segment deflected in the opposite direction of the QRS complex

- Treatment
  - Isolated PVCs are normally benign and not treated.

Ventricular Tachycardia (VT)

- Pathophysiology: VT is three or more PVCs in succession with ventricular rate > 150 with regular and wide QRS complexes.
- Rate: ventricular rate > 150 bpm.
- Treatment
  - Pulseless VT: immediate defibrillation (120–200 J biphasic, 360 J monophasic) and CPR
  - Unstable VT: synchronized cardioversion (100–200 J biphasic, 200 J monophasic)
    - Once NSR is obtained, start amiodarone or lidocaine drip to prevent recurrences.
  - Stable VT
    - Cardioversion with lidocaine, amiodarone, adenosine, or procainamide
    - Overdrive pacing

Torsades de Pointes (Twisting of the Points)

- Pathophysiology: polymorphic VT is due to early after depolarization with a prolonged QT segment. ECG has classic "twisting" appearance of ventricular complexes.
- Treatment
  - Unstable patient—defibrillation (120–200 J biphasic, 360 J monophasic)
  - Stable patient: electrical overdrive pacing and magnesium sulfate

Ventricular Fibrillation

- Pathophysiology: irregular and unsynchronized electrical activity throughout the ventricles that leads to no mechanical activity. ECG appears as fine/coarse zigzag line without discernible complexes.
- Treatment: defibrillation 120–200 J (biphasic) or 360 J (monophasic) and CPR.

Pulseless Electrical Activity

- Pathophysiology: pulseless electrical activity (PEA) also known as electromechanical dissociation. The monitor will show a rhythm, but there is no cardiac activity.
- Treatment
  - Treat the suspected etiology ("H's and T's"), epinephrine, and CPR

Asystole

- Pathophysiology: absence of ventricular muscle activity ("flat line" on ECG)
- Treatment
  - Epinephrine and CPR

Atrioventricular Blocks (AVB)

- Pathophysiology—occurs when conduction between the atria and ventricles is abnormal and delayed (in the atria, AV node, or proximal His–Purkinje system).

1st-Degree Block: Normal Conduction Is Slightly Prolonged

- P waves and QRS complexes are normal with a 1:1 relationship.
- PR interval is >0.2 seconds.
- No treatment needed.

2nd-Degree Blocks
- Mobitz I (Wenckebach)
- Pathophysiology: progressive increase in PR intervals until one P wave is not associated with a QRS complex (dropped beat)
- Treatment:
  - Asymptomatic patients—no specific therapy
  - For symptomatic patients—atropine and transcutaneous pacing
- Mobitz II
- Pathophysiology: block is below the AV node (His–Purkinje system), and random P waves do not conduct, so some QRS complexes are dropped. Conducted P waves will have consistent PR intervals.
- Treatment:
  - Transcutaneous or transvenous pacing and cardiology consultation

3rd-Degree Block
- Pathophysiology: no atrial impulses are conducted. Atria and ventricles beat independently of one another with complete AV dissociation. PP interval and RR intervals are constant.
- Block location determined by QRS:
  - Narrow QRS—above His–Purkinje system
  - Wide QRS—below His–Purkinje system
- Treatment: transvenous or transcutaneous pacing and cardiology consultation

Bundle-Branch Block (BBB)
- Pathophysiology—conduction abnormalities (not rhythm disturbances) where ventricles depolarize in sequence (not together) producing a wide QRS complex

Right Bundle-Branch Block (RBBB)
- Ventricles are activated by the left fascicle.
- Wide QRS (>0.12 seconds).
- Look for RSR complexes ("bunny ears") in V1.

Left Bundle-Branch Block (LBBB)
- Ventricles are activated by the right fascicle.
- Wide QRS (>0.12 seconds).
- Look for prominent R waves in the lateral leads (I, aVL, V5, and V6).
- T waves opposite the terminal deflection of QRS complexes

Paced Rhythm
- Paced rhythms on ECG depend on which chamber is being paced.
- A spike is seen on the ECG followed immediately by a P wave or a widened QRS complex.

Wolff–Parkinson–White Syndrome (WPW)
- Pathophysiology: tachyarrhythmia caused by re-entrant pathway that can bypass the AV node. It presents as SVT that can alternate with VT.
- Types:
  - Orthodromic—Conduction is anterograde through the AV node and retrograde through the accessory pathway.
  - Antidromic—Conduction is anterograde through the accessory pathway and retrograde through the AV node.

- ECG definition
  - Short PR interval (<0.12 seconds)
  - Delta wave—slurred upstroke of the beginning of the QRS complex
  - Wide QRS complex (>0.10 seconds)
  - Adult tachycardia > 200
- Treatment
  - Rate/rhythm control through synchronized cardioversion or procainamide IV.
  - Do not use: AV nodal blockers (beta-blockers, digoxin, calcium channel blockers).
    - Can create a severe, resistant tachycardia by activating the accessory pathway only

SUGGESTED READING

ECCguidelines.heart.org

3 Cardiovascular Emergencies: Arterial System

Enyo Ablordeppey

Abdominal Aortic Aneurysm (AAA)

GENERAL PRINCIPLES

Definition
- AAA is defined as a dilation of the aorta that is within the abdomen.

Epidemiology/Etiology
- AAA is more common in men than in women, with prevalence rates estimated up to 9% in men and up to 2% in women.
- Risk factors include smoking, male sex, age, hypertension, chronic obstructive pulmonary disease, hyperlipidemia, and family history of the disorder.

Pathophysiology
- AAA is linked to the degradation of the elastic media of the atheromatous aorta.
- There are many causes of aneurysmal dilatation, including trauma, acute infection (brucellosis, salmonellosis), chronic infection (tuberculosis), inflammatory diseases (Behçet, Takayasu disease), and connective tissue disorders (Marfan syndrome, Ehlers-Danlos type IV).

DIAGNOSIS

Clinical Presentation

History
- Nonruptured aneurysms are generally asymptomatic and diagnosed incidentally.
- Nonspecific symptoms include vague abdominal and back pain.
- Rupture of AAAs should be suspected by the triad of sudden-onset pain in the mid-abdomen or flank (that may radiate into the scrotum), shock, and pulsatile abdominal mass.

Physical Examination
- The examination for a pulsatile mass should be done by bimanual palpation of the supraumbilical area.

Differential Diagnosis
- Gastritis, appendicitis, cystitis, diverticulitis, pancreatitis, cholelithiasis, bowel obstruction, or PUD.

Diagnostic Criteria and Testing
- The normal diameter of the aorta is 30 mm or less. Anything larger is considered an aneurysm.

Laboratories
- There are no laboratory tests that diagnose an AAA.

Imaging
- Ultrasonography has a sensitivity of 99% in detecting an AAA.
- A CT scan is the most comprehensive imaging test and will provide visualization of the proximal neck (the transition between the normal and aneurysmal aorta), extension to the iliac arteries, patency of the visceral arteries, and presence of an intramural thrombus.
- MRI/MRA can also be used to characterize the AAA but is not ideal for unstable patients.

TREATMENT

Medications
- There are no medications that are specific for ED treatment of a stable AAA.

SPECIAL CONSIDERATIONS

Disposition
- Stable patients may be discharged home with follow-up with the PMD or a vascular surgeon.
- Patients with a new or expanding AAA should be admitted to the hospital.

Complications
- Leaking or rupture of the aneurysm, or death

Aortic Dissection

GENERAL PRINCIPLES

Definition
- Tears in the intimal layer results in separation of the inner and middle layers of the aorta
- Type A dissection involves the ascending aorta and the aortic arch and accounts for 60% of aortic dissections.
- Type B dissection begins beyond the brachiocephalic vessels.

Epidemiology/Etiology
- Most common in men and older individuals.
- Aortic dilatation is a well-established risk factor for thoracic aortic dissection; most ascending aortic dissections occur when aortic diameter is <5.5 cm.
- Other risk factors of rupture include a structural abnormality of the arterial wall (e.g., bicuspid or unicommissural aortic valve, aortic coarctation), systemic hypertension, or mechanical injury (postcardiac catheterization).
- Patients are at higher risks for rupture if they carry a concurrent diagnosis of an inherited disease (like Marfan syndrome, Ehlers-Danlos syndrome type IV, Turner syndrome, annuloaortic ectasia, and familial aortic dissection), infection (syphilis), arteritis such as Takayasu's or giant cell, aortic dilatation/aneurysm, wall thinning, and "crack" cocaine (abrupt catecholamine-induced hypertension).

Pathophysiology
- Blood enters the intima–media space and causes separation of the layers. Once the blood starts to cleave the vessel media, it can propagate forward or backward, as well as extending back into the true lumen or rupturing externally.
- Blood enters the media via:
  - Atherosclerotic ulcer leading to intimal tear
  - Disruption of vasa vasorum causing intramural hematoma
  - De novo intimal tear

DIAGNOSIS

Clinical Presentation
History
- Common presentation includes severe, sharp, acute-onset chest pain with radiation to the back or abdomen.

Physical Examination
- There may be a BP > 20 mm Hg difference in each arm or an absent pulse in an extremity.
- An aortic regurgitation murmur may be heard.

Differential Diagnosis
- Aortic stenosis, mechanical back pain, MI, PE, pleural effusion, pancreatitis

Diagnostic Criteria and Testing

Laboratories
- There are no specific laboratory tests to diagnose an aortic dissection.

Imaging
- Mediastinal widening or an abnormal aortic contour may be seen on chest radiography.
- Contrast CT is the preferred imaging modality to diagnose an aortic dissection.
- Transesophageal echocardiography and magnetic resonance imaging are other options but have time and availability limitations.

TREATMENT

Medications
- There is no medical management for type A dissection.
- Medical management for type B dissections is aimed at reducing shearing forces within the aorta.
- Beta-blockers (esmolol or labetalol) should be initiated to lower heart rate to <70 followed by vasodilators (nitroglycerin, nicardipine, or nitroprusside) for a target systolic BP < 120.
- Target acute decrease in BP to the lowest possible that still maintains end-organ perfusion (mentation, urinary output).

Other Nonpharmacologic Therapies
- Type A dissection is a surgical emergency. In patients with type B dissection, some will undergo percutaneous fenestration and/or stenting.

SPECIAL CONSIDERATIONS

Disposition
- The patient should be admitted to the hospital or ICU depending on clinical condition.

Arterial Occlusion

GENERAL PRINCIPLES

Definition
- Peripheral arterial disease (PAD) is an atherosclerotic process that causes stenosis and occlusion of noncerebral and noncoronary arteries.

Epidemiology/Etiology
- Risk factors include advancing age, smoking, diabetes, hypertension, dyslipidemia, and concomitant coronary and cerebrovascular disease.

Pathophysiology
- PAD is classified into four major stages with progression from an asymptomatic state to claudication, ischemic rest pain, and ulceration or gangrene.

DIAGNOSIS

Clinical Presentation

History
- There may be intermittent claudication progressing to pain at rest, ischemic ulceration, or gangrene (limb ischemia).

Physical Examination
- Pale or blue skin.
- Skin cool/cold to the touch.
- Weak or nonpalpable pulses.
- Ankle–brachial index (ABI) where the blood pressure in the ankle is compared to the blood pressure in the arm.
  - An abnormally low value of ABI is indicative of atherosclerosis in the leg. An ABI of ≤0.90 is commonly used to diagnose PAD.

Diagnostic Criteria and Testing

Laboratories
- There are no specific lab tests that help diagnose arterial occlusion.

Imaging
- Duplex ultrasound, computed tomographic angiography (CTA), and arteriography all may help diagnose arterial occlusion.

TREATMENT

Medications
- Anticoagulation, if not contraindicated, should be instituted as soon as the diagnosis of acute limb ischemia has been made.

Other Nonpharmacologic Therapies
- Catheter-directed thrombolysis, thrombectomy, angioplasty with/without stenting, endarterectomy, and open surgical revascularization such as peripheral bypass surgery are all options for acute arterial occlusion treatment.

SPECIAL CONSIDERATIONS

Disposition
- Disposition should be made in conjunction with a vascular surgeon.

Complications
- Complete occlusion may lead to the loss of a limb or muscle necrosis and sepsis.

SUGGESTED READINGS

Criqui MH, Aboyans V. Peripheral artery disease compendium: epidemiology of peripheral artery disease. *Circ Res* 2015;116:1509–26.

European Society of Cardiology. Diagnosis and management of aortic dissection. *Eur Heart J* 2001;22:1642–81.

Fink HA, Lederle FA, Roth CS, et al. The accuracy of physical examination to detect abdominal aortic aneurysm. *Arch Intern Med* 2000;160:833–6.

Glimaker H, Holmberg L, Elvin A, et al. Natural history of patients with abdominal aortic aneurysm. *Eur J Vasc Surg* 1991;5:125–30.

Golledge J, Eagle KA. Acute aortic dissection [review]. *Lancet* 2008;372(9632):55–66.

Hagan PG, Nienaber CA, Isselbacher EM, et al. The International Registry of Acute Aortic Dissection (IRAD): new insights into an old disease. *JAMA* 2000;283:897.

Johnston KW, Rutherford RB, Tilson MD, et al. Suggested standards for reporting on arterial aneurysms. Subcommittee on Reporting Standards for Arterial Aneurysms, Ad Hoc Committee on Reporting Standards, Society for Vascular Surgery and North American Chapter, International Society for Cardiovascular Surgery. *J Vasc Surg* 1991;13:452–8.

Lederle FA, Johnson GR, Wilson SE, et al. The aneurysm detection and management study-screening program: validation cohort and final results. *Arch Intern Med* 2000;160:1425–30.

Novo S, Coppola G, Milio G. Critical limb ischemia: definition and natural history. Current drug targets. *Cardiovasc Haematol Disord* 2004;4:219–25.

Ouriel K. Peripheral arterial disease. *Lancet* 2001;358(9289):1257–64.

Reed K, Curtis L. Aortic emergencies: part 1—thoracic dissections and aneurysms. *Emerg Med Pract* 2006;8(2):1–24.

Sakalihasan N, Limet R, Defawe OD. Abdominal aortic aneurysm. *Lancet* 2005;365(9470):1577–89.

Upadhye S, Schiff K. Acute aortic dissection in the emergency department: diagnostic challenges and evidence-based management [review]. *Emerg Med Clin North Am* 2012;30(2):307–27, viii.

4 Cardiovascular Emergencies: Venous System

Chien-Jung Lin and Stacey House

GENERAL PRINCIPLES

Definition

- Venous thromboembolism (VTE) encompasses deep vein thrombosis (DVT) and pulmonary embolism (PE).
  - Massive PE refers to those associated with systemic hypotension despite resuscitation.
  - Submassive PE refers to those causing significant cardiac dysfunction.[1]
- Venous thrombi are classified as proximal versus distal and deep versus superficial. Proximal vein DVT is defined as an occlusion of the popliteal vein and those proximal to it in the lower extremity or the axillary vein and those proximal to it in the upper extremity.

Epidemiology/Etiology

- Without treatment, half of the patients with proximal lower extremity DVT will develop PE.[2]
- Symptomatic DVT most commonly arises from the lower extremities. Most PE results from DVT in the pelvis and proximal lower extremities, although DVT in the upper extremity may also cause PE.
- Risk factors for VTE are stasis of blood flow, venous endothelial injury, and a hypercoagulable state (Virchow triad).
  - A dose–response relationship exists between travel and VTE: each 2-hour increase in travel duration increases risk of VTE by 18–26%.[3]

Pathophysiology

- VTE forms due to an imbalance of excessive clot production and inadequate clot resolution in the venous system. Intravascular deposition of fibrin and red blood cells, with platelet and leukocyte components, forms the basis for venous clots.

DIAGNOSIS

Clinical Presentation

History

- Presenting symptoms of DVT often involve leg pain and/or swelling that may increase as the DVT progresses.
- A history should include a family history of VTE, recurrent miscarriage, or any of Wells criteria (Table 4.1).

Physical Examination

- The classic symptoms of DVT include unilateral pain, tenderness, swelling, edema, discoloration, erythema, and warmth of the extremities. There may be palpable cords.
- Homan's sign (pain in the calf upon forceful and abrupt ankle dorsiflexion while the knee is extended) may be present.

Differential Diagnosis

- Venous insufficiency, postphlebitis syndrome, lymphedema, superficial thrombophlebitis, Baker cyst, cellulitis, myositis, muscle strain, hematoma, abscess, trauma

Diagnostic Criteria and Testing

- The history, symptoms, and signs, when used in isolation, are neither sensitive nor specific.[4] Along with a high suspicion for the diagnosis, a formalized clinical score, such as the Wells score (Table 4.1),[5] should be used to assess the pretest probability of DVT.

TABLE 4.1	The Wells Score
Clinical Feature	**Score**
Active cancer (treatment ongoing or within previous 6 mo or palliative)	1
Paralysis, paresis, or recent plaster immobilization of the lower extremities	1
Recently bedridden for more than 3 d or major surgery, within 4 wk	1
Localized tenderness along the distribution of the deep venous system	1
Entire leg swollen	1
Calf swelling by more than 3 cm when compared with the asymptomatic leg (measured 10 cm below tibial tuberosity)	1
Pitting edema (greater in the symptomatic leg)	1
Collateral superficial veins (nonvaricose)	1
Alternative diagnosis as likely or greater than that of deep vein thrombosis	−2

DVT is unlikely if score ≤1, likely if ≥2.

Laboratories
- A negative D-dimer test, in combination with a low pretest probability, provides sufficient negative predictive value to rule out DVT.[6] Further testing can be safely omitted. However, a negative D-dimer test, when combined with a moderate-to-high pretest probability (such as in cancer patients), does not adequately rule out DVT.[7]
- Adjusting the D-dimer cutoff value based on age (age × 10 µg/L in patients above 50 years old) may increase the specificity for diagnosing DVT.[5]
- A positive D-dimer test does not confirm the diagnosis of DVT. Such patients require further evaluation.

Electrocardiography
- There is no specific ECG finding in DVT. VTE resulting in PE most commonly shows sinus tachycardia, although findings of right heart strain may also be present.

Imaging
- Venous compression ultrasound identifies thrombosed veins by virtue of their noncompressibility.
- Ultrasonography has a sensitivity and specificity of above 90% for proximal DVT. The sensitivity for calf DVT is lower.[8]

TREATMENT

- Anticoagulation is indicated in proximal DVT and some selected cases of distal DVT unless contraindications exist.

Medications

- The initial anticoagulant for VTE treatment includes unfractionated heparin (UFH), low molecular weight heparin (LMWH), pentasaccharide (fondaparinux), or a nonwarfarin oral anticoagulant (Table 4.2). Longer-term anticoagulation is typically with warfarin or the novel oral anticoagulants (NOACs).

TABLE 4.2	Initial Treatment of Venous Thromboembolism
Drug	**Dosage**
UFH	Bolus 80 U/kg (maximum 6000 U), followed by infusion 18 U/kg/h, use IV heparin nomogram for infusion adjustments
Enoxaparin	1 mg/kg SC q12 h or 1.5 mg/kg SC q24 h
Tinzaparin	175 IU/kg SC daily
Dalteparin	200 IU/kg SC daily for month 1, followed by 150 IU/kg SC daily
Fondaparinux	5 mg SC daily for weight < 50 kg 7.5 mg SC daily for weight 50–100 kg 10 mg SC daily for weight > 100 kg
Apixaban	10 mg PO bid for 7 d, followed by 5 mg PO bid
Rivaroxaban	15 mg PO bid for 21 d, followed by 20 mg PO daily
Edoxaban	30 mg PO daily for <60 kg
	60 mg PO daily for >60 kg
Dabigatran	150 mg PO bid after LMWH SC or UFH IV for 5–11 d

- Heparins
  - UFH requires serial monitoring of anticoagulation.
  - LMWHs do not need for routine monitoring.
  - LMWHs require dose adjustments in patients with a CrCl of 15–30 mL/min and are contraindicated in patients undergoing dialysis.
  - LMWHs are the preferred agent for VTE treatment during pregnancy and in patients with cancer.[7]
    - In patients compliant on oral anticoagulants who develop recurrent VTE, a switch to LMWHs may be considered.[9]
    - In patients compliant on LMWHs who develop recurrent VTE, a dose escalation may be considered.[9]
- Warfarin
  - Warfarin is the classic long-term VTE management, especially in patients with renal insufficiency.
    - Warfarin should not be used as the sole initial agent without bridging with more rapid-acting anticoagulants (such as heparin or enoxaparin) until obtaining a therapeutic INR for 2 days. The dose should be titrated to a goal INR of 2–3.
- NOACs
  - NOACs provide a faster onset of anticoagulation, shorter half-life, wider therapeutic window, fixed dosing, and no need for therapeutic monitoring compared to warfarin.
  - Rivaroxaban and apixaban are approved for monotherapy, whereas dabigatran and edoxaban therapy should be overlapped with parenteral agents such as UFH, LMWH, or fondaparinux for at least 5 days.

Other Nonpharmacologic Therapies

- IVC filters should be considered in patients with contraindications to anticoagulation.
- Thrombolytic therapy, catheter embolectomy, and surgical thrombectomy may have roles in select patients, such as those with high clot burden, symptom <14 days, good functional status, life expectancy >1 year, and low risk for bleeding. Consultation with specialists is recommended.

SPECIAL CONSIDERATIONS

Disposition

- Patients that are stable with a low risk of bleeding, who can self-administer anticoagulants, contact their providers, and follow-up, may be safely discharged given no other inpatient indications exist.
  - The Choosing Wisely initiative recommends against reimaging DVT in the absence of a clinical change. However, the 2016 CHEST guideline suggests serial imaging of deep veins in 2 weeks in patients with isolated distal leg DVT not treated with anticoagulation[15].
- Inpatient management is appropriate for patients with massive DVT, phlegmasia cerulea dolens, concurrent symptomatic PE, high risk of bleeding, or other comorbid conditions that require inpatient management.

Complications

- Embolization of venous thrombi to other locations can occur although are much less common.

REFERENCES

1. Jaff MR, McMurtry MS, Archer SL, et al. Management of massive and submassive pulmonary embolism, iliofemoral deep vein thrombosis, and chronic thromboembolic pulmonary hypertension: a scientific statement from the American Heart Association. *Circulation* 2011;123:1788–830. doi:10.1161/CIR.0b013e318214914f.
2. Kearon C. Natural history of venous thromboembolism. *Circulation* 2003;107:I22–30. doi:10.1161/01.CIR.0000078464.82671.78.
3. Chandra D, Parisini E, Mozaffarian D. Meta-analysis: travel and risk for venous thromboembolism. *Ann Intern Med* 2009;151:180–90.
4. Goodacre S, Sutton AJ, Sampson FC. Meta-analysis: the value of clinical assessment in the diagnosis of deep venous thrombosis. *Ann Intern Med* 2005;143:129–39.
5. Schouten HJ, Geersing GJ, Koek HL, et al. Diagnostic accuracy of conventional or age adjusted D-dimer cut-off values in older patients with suspected venous thromboembolism: systematic review and meta-analysis. *BMJ* 2013;346:f2492. doi:10.1136/bmj.f2492.
6. Wells PS, Anderson DR, Rodger M, et al. Evaluation of D-dimer in the diagnosis of suspected deep-vein thrombosis. *N Engl J Med* 2003;349:1227–35. doi:10.1056/NEJMoa023153.
7. Lee AY, Julian JA, Levine MN, et al. Clinical utility of a rapid whole-blood D-dimer assay in patients with cancer who present with suspected acute deep venous thrombosis. *Ann Intern Med* 1999;131:417–23.
8. Goodacre S, Sampson F, Thomas S, et al. Systematic review and meta-analysis of the diagnostic accuracy of ultrasonography for deep vein thrombosis. *BMC Med Imaging* 2005;5:6. doi:10.1186/1471-2342-5-6.
9. Kearon C, Akl EA, Ornelas J, et al. Antithrombotic therapy for VTE disease: CHEST guideline and expert panel report. *Chest* 2016;149:315–52. doi:10.1016/j.chest.2015.11.026.

Cardiovascular Emergencies: Heart Failure and Cardiomyopathies

Rahul Chhana and Stacey House

GENERAL PRINCIPLES

Definition

- Heart failure can be characterized based on ejection fraction, cardiac output, location, and temporal nature:
  - Heart failure with reduced ejection fraction (HFrEF), also known as systolic heart failure, results from an impairment in ventricular contraction and is defined as occurring with an ejection fraction of <40%. It is commonly caused by ischemic heart disease, hypertension, cardiomyopathy, infiltrative disease, alcoholism, and certain medications.

- Heart failure with preserved ejection fraction (HFpEF), also known as diastolic heart failure, results from impairment in ventricular relaxation and filling and is defined as having an ejection fraction of >50%. It also results from the same causes as HFrEF.
- Low-output heart failure is heart failure with decreased cardiac output.
- High-output heart failure is heart failure with increased stroke volume and possibly increased cardiac output.
- Left-sided heart failure is heart failure caused by dysfunction of the left ventricle.
- Right-sided heart failure is heart failure caused by dysfunction of the right ventricle.
- Decompensated heart failure is an acute, sudden onset of symptoms of heart failure.
- Cardiogenic shock is hypotension, and end-organ dysfunction is caused by cardiac dysfunction.
- Cardiomyopathies are a group of acquired or inherited primary disease of the myocardium that may lead to various forms of heart failure.
  - Dilated cardiomyopathy is characterized by a decrease in ventricular contraction due to dilation of the cardiac chambers. It is the most common cardiomyopathy with etiologies that include idiopathic, primary (genetic), and secondary (myocarditis, chemotherapy agents such as doxorubicin, nutritional deficiencies, alcohol abuse, endocrine disorders, and autoimmune disorders).[1]
  - Hypertrophic cardiomyopathy is a genetic myocardial disorder characterized by asymmetric ventricular hypertrophy especially of the septal wall. Hypertrophic obstructive cardiomyopathy (HOCM) is characterized by a harsh crescendo–decrescendo systolic ejection murmur best heard at the left upper sternal border similar to that of aortic stenosis. HOCM places patients at risk of sudden cardiac death especially with strong exertion such as athletic activity.
  - Restrictive cardiomyopathy is characterized by nondilated, rigid ventricles with a normal thickness causing severe diastolic dysfunction.
  - Peripartum cardiomyopathy is characterized by left ventricular dysfunction that develops between the last month of pregnancy to 5 months postpartum.
- Takotsubo cardiomyopathy (also called stress cardiomyopathy) is a reversible cardiomyopathy more commonly found in postmenopausal women and in those with psychiatric and neurologic disorders. It is thought to be triggered by physical or emotional stress possibly through catecholamine excess, leading to vascular spasm resulting in myocardial stunning. It is characterized by left ventricular dysfunction mimicking myocardial infarction in the absence of obstructive coronary artery disease.[2,3]

Epidemiology/Etiology

- Heart failure is extremely common in the United States and increases with the increase in the elderly population.
- Heart failure is the leading cause of hospitalization among the elderly and carries a large burden of recurrent rehospitalization.

Pathophysiology

- Acute heart failure with pulmonary edema can result from a cycle of decreasing cardiac output and increasing systemic vascular resistance in the setting of a damaged myocardium that cannot adequately respond to hemodynamic alterations.
- In addition, activation of the renin–angiotensin–aldosterone system further elevates afterload leading to additional myocardial stress and worsened myocardial function.

DIAGNOSIS

Clinical Presentation

History
- Patients with acute or decompensated heart failure will normally have a history of prior heart failure, hypertension, or a valvular disorder.
- Volume overload causes lower extremity edema, paroxysmal nocturnal dyspnea, orthopnea, dyspnea, abdominal discomfort, and bloating.
- Patients may report dietary indiscretion, medication noncompliance/recent medication change, or symptoms of acute coronary syndromes.

Physical Examination
- Cardiac exam may reveal an S_3 heart sound. Murmurs are present with valvular dysfunction.
- Pulmonary exam may reveal rales. Decreased breath sounds at the lung bases may be present from pleural effusions. More severe acute heart failure may present with tachypnea and respiratory distress.
- JVD, hepatojugular reflex, and pitting lower extremity edema may be present.
- Patients with acute, decompensated heart failure are often severely hypertensive. Patients with cardiogenic shock will present with hypotension.

Differential Diagnosis
- Pneumonia, chronic obstructive pulmonary disease, pulmonary embolism, DVT, renal failure, acute coronary syndrome, aortic dissection, acute valvular compromise, arrhythmia, or cardiac tamponade.

Diagnostic Testing

Laboratories
- B-type natriuretic peptide (BNP) or amino-terminal pro-B–type natriuretic peptide (NT-proBNP) is highly sensitive and specific for the evaluation of heart failure.[4] These can be elevated in atrial fibrillation, renal disease, acute coronary syndrome, older age, or pulmonary embolism.[5,6]
- Troponin should be obtained to evaluate for myocardial infarction.
- A basic metabolic panel and magnesium can evaluate for renal disease or electrolyte abnormality.

Electrocardiography
- A 12-lead should be obtained to evaluate for ischemia and arrhythmias.

Imaging
- A chest plain radiograph can show signs of pulmonary venous congestion, pulmonary edema, pleural effusions, or cardiomegaly.
- A bedside cardiac ultrasound can be useful to evaluate for global cardiac function, pericardial effusion, cardiac tamponade, or right ventricular strain seen in severe pulmonary embolism. Severe valvular dysfunction may be observed.

TREATMENT

Medications
- Vasodilators such as nitroglycerin may be used to decrease preload. Initial therapy includes sublingual nitroglycerin (0.4 mg every 5 minutes), while intravenous

nitroglycerin (0.2–0.4 μg/kg/min) is being prepared. Vasodilators should be used with caution in patients with inferior ischemia or hypertrophic cardiomyopathy.

- Diuresis can help reduce volume overload. Options include furosemide (20–80 mg IV), bumetanide (1–3 mg IV), and torsemide (10–20 mg IV). The patient's home diuretic dosage and severity of volume overload should be considered when choosing the initial starting diuretic dose.
- Inotropic support is necessary in patients with cardiogenic shock. Dobutamine (0.5–1 μg/kg/min initially with titration to up to 40 μg/kg/min) increases inotropy and systemic vasodilation. Norepinephrine (0.01–3 μg/kg/min infusion) may result in vasoconstriction and increased afterload in addition to increased contractility.

Other Nonpharmacologic Therapies

- Optimization of respiratory status through the use of supplemental oxygen (if the patient is hypoxic) as well as patient positioning (typically best when sitting upright) should be performed.
- Ventilatory support with CPAP or BiPAP can be beneficial.
- Endotracheal intubation may be necessary.
- Urgent hemodialysis may be necessary in anuric patients with volume overload.

SPECIAL CONSIDERATIONS

Disposition

- Patients may be treated as an outpatient if they are hemodynamically stable with adequate symptom control. These patients need close follow-up with their cardiologist or primary care physician.
- Patients requiring inotropic agents or ventilatory support will require ICU admission.
- Patients that continue to be symptomatic after initial treatment but who do not require close airway or hemodynamic monitoring as well as patients with new diagnoses of heart failure should be admitted to the general floor for further management.

REFERENCES

1. Felker GM, Thompson RE, Hare JM, et al. Underlying causes and long-term survival in patients with initially unexplained cardiomyopathy. *N Engl J Med* 2000;342(15):1077–84.
2. Prasad A, Lerman A, Rihal CS. Apical ballooning syndrome (Tako-Tsubo or stress cardiomyopathy): a mimic of acute myocardial infarction. *Am Heart J* 2008;155(3):408–17.
3. Kurowski V, Kaiser A, von Hof K, et al. Apical and midventricular transient left ventricular dysfunction syndrome (Tako-Tsubo cardiomyopathy): frequency, mechanisms, and prognosis. *Chest* 2007;132(3):809–16.
4. Januzzi JL Jr, Chen-Tournoux AA, Moe G. Amino-terminal pro-B-type natriuretic peptide testing for the diagnosis or exclusion of heart failure in patients with acute symptoms. *Am J Cardiol* 2008;101(3a):29–38.
5. Maisel A, Mueller C, Adams K Jr, et al. State of the art: using natriuretic peptide levels in clinical practice. *Eur J Heart Fail* 2008;10(9):824–39.
6. Porta A, Barrabés JA, Candell-Riera J, et al. Plasma B-type natriuretic peptide levels are poorly related to the occurrence of ischemia or ventricular arrhythmias during symptom-limited exercise in low-risk patients. *Arch Med Sci* 2016;12(2):341–8.

6 Cardiovascular Emergencies: Hypertension

Nicole Messenger and Stacey House

GENERAL PRINCIPLES

Definition

- Normal blood pressure is defined as <120/80 mm Hg. Blood pressure from 120/80 to 139/89 mm Hg is defined as prehypertension. Stage 1 hypertension is defined as 140/90 to 159/99 mm Hg, whereas stage 2 hypertension is blood pressure ≥160/100 mm Hg.[1]
- Primary (essential) hypertension is persistently elevated blood pressure without a known secondary cause and is related to genetic and environmental factors.
- Secondary hypertension is elevated blood pressure from known sources such as medications endocrine disease, renal disease, and tumors.
- Hypertensive urgency refers to markedly elevated blood pressure (often arbitrarily chosen as ≥180/120 mm Hg) without end-organ dysfunction.
- Hypertensive emergency is acutely elevated blood pressure, which is associated with end-organ (brain, heart, kidneys, aorta, or eyes) dysfunction.

Epidemiology/Etiology

- One in five adults with hypertension is unaware that he or she has hypertension.[2]
- Only ~50% of patients with hypertension have adequately controlled blood pressure.[3]
- Stage 1 or 2 hypertension occurs in more than 40% of emergency department visits.[4]
- Risk factors include increased age, family history, African American race, obesity, smoking, high-salt diet, medication noncompliance, and alcohol abuse.

Pathophysiology

- Chronic hypertension leads to arterial wall changes resulting in the need for increased arterial pressure to maintain end organ blood flow.
- Additional damage occurs secondary to arterial wall stress, endothelial injury, platelet activation, activation of the renin/angiotensin system, vasoconstriction leading to ischemia, and cardiac hypertrophy and remodeling from increased afterload.

DIAGNOSIS

Clinical Presentation

History
- Patients may present asymptomatically or with signs of end organ dysfunction.
- Patients with hypertensive emergency may present with chest pain, shortness of breath, severe headache, neurologic deficit, or syncope (Table 6.1).

Physical Examination
- Patients with asymptomatic hypertension may not have any physical exam findings other than elevated blood pressure (Table 6.1), but a thorough physical exam should be performed to evaluate for signs of end organ damage.

TABLE 6.1   Hypertensive Emergencies: Diagnosis and Treatment

Diagnosis	Symptoms	Possible exam findings	Confirmatory diagnostic tests	BP goals/therapeutic agents
Intracerebral hemorrhage	Headache, neurologic deficit	AMS, neurologic deficit	Head CT	Decrease MAP < 110 mm Hg but caution in elevated ICP Nicardipine, labetalol, esmolol
Subarachnoid hemorrhage	Headache, neurologic deficit	AMS, neurologic deficit	Head CT, lumbar puncture	Decrease SBP < 160 mm Hg Nicardipine, labetalol, esmolol, clevidipine
Ischemic stroke	Neurologic deficit	Neurologic deficit	Head CT, brain MRI	Decrease BP < 185/110 mm Hg if fibrinolytic therapy planned or < 220/120 if no fibrinolytic Nicardipine, labetalol
Hypertensive encephalopathy, PRES	Headache, vomiting	AMS, papilledema	Head CT, brain MRI	Decrease MAP 20–25% Nicardipine, labetalol, clevidipine
Acute coronary syndrome	Chest pain, SOB, nausea	Diaphoresis, tachycardia	ECG, cardiac biomarkers	Reduce MAP by up to 25% Nitroglycerin, metoprolol, labetalol
Acute heart failure	SOB	Respiratory distress, rales/crackles on lung auscultation, peripheral edema	Chest plain radiograph, BNP	Reduce SBP by 20–30% Nitroglycerin, nicardipine, enalaprilat, nitroprusside
Aortic dissection	Chest pain, back pain	Unequal pulses or blood pressures in upper extremities, neurologic deficit	CT angiogram of chest and abdomen/pelvis	Reduce SBP to 100–120 mm Hg Esmolol, labetalol, nicardipine, nitroprusside

Eclampsia, preeclampsia	Headache, seizure	Seizure, AMS	Urinalysis	No specific BP goal Magnesium sulfate
HELLP	Abdominal pain	RUQ tenderness	Urinalysis, hepatic function panel, complete blood count	No specific BP goal Magnesium sulfate
Acute renal failure	Decreased urine output at later states, AMS if uremic	Typically no exam findings, can have AMS, flu d overload if severe	Basic metabolic panel, urinalysis	Reduce SBP by up to 20% Nicardipine, clevidipine
Hypertensive retinopathy	Visual changes	Decreased visual acuity, fundoscopic exam with retinal hemorrhages, cotton-wool spots, hard exudates, or sausage-shaped veins	Clinical diagnosis	No specific BP goal Caution in abruptly lower BP as may increase ischemia
Sympathetic crisis	Anxiety, agitation, palpitations	Tachycardia, diaphoresis, flushed skin	Drug screen (cocaine, PCP, amphetamines), 24 h urine	Reduce symptoms Benzodiazepines, nitroglycerin, phentolamine, nicardipine

AMS, altered mental status; BNP, brain natriuretic protein; CT, computed tomography; HELLP, hemolysis, elevated liver enzymes, low platelets; ICP, intracranial pressure; MAP, mean arterial pressure; PCP, phencyclidine; PRES, posterior reversible encephalopathy syndrome; RUQ, right upper quadrant; SBP, systolic blood pressure; SOB, shortness of breath.

Adapted from Baumann BM. Systemic Hypertension. In: Tintinalli JE, et al., eds. *Tintinalli's Emergency Medicine: A Comprehensive Study Guide.* 8th ed. New York: McGraw-Hill Education, 2016.

Differential Diagnosis
• Pain, anxiety, medication effect, or white coat hypertension.

Diagnostic Criteria and Testing[6,7]
Laboratories
• Laboratory evaluation should be focused on the hypertensive emergency state which is clinically suspected (Table 6.1).

Electrocardiography
• ECG should not routinely be performed for hypertension unless a hypertensive emergency such as acute coronary syndrome, aortic dissection, or acute heart failure is suspected.
• Patients with long-standing untreated or undertreated hypertension may commonly show signs of left ventricular hypertrophy on ECG.

Imaging
• Imaging is only necessary in patients with suspected hypertensive emergency (Table 6.1).

TREATMENT

Medications
• Hypertensive Emergency
  ○ Treatment of hypertensive emergencies typically involves parenteral antihypertensive therapy with continuous intravenous drips offering the ability to titrate therapy to specific blood pressure goals (Table 6.2).

TABLE 6.2	Dosing for Common Parenteral Antihypertensives
IV bolus dosing	
Hydralazine	10–20 mg
Phentolamine	5–15 mg
Labetalol	20–80 mg
Enalaprilat	0.625–1.25 mg
IV continuous infusion dosing	
Nicardipine	5–30 mg/h
Clevidipine	1–32 mg/h
Nitroprusside	0.3–2 µg/kg/min
Nitroglycerin	10–200 µg/min
Esmolol	0.5–1.0 mg/kg loading dose, followed by 50–300 µg/kg/min
Labetalol	1–2 mg/min
Nesiritide	2 µg/kg loading dose, followed by 0.01–0.03 µg/kg/min

- Hypertensive Urgency
  - Traditionally, patients with blood pressures ≥180/110 mm Hg often receive parenteral therapy to rapidly reduce blood pressure. Current approach to the management of hypertensive urgency calls for a more cautious approach to reduction of blood pressure over time with oral agents.[7,8]

| TABLE 6.3 | Initial Hypertension Therapy for Asymptomatic Patients |

Age	Diabetes	CKD	Race	BP goal	Initial therapy (choose one)
<60 y	–	–	Black	SBP < 140 mm Hg	Thiazide diuretic
				DBP < 90 mm Hg	Calcium channel blocker
			Nonblack	SBP < 140 mm Hg	Thiazide diuretic
				DBP < 90 mm Hg	ACE inhibitor
					Angiotensin receptor blocker
					Calcium channel blocker
≥60 y	–	–	Black	SBP < 150 mm Hg	Thiazide diuretic
				DBP < 90 mm Hg	Calcium channel blocker
			Nonblack	SBP < 150 mm Hg	Thiazide diuretic
				DBP < 90 mm Hg	ACE inhibitor
					Angiotensin receptor blocker
					Calcium channel blocker
All	+	–	Black	SBP < 140 mm Hg	Thiazide diuretic
				DBP < 90 mm Hg	Calcium channel blocker
			Nonblack	SBP < 140 mm Hg	Thiazide diuretic
				DBP < 90 mm Hg	ACE inhibitor
					Angiotensin receptor blocker
					Calcium channel blocker
All	+/–	+	All	SBP < 140 mm Hg	ACE inhibitor
				DBP < 90 mm Hg	Angiotensin receptor blocker

ACE, angiotensin-converting enzyme; BP, blood pressure; CKD, chronic kidney disease; DBP, diastolic blood pressure; SBP, systolic blood pressure.

Adapted from James PA, Oparil S, Carter BL, et al. 2014 Evidence-based guideline for the management of high blood pressure in adults: report from the panel members appointed to the Eighth Joint National Committee (JNC8). *JAMA* 2014;311(5):507–20.

- For asymptomatic patients with markedly elevated blood pressure ($\geq$180/110 mm Hg), repeat pressures should be obtained before initiating therapy.[9]
- Asymptomatic Hypertension
  - Initiation of medical therapy in the emergency department for asymptomatic patients with elevated blood pressure has not been shown to improve clinical outcomes.[8]
  - ACEP clinical guidelines state that initiating therapy for long-term blood pressure control may be performed in select patient populations (such as those with poor follow-up or limited access to outpatient care).[7]
  - Choice of initial therapeutic agent should be based on age, race, and comorbid conditions (see Table 6.3).

Other Nonpharmacologic Therapies

- Improved diet, especially reduction in salt and alcohol intake, increase in exercise, and smoking cessation can improve blood pressure.

SPECIAL CONSIDERATIONS

Disposition

- Patients with asymptomatic hypertension can be discharged from the emergency department with follow-up with a primary care physician.
- Patients with hypertensive urgency can often be discharged from the emergency department after a period of observation to ensure the blood pressure is adequately controlled and there is no end-organ damage.
- Patients with hypertensive emergency require inpatient admission.

REFERENCES

1. Chobanian AV, Bakris GL, Black HR, et al. Seventh report of the Joint National Committee on prevention, detection, evaluation, and treatment of high blood pressure. *Hypertension* 2003;42:1206–52. doi:10.1161/01.HYP.0000107251.49515.c2
2. Nwankwo T, Yoon SS, Burt V, Gu Q. Hypertension among adults in the United States: National Health and Nutrition Examination Survey, 2011–2012. *NCHS Data Brief* 2013:1–8.
3. Egan BM, Zhao Y, Axon RN. US trends in prevalence, awareness, treatment, and control of hypertension, 1988–2008. *JAMA* 2010;303:2043–50. doi:10.1001/jama.2010.650
4. Pitts SR, Niska RW, Xu J, Burt CW. National Hospital Ambulatory Medical Care Survey: 2006 emergency department summary. *National Health Statistics Reports* 2008:1–38.
5. Slovis CM, Reddi AS. Increased blood pressure without evidence of acute end organ damage. *Ann Emerg Med* 2008;51:S7–9. doi:10.1016/j.annemergmed.2007.11.005
6. Wolf SJ, Lo B, Shih RD, et al. Clinical policy: critical issues in the evaluation and management of adult patients in the emergency department with asymptomatic elevated blood pressure. *Ann Emerg Med* 2013;62:59–68. doi:10.1016/j.annemergmed.2013.05.012
7. Perez MI, Musini VM. Pharmacological interventions for hypertensive emergencies: a cochrane systematic review. *J Hum Hypertens* 2008;22:596–607. doi:10.1038/jhh.2008.25.
8. D, O'Flaherty M, Pellizzari M, et al. Hypertensive urgencies in the emergency department: evaluating blood pressure response to rest and to antihypertensive drugs with different profiles. *J Clin Hypertens* 2008;10:662–7. doi:10.1111/j.1751-7176.2008.00001.x.

Cardiovascular Emergencies: Pericarditis

Stacey House

GENERAL PRINCIPLES

Definition
- Acute pericarditis is inflammation of the pericardium, which can occur with or without pericardial effusion.

Epidemiology/Etiology
- 80–90% of cases are idiopathic (presumed viral).
- 10–20% of cases are postcardiac injury or related to connective tissue disease (especially systemic lupus erythematosus [SLE]) or malignancy.
- Risk factors for pericarditis include the following:
  - Recent viral infection or concurrent infection (TB, HIV, histoplasmosis, coccidioidomycosis).
  - Autoimmune disease—SLE, RA, and connective tissue disorders.
  - Metastatic cancer—breast cancer, lung cancer, leukemia, and Hodgkin lymphoma.
  - Myocardial injury—after acute myocardial infarction, 20% of patients develop pericarditis (Dressler syndrome).
  - Fluid retention states—uremia, congestive heart failure, and liver failure.
  - Recent cardiac procedure or surgery.

Pathophysiology
- Pericarditis is characterized by inflammation of the pericardial sac, which may be associated with the accumulation of pericardial fluid.
- Rubbing of the inflamed pericardial layers during the cardiac cycle is thought to cause the characteristic friction rub heard with auscultation of the heart.
- Accumulation of fluid within the fibrous pericardial sac can increase pressure surrounding the heart, leading to impaired diastolic filling and reduction in stroke volume.
- Cardiac tamponade can occur with small amounts of pericardial fluid in acute pericarditis. Larger amounts of fluid are necessary to cause hemodynamic compromise in patients with chronic pericarditis due to the ability of the pericardial sac to expand in capacity over long periods of time.

DIAGNOSIS

Clinical Presentation

History
- Patients with acute pericarditis will most commonly present with sharp or stabbing chest pain, which is retrosternal or precordial. It may radiate to the trapezius, neck, or left arm and is worsened with inspiration or movement. Chest pain is most severe when the patient is supine and relieved with sitting up and leaning forward.

- Other symptoms of pericarditis may include fever, dyspnea, or dysphagia (due to pericardial irritation of the esophagus).

Physical Examination
- A pericardial friction rub heard at the lower left sternal border is the most common physical exam finding. It is best heard when the patient is sitting and leaning forward but is often intermittent.

Differential Diagnosis
- ACS or MI, pulmonary embolism, pleurisy, musculoskeletal chest pain, or aortic dissection (rarely, due to bleeding into the pericardial sac)

Diagnostic Criteria and Testing
- The clinical diagnosis of pericarditis requires two of the following four criteria[1]:
  ○ Typical pericarditial chest pain, which is sharp, pleuritic, and improved by sitting up and leaning forward (occurs in 85–90% of cases)
  ○ Pericardial friction rub (occurs in ≤33% of cases)
  ○ ECG changes—diffuse ST elevation or PR depression (occurs in up to 60% of cases)
  ○ Pericardial effusion (occurs in up to 60% of cases)

Laboratories
- Laboratory values are not pathognomonic for pericarditis, but inflammatory markers may be drawn to monitor for resolution of disease.

Electrocardiography
- ST elevation is often diffuse but usually seen in leads I, V_5, and V_6 and is early in presentation. The ST elevation observed in pericarditis can be confused with that observed in benign early repolarization. If the ratio of the ST amplitude to the T-wave amplitude (in millivolts) is >0.25, pericarditis is more likely.[2]
- PR depression is most often seen in inferior and lateral leads.
- T-wave inversion is usually seen in leads I, V_5, and V_6 after ST changes have resolved.
- Electrical alternans and low-voltage QRS are typically only seen with large pericardial effusions.

Imaging
- Chest plain radiograph is most often normal since cardiomegaly is typically only seen with pericardial effusions >300 mL.[3]
- Transthoracic echocardiography can reveal the size of the associated pericardial effusion as well as early signs of cardiac tamponade.

TREATMENT

Medications
- Nonsteroidal anti-inflammatory drugs (ibuprofen 600 mg every 8 hours; indomethacin 25–50 mg every 8 hours) and aspirin (650 mg every 4 hours) therapy are first line.[1]
- Colchicine (0.6 mg twice a day) has recently been found to improve response to medical therapy and prevent recurrences.[4–6, 11]
- Immunosuppression with corticosteroids is the second-line therapy and should be limited to refractory or recurrent pericarditis.[7]

Other Nonpharmacologic Therapies
- Therapeutic pericardiocentesis may be required in patients with pericarditis who show signs of tamponade physiology.

SPECIAL CONSIDERATIONS

Disposition
- Most patients can be discharged unless they have a high fever, large pericardial effusions, tamponade, failure to respond to NSAIDs, immunosuppression, on anticoagulants, or have a concomitant myocarditis.[1,8]
- Patients should be instructed to restrict physical activity until resolution of symptoms.[9] Competitive athletes are typically restricted from returned to their sport until symptoms have resolved and diagnostic test such as inflammatory markers, ECG, and echocardiogram have returned to normal (usually 3 months).[9,10]

Complications
- The most life-threatening complication of pericarditis is cardiac tamponade, which can lead to hemodynamic collapse and cardiac arrest.

REFERENCES

1. Adler Y, Charron P, Imazio M, et al. 2015 ESC Guidelines for the diagnosis and management of pericardial diseases: The Task Force for the Diagnosis and Management of Pericardial Diseases of the European Society of Cardiology (ESC)Endorsed by: The European Association for Cardio-Thoracic Surgery (EACTS). *Eur Heart J* 2015;36:2921–64. doi:10.1093/eurheartj/ehv318.
2. Ginzton LE, Laks MM. The differential diagnosis of acute pericarditis from the normal variant: new electrocardiographic criteria. *Circulation* 1982;65:1004–9.
3. Imazio M, Adler Y. Management of pericardial effusion. *Eur Heart J* 2013;34:1186–97. doi:10.1093/eurheartj/ehs372.
4. Imazio M, Bobbio M, Cecchi E, et al. Colchicine in addition to conventional therapy for acute pericarditis: results of the COlchicine for acute PEricarditis (COPE) trial. *Circulation* 2016;112:2012–6. doi:10.1161/CIRCULATIONAHA.105.542738.
5. Imazio M, Bobbio M, Cecchi E, et al. Colchicine as first choice therapy for acute pericarditis. Results of the COPE trial. *Eur Heart J* 2005;26:110–1.
6. Alabed S, Cabello JB, Irving GJ, et al. Colchicine for pericarditis. *Cochrane Database Syst Rev* 2014;(8):CD010652. doi:Artn Cd01065210.1002/14651858.Cd010652.Pub2.
7. Imazio M, Brucato A, Cumetti D, et al. Corticosteroids for recurrent pericarditis: high versus low doses: a nonrandomized observation. *Circulation* 2008;118:667–71. doi:10.1161/CIRCULATIONAHA.107.761064.
8. Imazio M, Cecchi E, Demichelis B, et al. Indicators of poor prognosis of acute pericarditis. *Circulation* 2007;115:2739–44. doi:10.1161/CIRCULATIONAHA.106.662114.
9. Seidenberg PH, Haynes J. Pericarditis: diagnosis, management, and return to play. *Curr Sports Med Rep* 2006;5:74–9.
10. Pelliccia A, Corrado D, Bjørnstad HH, et al. Recommendations for participation in competitive sport and leisure-time physical activity in individuals with cardiomyopathies, myocarditis and pericarditis. *Eur J Cardiovasc Prev Rehabil* 2006;13:876–85. doi:10.1097/01. hjr.0000238393.96975.32.
11. Imazio M, Brucato A, Cemin R, et al. A randomized trial of colchicine for acute pericarditis. *N Engl J Med* 2013;369:1522–8. doi:10.1056/NEJMoa1208536.

8 Cardiovascular Emergencies: Valvular Heart Disease

Rahul Chhana

Aortic Stenosis (AS)

GENERAL PRINCIPLES

Epidemiology/Etiology
- The two most common causes of AS are congenital bicuspid aortic valve and senile calcification of the aortic valve.
- Bicuspid valvular disease has a peak incidence in the fifth or sixth decade and may be associated with rheumatic heart disease.

Pathophysiology
- Aortic sclerosis, or thickening of the aortic valve leaflets, may predispose patients to AS leading to left ventricle outflow obstruction.
  - Patients with severe or critical AS are preload dependent and may decompensate when preload is compromised.

DIAGNOSIS

Clinical Presentation
History
- Patients may present with angina, syncope, and dyspnea.

Physical Examination
- Crescendo–decrescendo systolic ejection murmur best heard at the second right intercostal space (right upper sternal border) and radiates to the carotids

Diagnostic Criteria and Testing
Electrocardiography
- LVH, atrial fibrillation, or repolarization abnormalities can be seen.

TREATMENT

Medications
- Diuresis can be used for patients that are grossly volume overloaded.
- Sodium nitroprusside decreases systemic vascular resistance and may be helpful.
- Dobutamine or phenylephrine will help maintain perfusion.
- Avoid vasodilators, as these may precipitate hypotension.

Other Nonpharmacologic Therapy
- Aortic valve replacement is the only effective treatment in severe AS

SPECIAL CONSIDERATIONS

Disposition
- All symptomatic patients should be admitted, and if symptoms are severe, should be admitted to an ICU.
- Patients should be cautioned to avoid strenuous physical activity and get prompt cardiology follow-up.

Aortic Insufficiency (AI)

GENERAL PRINCIPLES

Epidemiology/Etiology
- The most common cause of AI is a bicuspid aortic valve.
- It may be associated with other conditions including Marfan syndrome, syphilitic aortitis, reactive arthritis, and ankylosing spondylitis.
- Acute aortic insufficiency is a surgical emergency and may be caused by infectious endocarditis (IE), trauma, or aortic dissection.

Pathophysiology
- A portion of the stroke volume regurgitates back into the LV during diastole, decreasing diastolic blood pressure.
- SBP may be elevated as the forward stroke volume combined with the regurgitant volume ejected during systole causes an increase in total stroke volume.

DIAGNOSIS

Clinical Presentation
History
- Patients may present with acute decompensated heart failure or cardiogenic shock.
- Chronic AI may present with progressive dyspnea or symptoms of heart failure.

Physical Examination
- The murmur of chronic AI is described as a high-pitched, blowing, early diastolic, decrescendo murmur best heard at the left lower sternal border.[1]
- Widened pulse pressure.
- Chronic AI is associated with several physical findings (Table 8.1).

TABLE 8.1	Physical Findings in Chronic Aortic Insufficiency
Eponym	**Description**
Austin Flint murmur	A low-pitched diastolic rumble best heard at the apex
Watson water hammer pulse (Corrigan pulse)	Rapid rise and collapse of the carotid pulse
De Musset sign	Head bobbing with each pulse
Quinke sign	Pulsation of capillary nail bed
Traube sign	Pistol shot to-and-fro murmur heard over the femoral artery

Diagnostic Criteria and Testing

Imaging
- Chest plain radiograph may also show aortic dilation or widened mediastinum.
- Emergent echocardiogram should be obtained in acute AI.
- A CT or MRI can be performed when aortic root involvement is suspected.

Electrocardiography
- The ECG may show LVH, LAE, sinus tachycardia, or atrial fibrillation.

TREATMENT

Medications

- Chronic AI can be treated with calcium channel blockers, beta-blockers, or vasodilators if hypertension (SBP > 140 mm Hg) is present.[2]
- Sodium nitroprusside and dobutamine may help with forward flow in the acute setting.
- Beta-blockers should be avoided in acute decompensation.

Other Nonpharmacologic Therapy

- Emergent surgical consultation is needed in decompensated patients

SPECIAL CONSIDERATIONS

Disposition

- Decompensated patients should be admitted.

Mitral Stenosis (MS)

GENERAL PRINCIPLES

Epidemiology/Etiology

- Mitral valve involvement can be as high as 90% in patients with rheumatic fever and rheumatic heart disease (RHD).[3]
- Other less common causes include mitral valve calcification, congenital MS, and chemotoxic MS.

Pathophysiology

- Obstruction of blood flow through the mitral passage from the LA causes an increase in LA pressure. This leads to a compensatory dilation of the LA and eventually right-sided HF develops.[4]
- LV diastolic filling is reduced and cardiac output is diminished causing signs and symptoms of left-sided HF.
- The opening snap found in MS is due to an abrupt halt of the stenotic valve during diastole.
- Acute decompensation may occur in conditions that increase cardiac demand due to the inability to rapidly fill the left ventricle.

DIAGNOSIS

Clinical Presentation

History
- Patients may report dyspnea on exertion, orthopnea, and paroxysmal nocturnal dyspnea.
- Hoarseness may occur from the LA compressing the recurrent laryngeal nerve.
- Hemoptysis is a rare but emergent presentation.

Physical Examination
- The murmur of MS is described as a delayed, rumbling, late diastolic murmur best heard with the bell of the stethoscope at the apex.
- S_1 is loud and followed by a loud opening snap, which precedes the murmur.

Diagnostic Criteria and Testing

Electrocardiography
- LAE may cause atrial fibrillations and frequent PACs.
- Notched, bifid P waves from LAE.
- Right axis deviation and right ventricular hypertrophy may be present.

TREATMENT

- The definitive treatment for symptomatic disease is valvotomy, repair, or replacement.

Medications

- Anticoagulation (AC) is indicated in patients with atrial fibrillation, a history of prior embolic event, or LA thrombus.

SPECIAL CONSIDERATIONS

Disposition

- Symptomatic patients may require admission.

Mitral Regurgitation (MR)

GENERAL PRINCIPLES

Epidemiology/Etiology

- MR can be caused from the dysfunction of any part of the mitral valve apparatus.
- Causes include rupture of chordae tendineae, connective tissue disorders, and cardiomyopathy.

Pathophysiology

- With an acute rise in pressure, the LA pressure increases faster than the LA can accommodate, leading to pulmonary venous congestion.
- During systole, part of the cardiac output is regurgitated back into the LA causing hypotension and contributing to pulmonary edema.
- Chronically, there will be LVH and LV dysfunction.

Clinical Presentation
History
- Acute MR presents with respiratory failure, heart failure, or cardiogenic shock.
- Chronic MR is largely asymptomatic but may progress to worsening dyspnea, atrial fibrillation or pulmonary congestion, and heart failure.[5]
  - There may be acute decompensation when there is sudden dysfunction of the chordae tendineae or a papillary muscle.

Physical Examination
- The murmur of acute MR is a mid- or late systolic murmur that radiates to the base. There may be no associated murmur.
- The murmur of chronic MR is a holosystolic, high-pitched, blowing, systolic murmur that is loudest at the apex and radiates to the axilla.

Diagnostic Testing and Criteria
Electrocardiography
- May show LAE and P mitrale, LVH, or atrial fibrillation.

Echocardiogram (TTE)
- When acute MR is suspected, emergent TTE should be performed.

TREATMENT

- Acute MR is a medical emergency and requires urgent surgical consultation.

Medications

- Acute decompensation may be treated with nitroprusside, nitrates, and diuretics as tolerated by blood pressure.
- Attempts to slow tachycardia should be avoided as it may decrease forward flow and CO.
- Patients with atrial fibrillation may need anticoagulation.

SPECIAL CONSIDERATIONS

Disposition
- If stable, may be treated as an outpatient with cardiology follow-up.
- Symptomatic patients should be admitted for surgical evaluation or optimization of heart failure.

Mitral Valve Prolapse (MVP)

GENERAL PRINCIPLES

Etiology
- It may be associated with connective tissue disorders.[6]
- Patients are usually young and healthy.

Pathophysiology
- MVP is caused by the myxomatous degeneration of the mitral leaflet.
- The mitral click heard in MVP is caused by the sudden tensing of the chordae tendineae during systole.

DIAGNOSIS

Clinical Presentation

History
- Largely asymptomatic but may present with occasional palpitations or atypical chest pain not associated with exertion

Physical Examination
- The murmur is described as a midsystolic click followed by a late systolic murmur.

Diagnostic Criteria and Testing

Electrocardiography
- May show changes of LAE and atrial fibrillation if MR is present.

TREATMENT

Medications

- Low-dose beta-blockers may be used in symptomatic patients but is not recommended for asymptomatic patients.[7]

SPECIAL CONSIDERATIONS

Disposition

- Patients may be discharged home with cardiology follow-up.

Prosthetic Valves

- Bioprosthetic (porcine or bovine) valves do not require AC and last ~10 years. They have a lower thromboembolism risk and are less likely to fail.
- Mechanical valves (i.e., bileaflet St. Jude) carry a higher thromboembolism risk and must be treated with AC. They can last 20–30 years.
- Patients with a suspected prosthetic valve dysfunction should undergo emergent TTE.
- Aspirin is recommended for all prosthetic valves.

Complications

- Acute valve thrombosis symptoms range from asymptomatic to signs and symptoms of heart failure and cardiogenic shock.
- There is a risk of embolism from the thrombus.
  - Intravenous (IV) heparin should be started immediately.
  - Patients may need fibrinolysis or emergent surgery.
- Restenosis and regurgitation
  - May present with signs and symptoms of HF and will need admission
- Infectious endocarditis:
  - If suspected, TTE should be performed, blood cultures should be drawn, and broad-spectrum antibiotics should be started prior to admission.

REFERENCES

1. Biancaniello T. Innocent murmurs. *Circulation* 2005;111(3):e20–2.
2. Scognamiglio R, Rahimtoola SH, Fasoli G, et al. Nifedipine in asymptomatic patients with severe aortic regurgitation and normal left ventricular function. *N Engl J Med* 1994;331(11):689–94.

3. Bland EF, Duckett Jones T. Rheumatic fever and rheumatic heart disease: a twenty year report on 1000 patients followed since childhood. *Circulation* 1951;4(6):836–43.
4. Hugenholtz PG, Ryan TJ, Stein SW, Abelmann WH. The spectrum of pure mitral stenosis. Hemodynamic studies in relation to clinical disability. *Am J Cardiol* 1962;10:773–84.
5. Reed D, Abbott RD, Smucker ML, Kaul S. Prediction of outcome after mitral valve replacement in patients with symptomatic chronic mitral regurgitation. The importance of left atrial size. *Circulation* 1991;84(1):23–34.
6. Rybczynski M, Mir TS, Sheikhzadeh S, et al. Frequency and age-related course of mitral valve dysfunction in the Marfan syndrome. *Am J Cardiol* 2010;106(7):1048–53.
7. Tacoy G, Balcioglu AS, Arslan U, et al. Effect of metoprolol on heart rate variability in symptomatic patients with mitral valve prolapse. *Am J Cardiol* 2007;99(11):1568–70.

Dermatologic Disorders: Overview

Christopher Lawrence

GENERAL PRINCIPLES

Classification

- **Primary lesions**—The acute dermatologic changes composed of the first visible skin lesion or change.
  - Macules: nonpalpable circumscribed alteration in skin color <1 cm in size. There is no associated elevation or depression of the skin.
  - Patch: nonpalpable circumscribed alteration in skin color >1 cm in size. There is no associated elevation or depression of the skin.
  - Papules: palpable, discrete lesions that are <0.5 cm that may be isolated or grouped.
  - Nodules: palpable, discrete lesions that are >0.5 cm. A tumor can sometimes be described as a large nodule.
  - Plaques: >5 mm superficially raised fixed lesions that may be composed of a single discrete lesion or by a confluence of papules.
  - Telangiectasia: prominent dilated superficial blood vessels.
  - Petechiae: a small collection of blood in the skin <0.5 cm in diameter.
  - Purpura: reddish-purple lesions that do not blanch, can be macular or raised, and result from the extravasation of blood into the skin
  - Pustules: papules that contain pus, whereas vesicles are small (<5 mm) papules that contain serous material; bullae are large vesicles (>5 mm).
  - Wheals: irregularly elevated edematous areas of skin with well-defined but unstable borders; the lesion may grow or shrink over time and is often erythematous and pruritic.
- **Secondary lesions**—result as manipulation of the skin, infection, or a chronic change that occurs over time

○ Excoriation: superficial, typically linear, skin erosions that are due to localized trauma caused by scratching.

○ Lichenification: a more chronic thickening of the skin with associated induration and a surface pattern of skin lines due to chronic inflammation; can often occur due to scratching as well as other recurrent skin irritants.

○ Sclerosis: an alteration in the dermis due to accumulation of fluid, connective tissue, or metabolite, typically resulting in an inelastic feel of the dermis with altered skin wrinkling and texture.

○ Hypertrichosis: an area of excessive hair growth.

○ Hypotrichosis: an area of diminished hair growth.

○ Alopecia: absence of hair from a normally hair-bearing area.

○ Milium: a small white cyst containing keratin.

○ Edema: a generalized term for swelling due to water accumulation in the tissue.

○ Scaling: an accumulation of desquamated dead superficial epidermal cells (stratum corneum) that create a rough superficial layer over the surface of the skin.

○ Crust: an accumulation of dried exudate or blood, aka a "scab."

○ Fibrosis: a formation of excessive fibrous tissue.

○ Horn: an elevated projection of keratin.

○ Papilloma: a nipple-like mass coming off the surface of the skin.

○ Cyst: a closed cavity or sac with an epithelial, endothelial, or membranous lining containing fluid or semisolid material.

○ Ecchymosis: "bruise." A macular area of hemorrhage >0.5 cm in diameter.

○ Erythema: redness of the skin caused by vascular congestion or increased skin perfusion.

○ Eschar: an area of crust and tissue necrosis, often due to infection or burn.

○ Fistula: an abnormal passage from a deep structure to a more superficial structure.

○ Sinus: a cavity or track with a blind ending.

○ Target lesion: an area, typically <3 cm in diameter, and composed of three or more zones, typically with a central area of erythema or purpura, a middle zone of edema that is more pale in appearance, and a well-defined outer ring of erythema.

○ Impetiginization: a superficial honey-colored or purulent exudate, typically a sign of superficial infection such as in impetigo.

○ Gangrene: a sharply demarcated area of tissue death that may involve all three skin layers.

○ Fissure: a split or cleavage in the skin that can extend as deep as the dermis, typically occurring spontaneously without trauma. These are typically painful.

○ Erosion: a superficial depression due to focal loss of the epidermis, which will typically heal without scar formation. An ulceration extends into the dermis.

○ Necrosis: an area of dead tissue in a part or portion of a skin lesion.

○ Atrophy: a decrease in skin thickness and can occur from a multitude of sources. A scar is a collection of fibrous tissue that replaces normal skin tissue following injury.

○ Hyperpigmentation: an increase in skin pigmentation. Hypopigmentation is a decrease in pigmentation, and depigmentation refers to total loss of normal skin pigment. Achromia, or leukoderma, also refers to complete loss of skin color.

○ Burrow: a short, linear elevation of the horny layer of skin, characteristically due to the presence of a mite, such as in scabies, in the stratum corneum.

○ Comedone: an open (blackhead) or closed (whitehead) horny plug in the opening of the pilosebaceous duct.

History
- How long has the lesion been present?
- Any preceding sun, cold, dry air, or chemical exposure?
- How does it look now compared to when it first occurred?
- Where did it first appear, and has it spread?
- What treatment was tried and what response to treatment has occurred?
- What, if any, associated symptoms are there?
- Does anyone else in the family or work have similar skin findings?
- Has the patient ever had this lesion before? If so, how was it treated previously?
- Does the patient have any idea what caused the skin finding?
- Has anything new or different occurred recently (medication, hygiene products, occupational or recreational exposures of note?)
- Specific medical history questions
  - Any new medications or supplements?
  - Any increase in life stressors?
  - Any notable social history, including hobbies, recent travel, or high-risk occupation for any exposures?
  - Any pets?
  - Any risks factors for STI?

Physical Examination
- What type of lesion is it?
- Is there only one type or lesion, or are their multiple types?
- What morphology are the lesions?
- What is their configuration? (Scattered, grouped, linear, etc.)
- What distribution do they have? ("Christmas tree," extensor surface, flexor surface, photodistribution, etc.)
- What color and appearance do they have?
- What consistency and tactile qualities does it have?

Visual Inspection
- Should be performed under good lighting.
- Consider magnifying lens if necessary.
- Completely disrobe the patient to fully assess the distribution and number of lesions.
- Do not neglect examination of the nails, hair-bearing surfaces, and mucosa.
- Don't forget to palpate both the normal and the abnormal sections of skin.

Bedside Procedures for Workup
- Wood lamp examination
  - Useful for diagnosis of:
    - Tinea capitis—*Microsporum canis* and *Microsporum audouinii* fluoresce blue-green, though only account for ~20% of disease
    - Erythrasma: *Corynebacterium minutissimum* fluoresces coral red
    - Porphyria cutanea tarda: pink or orange-red fluorescence of urine
  - Technique
    - Examine in darkened room to achieve maximum fluorescence.
    - If patient recently bathed, may reduce fluorescence.
- Potassium hydroxide prep
  - Used to detect fungus or yeast from skin scrapings

○ Technique
  ▪ Clean the skin with alcohol prep pad.
  ▪ Specimen procurement: the skin can be scraped with a slide or blade and placed on slide with a few drops of KOH and coverslip prior to viewing under a microscope for bud and branching pattern.

SUGGESTED READINGS

Allen HB. *Dermatology Terminology*. London: Springer-Verlag, 2010.

Bolognia J, Schaffer J, Duncan K, Ko C. *Dermatology Essentials*. Oxford, Saunders: Elsevier, 2014.

Brady WJ, Perron AD, Martin ML. Approach to the Dermatologic Patient in the Emergency Department. In: Tintinalli JE, Kelen GD, Stapczynski JS, eds. *Emergency Medicine: A Comprehensive Study Guide*. 6th ed. NY: The McGraw Hill Companies, Inc, 2004:1507–13.

Burns T, Breathnach S, Cox N, eds. *Rook's Textbook of Dermatology*. Vol. 4. 8th ed. Hoboken: Wiley-Blackwell, 2010.

Buxton PK. ABC of dermatology. Introduction. *Br Med J (Clin Res Ed)*. 1987;295(6602):830–4.

Cox NH, Coulson IH. Diagnosis of Skin Disease. In: Burns T, Breathnach S, Cox N, Griffiths C, eds. *Rook's Textbook of Dermatology*. 8th ed. Oxford, UK: Wiley-Blackwell, 2010.

Gawkrodger DJ, Ardern-Jones MR. Terminology of Skin Lesions. In: *Dermatology: An Illustrated Colour Text*. 5th ed. Edinburgh: Elsevier, 2012.

Mann M, Berk DR, Bayliss SJ, Popkin D. *Handbook of Dermatology: A Practical Manual*. Hoboken: Wiley-Blackwell, 2009.

Rimoin L, Altieri L, Craft N, et al. Training pattern recognition of skin lesion morphology, configuration, and distribution. *J Am Acad Dermatol*. 2015;72:489.

Trozak DJ, Tenneshouse D, Russell J. *Dermatology Skills for Primary Care: An Illustrated Guide*. Totowa, NJ: Humana Press, 2006.

Wolff K. Fitzpatrick's Dermatology in General Medicine. 2008. Retrieved February 11, 2016. Available at: http://www.r2library.com/Resource/Title/0071466908

Zaidi Z, Lanigan SW. *Dermatology in Clinical Practice. Diagnosis of Skin Disease*. London: Springer-Verlag, 2010:25–35.

10 Dermatologic Emergencies: Dermatitis

Lauren O'Grady and SueLin M. Hilbert

GENERAL PRINCIPLES

Definition

• Dermatitis is a rash that develops after exposure and can be categorized as contact or allergic.

Epidemiology/Etiology

• Contact dermatitis affects about 20% of the adult population.
• Allergic dermatitis is most commonly caused by oleoresin from poison ivy, sumac, or oak plant.

- Clothing, jewelry, soaps, cosmetics, plants, and medications contain allergens that commonly cause allergic contact dermatitis.

Pathophysiology

- Allergic dermatitis is a type IV hypersensitivity reaction.
- Contact dermatitis is a direct effect of the offending irritant.
- Latex and some chemicals can produce an immunoglobulin E–mediated type I immediate hypersensitivity reaction resulting in contact urticaria, angioedema, and possibly anaphylactic shock.

DIAGNOSIS

Clinical Presentation

History

- The patient may or may not report a known exposure. The acute form can occur up to 2 weeks after exposure to irritant. The chronic form can by continuously or intermittently present for months or years.
- There will usually be report of itching and rash of varying severity and with attempts made to self-treat.
- History should include recent travel, exposure to plants, animals, soaps, lotions, powders, perfumes, make-up, and any occupational exposures.

Physical Examination

- Often seen is a pruritic papular erythematous dermatitis with indistinct margins, the distribution of which is determined by site of exposure
- Papules, vesicles, and bullae on an erythematous bed will frequently be present.
- Special attention should be paid to where on the body the rash appears (including what is covered by clothing, exposed to sun or chemicals, and overlying jewelry).

Differential Diagnosis

- Immunodeficiency, lichen simplex chronicus, mollusca contagiosa with dermatitis, mycosis fungoides, nummular dermatitis, plaque psoriasis, relative zinc deficiency, scabies, seborrheic dermatitis, or tinea corporis

Diagnostic Criteria and Testing

- Diagnosis is made based on history and physical examination.

Laboratories

- There are no specific laboratories that will confirm dermatitis in the ED.

Imaging

- There are no specific imaging studies that will confirm dermatitis in the ED.

Other Diagnostic Procedures

- Scrapings can be performed on the skin to rule out fungal elements.

TREATMENT

- Care is supportive.

Medications

- Dermatitis can be managed with topical and oral antihistamines such as hydroxyzine or diphenhydramine.
- Topical steroids (avoid in blistering areas) or oral steroid taper may be prescribed in severe cases.
- Oatmeal baths or calamine lotion can also offer symptomatic relief.

SPECIAL CONSIDERATIONS

Disposition

- Patients may be discharged to home unless evidence of superimposed infection or anaphylaxis is present. Referral to a dermatologist may be indicated in cases that do not respond to antihistamine or steroid treatment.

SUGGESTED READINGS

Marx JA, Hockberger RJ, Walls RM, et al, eds. *Rosen's Emergency Medicine: Concepts and Clinical practice*. 8th ed. Philadelphia: Saunders/Elsevier, 2014.
Tintinalli JE, Stapczynski JS, Cline DM, et al., eds. *Tintinalli's Emergency Medicine: A Comprehensive Study Guide*. New York: McGraw-Hill, 2011.

11 Dermatologic Emergencies: Infectious Disorders

Blake Bruton, Michael Willman, and Stephen Y. Liang

GENERAL PRINCIPLES

- Most skin and soft tissue infections (SSTIs) are caused by gram-positive organisms:
  - *Staphylococcus aureus*, group A, β-hemolytic *Streptococcus* (*S. pyogenes*), and *Enterococcus* sp.
- Some gram-negative organisms are common as well:
  - *Pseudomonas aeruginosa* and *Escherichia coli*

DISPOSITION

- Mild cases may be treated on an outpatient basis with appropriate follow-up and return precautions for worsening symptoms. Severe cases or those needing IV antibiotics should be observed for improvement for 24–72 hours.
- Antibiotic treatment may need to be modified if the patient is pregnant.

SPECIFIC INFECTIOUS DISEASES

Erysipelas

GENERAL PRINCIPLES

- Most common causative organism is β-hemolytic *Streptococcus*.
- Risk factors include impaired venous or lymphatic drainage, obesity, diabetes, and immune compromise.

DIAGNOSIS

- Most commonly affects the face (butterfly pattern), ears, and lower extremities
- Raised, erythematous areas with distinct lines of demarcation[1]
- Acute onset with systemic symptoms (e.g., fever, chills)

TREATMENT

- Keep affected area elevated to promote venous and lymphatic drainage. If applicable, compression stockings or diuretic therapy can be considered.[1]
- Systemic antibiotics are indicated.[1]
  - Amoxicillin 500 mg PO tid for 5–10 days[1]
  - Cephalexin 500 mg PO qid for 5–10 days[2]

    In severe cases, consider IV therapy:

  - Ceftriaxone 1000 mg IV every 24 hours for 5–10 days[1]

COMPLICATIONS

- Can recur in up to a third of patients

Abscesses

GENERAL PRINCIPLES

- A collection of pus within the dermis or subcutaneous tissue; also referred to as a furuncle, carbuncle, or boil.
- Risk factors include impaired venous or lymphatic drainage, immune compromise, poorly controlled diabetes, and IV drug use.

DIAGNOSIS

- Clinical diagnosis is made primarily by physical examination.
- Fever is uncommon.
- Affected areas will be erythematous, warm, and sometimes indurated.
  - Areas of fluctuance may be present. Ultrasound may aid in diagnosis.

TREATMENT

- Warm compresses may be adequate for very small abscesses.
- Incision and drainage (I&D) is the definitive treatment.[1,2]

○ Needle aspiration can be successful in some cases, but ultrasound should be used to ensure complete drainage. Proceed to I&D if not absolutely positive of complete drainage.[3]
• Most abscesses are successfully treated with I&D alone and do not require antibiotics.[1,2]
  ○ Consider antibiotics in patients who have extensive disease or systemic symptoms, are severely immune compromised, have failed previous treatment, or have frequent recurrences.
• If used, antibiotics should empirically cover for MRSA[2]:
  ○ Trimethoprim–sulfamethoxazole 2 double strength (DS) tabs PO bid for 7 days.[2,4]
    ▪ The addition of cephalexin to cover for group A streptococci is not necessary.[5]
  ○ Doxycycline 100 mg PO bid[1,2]

COMPLICATIONS

• Abscesses on the medial third of the face (e.g., nasal furuncles) are a risk factor for septic cavernous sinus thrombosis.

Cellulitis

GENERAL PRINCIPLES

• A bacterial SSTI involving the deeper layers of the dermis and subcutaneous tissue.
  ○ MRSA tends to cause purulent cellulitis or abscesses.
  ○ Diabetics are at greater risk for gram-negative and anaerobic infections.
• Certain cases of cellulitis are more commonly associated with particular pathogens, and therapy should be adjusted appropriately (Table 11.1).
• Risk factors include impaired venous or lymphatic drainage, obesity, poorly controlled diabetes, IV drug use, and immune compromise.

DIAGNOSIS

• Affected areas will be erythematous and warm. Some areas may have induration, or even purulent drainage, but no drainable collections of purulence.

TABLE 11.1	Cellulitis-Based Antibiotic Therapy	
Specific case	Specific pathogen	Specific therapy
Dog or cat bite	*Pasteurella multocida*	Augmentin 875 mg bid × 7 d
Fresh water exposure	*Aeromonas hydrophila*	Ciprofloxacin 500 mg bid × 7 d or TMP/SMX DS bid × 7 d
Salt water exposure	*Vibrio vulnificus*	Ciprofloxacin 500 mg bid × 7 d or doxycycline 100 mg bid × 7 d
IV drug use	Gram-negative rods (e.g., *Pseudomonas aeruginosa*)	With consultation by ID
	Anaerobes (e.g., *Clostridium* spp.)	

ID, infectious disease; TMP/SMX, trimethoprim/sulfamethoxazole.

- In contrast to erysipelas, cellulitis is not sharply demarcated.
  - Rapid progression should raise concern for necrotizing soft tissue infections.
- Vesicles/bullae, petechiae, or ecchymoses may also be seen.

TREATMENT

- Use a marking pen to delineate the affected area and aid in evaluation for disease progression. Rapid progression may warrant parenteral antibiotics and admission. It also raises the concern for necrotizing fasciitis.
- Keep the affected area elevated to promote venous and lymphatic drainage.[1]
- Severe infections warrant parenteral antibiotics and observation or admission.
- Systemic antibiotics are indicated.[1]

  If MRSA is not suspected:

  - Cephalexin 500 mg PO qid for 5–10 days[1,2] or
  - Clindamycin 300–450 mg PO qid for 5–7 days[1,2]

  If MRSA is suspected:

  - Trimethoprim–sulfamethoxazole 1–2 DS tabs PO bid for 5–7 days[1,2] or
  - Doxycycline 100 mg PO bid[1,2]

COMPLICATIONS

- Orbital cellulitis can lead to subperiosteal abscess, orbital abscess, brain abscess, or septic cavernous sinus thrombosis.

Necrotizing Soft Tissue Infection

GENERAL PRINCIPLES

- Fulminant infection caused by mixed aerobic and anaerobic bacteria with destruction of muscle, fascia, and fat.
  - Risk factors include recent surgery, peripheral vascular disease, diabetes, immune compromise, trauma, and IV drug abuse.

DIAGNOSIS

- Most commonly affects extremities but can also be seen on the neck, abdominal wall, and perineum and associated with postoperative wounds.
- Systemic toxicity (fever, hemodynamic instability) is common.
- Affected areas may have mild erythema initially. As the disease progresses, blisters and bullae may form, as well as skin crepitus and necrosis.
  - Plain radiographs may help assess for subcutaneous air.
  - CT should be performed to assess for gas in fascial planes and extent of disease.
- Pain out of proportion to the exam is common, especially in early stages with little overlying skin involvement initially.
  - Intense pain with movement, swelling, or taut skin should raise concern for compartment syndrome.
- Disease progression is rapid (hours in some cases).

TREATMENT

- Urgent surgical consultation is required for surgical debridement.
- Parenteral antibiotics are indicated.[1]
  - Vancomycin 15–20 mg/kg IV every 12 hours
    - Use renal dosing if the patient has renal disease.
    - Linezolid can be used instead for vancomycin-allergic patients.

  AND

  - Piperacillin–tazobactam 3.375 mg IV every 6 hours or 4.5 g IV every 8 hours
    - May also consider a carbapenem (e.g., imipenem–cilastatin)

  WITH or WITHOUT

  - Clindamycin (900 mg IV q 8 hours) for antitoxin effects

COMPLICATIONS

- High mortality rates—20–40%

DISPOSITION

- Admission, surgical debridement, and IV antibiotics

Toxic Shock Syndromes[6]

GENERAL PRINCIPLES

- Superantigen-mediated disease associated with life-threatening hemodynamic instability and multiorgan dysfunction.
- Classically caused by *S. aureus* exotoxins or *group A Streptococcus* (*S. pyogenes*) enterotoxins.
- Characterized by a nonspecific constellation of fever, diffuse macular rash, desquamation, hypotension, vomiting or diarrhea, myalgias, mucous membrane involvement, renal dysfunction, transaminitis, coagulopathy, thrombocytopenia, and altered mental status.
- Risk factors include retained foreign body (tampon, female barrier contraceptive, nasal packing), SSTI, varicella infection, surgery, trauma, childbirth, and influenza.

DIAGNOSIS

- Staphylococcal toxic shock syndrome (TSS):
  - Fever: temperature ≥38.9°C
  - Painless, diffuse, red, macular rash (resembles sunburn)
  - Desquamation: 1–2 weeks after onset of rash
  - Hypotension
  - Multiorgan involvement (≥3 organ systems)
- Streptococcal toxic-shock syndrome (STSS):
  - More commonly associated with necrotizing soft tissue infection.
  - Carries a significantly higher mortality.
  - Criteria include hypotension and multiorgan involvement (≥2 organ systems).
  - Rash and desquamation are uncommon.

- ○ Blood cultures are positive in up to 60% of STSS cases.
- ○ Commonly presents with pain out of proportion to exam.
- ○ CT and MRI may demonstrate necrotizing soft tissue destruction but should never delay urgent surgical consultation and surgical debridement.
- Obtain lab studies: CBC, CMP, PT/PTT, CPK, UA, blood cultures, wound cultures, culture of any removed foreign bodies, and lumbar puncture in patients with altered mental status.

TREATMENT

- Initial treatment is aimed at resuscitation of shock, infection source control, support of organ failure, and timely antibiotics.
  - ○ Emergent surgical consultation may be necessary for debridement of infected wounds or removal of foreign bodies.
  - ○ Empiric broad-spectrum antibiotics covering MRSA should be initiated as soon as possible following identification of sepsis syndrome.
    - Vancomycin, 15 mg/kg IV every 12 hours, or linezolid, 600 mg IV every 12 hours.
    - Plus β-lactamase inhibitor (e.g., pipercillin–tazobactam, 4.5 g IV every 6 hours) or carbapenem (e.g., meropenem, 1 g IV every 8 hours).
    - Plus clindamycin, 900 mg IV every 8 hours to limit toxin production.
    - IV immune globulin may be required if no improvement in first 6 hours. IV dose is 1–2 g/kg. Consult infectious disease.

DISPOSITION

- ICU admission.

Herpes Zoster ("Shingles")

GENERAL PRINCIPLES

- A painful, vesicular rash caused by reactivation of varicella-zoster virus (VZV).
- The reactivated virus travels down sensory nerve fibers resulting in a dermatomal distribution that does not cross midline. In immune compromised patients, there may be multiple dermatomes involved or the rash may be disseminated throughout the body.
- The rash commonly affects the trunk or face and is usually preceded by 2–4 days of pain or paresthesia.

DIAGNOSIS

- Diagnosis is made clinically. Typically, no labs are required.

TREATMENT

- Initial treatment is oral acyclovir or valacyclovir for 7 days.
- Treatment should begin within 24 hours of rash onset and is generally not effective if started after 72 hours.[7]
- Steroid use is controversial.
- Patients with severe infection or significant immune compromise may require IV antivirals and should be considered for therapy even after 72 hours.

COMPLICATIONS

- Postherpetic neuralgia: persistent pain over the affected area after resolution of the rash lasting 3 months or more. It can be severe or debilitating in some cases.

DISPOSITION

- Discharge home unless IV therapy required or the patient is immune compromised with multiple dermatomal involvement or disseminated zoster.

Fungal Infections[8]

GENERAL PRINCIPLES

- Tinea, a fungal infection caused by dermatophytes, is categorized by the location of infection.
- Exam is consistent with red, scaly patches or plaques, sometimes with central clearing.

  They can be spread through close physical contact.

DIAGNOSIS

- Diagnosis is made clinically. However, a scraping and KOH preparation can be used for confirmation.

TREATMENT

- Superficial cutaneous infections are typically treated with topical antifungal agents (azoles).
- Recalcitrant infections and those involving the scalp or nails require prolonged oral therapy.

REFERENCES

1. Ibrahim F, Khan T, Pujalte GGA, et al. Bacterial skin infections. *Prim Care Clin Office Pract* 2015;42:485–99.
2. Stevens DL, Bisno AL, Chambers HF, et al. Practice guidelines for the diagnosis and management of skin and soft tissue infections: 2014 update by the Infectious Diseases Society of America. *Clin Infect Dis* 2014;59:147.
3. Gaspari RJ, Resop D, Mendoza M, et al. Randomized controlled trial of incision and drainage versus ultrasonography guided needle aspiration for skin abscesses and the effect of methicillin-resistant *Staphylococcus aureus*. *Ann Emerg Med* 2011;57(5):483–91.
4. Talan DA, Mower WR, Krishnadasan A, et al. Trimethoprim-sulfamethoxazole versus placebo for uncomplicated skin abscess. *N Engl J Med* 2016;374:823–32.
5. Bowen AC, Lilliebridge RA, Tong SY, et al. Is *Streptococcus pyogenes* resistant or susceptible to trimethoprim-sulfamethoxazole? *J Clin Microbiol* 2012;50:4067–72.
6. Liang SY. Toxic Shock Syndromes. In: Tintinalli JE, Stapczynski J, Ma O, et al., eds. *Tintinalli's Emergency Medicine: A Comprehensive Study Guide*. 8th ed. New York: McGraw-Hill, 2016.
7. Friesen KJ, Alessi-Severini S, Chateau D, et al. The changing landscape of antiviral treatment of herpes zoster: a 17-year population-based cohort study. *Clinicoecon Outcomes Res* 2016;8:207–14.
8. Ely JW, Rosenfeld S, Seabury Stone M. Diagnosis and management of tinea infections. *Am Fam Physician* 2014;90(10):702–10.

12 Dermatologic Emergencies: Stevens-Johnson Syndrome/Toxic Epidermal Necrolysis

Lydia Luangruangrong and Caitlin Fuqua

GENERAL PRINCIPLES

Definition

- These mucocutaneous diseases are frequently drug related, characterized by separation of skin at the dermal–epidermal junction, and typically involve mucous membranes and systemic symptoms.
- The skin lesions can appear as dusky or red, flat, atypical, target-like confluent lesions.
- Classification is by body surface area (BSA):
  - SJS < 10%, SJS/TEN overlap 10–30%, and TEN > 30%

Epidemiology/Etiology

- Women are more affected than men.
- The elderly are at greater risk for developing SJS.
- Patients with HIV are at three times the risk of developing SJS/TEN.
- Mortality is affected by age, severity of reaction, preexisting severe liver or kidney disorder, recent malignancy, and recent infection.
- Associated primarily with medications (80–95%) and infections.
  - Most commonly associated medications: nevirapine, lamotrigine, sertraline, pantoprazole, tramadol, sulfonamides, allopurinol, carbamazepine, phenobarbital, phenytoin, and NSAIDs.
    - Symptoms typically start 1–3 weeks after administration of the medication.
  - *Mycoplasma pneumoniae* is frequently implicated and less frequently seen with CMV.
- Patients who are immune compromised (malignancy, HIV, SLE) or undergoing radiation therapy are at high risk for developing SJS/TENs.

Pathophysiology

- Immune response to antigenic complex of drug metabolites and host tissue
  - T-cell–mediated disease (the majority being CD8+ cytotoxic T cells) works with natural killer cells to induce apoptosis in keratinocyte cells.

DIAGNOSIS

Clinical Presentation

History

- >85% of patients with SJS/TEN will have an exposure to suspected medication and had initiated medication <8 weeks before onset of reaction.

- The patient may complain of fever, dysphagia, conjunctival irritation, and then a painful rash.

Physical Examination
- The acute phase lasts 8–12 days and is characterized by epidermal sloughing and fever.
- TEN is typically associated with higher fevers than SJS (often >39°C).
- Initially, erythematous or dusky-colored lesions appear irregular in size and shape and can coalesce.
- The rash is symmetric and painful and shows first on the trunk and then neck, face, and upper extremities.
  - >90% of cases involve buccal, ocular, and genital mucosa, so these should be examined.
  - Rarely involves the palms and soles.
- As skin necroses, the lesions can appear gray.
- The epidermis detaches from dermis and forms blisters.
  - The lesions may show a positive Nikolsky sign (epidermal shearing with gentle pressure) or Asboe-Hansen sign (pressure applied to skin causes extension of blistering).

Diagnostic Criteria
- Clinical diagnosis based on history, drug exposure, prodrome, and appearance of lesions
  - Can be confirmed by skin biopsy

Differential Diagnosis
- Erythema multiforme, erythematous drug eruptions, staphylococcal scalded skin syndrome, pemphigus vulgaris, or bullous pemphigoid

Diagnostic Testing
Laboratories
- A CBC and CMP may show anemia, leukopenia, transaminitis, hypoalbuminemia, increased blood urea nitrogen, or hyponatremia.
- Blood cultures and wound cultures should be obtained due to high susceptibility to infection.

TREATMENT

- Stop the suspected causative medication immediately.
  - Keep in mind the half-lives of offending agents.

Medications
- If caused by bacterial or viral infection, give the appropriate antibiotic or antiviral treatment.
- Consider IVIG, systemic corticosteroids, and cyclosporine A in severe cases, although none of these have been established as beneficial in a randomized trial.
  - Studies have found that systemic glucocorticoids are associated with increased morbidity and mortality (increased protein catabolism, decreased epithelialization).
  - TNF-alpha inhibitors have shown increased mortality and are not recommended.

Other Nonpharmacologic Therapies

Supportive care, fluid replacement, electrolyte repletion and monitoring, monitoring intake and output, monitoring for signs of sepsis, extensive wound care, and avoiding skin trauma should be provided. Surgical management may be required for secondary infections.

- Avoid aggressive debridement.
  - Use nonadherent dressings.
  - As topical treatment, use chlorhexidine as opposed to silver sulfadiazine until it can be proven that offending agent was not a sulfonamide.
  - Sitz baths and wet dressings are recommended for genital/urethral erosions.
  - Patients should be kept in warm rooms (30–32 degree Celsius) with pressure-alternating mattresses.
  - Fluid replacement requirements are around 70% of those for burn patients.
  - Sedation and pain therapy should be provided as necessary.

SPECIAL CONSIDERATIONS

Disposition

- Admission should be based upon the Score for Toxic Epidermal Necrolysis (SCORTEN) (Table 12.1).
  - Score of 0–1 can be on a nonspecialized ward.
  - Score of 2 or more should be in an ICU or burn unit.

Complications

- Sepsis and septic shock may occur and are typically caused by *Staphylococcus aureus* and *Pseudomonas aeruginosa*.

TABLE 12.1   SCORTEN Criteria

Risk Factors

Age > 40 years
Malignancy
Total body surface area affected > 10%
Heart rate > 120 beats per minute
Serum urea (blood urea nitrogen) > 28 mg/dL
Serum glucose > 250 mg/dL
Serum bicarbonate < 20 mEq/L

Criteria Present	Mortality Rate
0-1	3%
2	12%
3	35%
4	58%
>5	90%

SCORTEN, SCORe of Toxic Epidermal Necrosis. Adapted from Parker JR, Berkeley RP. Toxic epidermal necrolysis from a cigarette burn. *West J Emerg Med* 2010 May; 11(2): 205–207.

- The patient may experience acute renal failure, ARDS, bronchial mucosal sloughing, encephalopathy, or myocarditis.
- Abdominal compartment pressure should be monitored.
- Corneal involvement can lead to blindness.
- Genital tract involvement can lead to stenosis.
- Dry mouth as a consequence of oral cavity involvement.

SUGGESTED READINGS

Bolognia JL. *Dermatology*. 3rd ed. Saunders/Elsevier, 2012.

Buka RL, Uliasz A, Krishnamurthy K. In: *Buka's Emergencies in Dermatology*. New York: Springer-Verlag, 2013.

de Prost N, Ingen-housz-oro S, Duong T, et al. Bacteremia in Stevens-Johnson syndrome and toxic epidermal necrolysis. *Medicine* 2010;89(1). http://doi.org/10.1097/MD.0b013e3181ca4290

Khalaf D, Toema B, Dabbour N, Jehani F. Toxic epidermal necrolysis associated with severe cytomegalovirus infection in a patient on regular hemodialysis. *Mediterr J Hematol Infect Dis* 2011;3(1):1–4. http://doi.org/10.4084/MJHID.2011.004

Mockenhaupt M, Viboud C, Dunant A, et al. Stevens-Johnson syndrome and toxic epidermal necrolysis: assessment of medication risks with emphasis on recently marketed drugs. The EuroSCAR-study. *J Invest Dermatol* 2008;128(1):35–44. http://doi.org/10.1038/sj.jid.5701033

Buxton PK, Morris-Jones R. *ABC of Dermatology*. Oxford: Wiley-Blackwell, 2014.

Paul C, Wolkenstein P, Adle H, et al. Apoptosis as a mechanism of keratinocyte death in toxic epidermal necrolysis. *Br J Dermatol* 1996;134(4):710–4. Available at: http://www.ncbi.nlm.nih.gov/pubmed/8733377

Revuz J. *Life-Threatening Dermatoses and Emergencies in Dermatology*. Berlin: Springer, 2009.

Roujeau J-C, Guillaume J-C, Fabre J-P, et al. Epidermal necrolysis (Lyell syndrome). *Arch Dermatol* 1990;126.

Schwartz RA, McDonough PH, Lee BW. Toxic epidermal necrolysis: Part I. Introduction, history, classification, clinical features, systemic manifestations, etiology, and immunopathogenesis. *J Am Acad Dermatol* 2013;69(2):173.e1–13. http://doi.org/10.1016/j.jaad.2013.05.003

Sekula P, Dunant A, Mockenhaupt M, et al. Comprehensive survival analysis of a cohort of patients with Stevens-Johnson syndrome and toxic epidermal necrolysis. *J Invest Dermatol* 2013;133(5):1197–204. http://doi.org/10.1038/jid.2012.510

Struck MF, Illert T, Schmidt T, et al. Secondary abdominal compartment syndrome in patients with toxic epidermal necrolysis. *Burns* 2012;38(4):562–7. http://doi.org/10.1016/j.burns.2011.10.004

Wetter DA, Camilleri MJ. Clinical, etiologic, and histopathologic features of Stevens-Johnson syndrome during an 8-year period at Mayo Clinic. *Mayo Clin Proc* 2010;85(2):131–8. http://doi.org/10.4065/mcp.2009.0379

Endocrine Emergencies: Adrenal Disorders

Reuben D. Johnson

Cushing Syndrome: Hyperadrenalism (Hypercortisolism)

GENERAL PRINCIPLES

Definition

- Cushing's syndrome occurs when the body is chronically exposed to excess amounts of glucocorticoids either endogenously (Cushing disease) or exogenously.

Epidemiology/Etiology

- The median age of onset is 41 years with a female-to-male ratio of 3:1.
- Adrenocorticotropic hormone (ACTH)-dependent hypercortisolism is associated with 80% of cases (adenomas, malignancies).

Pathophysiology

- Excess cortisol is present either from excess ACTH production or from extrinsic or ectopic production resulting in a number or end-organ effects.

DIAGNOSIS

Clinical Presentation

History
- Patients often present with psychiatric symptoms (depression and psychosis), easy bruisability, weight gain, and decreased libido.

Physical Examination
- Common physical examination findings include obesity, hirsutism, fragility of skin, broad (>1 cm), purple striae, and proximal muscle weakness.

Differential Diagnosis

- Malignancy, polycystic ovarian syndrome, or exogenous steroid use

Diagnostic Criteria and Testing

- Formal diagnosis is made by an endocrinologist.

Laboratories
- There are no pathognomonic laboratory tests obtained in the ED.

Imaging
- CT or MRI after the diagnosis is made to find source of excess cortisol.

TREATMENT

- Most cases of hypercortisolism are treated by surgery. Medical management is reserved for unstable or nonsurgical candidates.

SPECIAL CONSIDERATIONS

Disposition
- Usually managed as an outpatient

Complications
- Hypercoagulability, infections, psychosis, diabetes, and osteoporosis

Adrenal Insufficiency (AI)

GENERAL PRINCIPLES

Definition
- AI is a condition caused by a lack of cortisol production due to either loss of adrenal function or suppression of the hypothalamic/pituitary regulation of adrenal cortisol synthesis.

Epidemiology/Etiology
- Primary AI is most commonly due to Addison's disease, adrenalectomy, and neoplasia. Primary AI is relatively rare. Secondary AI are pituitary adenomas followed by pituitary tumors, tuberculosis adrenalitis, and other infections. There are many medications that cause drug-induced AI including phenytoin, chlorpromazine, opiates, azoles, and etomidate.
- The most common causes for adrenal crisis are gastroenteritis and fever.

Pathophysiology
- The adrenal cortex secretes aldosterone, cortisol, and androgens. Aldosterone secretion is mediated by the renin/angiotensin and potassium levels so it is not associated with secondary AI. Cortisol production is regulated by corticotropin levels.

DIAGNOSIS

Clinical Presentation

History
- Nonspecific symptoms of AI include fatigue, loss of appetite, nausea, vomiting, and abdominal pain. Symptoms of adrenal crisis include altered mental status and weakness/syncope.

Physical Examination
- Physical examination may show skin hyperpigmentation and postural hypotension. In adrenal crisis, the patient may have altered mental status and hypotension.

Differential Diagnosis
- Sepsis, cardiogenic shock, tamponade, insulin shock, or dehydration

Diagnostic Criteria and Testing
- AI is diagnosed by abnormal response on a cosyntropin stimulation test.
- Adrenal crisis is AI in association with altered mental status and hypotension.

Laboratories
- Obtain ACTH
- Basic metabolic panel (BMP) may show hyponatremia and hyperkalemia.

- Cosyntropin stimulation test is not useful in the critically ill. Instead, obtain a random cortisol level. Cortisol levels in the body vary greatly throughout the day; a random cortisol level is not a definitive test for AI.
  - Cosyntropin stimulation test: draw cortisol level and then administer 250 mcg of cosyntropin. Measure cortisol levels at 30 and 60 minutes.

Imaging

- CT may be helpful in evaluation of the adrenal glands and the pituitary gland.

TREATMENT

- Adrenal crisis is a medical emergency. Patients require prompt aggressive fluid resuscitation in addition to steroid replacement

Medications

- Hydrocortisone 100 mg IV/IM followed by 200 mg total given over the next 24 hours either continuously or 50 mg IV q6 hours.

SPECIAL CONSIDERATIONS

Disposition

- patients in adrenal crisis should be admitted to the ICU.

SUGGESTED READINGS

Arlt W. Disorders of the adrenal cortex. In: Kasper D, Fauci A, Hauser S, et al., eds. *Harrison's Principles of Internal Medicine*. 19th ed. New York: McGraw-Hill, 2015. Available at: http://accessmedicine.mhmedical.com/content.aspx?bookid=1130&Sectionid=79752055 (last accessed 08/01/16).

Bancos I, Harner S, Tomlinson J, Arlt W. Diagnosis and management of adrenal insufficiency. *Lancet Diab Endocrinol* 2015;3:216–26.

Bornstein S, Allolio B, Arlt W, et al. Diagnosis and treatment of primary adrenal insufficiency: an endocrine society clinical practice guideline. *J Clin Endocrin Metab* 2016;101(2):364–89.

Charmandari E, Nicolaides N, Chousus G. Adrenal insufficiency. *Lancet* 2014;383:2152–67.

Lacroix A, Feelders RA, Stratakis CA, Nieman LK. Cushing's syndrome. *Lancet* 2015;386:913–27.

14 Endocrine Emergencies: Endocrine Tumors/ Pheochromocytoma

Reuben D. Johnson

GENERAL PRINCIPLES

- The majority of these tumors are benign and are increasingly found incidentally. Both benign and malignant tumors may be functional. Table 14.1 lists the common tumors. Treatment and evaluation of these tumors are beyond the scope of emergency medicine.

Organ	Tumor	Epidemiology	
Adrenal			
Medulla	Pheochromocytoma	3–4 cases/million/year	25% are found incidentally
Cortex	Adenoma	3–7% of adults (age > 50) on autopsy studies	
	Adrenocortical carcinoma	0.72 cases/million/year	1 in 4000 of adrenal masses are malignant
Pituitary	Prolactinoma	Most common pituitary tumor; 44 cases/100,000/year	25% are familial, 10:1 female-to-male ratio
Thyroid	Thyroid nodule	Unsure found in 19–35% of ultrasounds	Increasing in number (thought due to better diagnostics)
	Thyroid carcinoma	64,000 cases in US/year	
Pancreas	Insulinoma	1–4 cases/million/year	

TABLE 14.1 Common Endocrine Tumors

Pheochromocytoma

- Pheochromocytoma is a tumor arising from adrenomedullary chromaffin cells that commonly produces catecholamines: norepinephrine, epinephrine, or dopamine.

Epidemiology/Etiology

- They are most common in the fourth to fifth decades of life and equally common in men and women.
- They are exceedingly rare in the general population.

DIAGNOSIS

Clinical Presentation

History
- The "classic" triad of symptoms consists of episodic headache, diaphoresis, and palpitations.

Physical Examination
- Hypertension, pallor, tachycardia, tremor, and dyspnea may be seen.

Differential Diagnosis

- Hyperthyroidism/thyroid storm, infection, hypertensive crisis, stimulant abuse, autonomic dysfunction, or panic disorder

Diagnostic Criteria and Testing

Laboratories
- Diagnosis is made by elevated plasma free metanephrines or urinary fractionated metanephrines (not usually ordered from the ED).

- Vanillylmandelic acid has been recommended but has lower sensitivities than urinary tests.

Electrocardiography
- Looking for catecholamine-associated arrhythmias

Imaging
- CT to look for tumors only after the diagnosis has been established

TREATMENT

Medications
- Alpha-adrenergic blockers are used for blood pressure and heart rate control.
- Beta-blockade is indicated only after treatment with an alpha-blocker due to concerns for unopposed alpha activity.

SPECIAL CONSIDERATIONS

Disposition
- May need admission for symptomatic control

Complications
- Hypertensive crisis, psychosis, tachycardias, metastasis, and cardiomyopathy

SUGGESTED READINGS

Karuba R, Gallagher S. Current management on adrenal tumors. *Curr Opin Oncol* 2008;20:34–46.
Lenders J, Duh QY, Eisenhofer G, et al. Pheochromocytomas and paragangliomas: an endocrine society clinical practice guideline. *J Clin Endocrinal Metab* 2014;99:1915–42.

Endocrine Emergencies: Glucose Regulation

Matthew Greer and Brian T. Wessman

GENERAL PRINCIPLES

Definitions
- Diabetic ketoacidosis (DKA) is a metabolic state with an anion gap metabolic acidosis, ketosis, and elevated blood sugar.
- Hyperglycemic hyperosmolar state (HHS) is seen in patients with type 2 diabetes that is characterized by elevated osmolality and hyperglycemia leading to profound dehydration and metabolic derangement causing neurologic deficit.

- Hypoglycemic emergencies occur when blood sugar is below 50 mg/dL with the presenting spectrum of mild confusion to seizures and death.

Epidemiology/Etiology
- Risk factors for hyperglycemic emergencies[2]:
  - Lack of insulin: noncompliance or undertreatment.
  - Infection: urinary tract infection, pneumonia, abscess/cellulitis, sepsis, appendicitis, etc.
  - Ischemia: myocardial infarction, cerebrovascular accident, etc.
  - Ingestion: drugs (sympathomimetics, alcohol, etc.).
  - Other risk factors include pregnancy, pancreatitis, new-onset/initial presentation of DM, poor access to care/lower educational status, and lower socioeconomic status.[3]
- DKA occurs in patients with both insulin-dependent diabetes (IDDM) and non–insulin-dependent diabetes (NIDDM); more prevalent in younger patients with IDDM (though increasing in NIDDM patients).[1,3]
- HHS is more prevalent in NIDDM and in elderly/debilitated patients.[1,4]
- Hypoglycemic emergencies increase with age, dementia, vascular disease, renal failure, lack of food ingestion, EtOH use, and drug interactions.[5-7]

Pathophysiology
- DKA and HHS are the result of insulin deficiency/resistance causing increased hepatic glycolysis, gluconeogenesis, and impaired glucose utilization by peripheral tissues, leading to the hallmark of hyperglycemia. The hyperglycemia in both disorders causes an osmotic diuresis.
  - DKA
    - The presence of stress hormones leads to fasting state metabolism, lipolysis, and fatty acid oxidation causing production of ketone bodies and metabolic acidosis.
    - Excess glucose causes osmotic diuresis leading to dehydration.
    - Ketonemia causes nausea, vomiting, and worsening dehydration.
  - HHS
    - Limited lipolysis/fatty acid oxidation causes limited ketosis.
    - Hyperglycemia causes osmotic diuresis and dehydration.[1,8,9]
- Hypoglycemia is a complication of treatment with either insulin or longer-acting oral agents (i.e., sulfonylureas).
  - Renal clearance decreases with age, which can change the therapeutic insulin dose.[5,6]

DIAGNOSIS

Clinical Presentation

History
- DKA:
  - Patients may report the classic triad of polyuria, polydipsia, and weight loss. They may also mention fatigue, abdominal pain, and nausea/vomiting.
- HHS:
  - In addition to the triad mentioned above, the patient may notice that symptoms have increased over weeks, may report infection or debilitation, and may mention a neurologic deficit (limb weakness, sensory deficit).[1,4]
- Hypoglycemia:
  - Altered mental status, seizure, and coma[8]

Physical Examination

- Hyperglycemia:
  - Dry mucosa, poor skin turgor, tachycardia, or hypotension
  - Lethargy
- DKA = tachypnea, ketone breath, and abdominal tenderness
- HHS = mandatory neurologic deficit[1,8]
  - Labored breathing (Kussmaul respirations).
  - Dehydration: average of 3–6 L of volume depletion.
  - Patients may present seizing or in a coma.
- Hypoglycemia: Consider in all patients with altered mental status/neurologic complaints, seizure, or coma. Diaphoresis can also be present due to adrenergic response.[6,8]

Differential Diagnosis

- DKA:
  - Starvation or alcoholic ketoacidosis
  - Sepsis and infection (appendicitis, pneumonia)
  - Toxic ingestion (salicylate, toxic alcohols, acetaminophen)[8,9]
- HHS:
  - CVA, dementia, seizure (postictal), and dehydration[1,4]
- Hypoglycemia:
  - CVA, seizure, cardiogenic shock, adrenal crisis, sepsis, and insulinoma[5,6,8]

Diagnostic Criteria and Testing

Laboratories

- Bedside glucose (generally >250 mg/dL in DKA, >600 mg/dL for HHS).[9]
- Hypoglycemia ≤ 50 mg/dL.[5]
- Arterial or venous blood gas showing acidosis for DKA: pH ≤ 7.3.
- A BMP should also be drawn.[10]
  - Sodium will need to be corrected in hyperglycemia:[12]

$$[Na]_{corrected} = [Na]_{measured} + \frac{(2.4[Glu - 100])}{100}$$

  - Actual stores of potassium are low, and levels need to be monitored frequently.[1,8]
- Elevated serum ketones (β-hydroxybutyrate) and urine ketones (acetoacetate).[8,9]
  - HHS expected to have no ketones and no acidosis but increased serum osmolarity.
- Consider C-peptide in hypoglycemia to differentiate factitious hypoglycemia.[5]

Imaging

- There are no specific radiologic studies to diagnose glycemic emergencies.

TREATMENT

- Treatment should focus on reversal of the hyperglycemia with insulin and repleting volume and electrolytes. Hyperglycemia will resolve faster than acidosis in DKA.
- DKA and HHS:
  - Replace the intravascular volume with aggressive fluid boluses.
    - Fluid resuscitation: 20 mL/kg normal saline or lactated ringers bolus.
    - Repeat fluid bolus as necessary.
  - Replace total body water deficit over 12–24 hours.[1,8]
    - When glucose < 250 mg/dL, change all fluids to D5½NS (to provide a glucose source while awaiting correction of the acidosis).

- ○ Monitor and replace [K$^+$] as needed.
  - Add 20 mEq/L KCl/h for [K$^+$] < 4.0 mEq/L.[1]
  - Be cautious of administering insulin if [K$^+$] < 3.5 mEq/L.[3,4,8,9]
- ○ Insulin infusion (0.14 U/kg/h).
  - Decrease by 1/2 when changing to D5½NS.[1,9]
  - Goal: glucose 150–200 mg/dL until gap closes.
- ○ Goal: closed gap, pH > 7.30, HCO$_3$ > 18 mEq/L, and glucose < 250 mg/dL.
  - Patient tolerating oral intake.
  - To transition off the infusion, give long-acting insulin dose 60–120 minutes prior to stopping the insulin drip.[1,8]
- Hypoglycemia:
  - ○ If no intravenous access, administer glucagon IM.
  - ○ Administer dextrose 25 g.
    - Repeat as needed for improved mental status and glucose < 90 mg/dL.
  - ○ If oral route possible: provide simple and complex carbohydrates.[8]
  - ○ Consider octreotide for refractory hypoglycemia with sulfonylurea overdose/toxicity.[11]

SPECIAL CONSIDERATIONS

Disposition

- Correction of fluid and electrolyte deficits occurs over 18–24 hours, so admission is required, generally to an intensive care unit.[3,4]
  - ○ While in the ED, hourly glucose should be checked and chemistries can be repeated every 2–4 hours.
  - ○ May consider general floor if anion gap is closed, off insulin infusion, and able to tolerate oral intake.
- Hypoglycemia disposition based on etiology of episode and need for monitoring/treatment.
  - ○ Admit if no obvious cause, precipitated by oral hypoglycemic agent or long-acting insulin, or if there is persistent neurologic deficits.[8,9]

Complications

- Hyperglycemic emergencies:
  - ○ Most common: hypoglycemia (overcorrection) and hyperkalemia[2]
  - ○ Cerebral edema, volume overload/acute respiratory distress syndrome

REFERENCES

1. Corwell B, Knight B, Olivieri L, Willis GC. Current diagnosis and treatment of hyperglycemic emergencies. *Emerg Med Clin N Am* 2014;32:437–52.
2. Usher-Smith JA, Thompson MJ, Sharp SJ, Walter FM. Factors associated with the presence of diabetic ketoacidosis at diagnosis of diabetes in children and young adults: a systemic review. *Br Med J* 2011;343:d4092.
3. Chansky CL, Lubkin ME. Diabetic Ketoacidosis. In: Tintinalli JE, Stapczynski JS, Ma OJ, et al., eds. *Tintinalli's Emergency Medicine.* 7th ed. NY: McGraw-Hill, 2011:1432–8.
4. Graffeo CS. Hyperosmolar Hyperglycemic State. In: Tintinalli JE, Stapczynski JS, Ma OJ, et al., eds. *Tintinalli's Emergency Medicine.* 8th ed. NY: McGraw-Hill, 2016:1440–4.
5. Jalili M. Type 2 Diabetes Mellitus. In: Tintinalli JE, Stapczynski JS, Ma OJ, et al., eds. *Tintinalli's Emergency Medicine.* 7th ed. NY: McGraw-Hill, 2011:1430–2.
6. Smeeks F. Acute Hypoglycemia. Available at: http://emedicine.medscape.com/article/767359

7. Ha WC, Oh SJ, Kim JH, et al. Severe hypoglycemia is a serious complication and becoming an economic burden in diabetes. *Diab Metab J* 2012;36(4):280–4.
8. Beltran G. Diabetic emergencies: new strategies for an old disease. *Emerg Med Pract* 2014;16. Available at: www.ebmedicine.net
9. Van Ness-Otunnu R, Hack JB. Hyperglycemic crisis. *J Emerg Med* 2013;45:797–805.
10. Sinert R, Su M, Secko M, Zehtabchi S. The utility of routine laboratory testing in hypoglycaemic emergency department patients. *Emerg Med J* 2009;26(1):28–31.
11. Glatstein M, Scolnik D, Bentur Y. Octreotide for the treatment of sulfonylurea poisoning. *Clin Toxicol (Phila)* 2012;50(9):795–804.
12. Hillier TA, Abbott RD, Barrett EJ. Hyponatremia: evaluating the correction factor for hyperglycemia. *Am J Med* 1999;106(4):399–403.

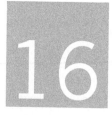

Endocrine Emergencies: Thyroid Disorders

Sara Manning, Chandra Aubin, and Reuben D. Johnson

Hypothyroid Disorders

GENERAL PRINCIPLES

Definition

- Hypothyroidism is a clinical syndrome caused by insufficient thyroid hormone production.
  - Subclinical hypothyroidism—elevated thyroid-stimulating hormone (TSH) in the setting of a normal serum free thyroxine (T4)
  - Myxedema crisis—severe, decompensated hypothyroid state characterized by mental status changes, hypothermia, and multiorgan system dysfunction
  - Primary hypothyroidism—dysfunction of the thyroid gland
  - Secondary and tertiary hypothyroidism—inadequate production of TSH or thyrotropin-releasing hormone (TRH)[17,19]

Epidemiology/Etiology

- Risk factors include female gender[11,12], caucasian race, and advanced age. The majority of cases are subclinical. Myxedema crisis is a rare complication of hypothyroidism occurring most commonly in acutely ill elderly women. More than 80% of cases occur in women over age 60.[1]
- All etiologies of hypothyroidism can be complicated by myxedema. Myxedema crises are often associated with an acute precipitant including infection, anesthesia, cold exposure, trauma, myocardial infarction, metabolic disturbances among others.[1,2]

Pathophysiology
- Due to the widespread metabolic effects of thyroid hormones, the signs and symptoms of thyroid dysfunction involve multiple organ systems.

DIAGNOSIS
- Myxedema crisis is a clinical diagnosis, and treatment should not be delayed for laboratory results.

Clinical Presentation

History
- Common complaints in hypothyroid states include fatigue, weakness, lethargy, weight gain, cold intolerance, dry skin, constipation, hair loss, sexual dysfunction, irregular menses, and low mood.
- Myxedema crisis may be preceded by a diagnosis of hypothyroidism, mild or subclinical symptoms consistent with hypothyroidism, or as a new presentation of disease. Sometimes a history of disorientation or psychiatric symptoms like depression, paranoia, or hallucinations may be elicited. Myxedema crisis is distinguished by acute mental status changes or coma, hypothermia. Decompensation into myxedema crisis is commonly precipitated by an acute trigger.

Physical Examination
- Findings consistent with hypothyroidism include hypothermia, nonpitting edema, periorbital edema, hoarseness, goiter, bradycardia, hypoventilation, decreased/absent bowel sounds, pallor, cool rough dry skin, loss of the outer third of the eyebrows, delayed reflexes, and peripheral neuropathy.

Differential Diagnosis
- Common general mimics of hypothyroidism include anemia, electrolyte disturbances, renal failure, infection, polypharmacy, primary psychiatric disease, and secondary hypothermia.
- The differential for abnormalities in thyroid hormone results (low T4 with or without elevated TSH) includes Hashimoto thyroiditis, iatrogenic (thyroidectomy, radioiodine therapy, external radiation, drug induced), postpartum thyroiditis, iodine deficiency, silent thyroiditis, subacute thyroiditis, pituitary or hypothalamic mass, infiltration or surgery, and iatrogenic pituitary or hypothalamic injury from surgery or radiation therapy.[3]
- The differential for the myxedema patient may include sepsis, acute stroke, central nervous system (CNS) infection, and overdose.

Diagnostic Criteria and Testing
- Hypothyroidism is a lab-based diagnosis, and myxedema crisis is a clinical diagnosis.

Laboratories
- Primary hypothyroidism is defined by a low T4 in the presence of an elevated or inappropriately normal TSH. Patients with secondary hypothyroidism will have low T4 with low TSH and occasionally low TRH.

Electrocardiography
- An ECG may show bradydysrhythmias or heart blocks.

Imaging
- MRI or CT imaging of the pituitary should be performed if there is a concern for secondary hypothyroidism.

TREATMENT

Medications

- Oral levothyroxine is used to treat hypothyroidism and can be started in conjunction with a PMD or endocrinology consult.[2,4]
- Myxedema Crisis Treatment
  - Acute stabilization—initial assessment and treatment should focus on adequate monitoring and critical supportive care including vasopressors (only after hormone replacement has been initiated).[2] Empiric broad-spectrum antibiotics should be administered to all myxedema patients due to the possible infectious causes underlying myxedema.[4,5]
  - Hormone replacement—hydrocortisone (100–200 mg IV) should be given prior to administration of replacement thyroid hormone.
    - Levothyroxine 4 μg/kg should be administered intravenously.
      □ Smaller doses should be considered in the elderly or those with known cardiac disease or history of tachydysrhythmias.
  - *Alternatively*
    - Triiodothyronine can be administered IV at a dose of 20 μg IV followed by 10 μg IV every 8 hours until the patient can tolerate oral dosing.
    - Lower dosing should be considered in the elderly and with caution in those with known cardiac disease.

SPECIAL CONSIDERATIONS

Complications

- Pregnancy—demand for thyroid hormone increases significantly due to increased maternal metabolism as well as fetal development. Women with preexisting hypothyroidism may require 30–50% dose increase with demands increasing sharply even early in the first trimester.[10]

Disposition

- Uncomplicated hypothyroidism can be safely discharged with primary care or endocrine follow-up. Concern for secondary hypothyroidism should prompt endocrine referral.
- Myxedema crisis is a critical illness with a high mortality. All patients with myxedema crisis should be admitted to an intensive care unit.

Hyperthyroid Disorders

GENERAL PRINCIPLES

Definition

- Subclinical hyperthyroidism—patients with low TSH and normal free T4 and T3, often asymptomatic
- Thyroid storm—rare endocrine emergency with life-threatening multiorgan system derangement in the setting of a known history of hyperthyroidism or laboratory values consistent with overt hyperthyroidism

- Primary hyperthyroidism—hyperthyroidism caused by excess thyroid hormone production from the thyroid gland
- Secondary hyperthyroidism—dysfunction of the pituitary or hypothalamus leading to inappropriately elevated levels of TSH and subsequent inappropriate production of excess thyroid hormone

Epidemiology/Etiology
- Nonwhite race, females, and advancing age are risk factors for hyperthyroidism.[6]
- Causes of hyperthyroid or thyrotoxic states include excess hCG production from trophoblastic disease, iatrogenic or other exogenous iodine intake, excess thyroid hormone supplementation, or radiation thyroiditis.[7]

Pathophysiology
- Hyperthyroidism is characterized by increased metabolic activity.
- Graves disease is an autoimmune condition in which the body develops antibodies that stimulate thyroid follicular cells.[7]
- Other causes of primary hyperparathyroidism include Hashimoto's, subacute painful, and painless thyroiditis. Typically, the hyperthyroid phase of these diseases is followed by a hypothyroid state.
- Secondary hyperparathyroidism can be caused by a thyrotropin-secreting pituitary adenoma.

DIAGNOSIS

Clinical Presentation
History
- Patients may complain of unintentional weight loss, increased appetite, heat intolerance, sweating, polydipsia, tremor, anxiety, fatigue, difficulty sleeping, dyspnea, diarrhea, nausea, vomiting, diplopia, eye pain, palpitations, hair loss, and/or irregular menses.[7,8]
  - Patients in thyroid storm will commonly report symptoms of thyrotoxicosis and may also report extreme lethargy, psychosis, confusion, GI pain and upset, and fever. Patients may be acutely altered at presentation.[7]
  - Pregnancy can be a trigger for development of thyroid storm.
- Elderly patients may present with atypical symptoms including confusion, memory loss, weight loss, dizziness, syncope with evidence of tachycardia, or atrial fibrillation. This is often referred to as apathetic thyrotoxicosis.

Physical Examination
- The signs associated with hyperthyroidism can be widespread and nonspecific but may include fever, goiter, exophthalmos, hypertension, atrial fibrillation, congestive heart failure (CHF), rales, abdominal tenderness, hair loss, warm moist skin, palmar erythema, pretibial myxedema, tremor, periodic paralysis, or altered sensorium.

Differential Diagnosis
- Common general mimics of hyperthyroidism include infections including CNS infections, acute coronary syndromes, myocarditis, pericarditis, pulmonary embolism, primary psychiatric disease, drug abuse or misuse, or medication side effects.

Diagnostic Criteria and Testing

Laboratories
- Primary hyperthyroidism is defined by elevated T4 with or without an elevated T3 in the presence of a low or inappropriately normal TSH. Patients with secondary hypothyroidism will have elevated T4 with or without T3 with high or normal TSH and occasionally high TRH.

Electrocardiography
- Sinus tachycardia, atrial fibrillation, PACs, or PVCs.

TREATMENT

- Antithyroid drugs such as methimazole should only be started in the emergency department (ED) in conjunction with a PMD or endocrinologist. Symptomatic treatment with β-blockers like propranolol can be started in the ED.[7]
- Thyroid storm is a life-threatening medical emergency. Treatment should be administered in a stepwise approach.
  - Acute stabilization—initial assessment should focus on adequate monitoring and critical supportive care including IV fluids, external cooling, and cardiac symptom control.[7]
  - Prevent thyroid hormone synthesis with thionamides.
    - Propylthiouracil 600–1000 mg PO or PR loading dose followed by 200–250 mg PO q4 hours (also inhibits conversion of T4 to T3), or methimazole 40 mg PO followed by 25 mg PO q4 hours
  - Prevent new hormone release.
    - Administer iodine therapies at least 1 hour after thionamide treatment
    - Lugol solution 8–10 drops PO q6–8 hours or potassium iodide 5 drops PO q6 hours or IV iopanoic acid 1 g q8 hours for the first 24 hours, then 500 mg bid or ipodate 0.5–3 g/d PO or lithium carbonate—if iodine allergic or has demonstrated agranulocytosis to thionamides in the past.
  - Peripheral symptom support with β-blockade.
    - Propranolol 1–2 mg IV q15 minutes until rate control achieved or esmolol 500 μg/kg IV bolus then 50–200 μg/kg/min continuous infusion titrated for rate control
    - Consider reserpine or guanethidine if contraindication to β-blocker use
  - Prevention of peripheral hormone conversion.
    - Hydrocortisone 100 mg IV then 100 mg TID until stable or dexamethasone 2 mg IV q6 hours

In pregnancy, propylthiouracil is favored over methimazole, as it less readily crosses the placenta.[9]

SPECIAL CONSIDERATIONS

Disposition
- Uncomplicated hyperthyroidism can be safely discharged with primary care or endocrine follow-up. If thionamides are prescribed, follow-up should be rapid to assess for potentially severe side effects of treatment.
- Thyroid storm is a critical illness with a high mortality requiring continuous monitoring and frequent titration of multiple medications. All patients with thyroid storm should be admitted to an intensive care unit.

REFERENCES

1. Klubo-Gwiezdzinska J, Wartofsky L. Thyroid emergencies. *Med Clin N Am* 2012;96:385.
2. Idrose AM. Chapter 228: Hypothyroidism. In: Tintinalli JE, ed. *Tintinalli's Emergency Medicine: A Comprehensive Study Guide*. 8th ed. NY: McGraw-Hill, 2016.
3. McDermott MT. In the clinic: hypothyroidism. *Ann Intern Med* 2009;151(11):ITC6-1.
4. Jonklaas J, Bianco AC, Bauer AJ, et al. Guidelines for the treatment of hypothyroidism: prepared by the American Thyroid Association Task Force on thyroid hormone replacement. *Thyroid* 2014;14(12):1670.
5. Dutta P, Bhansali A, Masoodi SR, et al. Predictors of outcome in myxoedema coma: a study from a tertiary care centre. *Crit Care* 2008;12(1):R1.
6. Aoki Y, Belin RM, Clickner R, et al. Serum TSH and total T4 in the United States population and their association with participant characteristics: National Health and Nutrition Examination Survey (NHANES 1999–2002). *Thyroid* 2007;17(12):1211.
7. De Leo S, Lee SY, Braverman LE. Hyperthyroidism. *Lancet* 2016;388(10047):906. doi:10.1016/S0140-6736(16)00278-6.
8. Pimentel L, Hansen K. Thyroid disease in the emergency department: a clinical and laboratory review. *J Emerg Med* 2005;28(2):201.
9. Yoshihara A, Noh JY, Yamaguchi T, et al. Treatment of Graves disease with antithyroid drugs in the first trimester of pregnancy and the prevalence of congenital malformation. *J Clin Endocrinol Metab* 2012;97:2396.
10. Cleary-Goldman J, Malone FD, Lambert-Messerlian G, et al. Maternal thyroid hypofunction and pregnancy outcome. *Obstet Gynecol* 2008;112(1):85.
11. Alexander EK, Marqusee E, Lawrence J, et al. Timing and magnitude of increases in levothyroxine requirements during pregnancy in women with hypothyroidism. *N Engl J Med* 2004;351:241.
12. Akamizu T, Satoh T, Isozaki O, et al. Diagnostic criteria, clinical features, and incidence of thyroid storm based on nationwide surveys. *Thyroid* 2012;22(7):661.
13. Chapter 58: Endocrine Disorders. In: Cunningham FG, Leveno KJ, Bloom SL, et al., eds. *Williams Obstetrics*. 24th ed. NY: McGraw-Hill, 2013.

Environmental Emergencies: Bites, Stings, and Envenomations

Lauren O'Grady and William Dribben

Mammalian Bites

GENERAL PRINCIPLES

Epidemiology/Etiology

- Dogs
  - Adults are more likely to be bitten on the extremities.
  - Most common mammalian bite.

  ○ Infections involve both aerobic and anaerobic bacteria.
  ○ Low risk for infection due to tearing of soft tissue resulting in open wound.
- Cats
  ○ Women are at higher risk.
  ○ Bites are usually from a family pet.
  ○ Higher risk for infection due to the slender, longer feline teeth that allow for deep penetration and inoculation.
  ○ Most common bacteria is *P. multocida*.
- Humans
  ○ 3/4 of human bites involve with upper extremity or hand to fight bites or closed fist injuries (CFI) and 2/3 involve the joint and bone and the majority get infected.
  ○ *Streptococcus anginosus* is the most common pathogen, followed by *S. aureus*.
  ○ Human bites to areas of the body besides the hand are at low risk for infection.

Pathophysiology

- Inoculation of bacteria occurs through a break in the skin with resultant growth secondary to an inability to fully fight the infection.

DIAGNOSIS

Clinical Presentation

History

- Most patients will report an animal bite, usually with resultant pain, erythema, or edema.
- Patients may not be forthcoming or may not remember being bit by another human or may have been involved in an altercation, hitting someone else's mouth without realizing it.

Physical Examination

- Erythema, edema, and a break in the skin are usually seen and a full neurologic exam of the proximal and distal joints (especially in the hand) should be performed.
- Careful exploration of the wound is important to ensure that foreign bodies are not retained.

Differential Diagnosis

- Fracture, cellulitis, local inflammation, joint disease, rheumatologic disorders

Diagnostic Criteria and Testing

Imaging

- A plain radiograph or ultrasound may locate a retained foreign body.

TREATMENT

Medications

- Tetanus should be updated on all patients.
- Antibiotics should be started on patients with cat or human bites or any patients with immunocompromise or bite to the hand.
  ○ Intravenous antibiotics to cover for presumed bacterial coverage may be started if the patient has signs of or is at risk for rapidly progressing infection.

○ Augmentin 875 mg PO bid for 14 days.
○ Moxifloxacin may be used if patients have a penicillin allergy.
○ Clindamycin may be used if *Pasteurella* is not of high concern.

Other Nonpharmacologic Therapies

• Wash all bites with soap and water (copious irrigation).
• Suturing should not be performed on any wounds except the face (if within 6 hours and without evidence of infection), although wounds may be loosely approximated.
• Surgical intervention may be necessary for involvement of the bone or joint or with flexor or extensor tendon involvement.

SPECIAL CONSIDERATIONS

Disposition

• Patients with an uncomplicated bite may be discharged home on oral antibiotics unless there are signs/symptoms of progressive infection or damage to underlying structures.

Complications

• Infection, tenosynovitis, loss of function of extremity

Hymenoptera

GENERAL PRINCIPLES

Epidemiology/Etiology

• 50% of deaths can occur in individuals with no previous systemic reaction.
• Apidae (honey bee and bumblebee) usually will only attack when provoked.
  ○ Africanized honeybees are aggressive and will respond to threats in great numbers.
• Vespidae (wasps, yellowjackets) are aggressive when disturbed and may sting multiple times.
  ○ Most cases of anaphylaxis caused by hymenoptera are secondary to Vespidae stings.
• Formiciae (ants, in particular fire ants) swarm when the nest is disturbed resulting in hundreds of stings.
  ○ The sting results in a raised papule that progresses to a pustule over the course of hours.

Pathophysiology

• Hymenoptera venom contains melittin, a membrane active polypeptide, which causes degranulation of mast cells and basophils.
• Cross-reactivity between different hymenoptera stings is common due to this shared polypeptide, with yellow jackets being the most potent sensitizer.

DIAGNOSIS

Clinical Presentation

History
• Patients will usually report being stung, or acute onset of pain followed by swelling and itching or burning.

Physical Examination
- Local Reaction
  - Urticaria at sting site, with patient experiencing localized pain, erythema, edema, and pruritus.
  - Oral stings may cause airway compromise from local edema.
  - Ocular stings can cause globe perforation and progressive ocular issues.
- Toxic Reaction
  - Massive envenomations from swarming stings can cause a systemic response.
  - Can look similar to anaphylaxis, though generally includes gastrointestinal disturbances.
  - Patients can develop complications of respiratory insufficiency, respiratory arrest, renal and/or hepatic failure, convulsions, DIC, and rhabdomyolysis.
- Anaphylaxis
  - Generally occur within the first 15 minutes following a sting and almost universally within the first 6 hours
- Delayed Reaction
  - A form of serum sickness characterized by fever, malaise, headache, urticaria, lymphadenopathy, and polyarthritis 1–2 weeks following stings

Differential Diagnosis
- Cellulitis, allergic reaction, or anaphylaxis

Diagnostic Criteria and Testing
Imaging
- Ultrasound may be able to locate stingers, whereas plain radiography does not.

TREATMENT

Medications
- Anaphylaxis should be treated immediately with epinephrine 0.3 mg IM.
- Tetanus prophylaxis should be updated.
- Hypotension should be treated with fluids and pressors as indicated.
- Diphenhydramine, ranitidine, corticosteroids, and inhaled beta agonists may be used for significantly symptomatic patients.
- Symptomatic treatment with NSAIDs and oral antihistamines are appropriate.

Other Nonpharmacologic Therapies
- Removal of the stinger, followed by thorough cleansing of the site with soap and water

SPECIAL CONSIDERATIONS

Disposition
- Patients may be discharged home if they are asymptomatic after several hours.
- Patients with an anaphylactic reaction should receive a prescription for an epinephrine auto-injector and instruction on use and follow-up with an allergist.
- Patients requiring ongoing management, or who suffered massive envenomation due to swarming insects, should be admitted.

Prognosis

- Patients who are exposed to envenomation have a higher risk of developing hypersensitivity reactions, which can be fatal so should be instructed to use their epinephrine auto-injector at the first sign of reaction in the future.

Arachnids (Spiders)

GENERAL PRINCIPLES

Epidemiology/Etiology

- Only a few types of spiders have fangs long enough to penetrate human skin and venom strong enough to severely affect a human being.
- Spiders are usually not aggressive, and most bites occur because a spider is trapped or unintentionally contacted.
- Black widow (*Latrodectus mactans*)
  - Most common in the southern and western areas of the United States.
  - Identified by the pattern of red coloration (hourglass) on the underside of their abdomen.
  - Black widow spiders build webs between objects, and bites usually occur when humans come into direct contact with these webs.
- Brown recluse (*Loxosceles reclusa*)
  - Predominately found in the south central states of the United States.
  - Identified by a dark brown violin-shaped spot on the back.
  - The brown recluse spider cannot bite humans without some form of counter pressure, for example, through unintentional contact that traps the spider against the skin.

Pathophysiology

- Black widow
  - The venom contains a potent neurotoxin (α-latrotoxin) that produces effects at cation-selective channels and depletion of presynaptic neurotransmitters resulting in neuromuscular blockade.
- Brown recluse
  - The venom contains a number of esterases, hyaluronidases, and proteases that are cytotoxic. Sphingomyelinase-D acts on red blood cells causing hemolysis.

DIAGNOSIS

Clinical Presentation

History
- Black widow
  - The patient may feel a sharp "pinprick" at the bite site and small white blister may develop. After approximately an hour, the patient can develop dull ache or crampy pain at the bite site that can spread to the chest and abdomen.
- Brown recluse
  - The bite can be painless or produce mild pain and tingling sensation. Due to minimal initial symptoms, identification of the spider is important for a proper diagnosis.

Physical Examination
- Black widow
  - A bite from a black widow can be distinguished from other insect bites by the two puncture marks it makes in the skin. The bite site may also develop some erythema with a reddish-blue border. Systemic signs include dizziness, nausea/vomiting, abdominal pain/rigidity, muscular fasciculations, and hypertension.
- Brown recluse
  - Bites can range from asymptomatic to both severe local and systemic symptoms. After 3–4 hours after the initial bite, pain can develop or worsen at the bite site followed by a ring of pallor surrounding the bite. A bleb can then develop in the center becoming an enlarging necrotic lesion. Systemic effects can include fever/chills, generalized rash, nausea/vomiting, and in severe cases, hypotension, hemolysis, DIC, and renal failure.

Differential Diagnosis
- Black widow
  - Pancreatitis, appendicitis, diverticulitis, or peptic ulcer disease
- Brown recluse
  - Stevens-Johnson syndrome, toxic epidermal necrolysis, purpura fulminans, skin ulcers (diabetic or vascular insufficiency), or dermatitis

Diagnostic Criteria and Testing
Laboratories
- There are no specific tests or studies to identify spider bites, but in patients with systemic symptoms, baseline labs should be performed including a complete blood count, electrolytes, coagulation studies, and urinalysis.

TREATMENT

Medications
- Black widow
  - Benzodiazepines and narcotic pain medication can be used for severe pain and muscle spasm.
  - Hypertension may require nitroprusside or nicardipine infusions.
  - Antivenom is available in the United States and should be reserved for severe cases.
  - Tetanus prophylaxis.
- Brown recluse
  - IV fluids and dopamine/norepinephrine may be administered for hypotension.
  - Antibiotics may be administered for bacterial superinfection.
  - Blood products may be necessary for coagulopathy or hemolysis.
  - Antivenom is not available in the United States.
  - Corticosteroids and dapsone have not been proven to be beneficial.

Other Nonpharmacologic Therapies
- Routine wound care, cool compresses

SPECIAL CONSIDERATIONS

Disposition
- Patients with moderate to severe symptoms should be admitted to the hospital.

Snakebites

GENERAL PRINCIPLES

Epidemiology/Etiology

- In North America, all venomous snakes belong to the family Viperidae (pit vipers) or Elapidae (coral snakes).
- From 2009 to 2013, there were only 2 deaths out of 7150 bites with 98% secondary to pit viper bites.
- At least one species of pit viper is found in each state of the contiguous US except for Maine and Rhode Island.
- Coral snakes are indigenous to the southeastern United States, Texas, and Arizona.

Pathophysiology

- Pit viper venom is a complex mixture of different proteins and enzymes that are cytotoxic and can affect almost every organ system, particularly the cardiovascular, hematologic, respiratory, and nervous systems.
- Coral snake venom is less proteolytic than pit viper venom; the primary component is a potent neurotoxin that blocks postsynaptic acetylcholine binding sites at the neuromuscular junction.

DIAGNOSIS

Clinical Presentation

History
- Typically, the bite is witnessed or felt.

Physical Examination
- Pit viper bites include the presence of one or more fang marks including punctures and scratches. Approximately 25% of bites are "dry" (no toxin injected), but if envenomation occurs, symptoms typically begin within 30–60 minutes. Findings include pain, edema, erythema, or ecchymosis at the site of the bite and in adjacent tissues. Compartment syndrome may be present depending on the location of the bite. Early systemic manifestations can include nausea, vomiting, perioral paresthesia, tingling of the fingertips and toes, myokymia, lethargy, and weakness. More severe systemic effects include hypotension, tachypnea, respiratory distress, tachycardia, and altered mental status.
- Coral snakes only effectively deliver their toxin ~40% of the time. Envenomation may produce little or no local pain but may result in tremors, salivation, nausea/vomiting, and altered mental status. Neurologic manifestations include cranial nerve palsies, dysarthria, dysphagia, dyspnea, and respiratory paralysis. The onset of neurotoxic effects may be delayed up to 12 hours.

Differential Diagnosis

- Envenomation, trauma, metabolic disorder, or botulism

Diagnostic Criteria and Testing

Laboratories
- Rattlesnake bites can result in hypofibrinogenemia, thrombocytopenia, hemolysis, and/or consumptive coagulopathy. Baseline labs should be obtained to include a

complete blood count, basic metabolic panel, coagulation studies including fibrinogen and fibrin split products, urinalysis, and a type/screen.

Imaging

• A plain film may be performed to assess for a retained fang, but this is rarely found.

TREATMENT

Medications

• Antivenom (Crotalidae Polyvalent immune Fab [CroFab]) should be administered to patients with a significant envenomation before the venom components are circulated and absorbed.
• Prophylactic antibiotics are usually not needed.
• Tetanus immunization should be given if indicated.

Other Nonpharmacologic Therapies

• Jewelry and restrictive clothing should be removed.
• Measures such as incision, suction, tourniquets, electric shock, ice, and alcohol are contraindicated.
• Baseline circumferential measurements at several points above and below the bite should be documented with serial measurements every 20 minutes until local swelling subsides.
• Wound management includes irrigation with saline and standard wound care and appropriate analgesia. If the bite involves an extremity, the limb should be kept above heart level to reduce swelling and monitored for compartment syndrome (although this is a rare complication).
• Currently, coral snake antivenom is not being produced, and supportive care with aggressive airway management is the mainstay of treatment.

SPECIAL CONSIDERATIONS

Exotic Snakes

• Although traditional zoos typically have safety measures and antivenom in place, private individuals may have exotic snakes as "pets." Initial management and supportive care would be similar as native North American species; a poison center should be contacted for the availability of antivenom.

Disposition

• Patients with pit viper bites may be discharged after 8 hours if asymptomatic. Patients with coral snake bites should be observed for 12–24 hours and may be discharged if asymptomatic. Patients with laboratory abnormalities or rapidly increasing swelling or bruising should be admitted.

SUGGESTED READINGS

Boyer LV, Binford GJ, Degan JA. Chapter 43: Spider Bites. In: *Wilderness Medicine*, Auerbach PS, Cushing TA, Harris NS, eds. 2017:993.

Cooper RA, Goldberg PL. Should x-rays be ordered to find a bee's stinger? *Pediatr Emerg Care* 1988;4(3):205–6.

Dellinger EP, Wertz MJ, Miller S, Coyle MB. Hand infections. Bacteriology and treatment: a prospective study. *Arch Surg* 1988;123:745–50.

Kwo S, Agarwal JP, Meletiou S. Current treatment of cat bites to the hand and wrist. *J Hand Surg Am* 2011;36:152–3.

Moran GJ, Talan DA, Abrahamian FM. Antimicrobial prophylaxis for wounds and procedures in the emergency department. *Infect Dis Clin North Am* 2008;22:117–43.

Medeiros I, Saconato H. Antibiotic prophylaxis for mammalian bites. *Cochrane Database Syst Rev* 2001;2.

Perron AD, Miller MD, Brady WJ. Orthopedic pitfalls in the ED: fight bite. *Am J Emerg Med* 2002;20:114–7.

Swanson DL, Vetter RS. Bites of brown recluse spiders and suspected necrotic arachnidism. *N Engl J Med* 2005;352:700–7.

Tintinalli JE, Stapczynski J, John Ma O, et al. *Tintinalli's Emergency Medicine: A Comprehensive Study Guide*. 8th ed. New York: McGraw Hill, 2015.

18 Environmental Emergencies: Drowning

P. Gabriel Miranda Gomez and Joan Noelker

GENERAL PRINCIPLES

Definition

- Drowning is defined as the process of experiencing respiratory impairment from submersion/immersion in liquid. Drowning may be used to include all manner of outcomes: death, morbidity, and life without morbidity. Modifiers of wet or dry drowning, active or passive drowning, primary or secondary drowning, near drowning, and silent drowning have all been discarded.

Epidemiology/Etiology

- The majority of drownings occur inland and ease of access to water is a major risk factor.
- Other key factors include male gender, preschool and school-aged children, lack of barriers around bodies of water, lack of adequate supervision of young children, the consumption of alcohol, flood disasters, and occupational exposures to water.

Pathophysiology

- The pathologic feature of drowning is asphyxiation from a combination of initial voluntary breath-holding followed by involuntary laryngospasm lasting up to several minutes.
- Eventual relaxation of the vocal muscles gives way to aspiration and cessation of gas exchange.
- Aspiration also contributes to late pulmonary injury via surfactant washout, atelectasis, and resultant V/Q mismatch and ongoing hypoxemia in the hospital setting. Lung compliance is often reduced and contributes to hypoventilation and further V/Q mismatch.

- The ill effects of tissue hypoxia may be somewhat mitigated by the bradycardia and peripheral vasoconstriction of the mammalian diving reflex, which reduce myocardial oxygen demand and shunt blood toward the heart and brain.
- Hypothermia, when present, reduces global tissue oxygen demand and is thought to be neuroprotective.

Clinical Presentation

History

- Patients who are alert should be prompted to provide a detailed history of any medical comorbidities or factors that may have contributed to drowning, including clues to syncope or other trauma as a proximate cause for drowning.
- Among patients who lose consciousness, the history relies heavily upon clues from witnesses and first responders.

Physical Examination

- Clinical presentation varies widely based upon patient characteristics and comorbidities, mechanism of immersion, duration of immersion, and the effects of any on-scene interventions made.
- Auscultation of the lungs may reveal wheezing, rales, and rhonchi or remain completely clear.

Differential Diagnosis

- Cardiogenic syncope, sudden cardiac death, traumatic brain injury (TBI), seizure, intoxication, stroke, or spine trauma

Diagnostic Criteria and Testing

Laboratories

- Initial screening tests of all patients should include rapid glucose, CBC, electrolytes, BUN, creatinine, and an ABG.
- Obtunded patients should also have lactate, liver enzymes, serum ethanol, and urine drug screen performed.

Imaging

- Obtain CXR in all patients.
- If trauma is suspected, obtain head and cervical spine CT as appropriate.

TREATMENT

Medications

- Bronchodilators may be useful to reverse cold-induced bronchospasm in patients with wheezing or who are difficult to bag ventilate.
- Isotonic crystalloid is the fluid of choice for volume resuscitation. In the setting of pulmonary edema and intracompartmental fluid shifts, volume expansion may help to correct acidosis.

Other Nonpharmacologic Therapies

- Correct acidosis and hypoxemia with the use of supplemental oxygen and noninvasive positive pressure ventilation and mechanical ventilation.
- Positive end-expiratory pressure (PEEP) should be considered in patients with poor lung compliance

- Extracorporeal membrane oxygenation should be considered in patients not responding to conventional mechanical ventilation.
- Hypothermia should also be treated.
- Routine prophylactic antibiotics for aspiration is not indicated.

SPECIAL CONSIDERATIONS

Disposition

- Any patient with persistent hypoxemia or obtundation (GCS < 13) should be admitted to an ICU. Asymptomatic patients should be observed for 6–8 hours before discharge.

Complications

- Hypoxic brain injury, cardiopulmonary arrest, pulmonary edema, acute respiratory distress syndrome, or acute kidney injury.

SUGGESTED READINGS

Centers for Disease Control and Prevention, National Center for Injury Prevention and Control. Web-based Injury Statistics Query and Reporting System (WISQARS). Available at: http://www.cdc.gov/injury/wisqars (last accessed 03/22/2016).

Ibsen L, Koch T. Submersion and asphyxia injury. *Crit Care Med.* 2002;30(11 Suppl):S402–S408.

Kim KI, Lee WY, Kim HS, et al. Extracorporeal membrane oxygenation in near-drowning patients with cardiac or pulmonary failure. *Scand J Trauma Resusc Emerg Med.* 2014;22:77.

Michelet P, Bouzana F, Charmensat O, et al. Acute respiratory failure after drowning: a retrospective multicenter survey. *Eur J Emerg Med.* 2015 Dec 17 [epub ahead of print].

Mott T, Latimer K. Prevention and treatment of drowning. *Am Fam Physician.* 2016;93(7):576–82.

Salomez F, Vincent JL. Drowning: a review of epidemiology, pathophysiology, treatment, and prevention. *Resuscitation.* 2004;63(3):261–68.

Schaller B, Cornelius JF, Sandu N, et al. Oxygen-conserving reflexes of the brain: the current molecular knowledge. *J Cell Mol Med.* 2009;13(4):644–47.

Schipke JD, Pelzer M. Effect of immersion, submersion, and scuba diving on heart rate variability. *Br J Sports Med.* 2001;35(3):174–80.

Suominen P, Baillie C, Korpela R, et al. Impact of age, submersion time, and water temperature on outcome in near-drowning. *Resuscitation.* 2002;52(3):247–54.

Van Beeck EF, Branche CM, Szpilman D, et al. A new definition of drowning: towards documentation and prevention of a global public health problem. *Bull World Health Organ.* 2005;83(11):853–56.

Environmental Emergencies: Dysbarism and Scuba

Kurt Eifling and Joan Noelker

GENERAL PRINCIPLES

Definition

- The term "diving-related medical conditions" refers to those diseases that are induced by the changes in ambient pressure, regardless of whether they occur in an aquatic environment or a hyperbaric atmosphere.

Classification

- Diving-related injuries are mostly classified by the physical events that induce injury and described according to the organ systems they impact.
- Decompression sickness is split into type 1 and type 2, which have shared physiology but different distribution and severity.

Epidemiology/Etiology

- Diving fatalities are predominantly male and occur disproportionately in older divers.[1]
- Divers with prior pneumothorax, COPD, and cystic pulmonary disease carry an elevated risk of diving-related pneumothorax.
- Inexperienced divers are at a greater risk of decompression sickness.
- Dive events with greater maximum depth, greater rate of ascent, and multiple dives in 1 day carry greater risks of decompression sickness.

Pathophysiology

- **Barotrauma**—the most common form of diving injury—occurs when the body is exposed to a change in ambient pressure and an air-filled body space fails to equilibrate with the environment. Gas expansion during ascent causes the majority of barotrauma.
  - Pulmonary barotrauma without air embolism has two forms, pneumomediastinum and pneumothorax, both secondary to gas expansion during ascent.
  - Ear barotrauma is the most common form.
    - Expanding gas in the middle ear during ascent can cause rupture of the tympanic membrane.
    - Shrinking gas in the middle ear during descent may cause hemorrhagic or serous effusion or allow the increasing environmental water pressure to rupture the tympanic membrane.

- Gastrointestinal barotrauma can occur due to compression of gas in the bowels during descent, leading to edema, microvascular rupture, and subsequent bleeding.
  - Sinus barotrauma, the second most common form, causes facial pain, headache, and potentially neurologic deficits related to pneumocephalus.
- Arterial gas embolism—a potentially fatal condition
  - Gas bubbles form de novo in the pulmonary veins then pass into the systemic circulation.
  - Gas emboli, too copious to be eliminated by the pulmonary capillaries, arrive at the heart and enter the systemic arterial circulation.
- Decompression sickness occurs during ascent as the result of dissolved gases forming bubbles in accordance with Henry's law.
  - The location and volume of the bubbles determine the clinical presentation.
  - Typically manifests in under 1 hour (75%), nearly all within 12 hours (90%), and very rarely over 24 hours after ascent.
  - Prodromal findings include anorexia, irritability, headache, fatigue, and malaise.
  - Decompression sickness is dichotomized by which organ systems are involved.
    - Type 1 is milder and characterized by peripheral symptoms.
      - Localized joint pain is the most common complaint in decompression illness. Pain may increase for 1–2 days then resolve. Elbows and shoulders are most commonly involved.
      - Localized erythema and mottling over the torso, usually resolving within 30 minutes.
      - Transient obstruction of lymphatic flow can cause localized edema.
    - Type 2 is more severe and characterized by CNS and pulmonary symptoms.
      - Neurologic symptoms (60% of decompression sickness) are due to bubbles forming within or traveling to the CNS.
        - Spinal cord involvement causes paraplegia, loss of bladder continence.
        - Cerebral involvement causes memory loss, ataxia, vision and speech deficits, and personality changes.
      - Pulmonary symptoms (5% of decompression sickness) are due to many small bubbles causing symptomatic venous gas embolism.
        - Findings may include dyspnea, chest pain, wheezing, and a choking sensation.
        - Right-sided heart failure ("air lock") may occur if pulmonary hypertension overwhelms the RV.
- Nitrogen narcosis is caused by increased burden of dissolved nitrogen in nervous system tissues, typically at depths >100 feet. It presents with impaired judgment, personality changes, inattention, and impaired motor skills. Hallucinations and syncope may occur at depths >300 feet.

DIAGNOSIS

- Clinical diagnosis is sufficient grounds for starting first-line therapy.

Clinical Presentation
History
- Individual factors include prior history of diving-related illnesses, comorbid medical conditions, and intoxication.
- Exposure factors: depth and duration of dive, number of dives per day, gas mixture used, descent profile, ascent profile, water temperature, protective devices used.

- Any patient who has been breathing compressed gases then surfaces unconscious or loses consciousness within 10 minutes of surfacing should be presumed to have an arterial gas embolism.

Physical Examination

- Cardiopulmonary exam should evaluate for work of breathing, presence of bilateral breath sounds, cardiac auscultation for a systolic crunch, and subcutaneous emphysema on neck and chest palpation.
- Head and ear exam should evaluate for tympanic membrane integrity, middle ear effusion or hemotympanum, epistaxis, CSF rhinorrhea, and mucosal pallor.
- Neurologic exam should evaluate cranial nerves including visual fields; sensory and skin exam should evaluate for mottling or pallor.

Differential Diagnosis

- Ischemic stroke for patients with focal neurologic deficits, MI for those with chest pain and dyspnea, orthopedic trauma and overuse in those with musculoskeletal pain, and hypothermia, hypoglycemia, or intoxication in those with generalized alteration of mental status.

Diagnostic Testing

Laboratories

- In cases of expected air embolism, consider urinalysis, basic metabolic panel, and cardiac enzymes.

Electrocardiography

- Pulmonary air embolism may cause regional ischemia.[2] A normal ECG does not rule out significant coronary involvement.[3]

Imaging

- Chest radiography may show pneumomediastinum.
- Neck radiography may show subcutaneous emphysema.
- CT of the head may reveal pneumocephalus in cases of sinus barotrauma.

TREATMENT

Air Embolism

- Immediate stabilization measures.
  - Administer 100% oxygen to all suspected air embolism patients in order to induce nitrogen washout and therefore increase the rate of reabsorption of air bubbles from the circulatory system.
  - Trendelenburg position decreases cerebral embolism but potentiates cerebral edema.
- Patients with persistent angina should undergo either urgent cardiac catheterization or hyperbaric therapy.
- Definitive treatment is with hyperbaric oxygen (HBO) treatment.[4–6,15]

Pneumothorax

- Diving-related pneumothorax responds to standard treatment of pneumothorax.
- Tube thoracostomy of pneumothorax must precede the use of hyperbaric oxygen therapy for any other indications.

Pneumomediastinum
- Administer 100% oxygen to increase reabsorption of air from tissue.[7]

Ear Barotrauma
- For the middle ear, supportive care for pain control and eustachian tube dysfunction may include topical and systemic decongestants, analgesics, and antihistamines.
- Antibiotics are only indicated for complicating purulent otorrhea. Avoid neomycin due to ototoxicity.
- For symptoms of disequilibrium or hearing loss though to be caused by inner ear barotrauma or air embolism, treat as type 2 decompression sickness.

Sinus Barotrauma
- Supportive care with analgesia and decongestants will ease recovery.
- Prophylactic antibiotics and close outpatient follow-up are warranted.[8,9]

Decompression Sickness
- Mild type 1 cases require no specific therapy and typically resolve within 48 hours.
- For type 2 or severe type 1 cases, immediate management is indicated.
  - Position the patient in the left lateral decubitus position with the head below the heart to allow air accumulation away from the ventricular outflow tracts.[10]
  - Hyperbaric oxygen is the mainstay of treatment of severe decompression sickness and should be initiated as soon as possible for patients with type 2 decompression illness.[6,11,12]

Nitrogen Narcosis
- Nitrogen narcosis typically resolves during ascent.

SPECIAL CONSIDERATIONS

Disposition
- Patients requiring immediate transfer to a HBO-capable facility include those with CNS deficits thought secondary to decompression or air embolism. Air transport is not appropriate for patients thought to be suffering from air embolism. Transfer should be in the supine position.
- Local intensive care unit placement may be appropriate for those patients with critical pneumomediastinum, pneumothorax, or severe craniofacial trauma.
- Floor admission may be appropriate for management of uncomplicated pneumothorax or pneumomediastinum, or for intravenous antibiotics in immunocompromised patients with sinus barotrauma that appears high risk for craniofacial infection.
- Patients with TM rupture, ongoing facial nerve palsy, or ongoing vertigo should have audiology and otolaryngology follow-up to rule out inner ear barotrauma and monitor the return of TM integrity and hearing.

Patient Education
- Air travel limitations
  - Air travel should be resumed after waiting 12 hours if making only one dive per day or 24 hours if taking multiple dives per day.[13,14]

- Diving limitations
  - No further diving is advised for patients with ruptured TM until it heals due to risk for caloric stimulation, nystagmus, and vomiting.
  - No diving is advised for 1 week after decompression for decompression sickness type 1 and for 4 weeks after hyperbarics for DCS type 2.
  - Diving-related conditions accepted as contraindications to future diving include arterial gas embolism, DCS type 2, and pneumothorax.

ADDITIONAL RESOURCES

The Undersea and Hyperbaric Medical Society maintains online resources at https://www.uhms.org.

The U.S. Navy Diving Manual is maintained online by the Office of the Director of Ocean Engineering, Supervisor of Salvage and Diving at http://www.supsalv.org.

REFERENCES

1. Navy Diving Manual. Revision 6. Available at: http://www.supsalv.org/00c3_publications.asp?destPage=00c3&pageId=3.9 (last accessed 03/23/2016)
2. Leitch DR, Hallenbeck JM. Electrocardiographic changes in serious decompression sickness. *Aviat Space Environ Med* 1985;56(10):966–71.
3. Doll SX, Rigamonti F, Roffi M, Noble S. Scuba diving, acute left anterior descending artery occlusion and normal ECG. *BMJ Case Rep* 2013;2013. pii: bcr2012008451.
4. Leitch DR, Green RD. Pulmonary barotrauma in divers and the treatment of cerebral arterial gas embolism. *Aviat Space Environ Med* 1986;57(10 Pt 1):931.
5. Murphy BP, Harford FJ, Cramer FS. Cerebral air embolism resulting from invasive medical procedures. Treatment with hyperbaric oxygen. *Ann Surg* 1985;201(2):242.
6. Moon RE. Hyperbaric oxygen treatment for decompression sickness. *Undersea Hyperb Med* 2014;41(2):151–7.
7. Raymond LW. Pulmonary barotrauma and related events in divers. *Chest* 1995;107(6):1648–52.
8. Fagan P, McKenzie B, Edmonds C. Sinus barotrauma in divers. *Ann Otol Rhinol Laryngol* 1976;85:61.
9. Jeong JH, Kim K, Cho SH, Kim KR. Sphenoid sinus barotrauma after scuba diving. *Am J Otolaryngol* 2012;33(4)477–80.
10. Tetzlaff K, Shank ES, Muth CM. Evaluation and management of decompression illness—an intensivist's perspective. *Intensive Care Med* 2003;29:2128.
11. Bennett MH, Lehm JP, Mitchell SJ, Wasiak J. Recompression and adjunctive therapy for decompression illness. *Cochrane Database Syst Rev* 2012;5:CD005277.
12. Melamed Y, Sherman D, Wiler-Ravell D, Kerem D. The transportable recompression rescue chamber as an alternative to delayed treatment in serious diving accidents. *Aviat Space Environ Med* 1981;52:480.
13. Sheffield PJ. Flying after diving guidelines: a review. *Aviat Space Environ Med* 1990;61:1130.
14. Freiberger JJ, Denoble PJ, Pieper CF, et al. The relative risk of decompression sickness during and after air travel following diving. *Aviat Space Environ Med* 2002;73:980.
15. Moon RE. Hyperbaric oxygen treatment for air or gas embolism. *Undersea Hyperb Med* 2014;41(2):159–66.

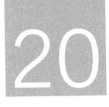

20 Environmental Emergencies: Electrical Injuries

P. Gabriel Miranda Gomez, Kurt Eifling, Joan Noelker, and David Seltzer

GENERAL PRINCIPLES

Definition

- Electrothermal injury occurs as the body joins an electrical circuit or when exposed to intense heat from a nearby electrical arc.
- Electrical injuries can be classified according to their source as high-voltage alternating current (AC), low-voltage AC, or direct current (DC).

Classification

- Classical exposures to electrical injury include:
  - High-voltage AC: contact with a conductor as it touches high-voltage overhead power lines. Also seen as an occupational exposure
  - Low-voltage AC: contact with an energized household appliance
  - DC: classically occurs by contact with a third rail of an electric railway system

Epidemiology/Etiology

- The typical household circuit breaker permits up to 30 mA of current; 16–20 mA causes skeletal muscle tetany; 20 mA may be sufficient to cause transient respiratory muscle paralysis and 50 mA can cause ventricular fibrillation.

Pathophysiology

- Damage can be caused by:
  - Direct contact with an electrical circuit, causing electrothermal burns at sites of source (entry), grounding (exit), and intervening deep tissues
  - Direct effects of electrical stimulation on nerve and muscle tissue, including seizure, respiratory arrest, cardiac dysrhythmia, and tetanic contraction of skeletal muscle
  - Blunt trauma from an associated fall
- Serious injury can occur from any electrical source.

Clinical Presentation

- Electrical injury can adversely affect almost any tissue in the body and can cause ongoing damage to multiple body tissues with delayed sequelae from unrecognized deep tissue injuries.

History

- Determine the source of injury, a high-voltage source (power lines, lightning) or low voltage (household appliances and wiring). The patient may complain of burns on the skin, though a multitude of signs and symptoms in other systems may exist.

Physical Examination
- Chest wall/respiratory: respiratory paralysis from tetany or central apnea from brainstem injury, pain and splinting causing atelectasis, circumferential eschar causing hypoventilation. Upper airway edema may be present.
- Neurologic: seizures from the injury, confusion, loss of consciousness, and spine trauma or radiculopathy
- HEENT: facial laceration, ocular trauma, globe rupture, corneal abrasion. tympanic membrane (TM) perforation[4]
- Skin and soft tissues: blunt trauma and various burns
  - Delayed: compartment syndrome from deep burns, compartment syndrome from deep burns and myofascial necrosis, rhabdomyolysis
- High-voltage electrothermal burns and arc burns:
  - Occur at entry/exit contact points (source and ground), typically appearing as painless, white, full-thickness burns. They are dry and have minimal bleeding.
- Low-voltage electrothermal burns:
  - Occur at sites of direct contact as well as secondary "flame" burns from ignited clothing or objects.
- "Flash" burns:
  - From an electrical arc traveling over and across, but not through, the body can affect large surface areas. Typically limited to partial thickness

Differential Diagnosis
- Dermatitis, arrhythmia, allergic reaction, trauma, or infection

Diagnostic Criteria and Testing
Laboratories
- Screening laboratory evaluation should be obtained including blood counts, chemistries, creatine kinase level, and urinalysis.

Electrocardiography
- Obtain an ECG to evaluate for arrhythmias.

Imaging
- Radiography should be performed looking for trauma.

TREATMENT
- Reversible cardiopulmonary arrest should be treated immediately with cardiopulmonary resuscitation (CPR) and defibrillation.
- Consider fiberoptic laryngoscopy to assess the extent of glottic swelling and intubate if necessary.
- Perform escharotomy of circumferential burns if causing vascular or respiratory compromise.
- Splint long bone fractures and obtain surgical consultation for compartment syndrome.

Medications
- Titrate IV fluids to 2 mL/kg/h urine output for renal protection.
- Pain medication should be provided.
- Prophylactic antibiotics are not necessary.

SPECIAL CONSIDERATIONS

Disposition

- Injuries are from a combination of the lightning itself and the blast wave that accompanies it, so patients can have electrical and blunt trauma mechanisms together. Injuries may include sudden cardiac death, severe burns, HEENT injury, long bone fractures, or no apparent injury at all. Outdoor exposures are most common, although indoor exposures around indoor swimming pools have been reported. A "ferning" pattern of burns on the skin is pathognomonic for lightning strike. Even when there is no apparent immediate injury, immediate medical evaluation is warranted to all persons affected.
- Patients should be admitted unless the exposure was for a very short time period from household current and there are no concerning physical exam features.

SUGGESTED READING

Strote J, Walsh M, Angelidis M, et al. Conducted electrical weapon use by law enforcement: an evaluation of safety and injury. *J Trauma* 2010;68(5):1239–46.

Koumbourlis AC. Electrical injuries. *Crit Care Med* 2002;30(11 Suppl):S424–30.

Hussmann J, Kucan JO, Russell RC, et al. Electrical injuries—morbidity, outcome and treatment rationale. *Burns* 1995;21(7):530–5.

Saffle JR, Crandall A, Warden GD. Cataracts: a long-term complication of electrical injury. *J Trauma* 1985;25(1):17–21.

21 Environmental Emergencies: High-Altitude Illness

Kurt Eifling and Joan Noelker

GENERAL PRINCIPLES

Definitions

- High-altitude illness (HAI)—a collective term for the cerebral and pulmonary syndromes that occur with rapidly moving from an area of low altitude to an area of high altitude (typically over 2800 m or 9200 feet) or moving rapidly from a high altitude to a greater altitude.
- Barometric hypoxia—low blood oxygen content due to low partial pressure of oxygen in the high-altitude environment
- Acute mountain sickness (AMS) and high-altitude cerebral edema (HACE)—a spectrum of illness caused by interstitial fluid collection within the brain.
  - The threshold for redesignating an AMS patient as having HACE is the onset of impaired neurologic function, commonly heralded by ataxia or confusion.

- High-altitude pulmonary edema (HAPE)—noncardiogenic pulmonary edema of acute onset coinciding with rapid ascent to high altitude, typically over 2500 m (8000 ft)
- Acclimatization is defined as the series of physiologic events that compensate for barometric hypoxia.

Epidemiology/Etiology

- HAI is observed in all ages though slightly less beyond age 50; both sexes though slightly more in women, and the likelihood of disease is most affected by rapidity and height of ascent.
- AMS is by far the most common entity among HAI.
- Risk factors include rapid ascent, high sleeping elevation, vigorous activity prior to acclimatization, history of HAI, respiratory depressants, and altitude reached.
  - <1500 m (5000 ft): unlikely to develop any HAI
  - 1500–2500 m (5000–8000 ft): mild AMS is possible but rare.
  - 2500–3000 m (8000–9800 ft): moderate AMS is common and HAPE is possible but rare.
  - 3000–4000 m (9800–13,000 ft): increased AMS and progressively increasing risk of severe HAI. HACE is possible at this elevation and usually accompanied by HAPE.
- HAPE is the most common cause of death from HAI.

Pathophysiology

- Barometric hypoxia, caused by a diminished oxygen absorption gradient at high altitude, serves as the inciting cause for all HAI. As altitude increases, PiO_2 decreases, and the gradient driving oxygen absorption decreases, resulting in tissue hypoxia.
- AMS and HACE are caused by changes in cerebrovascular blood flow secondary to compensatory mechanisms active in the setting of barometric hypoxia.
  - AMS is associated with changes in water distribution within the CNS.[1]
  - Death from HACE is from cerebral herniation secondary to increased intracranial pressure.
- HAPE is caused by pulmonary vascular constriction, increased capillary permeability, and increased sympathetic tone in the setting of barometric hypoxia.
  - Those areas with inadequate vasoconstriction develop regional hyperperfusion that causes progressive damage to the alveolar–capillary barrier.

DIAGNOSIS

Clinical Presentation

History

- Patients with AMS develop typical symptoms after ascending from low to high altitude, typically over 2000 m. Symptoms typically begin 6–12 hours after ascent, subside by day 2, and do not recur at the same altitude.
  - Common adult symptoms include headache, fatigue, anorexia, disturbed sleep, light-headedness, poor attention, and exertional dyspnea.
- Patients typically develop HACE after having already demonstrated AMS and/or HAPE at elevations over 3500 m.[2]
  - Neurologic manifestations: encephalopathy, ataxia, drowsiness, irritability, impaired thought, stupor, and coma.

- HAPE typically manifests insidiously 2–4 days after ascent with nonproductive cough and dyspnea on exertion, either of which could be normal findings at altitude.
  - The progression from dyspnea on exertion to dyspnea at rest heralds the development of HAPE.

Physical Examination
- AMS typically lacks distinct physical findings. Careful assessment for encephalopathy and ataxia should be performed before establishing the diagnosis.
- HACE causes broad deficits including altered consciousness and loss of finger–nose–finger and heel–shin coordination. Other focal neurologic deficits in a lucid patient would be atypical.
- HAPE causes tachycardia, tachypnea, crackles on chest auscultation, and hypoxia.
  - SpO_2 is typically 10 points below expected and rises with supplemental oxygen.
  - Rapid improvement with supplemental oxygen is typical of HAPE.
  - Peripheral cyanosis progresses to central cyanosis.

Differential Diagnosis

- AMS or HACE: carbon monoxide poisoning, hypothermia, intoxication, migraine headache, stroke, intracranial hemorrhage, and hypoglycemia
- HAPE: pneumonia, upper respiratory infection, reactive airway disease, cardiogenic pulmonary edema, myocardial infarction

Diagnostic Criteria and Testing
- These are clinical diagnoses.

Laboratories
- AMS/HACE—the white blood cell count may be elevated in HACE; arterial blood gas may show distinct hypoxemia.
- HAPE—arterial blood gas may show distinct hypoxemia and respiratory alkalosis. White blood cell count may be elevated. BNP is not elevated.

Electrocardiography
- While the ECG may show right heart strain in cases of HAPE, its main role in HAI to rule out alternative diagnoses.

Imaging
- Chest radiograph should show normal findings in lone AMS; pulmonary edema is expected in HAPE, with right-sided infiltrates presenting most commonly.[3]
- Ultrasound may reveal B-lines (comet tails) and right-sided heart strain in HAPE.
- CT of the head should be normal in AMS but can show cerebral edema with dense white matter in HACE.

TREATMENT

- Descent and oxygen administration are the most effective treatment for all HAI.
- HACE and HAPE are emergencies requiring immediate management.
  - The goal of treatment of HACE is reduction of intracranial pressure.
  - The goals of treatment of HAPE are oxygenation and reduction of PA pressure.

TABLE 21.1	Medical Management of High-Altitude Illness		
	AMS	**HACE**	**HAPE**
Prophylaxis	Acetazolamide	Dexamethasone	Nifedipine
	Dexamethasone		Tadalafil
			Sildenafil
			Dexamethasone
First-line treatment	Acetazolamide	Immediate descent	Immediate descent
	NSAIDs	Dexamethasone	Supplemental oxygen
	Antiemetics		Nifedipine
	Acetaminophen		
Second-line treatment	Dexamethasone	Acetazolamide	Tadalafil
		Mannitol if not hypovolemic	Sildenafil
		Supplemental oxygen	
Unclear benefit	Ginkgo biloba		Salmeterol

Medications (Table 21.1)

- AMS
  - Acetazolamide is the only available medication that accelerates acclimatization in addition to reducing symptoms of AMS.
  - Treat symptoms with NSAIDs, acetaminophen, and antiemetics. Consider adding dexamethasone if refractory or progressive.
  - Mild sleep aids, such as zolpidem, will not hinder acclimatization.
- HACE
  - First-line therapy is dexamethasone as 8 mg IV/IM/PO at the first sign of symptoms.
  - Furosemide and mannitol may have a role if the patient is not already hypovolemic.
- HAPE
  - If the patient requires supplemental oxygen, nifedipine may be indicated.[4,5] Dosing of nifedipine is 10 mg q4–6 h or 10 mg immediate release then 30 mg slow release q12 hours.

Oxygen

- Supplemental oxygen relieves the symptoms of AMS and can serve as an alternative to descent.

- In HAPE, supplemental oxygen is first-line therapy regardless of severity.[2,6,7,8]
  - In lone HACE, supplemental oxygen to support SpO_2 > 90% is sufficient to reduce primary hypoxic injury, yet descent remains mandatory.

Surgical Management

- Neurosurgic consultation may be sought for HACE patients who remain comatose despite maximal medical therapy.

SPECIAL CONSIDERATIONS

- Pregnant women are at no increased risk of HAI. They have higher SpO_2 at altitude due to respiratory stimulation from progesterone. Travel up to 2500 m appears safe. Acetazolamide is pregnancy class C, and it is excreted in breast milk.
- Elderly patients or those with comorbid cardiopulmonary disease may be more likely to suffer ischemic insults due to barometric hypoxia.
- Sickle cell disease may be exacerbated by hypoxemia at moderate altitudes over 1500 m.

ADDITIONAL RESOURCES

The Institute for Altitude Medicine, located in Telluride, Colorado, offers references for special populations such as athletes on their Web site, http://www.altitudemedicine.org

The International Society of Mountain Medicine provides free information for patients and health care providers, including a consensus statement concerning children at high altitude. Free resources available at http://issm.org

The Wilderness Medical Society maintains an evidence-based clinical practice guideline for high altitude illness, available through the journal Wilderness and Environmental Medicine or through their website, http://www.wms.org

REFERENCES

1. Lawley JS, Oliver SJ, Mullins PG, Macdonald JH. Investigation of whole-brain white matter identifies altered water mobility in the pathogenesis of high-altitude headache. *J Cereb Blood Flow Metab* 2013;33(8):1286–94.
2. Hackett PH, Roach RC. High-Altitude Medicine. In: Auerbach PS, ed. *Wilderness Medicine.* 6th ed. Philadelphia: Elsevier, 2012:2.
3. Vock P, Brutsche MH, Nanzer A, Bärtsch P. Variable radiomorphologic data of high altitude pulmonary edema. Features from 60 patients. *Chest* 1991;100:1306.
4. Hackett PH, Roach RC. High altitude cerebral edema. *High Alt Med Biol* 2004;5:136.
5. Oelz O, Maggiorini M, Ritter M, et al. Nifedipine for high altitude pulmonary oedema. *Lancet* 1989;2:1241.
6. Küpper T, Schöffl V, Netzer N. Cheyne stokes breathing at high altitude: a helpful response or a troublemaker? *Sleep Breath* 2008;12:123.
7. Marticorena E, Hultgren HN. Evaluation of therapeutic methods in high altitude pulmonary edema. *Am J Cardiol* 1979;43:307.
8. Zafren K, Reeves JT, Schoene R. Treatment of high-altitude pulmonary edema by bed rest and supplemental oxygen. *Wilderness Environ Med* 1996;7:127.

22 Environmental Emergencies: Hyperthermia and Hypothermia

Aurora Lybeck and Joan Noelker

GENERAL PRINCIPLES

Definition

- Thermal injuries are defined as any systemic illness or tissue damage that results from exposure to the extremes of temperature.
- Hyperthermia is defined as a core body temperature >37.5°C; heat stroke is often >40°C.
- Hypothermia is defined as a core body temperature <35°C.
  - Mild: 32–35°C
  - Moderate: 27–32°C
  - Severe/profound: <27°C

Classification

- Heat-related injuries
  - Mild: Sunburn, heat cramps, heat edema, heat syncope, or exhaustion
  - Severe: Heat stroke (exertional or nonexertional/classic)
- Cold-related injuries
  - Peripheral: Chilblains/pernio, trench foot, and frostbite
  - Systemic: Hypothermia

Epidemiology

- Heat- and cold-related injuries and illnesses are common worldwide and vary among climates and season.
  - Patients who are at higher risk for heat- and cold-related injuries are those with cardiovascular disease, neurologic or psychiatric disorders, obesity, anhydrosis, physical disability, extremes of age, and the use of recreational drugs, the use of alcohol, and patients on certain prescription drugs (anticholinergics or diuretics).
  - The mortality rate for heat stroke is up to 33%.
- Heat-related illness is the leading cause of morbidity and mortality among US high school athletes.

Pathophysiology

- The hypothalamus controls the body's temperature set point.
  - Hyperthermia occurs due to a rise in body temperature above the set point, when the heat-dissipating mechanisms are impaired or overwhelmed by external (environmental) or internal (metabolic) heat production.
  - Hypothermia occurs due to a drop in body temperature below the set point, when the warming and temperature maintenance mechanisms are impaired or overwhelmed by external (environmental) cold exposure.

DIAGNOSIS

- Diagnosis is made by measuring the core body temperature and/or by a history of extreme temperature exposure with concurrent physical exam findings.

Clinical Presentation

History

- Usually, a patient will give the history of being exposed to the environment for a long period of time, but may also give vague complaints that can range from skin complaints alone to stomach upset, muscle spasms, weakness, or altered mentation. A history of prolonged exposure to the environment should also be obtained.

Physical Examination

- Heat-related injury or illness
  - Sunburn: Sun-exposed areas of the body present with erythema of the skin, ranging from mild (superficial) to severe with edema and blistering (superficial partial thickness). In severe cases, systemic symptoms such as nausea, headache, vomiting, and fever may occur.
  - Heat cramps: Painful, self-limiting involuntary muscle spasms of any muscle associated with physical exertion in a warm or hot environment.
  - Heat edema: Edema of extremities associated with physical exertion in a warm or hot environment that improves with rest and elevation and is self-limiting.
  - Heat syncope or exhaustion: Transient light-headedness and brief loss of tone and consciousness associated with physical exertion in a warm or hot environment. Alone, it is a benign condition, though syncope can occur in more severe forms of heat illness.
  - Heat stroke: Hyperthermia and altered mental status or other central nervous system dysfunction occurring in the setting of exposure to a warm or hot environment in any range of patients from young healthy athletes (exertional heat stroke) to elderly or those with comorbid medical conditions (nonexertional/classic heat stroke). Severe cases can be associated with acute respiratory failure, ARDS, DIC, hypoglycemia, acute kidney injury, hepatic failure, rhabdomyolysis, seizures, and cardiac arrest.
- Cold-related injury or illness
  - Chilblains/pernio: Single or multiple lesions associated with exposure to a cold environment, typically on the dorsal fingers and toes, though can occur on nose, ears, other areas of the extremities, or buttocks. Symmetrically distributed, erythematous patches, plaques, or nodules may be associated with blisters or ulcers. They may be tender, pruritic, or burning. They usually appear within 24 hours of exposure and resolve over weeks.
  - Trench foot: Foot (and rarely hand) complaints associated with prolonged cold and wet/damp exposure; it may be worsened with tight-fitting boots and associated with edema, erythema, skin breakdown or sloughing, hemorrhagic bullae, numbness, or severe pain and often accompanied by infection.
  - Frostbite: Localized tissue edema and necrosis associated with exposure to a cold environment, often in peripheral extremities, nose, ears, or any exposed or inadequately covered skin. Prior to rewarming, area may be cold and numb, white or gray in color, and hard, feeling like leather or wax. During or after rewarming, severe pain and paresthesias may occur and clear or hemorrhagic blisters may develop. Mild self-limiting cases are known as frostnip.

○ Hypothermia: Systemic symptoms of varying degrees associated with prolonged exposure to a cold environment, ranging from shivering and tachycardia, confusion, and cold diuresis to more severe symptoms including hemodynamic instability, cardiac arrhythmias, coma, areflexia, and asystole/cardiac arrest.

Differential Diagnosis

- Heat-related injury or illness
  ○ Sunburn: Exaggerated sunburn reaction due to medications, phytophotodermatitis, bacterial infection, rash or viral exanthem, lupus, or solar urticaria
  ○ Heat cramps: Peripheral vascular disease, myalgias, tetany, or sickle cell crisis
  ○ Heat edema: Heart failure, cirrhosis, lymphedema, DVT, or nephrotic syndrome
  ○ Heat syncope or exhaustion: Vasovagal/neurocardiogenic syncope, orthostasis, cardiac syncope, cardiac syncope, hemorrhage, ruptured ectopic, pulmonary embolism, or seizure
  ○ Hyperthermia and heat stroke: Sepsis, thyroid storm, malignant hyperthermia, or neuroleptic malignant syndrome
- Cold-related injury or illness
  ○ Chilblains/pernio: Frostbite, Raynaud, cryoglobulinemia, or lupus
  ○ Trench foot: Frostbite, gangrene, or peripheral artery thrombosis/occlusion
  ○ Frostbite: Chilblains, Raynaud, cryoglobulinemia, or peripheral artery thrombosis/occlusion
  ○ Hypothermia: Sepsis, hypoglycemia, or hypothyroidism/myxedema coma

Diagnostic Criteria and Testing

- Core body temperature is the critical diagnostic step in suspected severe/systemic environmental injury.
  ○ Rectal temperature is considered the gold standard (a low temperature thermometer may be necessary for hypothermic patients). When not available or not practical, treat based off clinical suspicion.
  ○ In the hospital setting, a bladder catheter with temperature sensor may be used for continuous temperature monitoring.

Laboratories

- Most mild or peripheral thermal injuries do not require laboratory testing for diagnosis.
- A more thorough laboratory workup may be necessary for patients with extremes of temperature illness in order to diagnose and correct renal failure, DIC, hepatic dysfunction, and cardiac issues.

Electrocardiography

- No specific ECG findings aid in the diagnosis of hyperthermia.
- In hypothermia, the classic J wave often appears at core temps <33.8°C. In varying degrees of hypothermia, atrial fibrillation, junctional bradycardia, ventricular fibrillation, and asystole may be present.

TREATMENT

Medications

- Heat-related injury or illness
  ○ Sunburn: Topical aloe vera or topical benzocaine can be used for pain. Topical antimicrobials or sulfasalazine may be used for large areas of exposed blisters.

- ○ Heat cramps, heat edema, heat syncope or exhaustion: Oral (preferred) or IV rehydration.
- ○ Heat stroke: Avoid antipyretics. Active cooling measures that may include ice bath and IV rehydration with cooled (4°C) NS or D5NS are recommended.
- Cold-related injury or illness
  - ○ Chilblains/pernio: For refractory cases, consider nifedipine.
  - ○ Trench foot: Analgesia. Antibiotics may be prescribed for any concomitant skin infection.
  - ○ Frostbite: Analgesia and rewarming in a bath of water at 37–39°C until the skin becomes pliable and less painful is recommended. In severe frostbite cases, one can consider IV or intra-arterial TPA.
  - ○ Hypothermia: Replace cold diuresis/fluid losses with warmed D5NS IV boluses. In cardiac arrest, continue all advanced life support measures and medications and ensure normothermia before terminating resuscitative efforts.

Other Nonpharmacologic Therapies

- Heat-related injury or illness
  - ○ Remove the patient from the sun and warm/hot environment.
  - ○ Sunburn: Cool compresses, aloe vera–based lotion, or calamine lotion. Open blisters should be cleansed with soap and water.
  - ○ Heat cramps: Oral rehydration. Rest and stretch involved muscle(s).
  - ○ Heat edema: Oral rehydration. Elevate extremity, or use compression stocking as needed.
  - ○ Heat syncope: Oral rehydration. Lie supine, elevate legs, and rest.
  - ○ Heat stroke: Expose skin. Provide passive cooling (decrease ambient temperature in patient care area), evaporative or convective cooling (cool or ambient temp mist with fan blowing over patient), or cold water immersion therapy (ice water slurry) in appropriate patients. The goal is to maximize water–skin or water vapor–skin interface. Body cavity lavage (GI/bladder/thoracic) with cold fluids has been reported but has not been adequately studied. Intravascular cooling devices including ECMO can be considered in extreme cases when available.
- Cold-related injury or illness
  - ○ Remove the patient from the wet and cold environment.
  - ○ Chilblains/pernio, trench foot: Elevate affected part(s). Gentle rewarming. Keep area dry, clean, and loosely dressed.
  - ○ Frostbite: Never begin rewarming until the risk of refreezing is eliminated. Avoid rubbing or friction. Unroof/drain clear blisters; leave hemorrhagic blisters intact. Keep area dry, clean, and loosely dressed.
  - ○ Hypothermia: Remove wet/cold clothing. Rewarm by 0.5–1°C/h in most cases, with more aggressive warming in patients in cardiac arrest or multisystem organ failure. Provide passive rewarming (increase ambient temperature in room) or rewarming blankets or similar external devices when available. Body cavity lavage (GI/bladder/thoracic) with warm fluids has been reported, but not adequately studied. Intravascular rewarming devices including ECMO can be considered in extreme cases when available. In cardiac arrest, defibrillate V-fib and V-tach although arrhythmias may be refractory to electrical conversion. Ensure normothermia before terminating resuscitative efforts.

Surgical Management

- Early surgical consultation in cases of 4th degree/full-thickness frostbite is recommended.

SPECIAL CONSIDERATIONS

Disposition

- Patients with simple hyper- or hypothermia, whose temperature can be normalized, with normal laboratory values and a clear sensorium can likely be discharged safely from the hospital.
- Patients needing more intensive treatment should be admitted to the hospital, and patients in extremis should be admitted to the ICU.

SUGGESTED READINGS

Bergeron MF. Exertional heat cramps: recovery and return to play. *J Sport Rehabil* 2007; 16:190.

Brown DJ, Brugger H, Boyd J, Paal P. Accidental hypothermia. *N Engl J Med* 2012; 367:1930.

Capacchione JF, Muldoon SM. The relationship between exertional heat illness, exertional rhab-domyolysis, and malignant hyperthermia. *Anesth Analg* 2009;109:1065.

Centers for Disease Control and Prevention. (CDC). Heat illness among high school athletes—United States, 2005–2009. *MMWR Morb Mortal Wkly Rep* 2010;59:1009.

Fernandez Garza V, Valdez Delgado J. *Hypothermia: Prevention, Recognition and Treatment* [e-book]. Accidental Hypothermia, Chapter VI, pp 123–136. New York: Nova Science Pub-lishers, Inc, 2012. Available at: eBook Clinical Collection (EBSCOhost), Ipswich, MA (last accessed: 03/14/16).

Headdon WG, Wilson PM, Dalton HR. The management of accidental hypothermia. *BMJ* 2009;338:b2085.

Jardine DS. Heat illness and heat stroke. *Pediatr Rev* 2007;28:249.

Jurkovich GJ. Environmental cold-induced injury. *Surg Clin North Am* 2007;87:247.

Lipman GS, Eifling KP, Ellis MA, et al. Wilderness Medical Society practice guidelines for the prevention and treatment of heat-related illness: 2014 update. *Wilderness Environ Med* 2014;25:S55.

Murphy JV, Banwell PE, Roberts AH, McGrouther DA. Frostbite: pathogenesis and treatment. *J Trauma* 2000;48:171.

Pryor RR, Roth RN, Suyama J, Hostler D. Exertional heat illness: emerging concepts and ad-vances in prehospital care. *Prehosp Disaster Med* 2015;30:297.

Sawka M, O'Conner F. Disorders Due to Heat and Cold. In: Goldman L, ed. *Goldman-Cecil Medicine.* 25th ed. Philadelphia: Saunders Elsevier, 2016.

Sawka MN, Young AJ. Physiological Systems and their Responses to Conditions of Heat and Cold. In: Tipton CM, ed. *ACSM's Advanced Exercise Physiology.* Philadelphia: Lippincott Williams & Wilkins, 2006:535.

Soar J, Perkins GD, Abbas G, et al. European Resuscitation Council Guidelines for Resus-citation 2010 Section 8. Cardiac arrest in special circumstances: electrolyte abnormalities, poisoning, drowning, accidental hypothermia, hyperthermia, asthma, anaphylaxis, cardiac surgery, trauma, pregnancy, electrocution. *Resuscitation* 2010;81:1400.

Vano-Galvan S, Martorell A. Chilblains. *CMAJ* 2012;184:67.

World Health Organization. (1992). *The ICD-10 Classification of Mental and Behavioural Dis-orders: Clinical Descriptions and Diagnostic Guidelines.* Geneva, Switzerland: World Health Organization.

23 Gastrointestinal Emergencies: Abdominal Wall

Gregory M. Polites

GENERAL PRINCIPLES

Clinical Presentation

History
- A thorough history is fundamental in determining whether the abdominal pain is consistent with an abdominal wall or an intra-abdominal condition. Determining precipitating factors prior to the onset of pain, associated nausea, vomiting, constipation, or rash is also important.

Physical Examination
- In determining the nature of the abdominal pain, a thorough physical exam is crucial. The abdominal exam always begins with inspection, followed by auscultation, percussion, and palpation.
- A positive Carnett sign is increased or unchanged pain when the patient sits up and tenses the abdominal muscles or raises both legs off the table at the same time and is indicative of abdominal wall pain as opposed to an intra-abdominal etiology.[1-3]

Differential Diagnosis
- Trauma, infection, overuse syndrome, dermatitis, or hernia

Abdominal Wall Strain

PATHOPHYSIOLOGY

- Occurs when a muscle is stretched too far resulting in tearing of the muscle fibers or torn from its attachment. The muscles usually involved include the rectus abdominis and the internal or external obliques.

DIAGNOSIS

Clinical Presentation

History
- A history of overuse or trauma may be elicited.

Physical Examination
- Pain with palpation or movement of the involved area. Bruising may be present.

TREATMENT

- Rest, if appropriate, and NSAIDs

Abdominal Wall Hernias

PATHOPHYSIOLOGY

- A tearing or weakening of the abdominal wall musculature that may be genetic or due to overuse/strain allowing protrusion of bowel wall content
- **Groin hernias**—consist of inguinal and femoral hernias
  - Inguinal hernias are the most common type of abdominal wall hernia, may be direct or indirect, and are more common in males.
  - Femoral hernias—femoral hernias are less common than inguinal hernias and more common in females. They are more likely to incarcerate and strangulate.[4]
- **Ventral hernias**—occur in the anterior and lateral abdominal walls. Midline ventral hernias (e.g., umbilical, paraumbilical, epigastric, hypogastric) occur more commonly than paramedian (Spigelian) or lateral defects.
  - Umbilical—usually small and common in women. Congenital umbilical hernias rarely incarcerate.[5,6] Acquired umbilical hernias in adults are associated with obesity, pregnancy, and ascites. They frequently incarcerate.
  - Paraumbilical—large defects adjacent to the umbilicus in the linea alba region. These are usually related to diastasis of the rectus abdominis muscles.
  - Epigastric and hypogastric—occur above and below the umbilicus, respectively, in the linea alba region.
  - Paramedian or lateral defects—not as common as above. Usually, there are short segments of bowel or omentum that protrude through the abdominal wall defect. These are more likely to incarcerate.

DIAGNOSIS

Clinical Presentation

History
- The patient will likely report a bulge in the groin or abdominal wall and pain, most frequently with straining or Valsalva maneuvers.
- An incarcerated hernia will present as tender, possibly red or warm.

Physical Examination
- With the patient performing a Valsalva maneuver, a bulge will be noted in the groin or abdomen. These should be easily reducible. If unable to be reduced, this is most often a sign of incarceration.

Diagnostic Criteria and Testing

Imaging
- No imaging studies are needed unless the hernia cannot be reduced.
- In an incarcerated hernia, a CT scan is indicated.

TREATMENT

- Trusses and support binders may provide temporary relief.
- Outpatient follow-up with a surgeon and pain control is recommended for reducible hernias.
- Incarcerated hernias require surgical consultation and possible admission for reduction.

Abdominal Wall Hematomas

EPIDEMIOLOGY/ETIOLOGY

- Risk factors include systemic abdominal wall trauma, anticoagulation, older age, female sex, pregnancy, and impaired renal function.[7]

PATHOPHYSIOLOGY

- A potentially life-threatening condition caused by bleeding into the soft tissue.

DIAGNOSIS

Clinical Presentation

History
- There may be a history of recent procedure or complaints of bruising, swelling, and tenderness.
- A history of use of blood thinning/antiplatelet medication should be obtained.

Physical Examination
- Bruising may be significant and rapidly progressing.

Diagnostic Criteria and Testing

Laboratories
- A complete blood count (CBC) and coagulation studies are appropriate.

Imaging
- Depending on the size and spread of the hematoma, angiographic studies may be needed to evaluate active bleeding.

TREATMENT

- Surgical evaluation and consultation is appropriate for rapidly progressing hematoma.
- Reversal agents or blood products may be administered

REFERENCES

1. Meyer GW, Friedman LS, Gover S. Chronic abdominal wall pain. *UpToDate* 2016. Available at: http://www.uptodate.com/contents/chronic-abdominal-wall-pain?source=machine Learning&search=Abdominal+Wall+pain&selectedTitle=1%7E76&sectionRank=1&anchor=H6#H6
2. Gallagher EJ. Acute Abdominal Pain. In: Tintinalli JE, Kelen GD, Stapczynski JS, eds. *Emergency Medicine: A Comprehensive Study Guide.* 6th ed. NY: McGraw-Hill, 2004:497.
3. Carnett JB. Intercostal neuralgia as a cause of abdominal pain and tenderness. *Surg Gynecol Obstet* 1926;42:625.
4. Gallegos NC, Dawson J, Jarvis M, et al. Risk of strangulation in groin hernias. *Br J Surg* 1991;78:1171.
5. Skinner MA, Grosfeld JL. Inguinal and umbilical hernia repair in infants and children. *Surg Clin North Am* 1993;73:439.
6. Scherer LR, Grosfeld JL. Inguinal hernia and umbilical anomalies. *Pediatr Clin North Am* 1993;40:1121.
7. Nourbakhsh E, Anvari R, Nugent K. Abdominal wall hematomas associated with low-molecular weight heparins: an important complication in older adults. *J Am Geriatr Soc* 2011;59(8):1543–5.

24 Gastrointestinal Emergencies: Esophageal

Sonya Naganathan

GENERAL PRINCIPLES

Definition

- Esophagitis—inflammation of the esophagus
- Esophageal strictures—esophageal narrowing secondary to scar tissue from prior injury
- Diverticula (e.g., Zenker)—outpouchings of esophageal tissue
- Boerhaave rupture—a spontaneous, full-thickness laceration of the esophagus
- Mallory–Weiss tear—a partial-thickness laceration
- Gastroesophageal reflux disease (GERD)—reflux of gastrointestinal contents into the esophagus causing subsequent injury to the tissue

Epidemiology/Etiology

- Esophageal perforation is rare, though when it occurs, it is associated with a high morbidity and mortality of over 20%. Iatrogenic perforation is a leading cause, followed by spontaneous rupture (e.g., Boerhaave and Mallory–Weiss).
- Annual occurrence of variceal hemorrhage is 5–15% with a 40% spontaneous resolution in the bleed.
- Prevalence of eosinophilic esophagitis is the most common cause of food impaction.

Pathophysiology

- Medication-induced esophagitis is generally due to irritation of the esophageal mucosa, whereas eosinophilic esophagitis is due to histamine release and subsequent inflammation of the mucosa
- Variceal hemorrhage, Boerhaave, and Mallory–Weiss tears are all due to increased tension of the esophageal wall. Boerhaave ruptures are full-thickness lacerations while Mallory–Weiss tears are limited to the mucosa, most commonly seen at the gastroesophageal junction.
- GERD is most often associated with a weakened lower esophageal sphincter—episodes of relaxation of this muscle cause acid reflux.

DIAGNOSIS

Clinical Presentation

History
- The patient may present with complaints of pain and burning, and may or may not have relief with food ingestion. Chronicity is an important factor to consider. Strictures, achalasia, and diverticula oftentimes present with progressively worsening of dysphagia solids or liquids. Regurgitation of food may be a complaint with a Zenker diverticulum.

- Patients with gastritis may have additional history of HIV or potassium or bisphosphonate use.
- Variceal bleeds are generally associated with a history of alcoholism and/or alcoholic cirrhosis.
- A history of recent retching or violent vomiting may cause Boerhaave or Mallory–Weiss tears.
- The onset of GERD symptoms is classically associated with alcohol intake, spicy foods, or lying down soon after a meal and is generally described as a midsternal burning sensation, sometime associated iwth epigastric pain.

Physical Examination
- Thrush or ulcers in the oropharynx should be noted.
- Changes consistent with portal hypertension should be evaluated in the case of variceal bleeds.

Differential Diagnosis
- GERD, acute coronary syndrome (ACS), tumor, stricture, Zenker diverticulum, esophagitis (infectious vs. drug induced), foreign body, or food bolus impaction

Diagnostic Criteria and Testing
- Most diagnoses in this category will be made clinically, with imaging, or with endoscopy.

Laboratories
- There are no specific laboratories to diagnose esophageal disorders.

Imaging
- A chest plain radiograph may identify a foreign body, perforated mediastinum, nodules, or mass.

TREATMENT

Medications
- GERD: famotidine 10–20 mg bid, ranitidine 75–150 mg bid, omeprazole 20–40 mg daily.
- Esophagitis
  - Medication induced may benefit from a short course of PPI therapy.
- Variceal bleeding: start propranolol at 20 mg bid for risk reduction of primary variceal bleed; octreotide 50 µg IV bolus followed by 50 µg/h infusion for acute variceal hemorrhage
- Food bolus impaction: glucagon 1 mg IV; will induce vomiting, but has a risk of perforation.

Other Nonpharmacologic Therapies
- Emergent endoscopic removal is indicated in all objects causing complete obstruction or airway compromise, disc batteries, and any sharp objects lodged in the esophagus; urgent removal is indicated for magnets.
- Coins and other blunt objects may be observed for up to 24 hours before intervention.
- Endoscopic variceal ligation is the method of choice for the management of acute variceal hemorrhage.

SPECIAL CONSIDERATIONS

Disposition

• While a majority of these conditions can be managed as an outpatient (GERD, structural abnormalities), an ICU (or the OR) is necessary for patients with acute variceal hemorrhage as these patients may be at higher risk of decompensation. Floor is appropriate for those patients that are requiring observation (e.g., foreign body ingestion, new diagnosis of malignancy meeting criteria for inpatient admission).

SUGGESTED READINGS

ASGE Standards of Practice Committee, Ikenberry SO, Jue TL, et al. Management of ingested foreign bodies and food impactions. *Gastrointest Endosc* 2011;73:1085–91.

Dellon ES. Epidemiology of eosinophilic esophagitis. *Gastroenterol Clin North Am* 2014;43:201–18.

Dellon ES, Gonsalves N, Hirano I, et al. ACG clinical guideline: evidenced based approach to the diagnosis and management of esophageal eosinophilia and eosinophilic esophagitis (EoE). *Am J Gastroenterol* 2013;108:679–92.

Garcia-Tsao G, Sanyal AJ, Grace ND, Carey WD. Prevention and management of gastroesophageal varices and variceal hemorrhage in cirrhosis. *Am J Gastroenterol* 2007;102:2086–102.

Kahrilas PJ, Shaheen NJ, Vaezi MF, et al. American Gastroenterological Association Medical Position Statement on the management of gastroesophageal reflux disease. *Gastroenterology* 2008;135:1383–91.

Mendelson M. Esophageal Emergencies. In: Tintinalli JE, Stapczynski JS, John Ma O, et al., eds. *Tintinalli's Emergency Medicine.* 8th ed. McGraw-Hill Education, 2016.

Søreide JA, Viste A. Esophageal perforation: diagnostic work-up and clinical decision-making in the first 24 hours. *Scand J Trauma Resusc Emerg Med* 2011;19:66.

25 Gastrointestinal Emergencies: Anorectal

Mark D. Levine

Hemorrhoids

GENERAL PRINCIPLES

Definition

• Vascular structures that arise from the arteriovenous connective tissue and drain into the hemorrhoidal veins.
• External hemorrhoids are located distal to the dentate line.
• Internal hemorrhoids are located proximal to the dentate line.

Epidemiology/Etiology
- Equal prevalence in both sexes, most frequently in patients from 45 to 65 years of age.
- Cause of inflammation is usually due to age, diarrhea, pregnancy, tumors, prolonged sitting, straining, and constipation.

Pathophysiology
- Connective tissues that anchor hemorrhoids are thought to weaken, and the hemorrhoids then slide into the anal canal.
- During the passage of feces, hemorrhoids are pushed against the anal sphincter causing them to engorge.
- Abnormal dilation of hemorrhoidal venous plexus.

DIAGNOSIS

Clinical Presentation
History
- Patients may complain of bleeding, which can be on the stool or drip into the toilet with or without a bowel movement. There may be a complaint of itching, irritation, or discharge (mucous, watery, or fecal).

Physical Examination
- An exam of the anal and perianal region as well as a digital rectal exam should be performed to evaluate for masses or tenderness.
- A thrombosed hemorrhoid is tender to palpation, blue/black in color, and a firm mass may be felt in the center of the hemorrhoid.

Differential Diagnosis
- Anal fissures, polyps, rectal prolapse, cancer, or proctitis

Diagnostic Criteria and Testing
Laboratories
- There are no specific lab tests to diagnose hemorrhoids.
- A fecal occult test does not rule in or out the presence of hemorrhoids.

Imaging
- There are no emergent imaging studies to diagnose hemorrhoids.

TREATMENT

Medications
- Sitz baths, fiber-containing supplements, stool softeners, and over-the-counter analgesics/topical anti-inflammatories are most frequently recommended.

Other Nonpharmacologic Therapies
- Thrombosed hemorrhoids usually resorb and resolve in a few days but are very tender. Excision of the thrombosed hemorrhoid and removal of the clot can be performed under local anesthesia.

SPECIAL CONSIDERATIONS

Disposition
- Patients can be discharged home with PMD or colorectal surgery follow-up.

Perianal Abscess

GENERAL PRINCIPLES

Definition
- A collection of purulence that arises from glandular crypts in the anus or rectum

Epidemiology/Etiology
- The age range for patients is 20–60 years of age with males twice as likely to develop an abscess than females.

Pathophysiology
- An anal crypt gland becomes obstructed, allowing bacterial growth with abscess formation.

DIAGNOSIS

Clinical Presentation
History
- Patients present with constant pain in the anal/rectal region that is not relieved with a bowel movement.

Physical Examination
- Fever and purulent discharge may be present.
- Tenderness on rectal exam will be present. A mass may be felt on exam. There may be fluctuance, induration, or erythema present on the overlying skin.

Differential Diagnosis
- Anorectal fistula, hidradenitis suppurativa, hemorrhoid, pilonidal cyst, or abscess

Diagnostic Criteria and Testing
Laboratories
- No specific laboratory test will diagnose a perianal abscess.

Imaging
- A CT scan of the affected area will show presence, size, tracking, or anorectal abscess formation.

TREATMENT

Medications
- In patients who are immunocompromised or who would normally be treated with antibiotics (diabetics, valvular heart disease, cellulitis), provide coverage for skin and colonic flora.

Other Nonpharmacologic Therapies
- A simple perianal abscess can be drained in the ED, as a normal incision and drainage using a cruciate incision as close to the anal verge as possible.

SPECIAL CONSIDERATIONS

Disposition
- Patients with a simple perianal abscess may be drained and discharged home.

Complications
- Half of anal abscesses will develop a fistula from the gland to the skin, regardless of spontaneous or surgical drainage.

Rectal Foreign Body

EPIDEMIOLOGY/ETIOLOGY

- The majority of patients are male with an average age range of 30–50 years of age.

DIAGNOSIS

Clinical Presentation
History
- Patients may be embarrassed or reluctant to give an accurate history and may complain of anorectal or abdominal pain and only admit to a foreign body when directly asked.

Physical Examination
- Over and above the presence of a foreign body, there may be signs of trauma or bleeding from attempted self-extraction.
- Abdominal pain may be present on exam.
- Peritonitis may be present from perforation.
- Lack of palpation on digital rectal exam does not exclude the presence of a foreign body.

Diagnostic Criteria and Testing
Laboratories
- There are no laboratory values specific for this diagnosis.

Imaging
- Plain radiographs may delineate the foreign body and its location. An upright chest plain radiograph may also show free air from a perforation.
- A CT scan may be necessary for radiolucent materials.

TREATMENT

Other Nonpharmacologic Therapies
- Removal of the foreign body may be attempted in the ED with proper pain control, regional anesthesia, or sedation. There are multiple methods to remove an object. If successful, a repeat plain radiograph is recommended to evaluate for perforation that may have occurred during the procedure.
- Sharp objects increase the risk of perforation and removal should be performed by colorectal surgery.
- Special care should be taken in the removal of illicit drugs from body packers and body stuffers, as rupturing the packet can lead to systemic toxicity and death. These cases may be allowed to pass with the use of promotility agents.

SPECIAL CONSIDERATIONS

Disposition
- If the foreign body is removed intact at the bedside, the patient can be discharged home.

Complications
• Peritonitis, bleeding, or fecal incontinence

Anogenital Warts

See Chapter 46.

Anal Fissures

GENERAL PRINCIPLES

Definition
• A tear in the anal skin distal to the dentate line

Epidemiology/Etiology
• Most commonly found in middle-aged patients
• Usually caused by local trauma (hard stool passage, prolonged diarrhea, vaginal delivery, anal sex), inflammatory bowel disease, malignancy, STDs, and granulomatous diseases

Pathophysiology
• Tearing of the skin results from local stretch and trauma with the underlying muscle spasm, causing pain and pulling the edges apart, impeding healing.
• Lower regional blood flow leading to ischemia of the tissue or elevated anal pressures may also contribute to the disease process.

DIAGNOSIS

Clinical Presentation
History
• Patients may report pain with bowel movements, bright red blood per rectum, itching, or local skin irritation.

Physical Examination
• The posterior anal midline has a small laceration that may be superficial or deep.
• There may be fibrotic connective tissue present at the end of a chronic fissure.

Differential Diagnosis
• Ulceration, STD, fistula, and Crohn disease

Diagnostic Criteria and Testing
• There are no laboratory or radiographic studies that will diagnose an anal fissure.

TREATMENT

Other Nonpharmacologic Therapies
• Keeping the area clean and dry, preventing constipation with a high-fiber diet, treating diarrhea promptly, and avoiding trauma to the area

SPECIAL CONSIDERATIONS

Disposition
• Patients may be discharged home to follow up with their PMD or colorectal surgeon.
• If a fistula is present secondary to a fissure, refer for outpatient surgical repair.

SUGGESTED READINGS

Banov L Jr, Knoepp LF Jr, Erdman LH, Alia RT. Management of hemorrhoidal disease. *J S C Med Assoc* 1985;81:398.

Clarke DL, Buccimazza I, Anderson FA, Thomson SR. Colorectal foreign bodies. *Colorectal Dis* 2005;7:98.

Haas PA, Fox TA Jr, Haas GP. The pathogenesis of hemorrhoids. *Dis Colon Rectum* 1984;27:442.

Johanson JF, Sonnenberg A. The prevalence of hemorrhoids and chronic constipation. An epidemiologic study. *Gastroenterology* 1990;98:380.

MacRae HM, McLeod RS. Comparison of hemorrhoidal treatment modalities. A meta-analysis. *Dis Colon Rectum* 1995;38:687.

Rizzo JA, Naig AL, Johnson EK. Anorectal abscess and fistula-in-ano: evidence-based management. *Surg Clin North Am* 2010;90:45.

Rodríguez-Hermosa JI, Codina-Cazador A, Ruiz B, et al. Management of foreign bodies in the rectum. *Colorectal Dis* 2007;9:543.

Sainio P. Fistula-in-ano in a defined population. Incidence and epidemiological aspects. *Ann Chir Gynaecol* 1984;73:219.

Schouten WR, Briel JW, Auwerda JJ. Relationship between anal pressure and anodermal blood flow. The vascular pathogenesis of anal fissures. *Dis Colon Rectum* 1994;37:664.

Traub SJ, Hoffman RS, Nelson LS. Body packing—the internal concealment of illicit drugs. *N Engl J Med* 2003;349:2519. *Colorectal Dis* 2005;7:98.

Zaghiyan KN, Fleshner P. Anal fissure. *Clin Colon Rectal Surg* 2011;24:22.

26 Gastrointestinal Emergencies: Gallbladder and Biliary Tract

Martin H. Gregory and Daniel K. Mullady

Biliary Disease

GENERAL PRINCIPLES

Definitions

- Cholelithiasis
  - The presence of gallstones within the gallbladder
- Choledocholithiasis
  - The presence of gallstone(s) within the bile ducts
- Cholecystitis
  - Inflammation of the gallbladder, most commonly due to a gallstone becoming impacted at the cystic duct

- (Ascending) Cholangitis
  - Infection of the bile ducts often caused by an obstructing stone in the distal common bile duct (CBD).
- Primary sclerosing cholangitis (PSC) is a presumed autoimmune disorder characterized by inflammation of the intrahepatic and extrahepatic bile ducts that can progress to end-stage liver disease.
- Functional gallbladder disorder.
  - Patients with functional gallbladder disorder have classic biliary pain but no lab abnormalities and no gallstones.[1]
- Sphincter of Oddi (SOD) dysfunction.[1]
  - Biliary pain is suspected in patients who continue to have pain after cholecystectomy. Patients may or may not have biliary dilation or abnormal liver tests.[2]

Cholelithiasis

GENERAL PRINCIPLES

Epidemiology/Etiology

- Gallstones are more frequently found in patients who are female, pregnant, obese, and older and have a history of cirrhosis or Crohn's disease.[3]
- Patients who are on total parenteral nutrition (TPN), have experienced rapid weight loss (after bariatric surgery), are on certain medications (contraceptives, octreotide, ceftriaxone), are Hispanic or Native American, or have hemolytic anemia are also at high risk.

DIAGNOSIS

Clinical Presentation
History
- Most patients with gallstones are asymptomatic.[4]
- When a gallstone becomes impacted in the cystic duct, patients can develop pain in the right upper quadrant or epigastrium. The pain may radiate to the inferior portion of the scapula and may be accompanied by nausea and vomiting. Attacks of biliary pain are often precipitated by a fatty meal.

Physical Examination
- Mild tenderness in the right upper quadrant or epigastrium may be elicited. Jaundice suggests biliary obstruction.

Differential Diagnosis
- Choledocholithiasis, cholecystitis, ascending cholangitis, pancreatitis, peptic ulcer disease, gastroesophageal reflux disease (GERD), or myocardial ischemia

Diagnostic Criteria and Testing
Laboratories
- Laboratory studies are usually normal unless complications of cholelithiasis develop.
- Elevated alanine aminotransferase (ALP), bilirubin, and aspartate aminotransferase (AST) and ALT suggests choledocholithiasis.
- Leukocytosis may suggest cholecystitis.

Imaging
- Ultrasonography is the diagnostic test of choice.
  - Gallstones typically appear as echogenic, mobile objects with acoustic shadowing.
  - Gallbladder wall thickening to 5 mm or greater and pericholecystic fluid in combination with cholelithiasis suggest cholecystitis.[5]
  - A dilated CBD (greater than 6 mm) with cholelithiasis suggests choledocholithiasis.

TREATMENT

- Treatment is supportive unless the patient shows signs of acute cholecystitis.
- Consult general surgery for patients who present with acute cholecystitis.

SPECIAL CONSIDERATIONS

Disposition
- Patients with symptomatic cholelithiasis without complications can be referred to a general surgeon as an outpatient.

Complications
- Acute cholecystitis, choledocolithiasis, ascending cholangitis
- Gallstone pancreatitis—Migration of a gallstone into the CBD within the pancreas is one of the major causes of acute pancreatitis.
- Gallstone ileus—Large gallstones may erode through the gallbladder wall into the small intestine and lead to bowel obstruction.
- Mirizzi syndrome—This refers to a stone that becomes lodged in the cystic duct causing extrinsic compression of the CBD, leading to obstructive jaundice.

Choledocholithiasis

GENERAL PRINCIPLES

Classification
- Primary choledocholithiasis
  - This refers to formation of gallstones within the bile ducts.[4]
- Secondary choledocholithiasis
  - This refers to migration of gallstone from gallbladder into the bile ducts.

Epidemiology/Etiology
- Epidemiology/etiology is similar to that of uncomplicated cholelithiasis.[6]
- Risk factors are the same as those for cholelithiasis.

DIAGNOSIS

Clinical Presentation
History
- The pain is similar to that of uncomplicated symptomatic cholelithiasis, except that it persists for more than a few hours. The pain is usually in the right upper quadrant pain or epigastrium, is constant, and may be accompanied by nausea and vomiting.[7]

Physical Examination
- If fever is present, consider ascending cholangitis. Patients are usually tender in the right upper quadrant or epigastrium. Jaundice may be present.

Differential Diagnosis
- Same at cholelithiasis

Diagnostic Criteria and Testing
Laboratories
- AST, ALT, alkaline phosphatase, and bilirubin are typically elevated.[8] Leukocytosis may suggest ascending cholangitis.

Imaging
- Ultrasound
  ○ Choledocholithiasis is often inferred from dilation of the proximal bile duct.[6]
    ▪ Greater than 6 mm is usually considered dilated, but the normal duct diameter increases with age and prior cholecystectomy.[6]

TREATMENT

Medications
- Treatment is supportive with consultation by gastroenterology.

SPECIAL CONSIDERATIONS

- Pancreatitis
  ○ Patients with gallstone pancreatitis should only undergo endoscopic retrograde cholangiopancreatography (ERCP) if there is an obstructing stone seen on imaging and if there is evidence of persistent biliary obstruction (increasing bilirubin, transaminases), cholangitis (fever, sepsis), or clinical deterioration.[9]

Disposition
- Patients should be admitted to the hospital. If ascending cholangitis is suspected, broad-spectrum antibiotics should be administered and a gastroenterologist should be consulted.

Complications
- Pancreatitis, ascending cholangitis, hemobilia, bile leak, or bile duct injury

Cholecystitis

GENERAL PRINCIPLES

Classifications
- Acute calculous cholecystitis
  ○ Inflammation or infection within the gallbladder that arises from an impacted stone within the cystic duct
- Acalculous cholecystitis
  ○ Inflammation of the gallbladder in the absence of gallstones. This usually occurs in the setting of severe systemic illness or after a major operation.[8]

Epidemiology/Etiology
- For acute calculous cholecystitis, the risk factors are the same as those for cholelithiasis.
- For acalculous cholecystitis, the risk factors include critical illness and severe burns.

Pathophysiology[5]
- In calculous cholecystitis, a gallstone becomes impacted in the cystic duct. Inflammation of the gallbladder wall ensues superinfection, and necrosis can occur leading to perforation and sepsis.
- The pathogenesis of acalculous cholecystitis is not well understood.[8]

DIAGNOSIS

Clinical Presentation
History
- Patients typically develop right upper quadrant crampy pain. The diagnosis of acalculous cholecystitis should be considered in critically ill patients with sepsis and no clear cause.

Physical Examination
- Patients often have a fever, right upper quadrant tenderness, and Murphy sign.

Differential Diagnosis
- Same as cholelithiasis

Diagnostic Testing
Laboratories
- Leukocytosis is usually present. Mild elevation of bilirubin and transaminases may be present.

Imaging
- Ultrasound (US)
  - Thickening of the gallbladder wall (>5 mm), pericholecystic fluid, and gallstones indicate cholecystitis.[5] Tenderness when the probe is pushed against the gallbladder (ultrasonographic Murphy sign) indicates acute cholecystitis.[5]

TREATMENT
- Patients should be made NPO, given IV fluids, and started on antibiotics. Cholecystectomy is the treatment of choice in most circumstances.

Medications
- IV antibiotics are recommended when superimposed infection is suspected. Cefazolin, cefuroxime, or ceftriaxone is sufficient for patients with mild disease. Patients with severe disease or those at high risk for complications (older, immunosuppressed) should be covered with a carbapenem, piperacillin–tazobactam, or metronidazole in combination with a fluoroquinolone or cefepime[8] (Table 26.1).

TABLE 26.1	Initial IV Dosages of Antibiotics for Empiric Treatment of Complicated Intra-abdominal Infection
Antibiotic	**Adult dose**[a]
Piperacillin–tazobactam	3.375 g every 6 h[b]
Fluoroquinolones	
Ciprofloxacin	400 mg every 12 h
Levofloxacin	750 mg every 24 h
Moxifloxacin	400 mg every 24 h
Carbapenems	
Ertapenem	1 g every 8 h
Imipenem/cilastatin	500 mg every 6 h or 1 g every 8
Meropenem	1 g every 8 h
Cephalosporins	
Cefazolin	1–2 g every 8 h
Cefepime	2 g every 8–12 h
Cefotaxime	1–2 g every 6–8 h
Ceftazidime	2 g every 8 h
Ceftriaxone	1–2 g every 12–24 h
Cefuroxime	1.5 g every 8 h
Metronidazole	500 mg every 8–12 h
Vancomycin	15–20 mg/kg every 8–12 h[c]

[a]May need to be adjusted for renal or hepatic impairment.

[b]For *Pseudomonas aeruginosa* infection, dosage may be increased to 3.375 g every 4 h or 4.5 g every 6 h.

[c]Serum drug concentration monitoring should be considered for dosage individualization.

Adapted from Solomkin JS, Mazuski JE, Bradley JS, et al. Diagnosis and management of complicated intra-abdominal infection in adults and children: guidelines by the Surgical Infection Society and the Infectious Diseases Society of America. *Clin Infect Dis Off Publ Infect Dis Soc Am* 2010;50:133–64.

SPECIAL CONSIDERATIONS

Disposition

• Patients should be admitted, and general surgery consultation should be obtained as soon as the diagnosis is confirmed.

Complications

• Gallbladder gangrene
• Emphysematous cholecystitis
• Gallbladder perforation

Ascending Cholangitis

GENERAL PRINCIPLES

Epidemiology/Etiology

- Choledocholithiasis and malignant biliary obstruction are the most common cause of ascending cholangitis.[8]

Pathophysiology

- Obstruction of the bile ducts leads to elevated intraductal pressures that disrupt the tight junctions that normally reduce bacterial translocation into the biliary system.[8]
- Patients are at risk for ascending cholangitis if they have had biliary or pancreatic malignancy, manipulation of the biliary tree, a history of gallstones, biliary strictures, or PSC.

DIAGNOSIS

Clinical Presentation

History
- The patient may present with complaints of right upper quadrant pain, fever, and jaundice (Charcot triad), and it suggests ascending cholangitis.
- The addition of mental status changes and hypotension is called Reynolds pentad and indicates severe cholangitis.
- Previous biliary instrumentation is important to determine.

Physical Examination
- Fever is usually present. Right upper quadrant tenderness is commonly elicited.

Differential Diagnosis

- Choledocholithiasis, cholecystitis, pancreatitis, benign of malignant obstruction, intra-abdominal infection, or hepatitis

Diagnostic Criteria and Testing

Laboratories
- Leukocytosis and elevation of bilirubin and alkaline phosphatase are usually present. Transaminases are also often elevated. Blood cultures are often positive, usually with enteric gram-negative bacteria.

Imaging
- Ultrasound
  - Right upper quadrant ultrasound may reveal ductal dilation or CBD stones. Absence of ductal dilation does not rule out ascending cholangitis.
- Abdominal CT
  - CT can be performed if the diagnosis is in question or to assess for complications.

TREATMENT

Medications

- Broad-spectrum antibiotics with adequate gram-negative and anaerobic coverage should be started as soon as the diagnosis is suspected. Acceptable agents include fluoroquinolones, third- and fourth-generation cephalosporins, piperacillin–tazobactam, or carbapenems.[8] Anaerobic coverage with metronidazole is reasonable. Coverage for enterococcus should be considered in those with severe disease, previous biliary instrumentation, and the elderly and in those with compromised immune systems (Table 26.1).

SPECIAL CONSIDERATIONS

Disposition

• Gastroenterology should be consulted urgently once ascending cholangitis is suspected. Referral to a center with ERCP capability should be sought if the patient is stable for transfer.

Complications

• Sepsis and septic shock, hemobilia, or intra-abdominal abscess

Primary Sclerosing Cholangitis

GENERAL PRINCIPLES

Epidemiology/Etiology

• The disease is more common in males with the average age at diagnosis of 40.[10]

Pathophysiology

• Inflammation leads to fibrosis of the intra- and extrahepatic bile ducts. The process is focal, leading to dilation of the bile ducts proximal to strictures. This gives the classic "string of beads" appearance on cholangiography.[10]

DIAGNOSIS

Clinical Presentation

History

• Patients may present with pruritus, jaundice, and fatigue. Pruritus can be debilitating and it is usually worse at night and exacerbated by hot weather and can lead to excoriations.

Physical Examination

• Jaundice may be present. Excoriations can be seen from intractable pruritus. When advanced, patients may show stigmata of advanced liver disease (ascites, palmar erythema, spider angiomas).

Differential Diagnosis

• Cholangiocarcinoma, choledochal cyst, choledocholithiasis, ascending cholangitis, or AIDS cholangiopathy

Diagnostic Criteria and Testing

Laboratories

• Bilirubin and alkaline phosphatase are typically elevated.
• Transaminases may also be elevated.

TREATMENT

- Liver transplantation is the only curative therapy, though PSC may recur.[13]
- Supportive care is appropriate to help alleviate symptoms.

SPECIAL CONSIDERATIONS

Disposition

- Patients with suspected PSC should be admitted and referred to a gastroenterologist.

Complications

- Development of a dominant stricture causing obstruction, ascending cholangitis, or cirrhosis and its complications

ADDITIONAL RESOURCES

Gywali CP, ed. *The Washington Manual Gastroenterology Subspecialty Consult*. 3rd ed. Philadelphia: Lippincott Williams & Wilkins, 2012.

Sabiston DC, Townsend CM. *Sabiston Textbook of Surgery: The Biological Basis of Modern Surgical Practice*. 19th ed. Philadelphia: Elsevier Saunders, 2012.

REFERENCES

1. Silen W, Cope Z, eds. *Cope's Early Diagnosis of the Acute Abdomen*. 22nd ed. New York: Oxford University Press, 2010.
2. Behar J, Corazziari E, Guelrud M, et al. Functional gallbladder and sphincter of oddi disorders. *Gastroenterology* 2006;130:1498–509.
3. Stinton LM, Myers RP, Shaffer EA. Epidemiology of gallstones. *Gallbladder Dis* 2010;39:157–69.
4. Johnston DE, Kaplan MM. Pathogenesis and treatment of gallstones. *N Engl J Med* 1993;328:412–21.
5. Sheth S, Bedford A, Chopra S. Primary gallbladder cancer: recognition of risk factors and the role of prophylactic cholecystectomy. *Am J Gastroenterol* 2000;95:1402–10.
6. Jackson PG, Evans SRT. Biliary System. In: Sabiston DC, Townsend CM, eds. *Sabiston Textbook of Surgery*. 19th ed. Philadelphia: Elsevier Saunders, 2012:1476–514.
7. Sauter GH, Moussavian AC, Meyer G, et al. Bowel habits and bile acid malabsorption in the months after cholecystectomy. *Am J Gastroenterol* 2002;97:1732–5.
8. Barie PS, Eachempati SR. Acute acalculous cholecystitis. *Gastroenterol Clin North Am* 2010;39:343–57.
9. ASGE Standards of Practice Committee, Maple JT, Ben-Menachem T, Anderson MA, et al. The role of endoscopy in the evaluation of suspected choledocholithiasis. *Gastrointest Endosc* 2010;71:1–9.
10. Attasaranya S, Fogel EL, Lehman GA. Choledocholithiasis, ascending cholangitis, and gallstone pancreatitis. *Med Clin North Am* 2008;92:925–60.
11. Giljaca V, Gurusamy KS, Takwoingi Y, et al. Endoscopic ultrasound versus magnetic resonance cholangiopancreatography for common bile duct stones. *Cochrane Database Syst Rev* 2015;2:CD011549.
12. Fogel EL, Sherman S. ERCP for gallstone pancreatitis. *N Engl J Med* 2014;370:150–7.
13. Patel T. Increasing incidence and mortality of primary intrahepatic cholangiocarcinoma in the United States. Hepatol. Baltimore MD 2001;33:1352–7

27 Gastrointestinal Emergencies: Stomach

Joseph Brancheck, Stephen Hasak, and Robert Poirier

Peptic Ulcer Disease

GENERAL PRINCIPLES

Definition

- Peptic ulcers are breaks in the gastric or small intestinal mucosa that extend through the muscularis mucosae.[1]

Epidemiology/Etiology

- The epidemiology of peptic ulcer disease (PUD) reflects environmental factors, mainly *Helicobacter pylori* infection, smoking, and NSAID and aspirin use.[2] Age and concomitant steroid use also increase peptic ulcer disease risk.
- Peptic ulcer disease accounts for approximately half of all episodes of upper gastrointestinal (GI) bleeding.[3]
- Other less common causes of ulcers are acid hypersecretory states, infiltrating diseases, infections, critical illness, and medications.[4]

Pathophysiology

- Peptic ulcers are caused when normal mucosal barrier is disrupted, making it more susceptible to gastric acid.
- NSAID and aspirin inhibit COX-1 and COX-2, which impairs gastric mucosal protection.

DIAGNOSIS

Clinical Presentation

History
- Patients typically present with gnawing, dull, or achy epigastric pain that radiates to the upper quadrants or back. Pain usually is worse shortly after eating.[5]
- Patients may report nausea, hematochezia, melena, hematemesis, fatigue, or syncope.
- Significant worsening of pain heralds perforation.

Physical Examination
- Physical exam is frequently significant for epigastric tenderness to deep palpation. Patients with an acute or chronic bleed may have signs of shock and melena or gross blood on exam. Patients with perforation will present with a tense, rigid, diffusely tender abdomen.

Differential Diagnosis

- The differential is broad and includes gastroesophageal disease, gastritis, biliary tract disease, hepatitis, pancreatitis, gastroparesis, mesenteric ischemia, myocardial ischemia, or abdominal aortic aneurysm.

Diagnostic Criteria and Testing

Laboratories
- There is no specific blood test that is specific for peptic ulcer disease.

Imaging
- There is no study that is specific for peptic ulcer disease. If concern for perforation, a chest plain radiograph may show free air under the diaphragm.

Diagnostic Procedures
- Outpatient endoscopy is the definitive diagnostic test for peptic ulcer disease.

TREATMENT

- All peptic ulcer patients should be started on antisecretory therapy with an H_2 blocker. Patients should also be told to avoid NSAIDs, limit caffeine, and quit smoking.

SPECIAL CONSIDERATIONS

Disposition
- Patients without alarming symptoms, such as early satiety, can be discharged home, with gastroenterology follow-up.
- Patients suspected of having perforation need prompt surgical consultation, hospitalization, and surgery.

Gastroparesis

GENERAL PRINCIPLES

Definition
- Gastroparesis is a syndrome of delayed gastric emptying in the absence of mechanical obstruction.[6]

Epidemiology/Etiology
- There are many potential causes of gastroparesis.
  - Most common: idiopathic, diabetes mellitus, postsurgical
  - Neuromuscular disease: muscular dystrophy, Parkinson disease, amyloid neuropathy
  - Gastroesophageal disease: gastroesophageal reflux, gastritis, peptic ulcer disease, atrophic gastritis[1]
  - Rheumatologic: scleroderma
  - Surgical: post Roux-en-Y syndrome, gastrectomy, vagotomy
  - Other systemic illness: hypothyroidism, uremia, anorexia nervosa[1]
  - Viral: Norwalk virus, rotavirus, cytomegalovirus (CMV), Epstein-Barr virus (EBV), varicella-zoster virus (VZV), HIV
  - Medication: calcium channel blockers, alpha 2-adrenergic agonists, tricyclic antidepressants, dopamine agonists, opiates, cyclosporine, octreotide[1]

Pathophysiology
- Normal emptying requires coordination of the central nervous system, the enteric nervous system, the smooth muscles of the stomach, and chemical mediators.[1]
- Diabetes can lead to gastroparesis by causing excessive pyloric tone, autonomic neuropathy, and abnormal proximal gastric accommodation and contraction.[6]

DIAGNOSIS

History

- Patients most commonly report nausea, vomiting, abdominal pain, bloating, belching, and postprandial fullness. Vomit may contain undigested food. Abdominal pain is rarely the primary symptom.[7] Symptoms are typically worse after eating.

Physical Examination

- Physical exam may elicit a tender, distended abdomen; rigidity or guarding points to another cause of abdominal pain. They may have dry mucous membranes and poor skin turgor.
- Chronic gastroparesis patients may have signs of malnutrition and vitamin and electrolyte disturbances. Worn tooth enamel can be seen in chronic, recurrent vomiting.

Differential Diagnosis

- Mechanical obstruction, psychiatric disease, depression, rumination syndrome, cyclic vomiting syndrome, functional dyspepsia, or esophageal dysmotility

Diagnostic Criteria and Testing

Laboratories

- A basic metabolic panel (BMP) should be checked because electrolyte abnormalities can be severe.

Imaging

- Mechanical obstruction should be ruled out with CT or MRI.

TREATMENT

Medications

- Prokinetics such as metoclopramide and erythromycin have been shown to improve symptoms and increase gastric emptying.
- Nausea should be treated with serotonin antagonists, such as ondansetron. Prochlorperazine, promethazine, and diphenhydramine can also be used.
- Pain control can be treated with opiates or tricyclic antidepressants.[1]
- Treatment of hyperglycemia in those presenting with gastroparesis is important. Hyperglycemia is associated with delayed gastric emptying and gastric motor dysfunction.

Other Nonpharmacologic Therapies

- A nasogastric tube may be passed for decompression and treatment of malnutrition.

SPECIAL CONSIDERATIONS

Disposition

- If patients present with symptoms refractory to initial management, have severe metabolic disturbances, or present with chronic malnutrition, they should be admitted for further treatment.

- If discharged, patients should be instructed to eat frequent, smaller meals. High-fat food can delay gastric emptying. Diet should be advanced as tolerated.

Hiatal Hernia

GENERAL PRINCIPLES

Definition
- A hiatal hernia results from the herniation of abdominal viscera into the mediastinum through the esophageal hiatus of the diaphragm. It most commonly involves the stomach.

Epidemiology/Etiology
- Prevalence increases with increasing age and obesity.[7]

Pathophysiology
- It is thought that hiatal hernias may be secondary to age-related deterioration of the phrenoesophageal membrane, which anchors the GE junction to the diaphragm.[7]

DIAGNOSIS

Clinical Presentation
History
- Patients may have a widely varying presentation, including complaints of dysphagia, chest pain, postprandial discomfort, abdominal pain, dyspnea, GI blood loss, and symptoms of gastroesophageal reflux disease (GERD).

Physical Examination
- A full physical exam should be done, but the findings may be nonspecific, although epigastric tenderness may be present.

Differential Diagnosis
- GERD without hiatal hernia, acute coronary syndrome (ACS), or PUD

Diagnostic Criteria and Testing
Laboratories
- There are no specific laboratory tests that will diagnose a hiatal hernia.

Imaging
- Hiatal hernias can often be noted as a soft tissue density or air–fluid level in the retrocardiac area on a chest plain radiograph or via upper GI barium swallow studies and CT scans.[7]

TREATMENT

- Simple sliding hernias do not require treatment.[7]

Medications
- There are no specific medications that treat a hiatal hernia, but proton pump inhibitors (PPIs), H_2 blockers, and iron supplementation can be used to treat diseases associated with hiatal hernias.[7]

SPECIAL CONSIDERATIONS

- Disposition
  - Patients can often be discharged home unless a major complication such as GI bleed or volvulus is present, in which case admission is necessary.
- Complications
  - Complications of hiatal hernias include GERD, Cameron lesions (linear mucosal lesions, which may cause iron deficiency), and gastric volvulus (which is a life-threatening complication of paraesophageal hernia).[7]

Complications of Bariatric Surgery

GENERAL PRINCIPLES

Definition

- Bariatric surgery is weight loss surgery of which there are many different types and can be broadly categorized into restrictive, malabsorptive, and restrictive–malabsorptive subtypes.[8]

Epidemiology/Etiology

- Bariatric surgery is one of the fastest growing operative procedures performed worldwide, with an estimated >340,000 operations performed in 2011.[9]

Pathophysiology

- Early complications of bariatric surgery include marginal ulcers, stenosis, stomal obstruction, small bowel obstruction, enteric leaks, venous thromboembolism, GI bleeding, wound infections, pulmonary embolism, and pulmonary complications including pneumonia and respiratory failure.
- Late complications vary with the type of procedure but may include cholelithiasis, hernias, nutritional deficiencies, early and late dumping syndromes, band erosion, and neurologic and psychiatric complications.

DIAGNOSIS

Clinical Presentation

History

- Obtain the type of procedure, when it was performed, and a history of any prior postoperative complications.
- Patients may present with complaints of melena and abdominal pain secondary to marginal ulcer (ulcer at the anastomosis site), excessive nausea/vomiting from obstruction (stomal, small bowel obstruction), fever secondary to surgical infection, or dyspnea secondary to a pulmonary complication.

Physical Examination

- The physical exam should include a thorough inspection of any surgical incisions for signs of active infection or herniation.
- The abdominal exam may illicit tenderness, a distended abdomen (obstruction), rigidity, or guarding (perforation).
- Stool guaiac should be performed to rule out GI bleeding.

Diagnostic Criteria and Testing

Laboratories
- Laboratory workup includes a complete blood count (CBC), comprehensive metabolic panel (CMP), lipase, and urinalysis.[10,11]

Imaging
- A CT scan of the abdomen and pelvis can be helpful in evaluating pathology such as strictures, internal hernias, and intussusception.[11]

Diagnostic Procedures
- Endoscopy and nasogastric lavage should not be performed as they can distend newly created pouches and disrupt the surgical incisions.

TREATMENT

- The appropriate management of bariatric surgery complications will often require consultation with both surgical and gastroenterology services.

SPECIAL CONSIDERATIONS

Disposition
- Should be made in consultation with a bariatric surgeon or gastroenterologist

Nausea/Vomiting

GENERAL PRINCIPLES

Definition
- Nausea is the subjective feeling of desire to vomit, while vomiting is the oral expulsion of GI contents secondary to gut and thoracoabdominal wall musculature contractions.[12]

Pathophysiology
- Vomiting is a coordinated maneuver, which requires the interaction of multiple brainstem nuclei, dorsal vagal and phrenic nuclei, medullary nuclei (controlling respiration), and multiple other nuclei involved in pharyngeal movements.[12]
- Vomiting can be triggered by multiple neurotransmitters, which are selective for different anatomic sites throughout the body.[13]
- The area postrema, the location of the chemoreceptor trigger zone, may be activated by clinical stimuli such as medications, metabolic derangements, or radiation. This causes activation at dopamine, 5-HT$_3$, histaminergic H$_1$, muscarinic M$_1$, and vasopressin receptors.
- The labyrinths, which may be activated, for example, in motion sickness, can be activated by H$_1$ and M$_1$ receptor.
- Peripheral afferents, such as those present in the GI tract, activate 5-HT$_3$ receptors.

DIAGNOSIS

History
- It is important to determine the onset, duration, and timing of symptoms.
- Determining the frequency of episodes may help determine the severity of the illness and likelihood of the patient having complications of nausea and vomiting.[14]

- The quality of the emesis, such as undigested food, may be suggestive of an esophageal disorder, whereas partially digested food or feculent vomitus are suggestive of other disorders.[13]
- A review of current medications and obtaining history of ingestion, medication changes, or prior abdominal surgeries can be diagnostic.[14]
- Associated symptoms should be elicited.[12–14]

Physical Examination
- Initial assessment should involve evaluation for signs of dehydration.
- The physical exam may compliment the history already obtained. A general exam may illicit signs such as decayed enamel, lymphadenopathy, jaundice, absent bowel sounds, abdominal tenderness, papilledema, or focal neurologic deficits.[12–14]

Differential Diagnosis
- The differential diagnosis for nausea and vomiting is extensive.

TABLE 27.1	Antiemetics by Medication Class	
Medication class	**Example medications**	**General comments**
Antihistamines	Dimenhydrinate Diphenhydramine Meclizine	Useful in etiologies of nausea/vomiting that are vestibular in origin such as vertigo
Benzamides	Metoclopramide Trimethobenzamide	May be beneficial in suspected gastroparesis
Benzodiazepines	Alprazolam Diazepam Lorazepam	Used as an adjunct for chemotherapy-induced nausea and vomiting
Butyrophenones	Haldol	As with phenothiazines, monitor for extrapyramidal side effects
Corticosteroids	Dexamethasone	Used commonly for chemotherapy-induced nausea and vomiting
Phenothiazines	Compazine Promethazine	One study showed similar efficacy to ondansetron in adults in the emergency department[14]
Serotonin antagonists	Ondansetron Granisetron Palonosetron	Recommendation for ondansetron to be used as first-line therapy for undifferentiated nausea and vomiting given efficacy and safety profile[14]

Adapted from Hang BS, et al. Nausea and Vomiting. In: Tintinalli JE, et al., eds. *Tintinalli's Emergency Medicine: A Comprehensive Study Guide.* 8th ed. New York: McGraw-Hill, 2016.

Laboratories
- Dependent on the history and exam obtained, diagnostic labs can be obtained such as CBC, BMP, liver function tests, lipase, drug levels, thyroid function tests, urinalysis, and a urine pregnancy test.[14]

Electrocardiography
- An ECG should be obtained if there is concern for acute coronary syndrome or electrolyte abnormalities.

Imaging
- Imaging should be targeted to diagnosis suggested by the history and physical exam.

TREATMENT

- Treatment should be targeted to underlying etiology when possible.

Medications
- Symptomatic control can be provided by a number of medications (Table 27.1).
- IV fluid resuscitation and electrolyte repletion should be part of supportive management.

SPECIAL CONSIDERATIONS

- Disposition
  - Most patients can be discharged if symptoms are under control.
  - Surgery should be consulted when abdominal exam elicits peritoneal signs or history and physical exam is suggestive of surgical pathology.

REFERENCES

1. Lew E. Peptic Ulcer Disease. In: Greenberger NJ, Blumberg RS, Burakoff R, eds. *Current Diagnosis & Treatment: Gastroenterology, Hepatology, & Endoscopy.* 3rd ed. New York: McGraw-Hill, 2016.
2. Graham DY. Changing patterns of peptic ulcer disease; gastro-oesophageal disease and Helicobacter pylori: a unifying hypothesis. *Eur J Gastroenterol Hepatol* 2003;15(5):551.
3. Davis E, Powers K. Chapter 36: Gastrointestinal Emergencies. In: Humphries R, Stone E, eds. *Current Diagnosis and Treatment Emergency Medicine.* 7th ed. New York: McGraw Hill, 2011.
4. Malfertheiner P, Chan FK, McColl KE. Peptic ulcer disease. *Lancet* 2009;374:1449–61.
5. Barkun A, Leontiadis G. Systematic review of the symptom burden, quality of life impairment and costs associated with peptic ulcer disease. *Am J Med* 2010;123(4):358.
6. Kumar A, Attaluri A, Hashmi S, et al. Visceral hypersensitivity and impaired accommodation in refractory diabetic gastroparesis. *Neurogastroenterol Motil* 2008;20(6):635.
7. Richter JC, Friedenberg FK. Gastroesophageal Reflux Disease. In Feldman M, Friedman LS, Brandt LJ, eds. In: Sleisenger and Fordtran's Gastrointestinal and Liver Disease. 10th ed. Saunders/Elsevier. Philadelphia. p 733–754.
8. Kushner RF. Evaluation and Management of Obesity. In: Kasper D, et al., eds. *Harrison's Principles of Internal Medicine.* 19th ed. New York: McGraw-Hill, 2015. n. pag. AccessMedicine. Web. 18 April 2016.
9. Buchwald H, Oien DM. Metabolic/bariatric surgery worldwide 2011. *Obes Surg* 2013;23:427.
10. Wu JJ, Perugini RA. Chapter 68: Common Surgical Options for Treatment of Obesity. In: McKean SC, et al., eds. *Principles and Practice of Hospital Medicine.* New York: McGraw-Hill, 2012. n. pag.AccessMedicine. Web. 18 April 2016.

11. O'Brien MC. Acute Abdominal Pain. In: Tintinalli JE, et al., eds. *Tintinalli's Emergency Medicine: A Comprehensive Study Guide*. 8th ed. New York: McGraw-Hill, 2016. n. pag. AccessMedicine. Web. 18 April 2016.
12. Hasler WL. Nausea, Vomiting, and Indigestion. In: Kasper D, et al., eds. *Harrison's Principles of Internal Medicine*. 19th ed. New York: McGraw-Hill, 2015. n. pag. AccessMedicine. Web. 19 April 2016.
13. Quigley EM, Hasler WL, Parkman HP. AGA technical review on nausea and vomiting. *Gastroenterology* 2001;120:263.
14. Hang BS, et al. Nausea and Vomiting. In: Tintinalli JE, et al., Eds. *Tintinalli's Emergency Medicine: A Comprehensive Study Guide*. 8th ed. New York: McGraw-Hill, 2016. n. pag. AccessMedicine. Web. 20 April 2016.

28 Gastrointestinal Emergencies: Liver

Michael Weaver and Robert Poirier

GENERAL PRINCIPLES

Definition

- Cirrhosis is defined as progressive hepatic fibrosis that results in the destruction of normal hepatic architecture and is generally considered to be irreversible.
- Acute liver failure (ALF) is defined by acute hepatic injury, an elevated prothrombin time (PT)/international normalized ratio (INR) or hepatic encephalopathy in a patient without cirrhosis or prior liver disease.

Epidemiology/Etiology

- Risk factors for cirrhosis include nonwhite race, diabetes, alcohol abuse, hepatitis B virus (HBV) and C (HCV), male sex, and older age.
- The most common causes of ALF are drug-induced liver injury (DILI), viral hepatitis, autoimmune liver diseases, and shock/hypoperfusion.
- Hepatitis A, B, and C are the most common types of infectious hepatitis in the United States.
  - Risk factors for HBV and HCV include men who have sex with men (MSM), needlestick injuries, intravenous drug users, travel to endemic areas, and unprotected sexual contact with an infected individual.
  - Hepatitis A virus (HAV) is transmitted through the fecal–oral route.

Pathophysiology

- Cirrhosis
  - Is a late stage of hepatic fibrosis that is caused as hyperplasia of injured liver tissue regenerates and stimulates angiogenesis leading to portal vein pressure increase and ascites and compression of hepatic blood flow.

- ALF
  - Portosystemic encephalopathy most often caused by viruses, drugs, and toxins.
- Acute Viral Hepatitis
  - Inflammation of the liver caused by viral infiltration leading to hepatocyte destruction by cytotoxic cytokines and natural killer cells with resultant necrosis.

DIAGNOSIS

- ALF should be considered with new-onset mental status changes, jaundice, right upper quadrant abdominal pain, as well as generalized symptoms of malaise, nausea, and vomiting.
  - ALF diagnosis requires all of the following: elevated aminotransferases, hepatic encephalopathy, and INR > 1.5.
- Acute viral hepatitis should be suspected in all patients with aspartate aminotransferase (AST) and alanine aminotransferase (ALT) > 25 times the upper limit of normal.

Clinical Presentation

History
- The clinical manifestations of cirrhosis are often nonspecific.
  - Patients may present with generalized symptoms of anorexia, weakness, fatigue, and easy bruisability or may be completely asymptomatic with compensated cirrhosis.
  - The patient may also report signs and symptoms of decompensated hepatic cirrhosis including jaundice, pruritus, dark "cola"-colored urine, upper gastrointestinal bleeding, ascites, lower extremity edema, or hepatic encephalopathy.
- ALF also presents similarly to cirrhosis. By definition, signs of hepatic encephalopathy are required.
  - The patient history obtained in the emergency department (ED) should focus on a careful review of exposures to drugs, toxins, over-the-counter medicines, alcohol, acetaminophen ingestion, or viral infections.
- Viral hepatitis typically presents with signs and symptoms similar to ALF.
  - Generally, viral hepatitis presents with an insidious onset. The time to onset is typically 2–24 weeks following exposure.
  - Patients should be questioned for exposures including injection drug use, sexual activity, or recent travel to known endemic areas.

Physical Examination
- Patients with cirrhosis may have various physical exam findings.
  - Common findings include jaundice, spider angioma, gynecomastia, testicular atrophy, ascites, organomegaly, caput medusa, asterixis, and palmar erythema.
  - The severity of liver disease is directly associated with the number and size of spider angioma. The risk of variceal bleeding is increased with the number of spider angioma.
- In ALF, attention should be focused on the neurologic exam and other physical exam findings suggestive of ALF (jaundice, right upper quadrant abdominal pain, ascites).
  - Asterixis may be present in patients with hepatic encephalopathy.
- Physical exam findings in acute viral hepatitis may reveal a low-grade fever, jaundice, hepatomegaly, splenomegaly, or right upper quadrant pain/tenderness.
  - Jaundice and hepatomegaly are the two most common exam findings.
  - Less common exam findings include lymphadenopathy, rash, arthritis, lichen planus, or vasculitis.

Cirrhosis

DIAGNOSTIC CRITERIA AND TESTING

Laboratories

- Alkaline phosphatase is generally <2–3 times the upper limit of normal.
- Serum bilirubin levels can be normal in compensated cirrhosis.
- Hypoalbuminemia is often observed. Lower albumin levels correlate with worsening cirrhosis.
- Worsening coagulopathy correlates with the severity of cirrhosis.
- Hyponatremia is common and is related to total body water overload.

Imaging

- Abdominal ultrasound (US), CT, and MRI may have findings suggestive of cirrhosis. Radiologic findings include an irregular, nodular, shrunken liver, varices, and ascites.

Diagnostic Procedures

- Diagnostic paracentesis to rule out spontaneous bacterial peritonitis (SBP).
  - Early paracentesis (<12 hours from first physician encounter) has been shown to reduce in-hospital mortality, number of intensive care unit (ICU) days, number of hospital days, and 3-month mortality.
- Cirrhosis
  - Cirrhosis management in the ED should focus on the complications of cirrhosis including SBP, hepatic encephalopathy, and esophageal variceal bleeding.

SBP

- SBP is an infection of ascitic fluid in the absence of an intra-abdominal secondary source.

LABORATORIES

- SBP is established by the presence of a positive ascitic bacterial culture or the presence of >250/mm^3 neutrophils.

MEDICATIONS

- Broad-spectrum empiric antibiotic therapy should be started as soon as possible after ascitic fluid has been obtained.
  - A third-generation cephalosporin such as cefotaxime 2 g IV q8 hours or ceftriaxone 2 g IV q 24 hours
  - Alternatives to third-generation cephalosporins include fluoroquinolones.
- Intravenous albumin may decrease the risk of renal failure and mortality in patients with SBP.
  - Albumin should be given if creatinine is >1 mg/dL, blood urea nitrogen (BUN) is >30 mg/dL, or bilirubin is >4 mg/dL.

SPECIAL CONSIDERATIONS

- Disposition: All patients diagnosed with SBP should be admitted to the hospital for intravenous antibiotics and management of potential complications.

TABLE 28.1	Serologic Testing for Acute Hepatitis B Versus Chronic Hepatitis B					
Diagnosis	HbsAg	Anti-HBs	Anti-HBc	HBeAg	Anti-HBe	HBV DNA
Acute hepatitis	+		IgM	+		+
Window period			IgM	+/−	+/−	+
Recovery		+	IgG		+/−	
Immunization		+				
Chronic hepatitis (HBeAg+)	+		IgG	+		+
Chronic hepatitis (HBeAg−)	+		IgG		+	+

- Complications
  - Septic shock

ALF

LABORATORIES

- Common lab findings seen in ALF are anemia, renal failure, hypoglycemia, hyperammonemia, hyponatremia, hypokalemia, elevated lactate dehydrogenase (LDH), alkalosis leading to acidosis, and acute kidney injury. Thrombocytopenia and elevated INR, bilirubin, and liver enzymes are often seen.

IMAGING

- US with Doppler imaging is the preferred method for evaluating ALF due to the risk of renal failure with a contrast CT.

Acute Viral Hepatitis

LABORATORIES

- The acuity of a viral hepatitis can often be ascertained from aminotransferase levels.
  - Acute viral hepatitis will often have AST and ALT > 25 times the upper limit of normal.
  - Chronic HBV infections will have moderate elevations in aminotransferase levels often twice the upper limit of normal.
  - Acute HBV infection can reveal aminotransferase levels of 1000–2000 IU/L with an ALT predominance.
  - Acute versus chronic hepatitis B infection can be determined by hepatitis B serologies (Table 28.1).

IMAGING

- US findings in acute viral hepatitis may reveal hepatomegaly.

Hepatic Encephalopathy

TREATMENT

- Hepatic encephalopathy is a reversible impairment of neurologic function and its pathogenesis is poorly understood.
- Elevated ammonia levels are thought to play a role in pathogenesis.
- Current therapies are targeted toward decreasing ammoniagenic substances and inhibiting ammonia production.
- Identification and treatment of the underlying cause (gastrointestinal bleeding, infections, metabolic disturbances, and hypovolemia) are of utmost importance.

MEDICATIONS

- Lactulose is the mainstay of therapy to lower serum ammonia.
  ○ Lactulose 30–45 mL PO, via NG, or PR should be given two to four times per day.
- Rifaximin can be used to inhibit ammonia production by reducing gastrointestinal bacteria.
  ○ The dose of rifaximin is 400 mg tid or 500 mg bid.
  ○ Rifaximin should not be used as a substitute for lactulose.

OTHER NONPHARMACOLOGIC THERAPIES

- General supportive care is indicated for patients with hepatic encephalopathy.
- Restraints may be required if patients are a danger to themselves or others.

SPECIAL CONSIDERATIONS

- Disposition
  ○ Admission (floor or ICU) or discharge is dictated by patient status.

Esophageal Variceal (EV) Bleeding

- Esophageal varices are the source of bleeding in 50–90% of patients with cirrhosis and upper gastrointestinal bleeding.

MEDICATIONS

- Pharmacologic therapy begins with the administration of octreotide to reduce portal blood flow and should not be delayed in any patient suspected of having an EV bleed.
  ○ Octreotide can be given as a 50 μg IV bolus followed by 50 μg per hour drip.
- Bacterial infections are common in patients with cirrhosis and gastrointestinal bleeding.
  ○ Broad-spectrum antibiotics (ceftriaxone 1 g/d) should be given as soon as possible.

OTHER NONPHARMACOLOGIC THERAPIES

- Hemodynamic resuscitation, treatment of complications, and treatment of bleeding are the three primary goals of initial management in patients with EV bleeding.
  ○ Blood/platelet transfusions should be given to maintain a hemoglobin > 7 mg/dL if platelet counts drop below 50,000/mm³.
  ○ Fresh frozen plasma (FFP) should be given to normalize INR.

- Endotracheal intubation should be considered in all patients with massive EV bleeding for airway protection and to facilitate endoscopy.
- Balloon tamponade can be used as a temporary measure to obtain hemostasis but carries a high risk of rebleeding after deflation as well as esophageal necrosis and rupture.

SPECIAL CONSIDERATIONS

- Disposition
  - All patients with EV bleeding should be admitted to an ICU for close monitoring and expedited treatment.
- Complications
  - Complications of EV include aspiration, infection, hepatic encephalopathy, and renal failure.

SUGGESTED READINGS

Goldberg E, Chopra S. Cirrhosis in adults: etiologies, clinical manifestations, and diagnosis. 2015. Available at: www.uptodate.com (last accessed 07/31/16).

European Association for the Study of the Liver. EASL clinical practice guidelines: management of chronic hepatitis B virus infection. *J Hepatol* 2012;57:167.

Alter MJ. Epidemiology of viral hepatitis and HIV co-infection. *J Hepato* 2006;44:S6–S9.

Augustin S, Gonzalez A, Genesca J. Acute esophageal variceal bleeding: current strategies and new perspectives. *World J Hepatol* 2010;2:261–74.

Bailey C, Hern G. Hepatic failure: an evidence-based approach in the emergency department. *Emer Med Prac* 2010;12:1–24.

Bernal W, Auzinger G, Dhawan A, et al. Acute liver failure. *Lancet* 2010;376:190–201.

Giannini EG, Testa R, Savarino V. Liver enzyme alteration: a guide for clinicians. *CMAJ* 2005;172:367–79.

Gill RQ, Sterling RK. Acute liver failure. *J Clin Gastroenterol* 2001;33:191–98.

Holmberg SD, Spradling PR, Moorman AC, et al. Hepatitis C in the United States. *N Engl J Med* 2013;368:1859–61.

Klevens RM, Liu SJ, Roberts H, et al. Estimating acute viral hepatitis infections from nationally reported cases. *Am J Public Health* 2014;104:482–87.

Koff RS. Clinical manifestations and diagnosis of hepatitis A virus infection. *Vaccine* 1992;10: 1–15.

Lee WM. Etiologies of acute liver failure. *Semin Liver Dis* 2008;28:142–52.

Lee W, Larson A, Stravitz R. AASLD position paper: the management of acute liver failure: update 2011. *AASLD Position Paper* 2011:1–88.

McIntyre N. Clinical presentation of acute viral hepatitis. *Br Med Bull* 1990;46:533–47.

Runyon BA, AASLD. Introduction to the revised American Association for the Study of Liver Diseases Practice Guideline management of adult patients with ascites due to cirrhosis. *Hepatology* 2013;57:1651.

Runyon BA, McHutchison JG, Antillon MR, et al. Short-course versus long-course antibiotic treatment of spontaneous bacterial peritonitis. A randomized controlled study of 100 patients. *Gastroenterology* 1991;100:1737.

Stravitz RT. Critical management decisions in patients with acute liver failure. *Chest* 2008;134:1092.

Such J, Runyon BA. Spontaneous bacterial peritonitis. *Clin Infect Dis* 1998;27:669

Sudhamsu KC. Ultrasound findings in acute viral hepatitis. *Kathmandu Univ Med J* 2006;4:415–8.

Udell JA, Wang CS, Tinmouth J, et al. Does this patient with liver disease have cirrhosis? *JAMA* 2012;307:832–42.

Venkateshwarlu N, Gandiah P, Indira G, et al. Cardiac abnormalities in patients with cirrhosis. *Indian J L Sci* 2013;3:105–11.

Walsh SA, Creamer D. Drug reaction with eosinophilia and systemic symptoms (DRESS): a clinical update and review of current thinking. *Clin Exp Dermato* 2011;36:6–11.

Gastrointestinal Emergencies: Large Bowel

Mark D. Levine

Constipation

GENERAL PRINCIPLES

Definition

- Stool frequency of <3 per week. However, this definition has varied meanings for different people.

Epidemiology/Etiology

- Risk factors include female sex, age > 60 years, low income, little physical activity, and poor education.
- Causes may be due to neurologic and metabolic disorders of the gastrointestinal (GI) tract, obstructing lesions, and functional and psychiatric disorders.

Pathophysiology

- Neurologic innervation disturbances and hypothyroidism can cause hypomotility, dilation, and impaired defecation. There may be some psychosocial causes that lead to constipation, but these are not clearly understood.

DIAGNOSIS

Clinical Presentation

History
- Important historical items to ascertain are time course, caliber and type of stool, bleeding, and other potential causes of constipation including medications taken (including over the counter [OTC] or supplements).

Physical Examinationination
- Evaluation of the abdomen as well as rectal exam for neuro dysfunction and tenderness/mass/blood/stool should be performed. Rectal prolapse should also be evaluated.

Differential Diagnosis

- Dehydration, tumor, hypothyroidism, dietary causes, iatrogenic mediation ingestion, narcotic use

Diagnostic Criteria and Testing

- The Rome IV criteria for functional constipation must include two of the following:
  - Straining during more than 25% of defecations.
  - Lumpy or hard stools in more than 25% of defecations.
  - Sensation of incomplete evacuation in more than 25% of defecations.

- ○ Manual maneuvers to facilitate movement in more than 25% of defecations.
- ○ Sensation of anorectal obstruction/blockage for more than 25% of defecations.
- ○ Fewer than three spontaneous bowel movements per week.

and
- ○ Loose stools are rarely present without the use of laxatives.
- ○ There are insufficient criteria to diagnose irritable bowel syndrome (IBS).

Laboratories
- There are no specific laboratory values that will diagnose constipation, although electrolytes and thyroid studies may direct toward a cause.

Imaging
- Plain films of the abdomen may show large amounts of stool or evidence of megacolon.
- A CT scan of the abdomen may show other causes of acute or chronic constipation.

TREATMENT

Medications
- Bulk-forming laxatives, fiber supplementation, osmotic agents, stimulant laxatives, and surfactants may all help with relief of the constipation.

Other Nonpharmacologic Therapies
- Patients who are distally impacted, may benefit from a manual disimpaction.

SPECIAL CONSIDERATIONS

Disposition
- The majority of these patients can be discharged home with a bowel regimen and expectant management. Patients with atonic bowel should be admitted to the hospital.

Complications
- Chronic constipation may occur, and patients with atonic bowel (Hirschsprung) are at risk for perforation.

Diverticulitis

GENERAL PRINCIPLES

Definition
- Inflammation of diverticulum in the colonic wall, usually secondary to microperforation

Epidemiology/Etiology
- Diverticulitis is usually seen in patients >45 years of age (more males under 50 years of age) and is more frequently found in the sigmoid colon.
- Risk factors include diet low in fiber and high in red meat/total fat, obesity, lack of exercise, and smoking.

Pathophysiology
- Diverticula develop at points where the vasa recta penetrate the circular muscle layer of the colon. Increased intraluminal pressure causes herniation of the mucosa and submucosa. Diverticulitis occurs when there is micro- or macroperforation of the

diverticula and the inflammation is walled off by pericolic fat and mesentery and can lead to an abscess, fistula, obstruction, or peritonitis.

DIAGNOSIS

Clinical Presentation
History
- Left lower quadrant abdominal pain for several days is the most common complaint in diverticulitis. Some patients may report nausea and vomiting. A low-grade fever may be present. Urinary urgency, frequency, or dysuria may be reported as a result of irritation of the bladder from the inflamed sigmoid. Hematochezia is rare.

Physical Examination
- Rectal exam may reveal a mass, tenderness, or blood. Shock, fever, and peritoneal signs may only be present in the case of peritonitis.

Differential Diagnosis
- Cancer, appendicitis, IBS, colitis, mesenteric ischemia, volvulus, or gynecologic pathology

Diagnostic Criteria and Testing
Laboratories
- There are no specific laboratory tests that will diagnose diverticulitis.

Imaging
- A CT scan of the abdomen can show bowel thickening, diverticula, and complications of diverticulitis.

TREATMENT

Medications
- Ciprofloxacin 500 mg PO bid plus metronidazole 500 mg PO q8 hours for 7–10 days OR
- Trimethoprim–sulfamethoxazole 1 DS tablet q12 hours plus metronidazole 500 mg PO q8 hours for 7–10 days OR
- Amoxicillin–clavulanate 875 mg q12 hours for 7–10 days OR
- Moxifloxacin 400 mg PO daily for 7–10 days

SPECIAL CONSIDERATIONS

Disposition
- Patients should be admitted for perforation, obstruction, abscess/fistula formation, high fever, peritonitis, noncompliance, immunosuppression, inability to eat/drink, or failure of outpatient treatment.

Ulcerative Colitis

GENERAL PRINCIPLES

Definition
- Inflammation of the mucosal layer of the colon and rectum

Epidemiology/Etiology
- Age of onset is bimodal at ages 15–40 and 50–80.
- Risk factors include male sex, Jewish heritage, dietary fat intake, and white population. There may be a genetic component to the disease as well. Smoking may be protective against developing ulcerative colitis.

Pathophysiology
- The mucosa and submucosa become inflamed and lose the normal vascular pattern, leading to petechiae and bleeding. Edema then causes the bowel to lose its protective mucosal layer, leading to abscesses.

DIAGNOSIS

Clinical Presentation

History
- Patients usually present with complaints of diarrhea, sometimes with blood. There may be colicky abdominal pain, urgency, tenesmus, and incontinence. There may also be complaints of mucus discharge.
- History consistent with other causes of colitis including parasitic infections, recent antibiotic use, proctitis, and NSAID use should be obtained.

Physical Examination
- There may be abdominal tenderness, hypotension, tachycardia, and fever. Rectal examination may reveal blood. Signs of malnutrition may be present.
- Arthritis, uveitis, erythema nodosum, pyoderma gangrenosum, primary sclerosing cholangitis, liver disease, thromboembolism, and pulmonary complications may also be present in patients with ulcerative colitis.

Differential Diagnosis
- Crohn disease, infectious colitis, radiation colitis, graft versus host disease, diverticular colitis, or medication-associated colitis.

Diagnostic Criteria and Testing

Laboratories
- There are no specific laboratory tests that will diagnose ulcerative colitis.
- Stool culture for ova and parasites should be sent.

Imaging
- A plain film of the abdomen may show mucosal thickening or "thumbprinting" and colonic dilation.
- A CT may show thickening of the bowel wall but is nonspecific.
- A double-contrast barium enema may show microulcerations, shortening of the colon, loss of haustra, and narrowing of the lumen but may cause ileus in patients with toxic megacolon.

TREATMENT

Medications
- 5-ASA therapies can be prescribed to patients, but route and dosing should be discussed with a gastroenterologist.

- Over-the-counter antidiarrheal agents may also be used in patients who do not have signs of systemic toxicity.
- Cramping can be controlled with dicyclomine or hyoscyamine in patients who do not have signs of systemic toxicity.

SPECIAL CONSIDERATIONS

Disposition

- Patients with mild disease may be discharged home to follow up with their primary physician or gastroenterologist. Patients with fever, perforation, or cardiovascular instability should be admitted.

Complications

- Strictures, dysplasia, colorectal cancer, severe bleeding, toxic megacolon, and perforation may occur.

Appendicitis

GENERAL PRINCIPLES

Definition

- Inflammation of the vermiform appendix

Epidemiology/Etiology

- Most frequently seen in the 20s and 30s with a male predominance

Pathophysiology

- Obstruction of the appendix frequently leads to increased pressure and inflammation. This inflammation of the appendiceal wall leads to ischemia and perforation and formation of an abscess. This abscess may rupture, leading to spillage of bowel contents into the peritoneum and peritonitis.

DIAGNOSIS

Clinical Presentation

History

- The patient will frequently complain of abdominal pain, sometimes beginning periumbilical and then radiating to the right lower quadrant. The patient may also report anorexia or nausea/vomiting (following the onset of pain).

Physical Examination

- Fever may be present, and initially, the exam may be unremarkable. As appendicitis increases, there is usually tenderness in the right lower quadrant. A retrocecal appendix may only have tenderness on a pelvic or rectal exam. And pregnant patients may have tenderness along the right middle abdomen or even right upper quadrant.
- McBurney point tenderness, Rovsing sign, and a psoas or obturator sign are classic findings, but their presence or absence alone is not enough to make a diagnosis.

Differential Diagnosis

- Bowel/appendix perforation, diverticulitis, gynecologic disorders, Crohn disease, renal colic, and testicular torsion/epididymitis

Diagnostic Criteria and Testing

Laboratories
- A leukocytosis with left shift will frequently be present, but there are no laboratory values that are diagnostic for appendicitis.

Imaging
- A CT scan of the abdomen/pelvis is the imaging study of choice for diagnosis.

TREATMENT

Medications
- Nonperforated
  - Cefoxitin 1–2 g IV or
  - Ampicillin/sulbactam 3 g IV or
  - Cefazolin 2–3 g IV plus metronidazole 500 mg IV or
  - Clindamycin plus ciprofloxacin, levofloxacin, gentamicin, or aztreonam
- Perforated
  - Piperacillin–tazobactam 4.5 g IV or
  - Ceftriaxone 1 g IV plus metronidazole 500 mg IV

Other Nonpharmacologic Therapies
- Although some recent studies are advocating antibiotic treatment alone for certain subsets of patients, surgical consultation is necessary for all patients with appendicitis.

SPECIAL CONSIDERATIONS

Disposition
- Patients with appendicitis should be admitted to the hospital.

Complications
- Perforation, infection, and sepsis

SUGGESTED READINGS

Addiss DG, Shaffer N, Fowler BS, Tauxe RV. The epidemiology of appendicitis and appendectomy in the United States. *Am J Epidemiol* 1990;132:910.

Aldoori WH, Giovannucci EL, Rimm EB, et al. A prospective study of alcohol, smoking, caffeine, and the risk of symptomatic diverticular disease in men. *Ann Epidemiol* 1995;5:221.

Bharucha AE, Pemberton JH, Locke GR III. American Gastroenterological Association technical review on constipation. *Gastroenterology* 2013;144:218.

Birnbaum BA, Balthazar EJ. CT of appendicitis and diverticulitis. *Radiol Clin North Am* 1994;32:885.

Etzioni DA, Mack TM, Beart RW Jr, Kaiser AM. Diverticulitis in the United States: 1998–2005: changing patterns of disease and treatment. *Ann Surg* 2009;249:210.

Floch MH, Wald A. Clinical evaluation and treatment of constipation. *Gastroenterologist* 1994;2:50.

Hanauer SB. Inflammatory bowel disease. *N Engl J Med* 1996;334:841.

Higuchi LM, Khalili H, Chan AT, et al. A prospective study of cigarette smoking and the risk of inflammatory bowel disease in women. *Am J Gastroenterol* 2012;107:1399.

Jaffe BM, Berger DH. The Appendix. In: Schwartz, SI, Brunicardi CF, eds., *Schwartz Principles of Surgery*. 8th ed. New York: McGraw-Hill Health Publication Division, 2005.

Novacek G, Weltermann A, Sobala A, et al. Inflammatory bowel disease is a risk factor for recurrent venous thromboembolism. *Gastroenterology* 2010;139:779.

Parks TG. Natural history of diverticular disease of the colon. *Clin Gastroenterol* 1975;4:53.

Rao PM, Rhea JT, Novelline RA. Sensitivity and specificity of the individual CT signs of appendicitis: experience with 200 helical appendiceal CT examinations. *J Comput Assist Tomogr* 1997;21:686.

Rege RV, Nahrwold DL. Diverticular disease. *Curr Probl Surg* 1989;26:133.

Safdi M, DeMicco M, Sninsky C, et al. A double-blind comparison of oral versus rectal mesalamine versus combination therapy in the treatment of distal ulcerative colitis. *Am J Gastroenterol* 1997;92:1867.

Salminen P, Paajanen H, Rautio T, et al. Antibiotic therapy vs. appendectomy for treatment of uncomplicated acute appendicitis: the APPAC randomized clinical trial. *JAMA* 2015;313:2340.

Salzman H, Lillie D. Diverticular disease: diagnosis and treatment. *Am Fam Physician* 2005;72:1229.

Sandler RS, Jordan MC, Shelton BJ. Demographic and dietary determinants of constipation in the US population. *Am J Public Health* 1990;80:185.

Silverberg MS, Satsangi J, Ahmad T, et al. Toward an integrated clinical, molecular and serological classification of inflammatory bowel disease: report of a Working Party of the 2005 Montreal World Congress of Gastroenterology. *Can J Gastroenterol* 2005;19(Suppl A):5A.

Stollman N, Smalley W, Hirano I; AGA Institute Clinical Guidelines Committee. American Gastroenterological Association Institute guideline on the management of acute diverticulitis. *Gastroenterology* 2015;149:1944.

Strate LL, Liu YL, Aldoori WH, et al. Obesity increases the risks of diverticulitis and diverticular bleeding. *Gastroenterology* 2009;136:115.

Tehrani HY, Petros JG, Kumar RR, Chu Q. Markers of severe appendicitis. *Am Surg* 1999;65:453.

Thompson WG, Patel DG. Clinical picture of diverticular disease of the colon. *Clin Gastroenterol* 1986;15:903.

Tramonte SM, Brand MB, Mulrow CD, et al. The treatment of chronic constipation in adults. A systematic review. *J Gen Intern Med* 1997;12:15.

Wald A. Approach to the Patient with Constipation. In: Yamada T, ed. *Textbook of Gastroenterology*. 2nd ed. Philadelphia: JB Lippincott, 1995:864.

Yamada T, Alpers DH, Kaplowitz N, et al., eds., *Textbook of Gastroenterology*. Philadelphia: Lippincott Williams & Wilkins, 2003.

30 Gastrointestinal Emergencies: Pancreatitis

David Page and Brian T. Wessman

GENERAL PRINCIPLES

Definition

- Acute pancreatitis is an inflammatory process of the pancreas with potential for autodigestion, edema, necrosis, and hemorrhage of pancreatic tissue.

Epidemiology/Etiology

- Acute pancreatitis is common.[1]
- Alcoholic and gallstone pancreatitis account for vast majority in the United States.

- Other common pancreatitis causes include medication-induced, hypertriglyceridemia, trauma, surgery, infectious, autoimmune, malignancy, hypercalcemia, and endoscopic retrograde cholangiopancreatography (ERCP).[2]

Pathophysiology

- Trypsinogen is inappropriately converted to trypsin inside the pancreas, which leads to inappropriate activation of other proenzymes as well as further cleavage of trypsinogen.[1]

DIAGNOSIS

- Diagnosis requires two of the following[2]:
  ○ Characteristic abdominal pain
  ○ Elevated serum lipase/amylase (usually 3× the upper limit of normal)
  ○ Imaging findings consistent with pancreatitis

Clinical Presentation

History

- The patient classically experiences persistent epigastric pain of varying intensity radiating to the back with associated nausea and vomiting that is worse with oral intake.[3]

Physical Examination

- Focal epigastric tenderness with or without guarding and/or rebound.
- Cullen and Grey Turner signs occur rarely and suggest retroperitoneal hemorrhage.[2]
- Cachexia is associated with chronic or a malignant cause of pancreatitis.

Differential Diagnosis

- Acute cholecystitis, gastritis, perforated ulcer, bowel ischemia, myocardial ischemia, pulmonary embolus, or aortic pathology

Laboratory

- Elevated lipase is characteristic. Lipase is more sensitive and specific than amylase.[4] Lipase may not be elevated in chronic pancreatitis.

Imaging

- Not required for diagnosis if history, exam, and labs consistent with pancreatitis.
- CT may be normal in early disease but is used to evaluate hemorrhage or pseudocyst.
- Ultrasound of the RUQ may show gallstones concerning for gallstone pancreatitis.
- KUB may show pancreatic calcifications as a sequelae of chronic pancreatitis.

TREATMENT

- Provide aggressive analgesia (no literature exists demonstrating opiate-induced sphincter of Oddi spasm).[5]
- NPO if ill while in ED; otherwise liquids as tolerated (literature shifting away from NPO and toward early enteral feeding).
- Appropriate supportive care[3,7]
  ○ Some patients require massive volume isotonic fluid administration.
- Identifying a surgical etiology of pancreatitis is imperative.[8]
  ○ Can be caused by posterior gastric ulcer perforation requiring emergent surgery.
  ○ Pancreatitis associated with cholangitis is an emergency requiring broad empiric antibiotics and urgent GI or surgical consultation.[2,6]

TABLE 30.1	Ranson Criteria

- 0 h
  - Age > 55 years
  - White blood cell count > 16,000/mm³
  - Blood glucose > 200 mg/dL
  - Lactate dehydrogenase > 350 U/L
  - Aspartate aminotransferase > 250 U/L
- 48 h
  - Hematocrit fall by >10%
  - Blood urea nitrogen increase by >5 mg/dL
  - Serum calcium < 8 mg/dL
  - pO_2 (partial pressure of oxygen) < 60 mm Hg
  - Base deficit > 4 mEq/L
  - Fluid sequestration > 6 L

SPECIAL CONSIDERATIONS

Disposition

- Mild pancreatitis can be treated at home with pain medication, anti-emetics and a bland, low fat diet; otherwise admit for IV fluids and pain control if the patient is unable to tolerate PO or manage pain in ED.
- Admit to ICU if severe illness or expected clinical decompensation (Ranson criteria, see Table 30.1).[3]

REFERENCES

1. Dennis Kasper AF, Hauser S, Dan Longo D, et al. *Harrison's Principles of Internal Medicine.* 19th ed. New York: McGraw-Hill, 2015.
2. Jesse Hall GS, Kress J. *Principles of Critical Care.* 4th ed. New York: McGraw-Hill, 2015.
3. Tintinalli JE, John Ma O, Yealy DM, et al. *Tintinalli's Emergency Medicine: A Comprehensive Study Guide.* 8th ed. New York: McGraw-Hill, 2015.
4. Keim V, Teich N, Fiedler F, et al. A comparison of lipase and amylase in the diagnosis of acute pancreatitis in patients with abdominal pain. *Pancreas* 1998;16(1):45–9.
5. Thompson DR. Narcotic analgesic effects on the sphincter of Oddi: a review of the data and therapeutic implications in treating pancreatitis. *Am J Gastroenterol* 2001;96(4):1266–72.
6. Fogel EL, Sherman S. ERCP for gallstone pancreatitis. *N Engl J Med* 2014;370(2):150–7.
7. Isenmann R, Runzi M, Kron M, et al. Prophylactic antibiotic treatment in patients with predicted severe acute pancreatitis: a placebo-controlled, double-blind trial. *Gastroenterology* 2004;126(4):997–1004.
8. Hartwig W, Maksan SM, Foitzik T, et al. Reduction in mortality with delayed surgical therapy of severe pancreatitis. *J Gastrointest Surg* 2002;6(3):481–7.

31 Gastrointestinal Emergencies: Small Bowel

Mark D. Levine

Small Bowel Obstruction (SBO)

GENERAL PRINCIPLES

Definition
- A functional or mechanical interruption of the normal passage of contents through the GI tract

Epidemiology/Etiology
- Males and females have equal incidence, and the average age of patients is ~64 years of age.
- Risk factors include prior abdominal surgery (most common), hernia of the abdominal wall or groin, cancer, irradiation, history of foreign body ingestion, prior obstruction, or inflammation of the small bowel.

Pathophysiology
- Obstruction occurs from an interruption of the flow of contents that can be external to the bowel or within the wall of the bowel. Obstructions may be partial or complete.
- The obstruction leads to accumulation of air and gas, the bowel wall becomes swollen, and fluid accumulates in the lumen stretching the wall until perfusion of the wall is compromised.

DIAGNOSIS

Clinical Presentation

History
- Patients will often report sudden onset of abdominal pain, nausea, vomiting, and distention, all of which may be on an intermittent basis that will reoccur. If the pain remains constant, perforation should be considered.
- Obstipation may or may not be present, but passage of stool and flatus may continue 12–24 hours after the onset of symptoms.

Physical Examination
- Signs of dehydration, abdominal distention, and hyperresonance on percussion will usually be present. Bowel sounds are usually characterized as high pitched, "tinkling", or hypoactive/absent.

Differential Diagnosis
- Ileus, pseudoobstruction, large bowel obstruction, tumor, volvulus, trauma, intussusception, infection, or mesenteric ischemia

Diagnostic Criteria and Testing

Laboratories
- There are no specific laboratory values that are diagnostic for obstruction.

Imaging
- Plain radiographs of the abdomen (obstructive series) may quickly confirm the diagnosis with dilated loops of bowel with air–fluid levels.
- A CT scan can show the transition point and confirm the diagnosis along with a causative etiology.

TREATMENT

Medications
- Fluid resuscitation, antiemetics, and pain control are mainstays of treatment for small bowel obstruction (SBO).

Other Nonpharmacologic Therapies
- The majority of patients should be made NPO, but some patients may tolerate limited amounts of liquids.
- Gastric decompression with a nasogastric tube is scenario dependent. It is recommended for patients with significant distention, vomiting, or high-grade obstruction.
- Surgical consultation is necessary.

SPECIAL CONSIDERATIONS

Disposition
- Patients with an SBO should be admitted to the hospital.

Gastroenteritis

GENERAL PRINCIPLES

Definition
- Acute gastroenteritis is defined as vomiting accompanied by three or more episodes of diarrhea (200 g or more of stool) daily that lasts <2 weeks.

Epidemiology/Etiology
- Main causes of viral gastroenteritis are *Rotavirus, Norovirus, Astrovirus,* and enteric adenovirus. Transmission is usually through the fecal–oral route or through food/water transmission. Norovirus can be spread person-to-person. Spring and winter are the usual peak time periods for viral gastroenteritis.
- The most common causes of bacterial gastroenteritis include *Campylobacter, Salmonella, Shigella, Vibrio, Yersinia, Clostridium, Bacteroides fragilis,* and *Escherichia coli* with *E. coli* O157:H7 being the most common cause of bloody diarrhea. Bacterial gastroenteritis is most commonly seen in the summer months and through ingestion of contaminated food products.
- *Cryptosporidium, Giardia, Cyclospora,* and *Entamoeba histolytica* are the common causes for diarrhea caused by parasites. Person-to-person and contaminated food/water are the common routes of transmission.

Pathophysiology
- Interference in regulation of fluid absorption and secretion leads to diarrhea.
- The exact pathophysiology of vomiting in gastroenteritis is not clear.

DIAGNOSIS

Clinical Presentation
History
- Patients will report diarrhea and may have associated nausea, vomiting, abdominal pain, or fever. Presence of the blood in the stool may be reported.
- Questions relating to exposure to potentially contaminated food or water, travel or recreation with waterborne activities, pets, and time course of the vomiting/diarrhea should all be elicited.

Physical Examination
- The exam should focus on focal tenderness and for occult blood in the stool.

Differential Diagnosis
- Cancer, irritable bowel syndrome, inflammatory bowel disease, colitis, malabsorption syndromes, medication or postcholecystectomy-related causes, medication abuse, or withdrawal symptoms

Diagnostic Criteria and Testing
Laboratories
- There are no specific laboratory tests that will diagnose gastroenteritis.
- Stool cultures should be performed for infectious or parasitic sources if indicated or if there is bloody diarrhea, fever, immune compromise, pregnancy, potential for sexual transmission or the patient is >70 years old.
- A stool guaiac may be performed if there is concern for blood in the stool.

Imaging
- Routine imaging is not recommended for gastroenteritis.

TREATMENT

Medications
- Fluid resuscitation through PO or IV routes is acceptable. Soft drinks and fruit juices should be avoided. Sports drinks and oral rehydration solutions are acceptable.
- Antiemetics may be administered.
- Empiric antibiotics are not recommended unless the patient has severe disease (fever, >6 stools/day, hospitalization, bloody diarrhea, or symptoms >1 week without improvement).
- Ciprofloxacin 500 mg PO twice daily or levofloxacin 500 mg PO daily for 3–5 days are acceptable treatments as is azithromycin 500 mg PO daily for 3 days or erythromycin 500 mg PO bid for 5 days.
- Antiparasitic agents may be administered if the diagnosis is likely or confirmed.
- Antimobility agents such as loperamide or diphenoxylate can be used if there is no fever and bloody or mucoid stools unless antibiotics are administered concurrently. Bismuth salicylate is an acceptable alternative (caution in patients already taking salicylates) in patients that other antimotility agents may be relatively contraindicated.

SPECIAL CONSIDERATIONS

Disposition

- Most patients may be discharged home with conservative treatment, but hospitalization should be considered for severely affected, immune compromised, or older, frail adults.

Intestinal Ischemia (Mesenteric Ischemia)

GENERAL PRINCIPLES

Definition

- A reduction or occlusion of intestinal blood flow that leads to ischemia or infarction of the bowel

Epidemiology/Etiology

- Causes of ischemia are arterial embolism, arterial thrombosis, venous thrombosis, and intestinal hypoperfusion.
  - These causes may be secondary to volvulus, SBO, hypercoagulable states, hypoperfusion, vasoconstriction, or mechanical obstruction.
- Risk factors include cardiac disease, aortic instrumentation/surgery, peripheral artery disease, medication, low flow states, hereditary or acquired hypercoagulability, mass effect, or inflammation/infection.

Pathophysiology

- Vascular occlusion leads to ischemia or infarction of the bowel, with resultant translocation of bacteria, leading to sepsis.

DIAGNOSIS

Clinical Presentation

History

- Patients usually present with abdominal pain "out of proportion to the exam." The time course may vary depending on collateral circulation. A history or family history of occlusive disease should be obtained. Patients may report postprandial pain.

Physical Examination

- The exam may initially be normal and then have distention, decreased bowel sounds, and peritonitis as the ischemia progresses. A feculent odor on the breath may be noted.

Differential Diagnosis

- The differential includes most causes for abdominal pain.

Diagnostic Criteria and Testing

Laboratories

- There are no laboratory tests that are specific for mesenteric ischemia. Leukocytosis, elevated lactate, and elevated amylase levels may be present but do not rule out mesenteric ischemia.

Imaging

- Plain radiographs may be normal. Ileus, bowel distention, and bowel wall thickening or pneumatosis intestinalis may be present.

- A CT angio of the abdomen may be more diagnostic for changes consistent with bowel ischemia.

TREATMENT

Medications
- Fluid resuscitation and correction of electrolytes should be undertaken.
- Broad-spectrum antibiotics should be initiated.
- If vasopressors are necessary, dobutamine, low-dose dopamine, or milrinone is recommended.
- Pain control should be administered.
- Unless the patient is actively bleeding or going right to the operating room, systemic anticoagulation should be started to prevent thrombus formation.

Other Nonpharmacologic Therapies
- Gastric decompression is frequently indicated.
- Surgical consultation is necessary for potential laparotomy or embolectomy.

SPECIAL CONSIDERATIONS

Disposition
- Patients should be admitted to the hospital, with unstable patients admitted to an intensive care unit.

Complications
- Bowel perforation, sepsis, and death

Crohn's Disease

GENERAL PRINCIPLES

Definition
- A disorder characterized by transmural inflammation and skip lesions of the GI tract and can be present from the mouth to the anus.

Epidemiology/Etiology
- Risk factors include age from 15 to 40 years of age with a second peak from 50 to 80 years of age, Jewish ancestry, white race, genetic predisposition, tobacco use, and obesity.

Pathophysiology
- Inflammation leads to fibrosis and strictures, causing microperforations that lead to fistula and abscess formation.

DIAGNOSIS

Clinical Presentation
History
- Patients may report prolonged fatigue, diarrhea, abdominal pain, weight loss, fever, and blood in the stool. Crampy pain is a common complaint.
- Patients may also report aphthous ulcers, odynophagia, and dysphagia.

Physical Examination
- Perianal skin tags, sinus tracts, and abdominal tenderness may be present.
- Dermatologic, ocular, joint, and pulmonary involvement may also be present, and abnormalities may be found on examination.

Differential Diagnosis
- Irritable bowel syndrome, lactose intolerance, infectious or ulcerative colitis, appendicitis, diverticulitis, tumor, carcinoid, or endometritis

Diagnostic Criteria and Testing
Laboratories
- There are no specific laboratory tests that will diagnose Crohn disease.

Imaging
- A CT scan may diagnose inflammation or abscess.
- MRI may be a safer imaging modality, as these patients have multiple CT scans performed throughout their life.

Diagnostic Procedures
- Endoscopy or colonoscopy is the diagnostic modality of choice.

TREATMENT

Medications
- Medications including triamcinolone acetonide for oral lesions, prednisone (40–60 mg/d), or 5-ASA (sulfasalazine or mesalamine) may be started in consultation with a gastroenterologist.
- Loperamide for diarrhea may be recommended.

Other Nonpharmacologic Therapies
- Diet control including lactose avoidance is recommended.

SPECIAL CONSIDERATIONS

Disposition
- Patients with mild to moderate disease may be able to be discharged to follow up with their primary physician or gastroenterologist. Patients with significant pain and change in bowel habits or needing resuscitation should be admitted to the hospital. Disposition in conjunction with a gastroenterologist is recommended.

Complications
- Abscess, fistula, hemorrhage, dehydration, and chronic pain

SUGGESTED READINGS

Catena F, Di Saverio S, Kelly MD, et al. Bologna Guidelines for Diagnosis and Management of Adhesive Small Bowel Obstruction (ASBO): 2010 Evidence-Based Guidelines of the World Society of Emergency Surgery. *World J Emerg Surg* 2011;6:5.

Diaz JJ Jr, Bokhari F, Mowery NT, et al. Guidelines for management of small bowel obstruction. *J Trauma* 2008;64:1651.

Drożdż W, Budzyński P. Change in mechanical bowel obstruction demographic and etiological patterns during the past century: observations from one health care institution. *Arch Surg* 2012;147:175.

Hanauer SB, Sandborn W; Practice Parameters Committee of the American College of Gastro-enterology. Management of Crohn's disease in adults. *Am J Gastroenterol* 2001;96:635.

Lichtenstein GR, Hanauer SB, Sandborn WJ; Practice Parameters Committee of American College of Gastroenterology. Management of Crohn's disease in adults. *Am J Gastroenterol* 2009;104:465.

Lopman BA, Reacher MH, Vipond IB, et al. Clinical manifestation of norovirus gastroenteritis in health care settings. *Clin Infect Dis* 2004;39:318.

McKinsey JF, Gewertz BL. Acute mesenteric ischemia. *Surg Clin North Am* 1997;77:307.

Mekhjian HS, Switz DM, Melnyk CS, et al. Clinical features and natural history of Crohn's disease. *Gastroenterology* 1979;77:898.

Miller G, Boman J, Shrier I, Gordon PH. Etiology of small bowel obstruction. *Am J Surg* 2000;180:33.

Miller G, Boman J, Shrier I, Gordon PH. Natural history of patients with adhesive small bowel obstruction. *Br J Surg* 2000;87:1240.

Mucha P Jr. Small intestinal obstruction. *Surg Clin North Am* 1987;67:597.

Nugent FW, Roy MA. Duodenal Crohn's disease: an analysis of 89 cases. *Am J Gastroenterol* 1989;84:249.

Reinus JF, Brandt LJ, Boley SJ. Ischemic diseases of the bowel. *Gastroenterol Clin North Am* 1990;19:319.

Sandborn WJ, Feagan BG, Lichtenstein GR. Medical management of mild to moderate Crohn's disease: evidence-based treatment algorithms for induction and maintenance of remission. *Aliment Pharmacol Ther* 2007;26:987.

Scallan E, Griffin PM, Angulo FJ, et al. Foodborne illness acquired in the United States—unspecified agents. *Emerg Infect Dis* 2011;17:16.

Siddiki HA, Fidler JL, Fletcher JG, et al. Prospective comparison of state-of-the-art MR enterography and CT enterography in small-bowel Crohn's disease. *AJR Am J Roentgenol* 2009;193:113.

Thielman NM, Guerrant RL. Clinical practice. Acute infectious diarrhea. *N Engl J Med* 2004;350:38.

Geriatric Evaluation

Christopher R. Carpenter

GENERAL PRINCIPLES

Definition

- Synonyms for "geriatric"[1,2] include older adult, aging population, or senior citizen, whereas the term "elderly" implies a subset of frail adults of advanced age in many contexts, so is reserved for that connotation.
- Aging adults are not one homogeneous subset of the population but instead represent a diverse spectrum of society.
- Chronologic age alone should not define any individual's sense of wellness or goals of care.

Epidemiology/Etiology

- From 2000 to 2010, the population over age 65 years old has expanded faster than all other age groups, and overall ED visits by those over age 65 years increased from 108 million to 136 million between 2001 and 2009, a 26.6% increase, and older adult intensive care unit admissions grew by 131%.[3]

- Seniors are not simply older versions of the young adult, and the traditional ED management approach is often inadequate for some geriatric patients who may require a holistic approach.[4]
- Older adults often lack a reliable social safety net, which can lead to preventable ED returns.[5] In addition, they often suffer from unrecognized malnutrition[6] cognitive impairment,[7] elder abuse of many forms,[8] and misunderstanding of ED care received.[9]

Pathophysiology

- Each organ system experiences age-related changes that can compromise the physiologic response to acute illness or injury.[10]
- Osteoporosis reduces the capacity of the skeletal system to withstand minor blunt trauma like standing-level falls that frequently cause fractures.[11,12]
- Immune senescence reduces the capacity to develop long-standing immunity in response to vaccines and predisposes aging adults to atypical presentations of infectious illness.[13]
- Alveoli compliance is decreased and tidal volume is diminished increasing the risks for respiratory compromise with rib fractures and pneumothorax with mechanical ventilation.[14]
- Cardiac output is often decreased, while both intrinsic conduction system changes and common chronotropic medications impair the aging individual's ability to respond to hemodynamic stressors.

DIAGNOSIS

- Atypical presentations of common diseases such as acute coronary syndrome, stroke, and pulmonary embolism are common in the older adult.[10]
- Emergency providers often display a low threshold for diagnostic testing in older adults to avoid diagnostic error related to atypical presentations.
- Little empiric evidence exists to support indiscriminant diagnostic testing with labs, advanced imaging, and ECGs in older adults.[9] In fact, diagnostic test results can mislead clinicians.

Clinical Presentation

Falls

- 30–40% of senior citizens who live at home suffer a fall and the percent increases with each year of life. Over 50% of those over age 80 suffer a fall annually.[12]
- Most falls are noninjurious, but even these minor falls cause 3-month functional decline in up to 33% of older adults.[15,16]
- Aging physiology results in multiple intrinsic and extrinsic risk factors for older adult falls. Discussions should be had with patients and caregivers to identify opportunities to prevent future injurious falls such as household hazards (loose rugs to tape down, stairs to avoid, loose fitting clothing, furniture placement).
- Patients with nonhealing foot sores, falls in the last year, depression, or inability to cut own toenails provides the most accurate fall risk prediction instrument derived in ED settings.[17]
- Referrals to fall clinics, PT/OT, ophthalmology, PMD (for elimination of vasoactive medications) are all methods of fall prevention that can be done through the ED.[12]

Cognitive Impairment

- Delirium and dementia are frequently encountered in the ED management of older adults.

- Delirium has two subtypes: hyperactive and hypoactive.
  - Hypoactive delirium is more common among elderly ED patients.[18]
  - Delirium is an independent predictor of ED returns and 6-month mortality.[19,20]
- The Brief Confusion Assessment Method (bCAM) (Fig. 32.1) is useful to rule in delirium,[21] but the Richmond Agitation Sedation Scale (RASS; Table 84.3) also appears to be a sensitive ultrabrief screening instrument.[22]
- Multiple dementia instruments of varying complexity have been evaluated in ED settings.[7,23] The Ottawa 3DY assesses day, date, year, and the ability to spell "world" backward (a single incorrect response implies cognitive impairment) and is one of the simplest instruments to use.
  - Nonpharmacologic approaches to acute delirium are preferred to pharmacologic management.[24]
  - Positive dementia screening results should prompt referral to primary care or dementia centers for confirmatory dementia testing.[25,26]

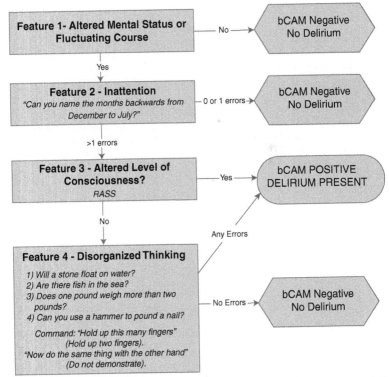

Figure 32.1. A Brief Confusion Assessment Method (bCAM) delirium screen. RASS, Richmond Agitation Sedation Scale. (Reproduced with permission from Han JH et al. Diagnosing delirium in older emergency department patients: validity and reliability of the Delirium Triage Screen and the Brief Confusion Assessment Method. *Ann Emerg Med* 2013;62: 457–465.)

Polypharmacy

- The combination of age-related physiologic changes and the decentralized nature of modern medical practice lead to polypharmacy.
- There is a "prescribing cascade" in which an adverse drug reaction interpreted as a new disease precipitates additional medication prescribing.[27,28]
- The GED Guidelines recommend that providers both recognize adverse effects of medications secondary to polypharmacy and avoid causing these adverse effects.[2,29]

SPECIAL CONSIDERATIONS

Disposition

- Effective medical management of older adults is a team-based endeavor that often requires coordination between ED providers and hospitalists, outpatient clinics, case managers, physiotherapy, pharmacy, and home health, among others.[30]
- The elements of effective case management include collaboration with clinical nurse leadership teams, focused geriatric assessments, and the initiation of interprofessional discharge planning prior to ED discharge.[31]

Patient Education

- Efficient patient education requires screening for dementia and delirium, as well as providing health literacy–appropriate written discharge instructions with vision-appropriate font, communicating the impression and follow-up plan with primary care providers, while ensuring that caregivers are both capable of providing medical and mobility assistance and understanding all components of the discharge instructions.[2,30]

REFERENCES

1. Carpenter CR, Bromley M, Caterino JM, et al. Optimal older adult emergency care: Introducing multidisciplinary geriatric emergency department guidelines from the American College of Emergency Physicians, American Geriatrics Society, Emergency Nurses Association, and Society for Academic Emergency Medicine. *J Am Geriatr Soc* 2014;62(7):1360–63.
2. Rosenberg M, Carpenter CR, Bromley M, et al. Geriatric emergency department guidelines. *Ann Emerg Med* 2014;63(5):e7–e25.
3. Pines JM, Mullins PM, Cooper JK, et al. National trends in emergency department use, care patterns, and quality of care of older adults in the United States. *J Am Geriatr Soc.* 2013;61(1):12–17.
4. Carpenter CR, Platts-Mills TF. Evolving prehospital, emergency department, and "inpatient" management models for geriatric emergencies. *Clin Geriatr Med* 2013;29(1):31–47.
5. Hastings SN, George LK, Fillenbaum GG, et al. Does lack of social support lead to more ED visits for older adults? *Am J Emerg Med* 2008;26(4):454–61.
6. Pereira GF, Bulik CM, Weaver MA, et al. Malnutrition among cognitively intact, noncritically ill older adults in the emergency department. *Ann Emerg Med* 2015;65(1):85–91.
7. Carpenter CR, DesPain B, Keeling TK, et al. The Six-Item Screener and AD8 for the detection of cognitive impairment in geriatric emergency department patients. *Ann Emerg Med* 2011;57(6):653–61.
8. Rosen AB, Hargarten S, Flomenbaum NE, Platts-Mills TF. Identifying elder abuse in the emergency department: toward a multidisciplinary team-based approach. *Ann Emerg Med* 2016;68(3):378–82.
9. Hastings SN, Barrett A, Weinberger M, et al. Older patients' understanding of emergency department discharge information and its relationship with adverse outcomes. *J Patient Saf* 2011;7(1):19–25.
10. Rhodes SM, Sanders AB. General Approach to the Geriatric Patient. In: Kahn JH, Magauran BG, Olshaker JS, eds. *Geriatric Emergency Medicine: Principles and Practice.* Cambridge: Cambridge University Press, 2014:20–30.

11. Carpenter C, Taleghani N. Older Adults in the Wilderness. In: Auerbach PS, ed. *Wilderness Medicine*. 7th ed. Philadelphia: Elsevier-Mosby, 2016:2157–72.

12. Carpenter CR. Falls and Fall Prevention in the Elderly. In: Kahn JH, Magauran BG, Olshaker JS, eds. *Geriatric Emergency Medicine Principles and Practice*. Cambridge: Cambridge University Press, 2014:343–50.

13. Katz ED, Carpenter CR. Fever and Immune Function in the Elderly. In: Meldon SW, Ma OJ, Woolard R, eds. *Geriatric Emergency Medicine*. New York: McGraw-Hill, 2004:55–69.

14. Carpenter CR, Rosen PI. Trauma in the Geriatric Patient. In: Mattu A, Grossman SA, Rosen PI, et al., eds. *Geriatric Emergencies: A Discussion-Based Review*. Oxford: Wiley-Blackwell, 2016:277–301.

15. Sirois MJ, Emond M, Ouellet MC, et al. Cumulative incidence of functional decline following minor injuries in previously independent older Canadian emergency department patients. *J Am Geriatr Soc* 2013;61(10):1661–68.

16. Carpenter CR. Deteriorating functional status in older adults after emergency department evaluation of minor trauma-opportunities and pragmatic challenges. *J Am Geriatr Soc* 2013;61(10):1806–07.

17. Carpenter CR, Scheatzle MD, D'Antonio JA, et al. Identification of fall risk factors in older adult emergency department patients. *Acad Emerg Med* 2009;16(3):211–9.

18. Han JH, Zimmerman EE, Cutler N, et al. Delirium in older emergency department patients: recognition, risk factors, and psychomotor subtypes. *Acad Emerg Med* 2009;16(3):193–200.

19. Han JH, Shintani A, Eden S, et al. Delirium in the emergency department: an independent predictor of death within 6 months. *Ann Emerg Med* 2010;56(3):244–52.

20. Han JH, Bryce SN, Ely EW, et al. The effect of cognitive impairment on the accuracy of the presenting complaint and discharge instruction comprehension in older emergency department patients. *Ann Emerg Med* 2011;57(6):662–71.

21. Han JH, Wilson A, Vasilevskis EE, et al. Diagnosing delirium in older emergency department patients: validity and reliability of the delirium triage screen and the brief confusion assessment method. *Ann Emerg Med* 2013;62(5):457–65.

22. Han JH, Vasilevskis EE, Schnelle JF, et al. The Diagnostic Performance of the Richmond Agitation Sedation Scale for Detecting Delirium in Older Emergency Department Patients. *Acad Emerg Med* 2015;22(7):878–82.

23. Carpenter CR, Bassett ER, Fischer GM, et al. Four sensitive screening tools to detect cognitive impairment in geriatric emergency department patients: Brief Alzheimer's Screen, Short Blessed Test, Ottawa3DY, and the Caregiver Administered AD8. *Acad Emerg Med* 2011;18(4):374–84.

24. Flaherty JH, Little MO. Matching the environment to patients with delirium: lessons learned from the delirium room, a restraint-free environment for older hospitalized adults with delirium. *J Am Geriatr Soc* 2011;59(Suppl 2):S295–300.

25. Schnitker LM, Martin-Khan M, Burkette E, et al. Process quality indicators targeting cognitive impairment to support quality of care for older people with cognitive impairment in emergency departments. *Acad Emerg Med* 2015;22(3):285–98.

26. Carpenter CR. Dementia and the rural emergency department. *J Rural Emerg Med* 2014;1(1):32–40.

27. Rochan PA, Gurwitz JH. Optimising drug treatment for elderly people: the prescribing cascade. *BMJ* 1997;315(7115):1096–99.

28. Budnitz DS, Shehab N, Kegler SR, Richards CL. Medication use leading to emergency department visits for adverse drug events in older adults. *Ann Intern Med* 2007;147(11):755–65.

29. American Geriatrics Society 2015 Updated Beers Criteria for Potentially Inappropriate Medication Use in Older Adults. *J Am Geriatr Soc* 2015;63(11):2227–46.

30. Kessler C, Williams WC, Moustoukas JN, Pappas C. Transitions of care for the geriatric patient in the emergency department. *Clin Geriatr Med* 2013;29(1):49–69.

31. Sinha SK, Bessman ES, Flomenbaum N, Leff B. A systematic review and qualitative analysis to inform the development of a new emergency department-based geriatric case management model. *Ann Emerg Med* 2011;57(6):672–82.

Ear Emergencies

Mark D. Levine

Cerumen Impaction

GENERAL PRINCIPLES

Epidemiology/Etiology
- Relatively common in the adult population and affects up to 30% of older adults

Pathophysiology
- A breakdown of the epithelial migratory pattern out of the ear leading to an increase of skin, sebaceous and ceruminous material, water, and normal flora due to ear canal disease, narrowing of the ear canal, or overproduction of cerumen

DIAGNOSIS

Clinical Presentation
History
- Patients may complain of hearing loss, tinnitus, dizziness, fullness, or pain.

Physical Examination
- Evaluation of the ear canal will show occlusion. Cerumen may vary in color and texture.

Differential Diagnosis
- Foreign body, otitis externa, mastoiditis, Ménière disease, benign positional vertigo, and acoustic neuroma

Diagnostic Criteria and Testing
- There are no laboratory values, imaging studies, or diagnostic tests that diagnose cerumen impaction.

TREATMENT

- Patients who are asymptomatic should not have cerumen removed.

Medications
- Cerumenolytics may be used if there is no history of infection, perforation, or ear surgery.
  - Docusate, mineral oil, hydrogen peroxide, and carbamide peroxide have all been used, but there is no significant difference in efficacy.

Other Nonpharmacologic Therapies
- Gentle irrigation (may not be effective for hard impaction)
  - Immunocompromised patients should have 2% acetic acid solution or boric acid powder to discourage bacterial growth and water retention.
- Manual removal

SPECIAL CONSIDERATIONS

Disposition
- Patients may be discharged home. Patients should be referred to ENT if there is perforation of the tympanic membrane (TM).

Complications
- Eardrum rupture, infection, bleeding/irritation of ear canal, and dizziness/vertigo

Otitis Externa

GENERAL PRINCIPLES

Definition
- Inflammation of the external auditory canal

Epidemiology/Etiology
- More likely to occur in the summer months and in younger adults
- Infectious (bacterial), allergic, or due to other dermatologic causes
- Trauma (cleaning or scratching), swimming (water exposure), contact dermatitis, and devices that occlude the ear canal all predispose to otitis externa.
- *P. aeruginosa*, *S. epidermidis*, *S. aureus*, and *Candida* are the most common responsible organisms.

Pathophysiology
- Breakdown of the cerumen barrier of the ear canal leads to inflammation, edema, pruritus, and obstruction. The pH of the ear canal increases, leading to overgrowth of bacterial organisms and subsequent breakdown of epithelial migration.

DIAGNOSIS

Clinical Presentation
History
- The patient usually complains of pain, discharge, and hearing loss.
- A history of prior ear infections, prior ear surgery, trauma/instrumentation, and water exposure should be obtained.

Physical Examination
- Manipulation of the external ear canal by either tragal pressure or pulling of the auricle can cause tenderness.
- Debris may be noted in the ear canal that can vary in color and texture. TM rupture should be ruled out.

Differential Diagnosis
- Psoriasis, fungal infection, carcinoma, dermatitis, and allergic reaction

Diagnostic Criteria and Testing
- There are no specific laboratory or imaging studies to diagnose otitis externa.

TREATMENT

Medications

- Topical fluoroquinolones (ofloxacin, ciprofloxacin), polymyxin B, neomycin, and aminoglycosides (tobramycin, gentamicin) are all effective and may be given 3–4×/ day (fluoroquinolones are dosed 2×/day).
- Topical glucocorticoids (hydrocortisone, prednisolone, dexamethasone) help decrease pain and pruritus.

Other Nonpharmacologic Therapies

- The ear canal should be cleaned with a loop or swab to remove debris prior to antibiotic administration.
- Wicks may be placed to allow medicine to reach the affected area but should be replaced every 1–3 days and can be removed once swelling subsides.

SPECIAL CONSIDERATIONS

Disposition

- Patients may be discharged home to follow up with their PMD or otolaryngologist.

Complications

- Periauricular cellulitis and malignant otitis externa

Otitis Media

GENERAL PRINCIPLES

Definition

- Infection or inflammation of the middle ear. If there is middle ear fluid without inflammation or infection, it is referred to as otitis media with effusion (OME).
- If pus enters the mastoid air cells and infects the bone, this is referred to as mastoiditis.

Epidemiology/Etiology

- Mainly in pediatric populations and caused by obstruction of the eustachian tube
- Common causes include inflammation, ciliary dysfunction, muscle dysfunction, or mass effect.
- S. pneumonia and H. influenza are common infectious causes.

Pathophysiology

- The eustachian tube descends as a child grows, improving patency and decreasing obstruction, although changes may persist. Also, negative pressure in the middle ear leads to lack of air movement and accumulation of materials that are conducive to development of otitis media.

DIAGNOSIS

Clinical Presentation

History

- Patients may complain of pain, decreased hearing, and an antecedent upper respiratory tract infection. Sometimes, the patient may report feeling off balance.

Physical Examination
- A bulging TM is usually seen, sometimes with an air–fluid level. The TM may be opacified or erythematous.
- There may be conductive hearing loss noted with the Weber test.

Differential Diagnosis
- Otitis externa, infection, mass effect, and eustachian tube dysfunction

Diagnostic Criteria and Testing
- There are no specific laboratory or imaging studies to diagnose otitis media.
- Mastoiditis may be seen on CT scan or MRI.

TREATMENT

Medications
- Amoxicillin 500 mg PO q12 hours for 5–10 days for mild disease or q8 hours for severe disease
  - For patients with allergy to β-lactam antibiotics, erythromycin, azithromycin, and clarithromycin can be used.
- If there is a rupture of the TM, ototopic medications such as ofloxacin otic (5 drops bid × 3–5 days) are preferred, and neomycin–polymyxin B–hydrocortisone should not be used.
- If mastoiditis is suspected, IV antibiotics should be started that cover *S. pneumonia* and *H. influenzae*.

SPECIAL CONSIDERATIONS

Disposition
- Patients with uncomplicated otitis media may be discharged home.
- Patients with presumed mastoiditis should be admitted to the hospital.

SUGGESTED READINGS

Amsden GW. Tables of Antimicrobial Agent Pharmacology. In: Mandell GL, Bennett JE, Dolin R, eds. *Principles and Practice of Infectious Diseases.* 7th ed. Philadelphia: Churchill Livingstone, 2010:718.

Beers SL, Abramo TJ. Otitis externa review. *Pediatr Emerg Care* 2004;20:250.

Burton MJ, Doree C. Ear drops for the removal of ear wax. *Cochrane Database Syst Rev* 2009:CD004326.

Gates GA. Acute Otitis Media and Otitis Media with Effusion. In: Cummings C, Frederickson J, Harker L, eds. *Otolaryngology: Head & Neck Surgery.* Baltimore: Mosby, 1998:461.

Hand C, Harvey I. The effectiveness of topical preparations for the treatment of earwax: a systematic review. *Br J Gen Pract* 2004;54:862.

Jones RN, Milazzo J, Seidlin M. Ofloxacin otic solution for treatment of otitis externa in children and adults. *Arch Otolaryngol Head Neck Surg* 1997;123:1193.

Kaushik V, Malik T, Saeed SR. Interventions for acute otitis externa. *Cochrane Database Syst Rev* 2010:CD004740.

Kelly KE, Mohs DC. The external auditory canal. Anatomy and physiology. *Otolaryngol Clin North Am* 1996;29:725.

Mitka M. Cerumen removal guidelines wax practical. *J Am Med Assoc* 2008;300:1506.

Osguthorpe JD, Nielsen DR. Otitis externa: review and clinical update. *Am Fam Physician* 2006;74:1510.

Roland PS, Smith TL, Schwartz SR, et al. Clinical practice guideline: cerumen impaction. *Otolaryngol Head Neck Surg* 2008;139:S1.

Roland PS, Stroman DW. Microbiology of acute otitis externa. *Laryngoscope* 2002;112:1166.

Schwartz LE, Brown RB. Purulent otitis media in adults. *Arch Intern Med* 1992;152:2301.

34 Eye Emergencies

Tracy Cushing and Mark D. Levine

GENERAL PRINCIPLES

History

- Determine time course and chronicity of symptoms.
- Determine if condition is unilateral or bilateral; inquire as to the type and amount of drainage.
- Inquire about the presence of ocular pain, photophobia, change in vision, foreign body sensation/itching/burning, and eye discharge and type.
- Inquire about personal and family history of hay fever, allergic rhinitis, and other contacts with conjunctivitis.
- Obtain past medical and medication history, specifically ask about ocular medications.

Physical Examination

- Evaluate visual acuity, visual fields, papillary function, and extraocular movements.
- Evert and examine eyelids for inflammation, tenderness, or foreign body.
- Examine sclera and conjunctiva for hyperemia and edema; check cornea for clarity.
- Examine the cornea for irregularities.
- Examine the pupils for size, shape, and reaction to light.
- Determine type of discharge.
- Palpate for regional lymphadenopathy.

Slit-Lamp Examination

- The use of a topical anesthetic such as proparacaine or tetracaine may help enable slit-lamp examination. Severe photophobia that causes blepharospasm may require instillation of a cycloplegic agent (such as cyclopentolate or homatropine) 20–30 minutes prior to examination.
- Perform fluorescein instillation and examination with blue light. Fluorescein can permanently stain soft contact lenses. Do not forget to remove lenses before applying the stain.
- Fluorescein is applied using a paper strip applicator that is gently placed over the inferior cul-de-sac of the eye and allowing saline or anesthetic solution to drop into the eye. Once the patient blinks, the dye is spread over the cornea.

- Fluorescein stains basement membrane that has been exposed by damage to the corneal epithelium. This causes injuries to appear green using cobalt blue light or a Wood lamp.

Differential Diagnosis
- Infection, inflammation, trauma, acute angle closure glaucoma, or thrombosis

Corneal Abrasion

GENERAL PRINCIPLES

Pathophysiology
- Disruption of the epithelium on the cornea by mechanical or chemical factors results in corneal abrasion.
- Because the epithelium is richly innervated with sensory nerve endings, even minor injuries are painful.

Clinical Presentation
- The degree of pain is generally related to the amount of epithelial disruption and motion of the eyeball, and blinking increases the pain and foreign body sensation.
- Redness of the eye follows corneal insult due to the reactive conjunctival vasodilation.
- Photophobia is often present.
- When illuminated, an abrasion may be noted by a shadow that is cast on the iris from a surface defect. Likewise, there may be fluorescein uptake.

TREATMENT

- Instill antibiotic ointment (erythromycin ophthalmic ointment [1" ribbon, 6×/day, 7–10 days] or gentamicin ophthalmic [1" ribbon bid or tid or 1–2 drops q4h until improvement]).
- Advise to avoid bright lights/sunlight. Wear sunglasses to help with the associated light sensitivity.

Subconjunctival Hemorrhage

GENERAL PRINCIPLES

Pathophysiology
- A subconjunctival hemorrhage can occur spontaneously, with raised venous pressure from a forced Valsalva maneuver (coughing or sneezing).
- It may occur with major or minor (nondetectable) trauma to the front of the eye.

Clinical Presentation
- A flat, deep-red hemorrhage is noted under the conjunctiva that may cause chemosis to expand over the lid margin.
- Subconjunctival hemorrhage is usually asymptomatic.
- The pupils should be normal.

TREATMENT

- With the absence of other signs and symptoms, no treatment is required and the blood will clear in 2–3 weeks.
- Moisturizing eye drops may be used for comfort.

Conjunctivitis

GENERAL PRINCIPLES

Definition

- Inflammation of the conjunctiva characterized by vascular dilation, cellular infiltration, and exudate.

Viral Conjunctivitis

GENERAL PRINCIPLES

Pathophysiology

- Adenovirus is usually the causative organism.
- It can develop during or after a respiratory tract infection.
- Adenovirus is highly contagious and is the leading cause of conjunctivitis.

Clinical Presentation

- Conjunctivitis acutely presents with conjunctival hyperemia, edema, and a watery discharge.
- Vision is usually not affected; watery discharge can cause transient blurring of the vision and photophobia is uncommon.

TREATMENT

- Viral conjunctivitis is usually self-limited; treatment with a topical antibiotic may make the patient feel more comfortable
  - The rationale for treatment is to prevent bacterial superinfection.
  - Treat with broad-spectrum topical eye drops, polymyxin B–trimethoprim combination (1–2 drops qid for 7 days). No topical antiviral is indicated.

Bacterial Conjunctivitis

GENERAL PRINCIPLES

Pathophysiology

- Gram-positive organisms are the predominate cause.
- *Staphylococcus aureus* is the most common cause of bacterial conjunctivitis.

Clinical Presentation

- Bilateral irritation and discharge, with matting of the eyelids.
- The patient will usually report irritation and tearing starting in one eye initially and spreading to the other eye within 48 hours, followed by a mucopurulent discharge.

- Eyelids and conjunctiva become edematous with debris at the base of the lashes and matting of the eyelids upon wakening.

TREATMENT

- Gentamicin or tobramycin 0.3% ophthalmic drops are instilled in the affected eye qid for 7–10 days.
- Topical fluoroquinolones (ciprofloxacin and ofloxacin) are effective but reserved for severe infections.

Hyperacute Bacterial Conjunctivitis

GENERAL PRINCIPLES

Pathophysiology

- Most commonly, this is caused by *Neisseria gonorrhoeae* (less often by *Neisseria meningitides*). This occurs through autoinoculation from infected genitalia.
- Adults transmit the infection from genitalia to the hands and then the eyes.

Clinical Presentation

- An abrupt onset of copious yellow-green purulent discharge to both eyes with lid edema, erythema, and chemosis is the typical presentation.

Diagnostic Testing

- Culture and gram stain of the discharge is appropriate.

TREATMENT

- Because this is a rapidly progressive, sight-threatening ocular infection, immediate consultation by ophthalmology is required.

Ocular Chlamydial Conjunctivitis

GENERAL PRINCIPLES

Pathophysiology

- *Chlamydia trachomatis* is the cause of ocular chlamydial infections.

Clinical Presentation

- It presents in sexually active patients, and symptoms may be present for a long period of time prior to seeking medical assistance.
- Presentation is usually unilateral.
- Infection is usually indolent and is characterized by a thin, mucoid discharge.
- Photophobia and enlarged, tender periauricular nodes may be present.

TREATMENT

- Oral doxycycline 100 mg twice a day for 14 days.
- Oral erythromycin 250 mg four times a day for 21 days in pregnant and lactating women.
- This diagnosis should prompt a sexually transmitted disease (STD) workup in patients.

Allergic Conjunctivitis

GENERAL PRINCIPLES

Pathophysiology

- Seasonal allergic conjunctivitis is a type 1 IgE-mediated hypersensitivity to certain allergens (ragweed, pollen) and is the most common form of ocular allergy.
- Perennial allergic conjunctivitis is similar to the seasonal type, but symptoms are less severe and happen year round due to the nonseasonal nature of the antigens.
- Conjunctivitis medicamentosa is an allergic response that occurs as a reaction to the use of ocular medications.

Clinical Presentation

- Seasonal allergic conjunctivitis
  - Itching, watery eyes, rhinitis or allergic pharyngitis, eyes with mild lid edema, fine papillary hypertrophy, and bulbar conjunctival hyperemia.
  - Corneal involvement is rare.
- Perennial allergic conjunctivitis
  - Itching, burning, and tearing
  - Normal-appearing eyes (symptoms are less severe than in seasonal allergic conjunctivitis)
- Conjunctivitis medicamentosa
  - Bilateral dilation of the conjunctival blood vessels with eyelid edema, erythema, and scaling in a patient using topical ophthalmic medication.

TREATMENT

- Remove offending allergen or dilute it by using artificial tears every 2–3 hours during the acute phase.
- Ocular
  - Levocabastine hydrochloride (0.05%)—one drop in both eyes qid
  - Olopatadine HCl (0.1%)—one drop in affected eye bid
- Systemic
  - Fexofenadine 60 mg bid
- Chronic perennial conjunctivitis
  - Cromolyn sodium ophthalmic solution—1–2 drops qid

Keratitis

GENERAL PRINCIPLES

Pathophysiology

- Corneal defects seen as a cause of multiple sources, including dry eye, blepharitis, trauma, topical drug toxicity, and ultraviolet burns (welders or sun lamps)

Clinical Presentation

- Pain, photophobia, foreign body sensation with conjunctival injection, and a watery discharge
- Pinpoint corneal epithelial defects are seen on fluorescein exam.

TREATMENT

- Artificial tears and erythromycin ointment or drops 2–3×/day for 4 days. A cycloplegic may be used for pain.
- If a contact lens wearer, discontinue use and use tobramycin drops 4–6×/day and qHS. A cycloplegic may be used for pain.

Chalazion/Hordeolum (Stye)

GENERAL PRINCIPLES

Pathophysiology
- A blockage in the meibomian gland on the eyelid that becomes enflamed and if infected is classified as a hordeolum

Clinical Presentation
- A visible and palpable well-defined nodule in the eyelid, sometimes with associated eyelid swelling and erythema

TREATMENT

- Warm compresses for 15–20 minutes, qid.
- Bacitracin or erythromycin ointment may be used bid.
- Gentle massage over the lesion several times a day may help clear blockage.
- May be removed surgically as an outpatient.

Acute Closed Angle Glaucoma

GENERAL PRINCIPLES

Pathophysiology
- The iris flattens out and blocks the drainage of aqueous humor from the trabecular channels and causes increased ocular pressure. It may occur secondary to mydriatics, anticholinergics, or low light.

Clinical Presentation
- Pain, blurry vision, halo around lights, headache, nausea, and vomiting

TREATMENT

- Topical beta-blocker (timolol 0.5%, one drop).
- Topical steroid (prednisolone acetate 1%) q15–30 minutes for four doses and then hourly.
- Acetazolamide (250–500 mg IV).
- Osmotic agent (mannitol 1–2 g/kg IV over 45 minutes).
- Emergent ophthalmologic consultation. The patient may be discharged as an outpatient with medication recommendations or may be admitted for laser iridectomy.

Central Retinal Artery Occlusion

GENERAL PRINCIPLES

Pathophysiology
• Embolus/thrombosis of the arterioles of the eye

Clinical Presentation
• Acute painless unilateral acute loss of vision.
• Afferent pupillary defect.
• Fundoscopic exam shows a cherry-red spot in the center of the macula and whitening of the retina.
• Segmented "boxcar" of the retinal arterioles.

TREATMENT

• Ocular massage
• Acetazolamide (500 mg IV)
• Timolol (0.5% drop bid)
• Emergent ophthalmologic consultation

Central Retinal Vein Occlusion

GENERAL PRINCIPLES

Pathophysiology
• Caused by blockage of the main retinal vein causing extravasation of blood and fluid into the retina. Vision is blurred because of fluid collecting in the macula.

Clinical Presentation
• Painless unilateral loss of vision
• Cotton-wool spots, disc edema, and hemorrhages on the fundoscopic exam
• Neovascularization of the optic disc, retina, and iris

TREATMENT

• Topical beta-blocker (timolol 0.5%, one drop)
• Pilocarpine (0.5–1% qid)
• Ophthalmologic consulation is recommended

Retinal Detachment

GENERAL PRINCIPLES

Pathophysiology
• The retina becomes detached (flap or tear) from posterior surface of the eye.

Clinical Presentation
• Flashes of light, floaters, or a curtain/shadow moving over the field of vision with a field deficit or vision loss
• Can be seen on direct ophthalmologic exam or with the use of ultrasound

TREATMENT
- If the retina is covering the macula, bed rest with bilateral patching until surgical repair.
- Ophthalmologic consultation is required.

Iritis/Uveitis

GENERAL PRINCIPLES

Pathophysiology
- Trauma and inflammation or infection (anterior); infection (posterior)

Clinical Presentation
- Pain and red eye with photophobia and some mild decreased vision and tearing.
- Cells and flare in the anterior chamber, miosis, and usually low intraocular pressure.
- Posterior uveitis may have blurred vision and floaters, disc swelling, and retinal hemorrhages.

TREATMENT

- Cyclopentolate 1–2% tid
- Prednisolone acetate 1% q1–6 hours
- Ophthalmology consultation for outpatient management or intralesional injection

SPECIAL CONSIDERATIONS

- In any patient who presents with any eye complaint and wears contact lenses, make sure the antibiotic coverage is broadened to include coverage for *Pseudomonas*.
- Any corneal ulceration, herpetic lesion, potential disruption of the globe, or acute closed angle glaucoma should be referred to an ophthalmologist emergently.
- Refer all cases to an ophthalmologist within 24 hours.
- Infections are easily spread to unaffected eye and other household members, so frequent handwashing should be done to limit the spread of infection.
- Eye secretions are contagious 24–48 hours after the onset of therapy.
- Viral infections are contagious for at least 7 days after onset.

SUGGESTED READINGS

Azar AA, Barney NP. Conjunctivitis: a systematic review of diagnosis and treatment. *J Am Med Assoc* 2013;310(16):1721–8.

Ball JW, Dains JE, Flynn JA, et al. *Seidel's Guide to Physical Examination*. 8th ed. St. Louis: Elsevier Mosby, 2015.

Bodor FF, Marchant CD, Shurin PA, Barenkamp SJ. Bacterial etiology of conjunctivitis-otitis media syndrome. *Pediatrics* 1985;76(1):26–8.

Cullom RD, Chang B. *The Wills Eye Manual: Office and Emergency Room Diagnosis and Treatment of Eye Disease*. Philadelphia: JB Lippincott Co., 1994.

Keim SM, Gomella LG. *Emergency Medicine on Call*. New York: McGraw Hill, 2004.

Lanternier ML. Ophthalmology. In: Graber MA, Lanternier ML, eds. *University of Iowa: The Family Practice Handbook*. St. Louis: Mosby, 2002:699–711.

Leibowitz HM. The red eye. *N Engl J Med* 2000;343:345–51.

McManaway JA, Frankel CA. Red Eye. In: Hoekelman RA, Adams HM, Nelson NM, et al., eds. *Pediatric Primary Care*. St. Louis: Mosby, 2001:1240–6.

Pavan-Langson D. Cornea and External Disease. In: Pavan-Langson D, ed. *Manual of Ocular Diagnosis and Therapy*. Philadelphia: Lippincott Williams & Wilkins, 2002:1–20.

Oropharyngeal Emergencies

Mark D. Levine

Peritonsillar Abscess (PTA)

GENERAL PRINCIPLES

Definition
• A collection of pus between the palatine tonsil and pharyngeal muscles

Epidemiology/Etiology
• Most frequently seen in young adults.
• Usually preceded by tonsillitis or pharyngitis.
• Smoking is a risk factor for PTA.

Pathophysiology
• Thought to be due to blockage of the Weber glands
• Polymicrobial in nature, with *Streptococcus pyogenes, Streptococcus anginosus,* and *Staphylococcus aureus* as the most frequent pathogens

DIAGNOSIS

Clinical Presentation
History
• Patients will usually complain of a sore throat, fever, and a muffled voice ("hot potato" voice). They may report not being able to open their mouths widely. They may complain of ear pain or neck swelling and report not being able to eat.

Physical Examination
• Normally, a swollen, unilateral, fluctuant tonsil is seen with uvular deviation. There may also be fullness of the posterior soft palate. Adenopathy and trismus may be present.

Differential Diagnosis
• Parotiditis, TMJ dislocation, vascular trauma, dental space infection, deep space infection, Ludwig angina, epiglottitis, or retropharyngeal abscess

Diagnostic Criteria and Testing
Laboratories
• No laboratory values are specific for PTA, but if the abscess is drained, the pus should be sent for Gram stain and culture.

Imaging
- An ultrasound can distinguish between cellulitis/phlegmon and abscess and guide aspiration.
- CT is another modality to identify abscess and deep space infection.

TREATMENT

- Airway compromise and control should be considered early in any patient with an oropharyngeal issue.

Medications
- Ampicillin/sulbactam 3 g IV q6 hours or
- Clindamycin 600 mg IV q6–8 hours.
  - Coverage for MSRA should be considered.
  - In patients who have a fever >39°C, drooling, and /or respiratory distress, he or she should receive additional coverage of vancomycin or linezolid.
- After clinical improvement, the patient may be started on amoxicillin–clavulanate 875 mg PO q12 hours for 10 days or clindamycin 300–450 mg PO q6 hours for 10 days.
- If MRSA is suspected, administer linezolid 600 mg PO BID for 10 days.

Other Nonpharmacologic Therapies
- Drainage is the ideal treatment for PTA.

SPECIAL CONSIDERATIONS

Disposition
- Patients may be managed as an outpatient if they are able to eat/drink, their pain is controlled, and there is a low risk of obstruction/complication.

Complication
- Spread of infectious process or carotid injury during I&D

Pharyngitis

GENERAL PRINCIPLES

Definition
- Inflammation of the pharynx or a "sore throat"

Epidemiology/Etiology
- Viral etiologies are the most common and include influenza, Epstein–Barr, cytomegalovirus, HIV, and herpes simplex.
- Bacterial etiologies include group A streptococcus, *Arcanobacterium haemolyticum, Corynebacterium diphtheriae, Neisseria gonorrhoeae, Chlamydophila pneumoniae, Mycoplasma pneumoniae, and tularemia.*

Pathophysiology
- Local invasion of the mucosa leads to an immune response including inflammation and irritation.

DIAGNOSIS

Clinical Presentation

History
- Patients usually report a sore throat and pain with swallowing. Fever and malaise may be present with a bacterial infection. Many patients also report congestion, cough, hoarseness, and ear/sinus pain.

Physical Examination
- Pharyngeal edema and erythema as well as tonsillar exudate may be present. There may be cervical adenopathy. The uvula may be erythematous or minimally swollen.

Differential Diagnosis
- PTA, parotiditis, TMJ dislocation, vascular trauma, dental space infection, deep space infection, Ludwig angina, epiglottitis, or retropharyngeal abscess

Diagnostic Criteria and Testing
- The Centor criteria are used as a clinical decision tool for GAS. Patients with fewer than three criteria are unlikely to have GAS and do not need further testing or treatment. The criteria are:
  - Tonsillar exudates
  - Tender anterior cervical adenopathy
  - Fever by history
  - Absence of cough

Laboratories
- The rapid antigen detection test (RADT) may be used to test for GAS.

Imaging
- There is no radiologic study that will diagnose pharyngitis.

TREATMENT

Medications
- OTC lozenges and sprays have some anesthetic properties.
  - In 2006, the FDA issued an advisory regarding the risk of methemoglobinemia associated with benzocaine sprays.
- Acetaminophen and NSAIDs have been shown to decrease pain in pharyngitis.
- Glucocorticoids should only be used in patients with severe throat pain and inability to swallow.
  - Options include: Dexamethasone 20 mg IM or PO, betamethasone 8 mg IM, and prednisone 60 mg PO × 1–2 days are the recommended dosing for steroids, if used.

Other Nonpharmacologic Therapies
- Gargles, tea, and other home remedies have weak evidence of efficacy.

SPECIAL CONSIDERATIONS

Disposition
- Most patients can be discharged home as long as they can take food/drink by mouth.

Deep Space Infection (Retropharyngeal Abscess, Ludwig's Angina)

GENERAL PRINCIPLES

Definition

- Infection that occurs in the deeper structures of the neck/mouth secondary to a spread from teeth, tonsils, ear, or sinuses
  - Retropharyngeal abscess—infection behind the constrictor muscles of the neck near the carotid sheaths
  - Ludwig angina—submandibular infection that can occlude airway and spread to the mediastinum

Epidemiology/Etiology

- Usually polymicrobial in nature but *Streptococcus viridans* is most common. Oral anaerobes are also frequently isolated bacteria.

Pathophysiology

- Bacteria spread via local or hematogenous seeding into the loose connective tissues that may have been compromised from comorbid conditions, antecedent surgery, trauma, radiation, or immunocompromise and rapidly multiply potentially compromising the airway, oropharyngeal, and mediastinal structures.

DIAGNOSIS

Clinical Presentation

History

- The presentation of deep space infections varies but will usually include fever, swelling in the neck or submandibular regions, trismus, and difficulty talking or swallowing, and the patient may report respiratory distress.

Physical Examination

- Since deep space infections may not be easily visible on exam, a full evaluation of the head and neck, including submandibular spaces, should be evaluated. There may be areas of fluctuance in the neck or oral cavity. Trismus may be present.
- Dysphagia and odynophagia and pooling of saliva may be noted.
- Dysphonia, hoarseness, tongue paresis, and stridor or dyspnea are signs of impending airway compromise.
- Ludwig's angina typically presents as a swelling under the tongue and "woody" cellulitis without lymphadenopathy.

Differential Diagnosis

- Parotitis, TMJ dislocation, vascular trauma, dental space infection, meningitis, Pott disease, or tendonitis of the neck

Diagnostic Criteria and Testing

Laboratories
- A CBC, BMP, lactate, type and cross should all be drawn.

Imaging
- CT scan is the imaging modality of choice to evaluate the location and extension of infection.

TREATMENT

Medications

- Retropharyngeal abscess
  - Immunocompetent: ampicillin/sulbactam 3 g IV q6 hours OR penicillin G 2–4 million units IV q4–6 hours plus metronidazole 500 mg IV q6–8 hours OR clindamycin 600 mg IV q6–8 hours
  - Immune compromised: cefepime 2 g IV q12 hours plus metronidazole 500 mg IV q6–8 hours OR imipenem 500 mg IV q6 hours or meropenum 1 g IV q8 hours OR piperacillin-tazobactam 4.5 g IV q6 hours
- Ludwig angina
  - Immunocompetent: ampicillin/sulbactam 3 g IV q6 hours OR penicillin G 2–4 million units IV q4–6 hours plus metronidazole 500 mg IV q6–8 hours OR clindamycin 600 mg IV q6–8 hours
  - Immune compromised: cefepime 2 g IV q12 hours plus metronidazole 500 mg IV q6–8 hours OR imipenem 500 mg IV q6 hours or meropenem 1 g IV q8 hours OR piperacillin–tazobactam 4.5 g IV q6 hours

Other Nonpharmacologic Therapies

- Surgical drainage of any loculation is the treatment of choice.

SPECIAL CONSIDERATIONS

- Emergent surgery consultation is required.

Disposition

- These patients should be admitted to the ICU as there is a risk for airway compromise and sepsis.

Complications

- Mediastinitis, sepsis, and death

Salivary Gland Stones (Sialolithiasis)

GENERAL PRINCIPLES

Definition

- The presence of calculi in the salivary glands/ducts

Epidemiology/Etiology

- Most stones arise from submandibular and parotid glands. There is a male predominance. The stones are mainly calcium in nature.
- Risk factors include dehydration, trauma, gout, smoking, a history of kidney stones, periodontal disease, or use of diuretics or anticholinergic medications.
- *S. aureus* is the most commonly found bacteria in suppurative sialolithiasis.

Pathophysiology

- Inflammation or trauma to the ductal system or glandular inflammation causes slowing of saliva (which is alkaline, high in calcium and mucin content)

DIAGNOSIS

Clinical Presentation

Physical Examination
- The patient frequently complains of pain and swelling in the face in the area of the involved gland and it may be aggravated by salivating or eating. Symptoms may vary in intensity and time course.
- Small stones may be seen at either Wharton's duct or Stensen's duct on exam, and clear saliva should normally flow when the gland is pressed. The gland may be tender to exam.
- With sialolithiasis, pain, swelling, and erythema will be noted near the gland, and pus may drain from the duct.

Differential Diagnosis
- Infection, inflammation, neoplasm, trauma, mumps, HIV, and Sjögren syndrome

Diagnostic Criteria and Testing

Laboratories
- There are no specific laboratory tests for sialolithiasis.

Imaging
- A plain film can detect a radiopaque stone in most cases.
- Ultrasound can be detected if the stone is >2 mm.
- CT is the modality of choice, but fine cuts must be performed.

Diagnostic Procedures
- Milking of the duct may express the stone or purulence.

TREATMENT

Medications
- Pain can be usually controlled with NSAIDs.
- If superinfection is present, dicloxacillin or cephalexin 500 mg PO QID for 7–10 days can be prescribed.

Other Nonpharmacologic Therapies
- Sialogogues, such as lemon drops, as well as hydration and warm moist heat to the area while milking the duct are the most common conservative approaches. Medications such as anticholinergics should be discontinued if possible.

SPECIAL CONSIDERATIONS

Disposition
- These patients can be discharged home to follow up with an otolaryngologist unless there is concern for airway compromise.

Epiglottitis

GENERAL PRINCIPLES

Definition
- Inflammation of the epiglottis and adjacent structures

Epidemiology/Etiology

- May be caused by bacterial, viral, or fungal pathogens, but *Haemophilus influenzae* type b (HiB) is the most common cause in immunocompetent adults.
- In immune compromised hosts, epiglottitis may be caused by *Pseudomonas aeruginosa* or *Candida*.
- Epiglottitis is less common since the HiB vaccine was introduced and is now rare in the immunized adult population.
- Risk factors include immune deficiency and incomplete or lack of immunization.

Pathophysiology

- Cellulitis of the epiglottis and surrounding structures occurs from bacterial invasion, leading to swelling and occlusion of the upper airway.

DIAGNOSIS

Clinical Presentation

History

- Adults usually present with fever and pain on swallowing that has occurred over the course of 2 days to 1 week.

Physical Examination

- Airway compromise is less common than in children, but the patient may have a fever >37.5°C, muffled voice, drooling, stridor, or hoarseness.
- Some patients may not be able to handle their secretions.
- The laryngeal area including the hyoid bone may be tender to palpation.
- Inflammation and edema of the supraglottic structures will usually be present.

Differential Diagnosis

- Croup, uvulitis, tracheitis, foreign body, RPA, PTA, angioedema, diphtheria, or trauma

Diagnostic Criteria and Testing

- Visualization of the epiglottis is the accepted standard for diagnosis but should be done with the awareness that a loss of the airway may occur. Any laboratory testing should be performed after the airway is secure, as pain and agitation may lead to airway loss.

Laboratories

- There are no laboratory tests specific for epiglottitis, but an epiglottal culture may be taken if the patient is intubated. Blood cultures may lead to a causative organism.

Imaging

- Soft tissue films of the neck usually show a swollen epiglottis or "thumb sign."

Diagnostic Procedures

- Visualization of an erythematous edematous epiglottis with a flexible nasopharyngeal scope is the gold standard for diagnosis.

TREATMENT

- Emergent control of the airway should be undertaken if needed.

Medications

- Ceftriaxone 2 g IV daily OR
- Cefotaxime 2 g IV q4–8 hours plus vancomycin 1 g IV q12 hours OR
- Clindamycin 600–900 mg IV q8 hours OR
- Oxacillin 1–2 g IV q4–6 hours OR
- Nafcillin 2 g IV q4 hours OR
- Cefazolin 1–2 g IV q6 hours

SPECIAL CONSIDERATIONS

Disposition

- These patients should be admitted to an ICU setting.

Complications

- Respiratory compromise, sepsis, and death

SUGGESTED READINGS

Barton ED, Bair AE. Ludwig's angina. *J Emerg Med* 2008;34:163.

Blaivas M, Theodoro D, Duggal S. Ultrasound-guided drainage of peritonsillar abscess by the emergency physician. *Am J Emerg Med* 2003;21:155.

Boscolo-Rizzo P, Da Mosto MC. Submandibular space infection: a potentially lethal infection. *Int J Infect Dis* 2009;13:327.

Brook I. Microbiology and principles of antimicrobial therapy for head and neck infections. *Infect Dis Clin North Am* 2007;21:355.

Chow AW. Life-Threatening Infections of the Head, Neck, and Upper Respiratory Tract. In: Hall JB, Schmidt GA, Wood LD, eds. *Principles of Critical Care*. New York: McGraw-Hill, 1998:887.

Galioto NJ. Peritonsillar abscess. *Am Fam Physician* 2008;77:199.

Gerber MA, Shulman ST. Rapid diagnosis of pharyngitis caused by group A streptococci. *Clin Microbiol Rev* 2004;17:571.

Glezen WP, Clyde WA Jr, Senior RJ, et al. Group A streptococci, mycoplasmas, and viruses associated with acute pharyngitis. *JAMA* 1967;202:455.

Glynn F, Fenton JE. Diagnosis and management of supraglottitis (epiglottitis). *Curr Infect Dis Rep* 2008;10:200.

Goldstein NA, Hammerschlag MR. Peritonsillar, Retropharyngeal, and Parapharyngeal Abscesses. In: Feigin RD, Cherry JD, Demmler-Harrison GJ, Kaplan SL, eds. *Textbook of Pediatric Infection Diseases*. 6th ed. Philadelphia: Saunders, 2009:177.

Guldfred LA, Lyhne D, Becker BC. Acute epiglottitis: epidemiology, clinical presentation, management and outcome. *J Laryngol Otol* 2008;122:818.

Huoh KC, Eisele DW. Etiologic factors in sialolithiasis. *Otolaryngol Head Neck Surg* 2011;145:935.

Myer CM III. Candida epiglottitis: clinical implications. *Am J Otolaryngol* 1997;18:428.

Passy V. Pathogenesis of peritonsillar abscess. *Laryngoscope* 1994;104:185.

Reynolds SC, Chow AW. Life-threatening infections of the peripharyngeal and deep fascial spaces of the head and neck. *Infect Dis Clin North Am* 2007;21:557.

Scott PM, Loftus WK, Kew J, et al. Diagnosis of peritonsillar infections: a prospective study of ultrasound, computerized tomography and clinical diagnosis. *J Laryngol Otol* 1999;113:229.

Shulman ST, Bisno AL, Clegg HW, et al. Clinical practice guideline for the diagnosis and management of group A streptococcal pharyngitis: 2012 update by the Infectious Diseases Society of America. *Clin Infect Dis* 2012;55:1279.

Snow V, Mottur-Pilson C, Cooper RJ, et al. Principles of appropriate antibiotic use for acute pharyngitis in adults. *Ann Intern Med* 2001;134:506.

Solomon P, Weisbrod M, Irish JC, Gullane PJ. Adult epiglottitis: the Toronto Hospital experience. *J Otolaryngol* 1998;27:332.

Tebruegge M, Curtis N. Infections Related to the Upper and Middle Airways. In: Long SS, Pickering LK, Prober CG, eds. *Principles and Practice of Pediatric Infectious Diseases.* 4th ed. New York: Elsevier Saunders, 2012:205.

Thomas M, Del Mar C, Glasziou P. How effective are treatments other than antibiotics for acute sore throat? *Br J Gen Pract* 2000;50:817.

van den Akker HP. Diagnostic imaging in salivary gland disease. *Oral Surg Oral Med Oral Pathol* 1988;66:625.

Williams MF. Sialolithiasis. *Otolaryngol Clin North Am* 1999;32:819.

Work WP, Hecht, DW. Inflammatory Diseases of the Major Salivary Glands. In: Papparella MM, Shumrick DF, eds. *Otolaryngology*. Philadelphia: WB Saunders, 1980:2235.

36 Hematologic Emergencies: Hemophilia

Mark D. Levine

GENERAL PRINCIPLES

Definition

• Abnormal bleeding secondary to a hereditary lack of clotting factors

Classification

• Hemophilia A—inherited deficiency of factor VIII
• Hemophilia B (Christmas disease)—inherited deficiency of factor IX
• Hemophilia C (Rosenthal syndrome)—inherited deficiency of factor XI

Epidemiology/Etiology

• Almost all patients with the disease will be male, but there are some females who are heterozygote carriers and may have mild disease.
• Hemophilia A—X-linked recessive, 1:5000 live male births.
• Hemophilia B—X-linked recessive, 1:30,000 live male births.
• Hemophilia C—autosomal recessive, common in Ashkenazi Jews (from Eastern Europe).
• Mild hemophilia may not appear until later in life and generally only in response to trauma or surgery. Joints and muscles are the most common sites of bleeding in adults.

Pathophysiology

• Mild hemophilia—factor activity level between 5% and 40% of normal (>0.05 and <0.40 IU/mL)

- Moderate hemophilia—factor activity level between 1% and 5% of normal (>0.01 and <0.05 IU/mL)
- Severe hemophilia—factor activity level <1% of normal (<0.01 IU/mL)

DIAGNOSIS

Clinical Presentation

History
- Patients can frequently report spontaneous bleeding, and it may be severe. Delayed bleeding after trauma may be reported, and it may take a very long time for small cuts to stop bleeding or heal. Questions regarding abnormal bleeding with menstrual cycles, dental extractions, trauma, and surgical interventions should be asked. A family history of bleeding disorders should also be ascertained.

Physical Examination
- A full examination should be performed, with special attention paid to areas that have experienced even minor trauma. Bruising, hematoma formation, or active bleeding may be noted. The neurologic exam may also raise concerns for spontaneous intracranial hemorrhage.

Differential Diagnosis

- von Willebrand disease, other factor deficiencies, trauma, liver failure, heparin-induced thrombocytopenia (HIT), thrombocytopenia, or disseminated intravascular coagulation (DIC)

Diagnostic Criteria and Testing

Laboratories
- A complete blood count and a prothrombin time (PT)/activated partial thromboplastin time (aPTT) panel should be drawn, as well as factor activity level. There will be a prolonged aPTT; however, aPTT may be normal if factor activity level is >15%. Platelet counts and PT will be normal in hemophilia.
- Initial peak factor activity level should be checked about 10 minutes after the first dose of factor administration, and a trough level should be measured at ~4–6 hours for factor VIII and 8–12 hours for factor IX.

Imaging
- There is no imaging study that will diagnose hemophilia, although ultrasound or CT scans may help evaluate hematoma or active extravasation.

TREATMENT

- The immediate goal is to increase the factor activity to achieve hemostasis. If there is serious or life-threatening bleeding, treatment should be initiated before the assessment is completed. The patient may know his or her factor level and how much factor the patient will need.

Medications

Severe or moderate hemophilia
- Severe bleeding—factor activity should be maintained above 50%, and dosage should be given to raise the level to 80–100%.
  - Hemophilia A—give an initial dose of 50 units/kg of factor VIII. Dosing— pt weight (kg) × desired rise in factor level (as a whole number to get to 100) × 0.5.

Repeat dosing should be done at the time of one-half life. An initial bolus can be given followed by an infusion of 4 units/kg/h.

- ○ Hemophilia B—give an initial dose of factor IX of 100–120 units/kg. Dosing— pt weight (kg) × desired rise in factor level (as a whole number to get to 100) × 0.6. Repeat dosing should be done at the time of one-half life. An initial bolus can be given followed by an infusion of 6 units/kg/h.
- Joint bleeds—factor replacement should be given within 2 hours of identification of bleed.
  - ○ Hemophilia A—give an initial dose of 25 units/kg of factor VIII. Dosing— pt weight (kg) × desired rise in factor level (as a whole number to get to 50) × 0.5
  - ○ Hemophilia B—give an initial dose of factor IX of 100–120 units/kg. Dosing— pt weight (kg) × desired rise in factor level (as a whole number to get to 50) × 0.6
- Minor bleeding—can be managed with local pressure, ice, elevation, or local anti-fibrinolytic agents.

Mild hemophilia

- Severe bleeding—should be treated similarly to those with severe hemophilia
- Minor bleeding
  - ○ Hemophilia A—may be treated with DDAVP after a test dose has been given and the patient has shown response. The dose is 0.3 µg/kg (maximum dose 20 µg) IV or SC. It is not indicated for patients with severe or moderate hemophilia A or if a delay of 30–60 minutes prior to treatment is unacceptable. An intranasal formulation is also available and may be given as 150 µg for patients <50 kg and 300 µg (one puff of 150 µg per nostril) for patients >50 kg.
  - ○ Hemophilia B—may be treated with factor IX.
  - ○ If there is no purified factor available, fresh frozen plasma (FFP) may be use. Cryoprecipitate may be used in hemophilia A.
  - ○ Cryoprecipitate contains ~3–5 units/mL of factor VIII.
  - ○ FFP contains one unit of factor activity (a dose of 15–20 mL/kg will raise factor VIII by about 30–40% and factor IX by ~15–20%).
  - ○ Tranexamic acid (TXA) (25/mg/kg q6–8h) and epsilon aminocaproic acid (EACA) (75–100 mg/kg q6h [max 3–4 g]) may be used for mucosal bleeding but should not be given simultaneously with activated prothrombin complex concentrate.

SPECIAL CONSIDERATIONS

Disposition

- These patients should be admitted to the hospital to monitor factor levels and hemostasis.

Complications

- Patients who are on factor inhibitors should be managed in consultation with a hematologist.
- DDAVP can cause hyponatremia as it has antidiuretic properties. Headache, nausea, and tingling are sometimes encountered with the administration of DDAVP for the future.

von Willebrand Disease (VWD)

GENERAL PRINCIPLES

Definition

- A lack of von Willebrand factor (VWF) causing a decreased ability to clot

Epidemiology/Etiology
- Mutations or genetic inheritance may cause VWD.
- One percent of the population may be affected, as VWD is the most common inherited bleeding disorder.

Pathophysiology
- von Willebrand factor binds platelets and endothelium and contributes to the fibrin clot formation. Mutations cause damage to this factor and decreases the ability of the body to clot.

DIAGNOSIS

Clinical Presentation
History
- Patients may report easy bruising, prolonged bleeding from minor wounds, or prolonged bleeding from mucosal surfaces. Patients can become symptomatic at any age. Patients may have spontaneous bleeding after ingestion of aspirin or NSAIDs. A careful family history is important. A negative bleeding history does not rule out VWD.

Physical Examination
- Careful attention should be paid to any bruises, bleeding from mucosal surfaces, hematoma, or prolonged oozing from areas of minor trauma.

Differential Diagnosis
- Hemophilia, trauma, HIT, thrombocytopenia, DIC, and other factor deficiencies

Diagnostic Criteria and Testing
Laboratories
- Platelet and coagulation studies should be drawn, as well as von Willebrand factor antigen (vWF Ag) and von Willebrand factor activity level. Bleeding time should also be ordered, although may be normal in mild or moderate disease.

Imaging
- There are no imaging studies that will diagnose VWD, although ultrasound and CT scans may help identify hematoma or active extravasation.

TREATMENT

Medications
- A DDAVP trial should be undertaken prior to the patient actively bleeding.
- 0.3 µg/kg (max 20 µg) can be given, and a three- to fivefold increase in VWF can be seen in 30–60 minutes and will last for ~6–12 hours. A repeat dose may be given in 8–12 hours if needed.
- Intranasal therapy is also available (150 µg for patients <50 kg and 300 µg for patients >50 kg).
- Replacement of VWF-containing concentrates can be used if DDVAP administration is ineffective.
- IVIG 1 g/kg/d may be used in patients with acquired VWD or a monoclonal gammopathy.

SPECIAL CONSIDERATIONS

Disposition

• These patients should usually be admitted to the hospital to monitor bleeding and factor levels.

Complications

• DDAVP can cause hyponatremia as it has antidiuretic properties. Headache, nausea, and tingling are sometimes encountered with the administration of DDAVP.

SUGGESTED READINGS

Aledort LM. Treatment of von Willebrand's disease. *Mayo Clin Proc* 1991;66:841.

Aviña-Zubieta JA, Galindo-Rodriguez G, Lavalle C. Rheumatic manifestations of hematologic disorders. *Curr Opin Rheumatol* 1998;10:86.

Blanchette VS, Key NS, Ljung LR, et al. Definitions in hemophilia: communication from the SSC of the ISTH. *J Thromb Haemost* 2014;12:1935.

Franchini M, Favaloro EJ, Lippi G. Mild hemophilia A. *J Thromb Haemost* 2010;8:421.

Franchini M, Mannucci PM. Hemophilia A in the third millennium. *Blood Rev* 2013;27:179.

Hoots KW. Emergency Management of Hemophilia. In: Lee CA, Berntorp EE, Hoots WK, eds. *Textbook of Hemophilia*. 3rd ed. John Wiley & Sons, Ltd., 2014.

Noble S, Chitnis J. Case report: use of topical tranexamic acid to stop localised bleeding. *Emerg Med J* 2013;30:509.

Ruggeri ZM, Ware J. von Willebrand factor. *FASEB J* 1993;7:308.

Srivastava A, Brewer AK, Mauser-Bunschoten EP, et al. Guidelines for the management of hemophilia. *Haemophilia* 2013;19:e1.

Steven MM, Yogarajah S, Madhok R, et al. Haemophilic arthritis. *Q J Med* 1986;58:181.

The Diagnosis, Evaluation and Management of von Willebrand Disease—2008 Clinical Practice Guidelines. National Heart, Lung and Blood Institute. Available at: www.nhlbi.nih.gov/guidelines/vwd (last accessed 07/25/11).

37 Hematologic Emergencies: Idiopathic Thrombocytopenic Purpura

Amanda Poskin and Christopher Brooks

GENERAL PRINCIPLES

Definition

• Idiopathic thrombocytopenic purpura (ITP) is an process in which antiplatelet antibodies result in rapid platelet destruction and inhibition of platelet production resulting in profound thrombocytopenia and bleeding.[1]

Epidemiology/Etiology
• The median age is 56 years with a slightly higher incidence in females.[2]

Pathophysiology
• Antiplatelet antibodies bind to antigens on megakaryocytes and proplatelets inhibiting platelet production. The IgG-rich coating of the platelets predisposes them to phagocytosis by macrophages in the spleen and Kupffer cells in the liver.[3]

DIAGNOSIS

History
• The patient may complain of fatigue, easy bruising and bleeding.

Physical Examination
• On exam, epistaxis, gingival bleeding, petechiae, purpura, and ecchymosis may be seen. Spontaneous intracerebral hemorrhage (ICH) is possible as is hematuria or menorrhagia.

Differential Diagnosis[4]
• Exposure (drugs, foods, herbs), pseudothrombocytopenia, giant platelet disorder, familial inherited thrombocytopenia, systemic lupus erythematosus (SLE), HIV, B-cell malignancies, antiphospholipid syndrome, or thrombotic thrombocytopenic purpura (TTP)

Diagnostic Testing and Criteria
Diagnostic Criteria
• ITP is a diagnosis of exclusion but must fit the following criteria:
  ○ Thrombocytopenia with platelet count < 100,000/μL
  ○ Other normal blood counts
  ○ Normal peripheral blood smear
  ○ No evidence of hemorrhage to account for consumption of platelets
  ○ Exclusion of other causes of thrombocytopenia

Laboratories
• A peripheral smear and CBC should be obtained.

TREATMENT

• Treatment is typically reserved for patients with bleeding or determined to be at high risk of bleeding based on platelet count of <30,000/μL.[5]
• Patients at risk for injury (athletes, elderly) are treated at higher platelet counts than those without these risk factors.

Medications
• First line
  ○ High-dose methylprednisolone (1 mg/kg/day)
  ○ IVIG (1 g/kg/day) for 1–2 days[4]
    ▪ IV anti-D can be substituted for corticosteroid in the patient that is Rh-positive and DAT (direct antithrombin negative).
• Second line
  ○ There is no defined second-line treatment for ITP aside from consideration of splenectomy.[5] Chemotherapy and stem cell transplant may be considered and used for steroid/IVIG refractory ITP.[6]

Other Nonpharmacologic Therapies
- Platelet transfusions
- Factor VIIa

SPECIAL CONSIDERATIONS

Disposition

- These patients should be admitted. Hematology should be consulted.

REFERENCES

1. Cines DB, McMillan R. Pathogenesis of chronic immune thrombocytopenic purpura. *Curr Opin Hematol* 2007;14(5):511–4.
2. Frederiksen H, Schmidt K. The incidence of idiopathic thrombocytopenic purpura in adults increases with age. *Blood* 1999;94:909–13.
3. Schwartz RS. Immune thrombocytopenic purpura—from agony to agonist. *N Engl J Med* 2007;357(22):2299–301. doi:10.1056/NEJMe0707126. PMID 18046034.
4. Cines DB, Blanchette VS. Immune thrombocytopenic purpura. *N Engl J Med* 2002;346(13):995–1008. doi:10.1056/NEJMra010501.PMID11919310.
5. Ghanima W, Godeau B, Cines B, et al. How I treat immune thrombocytopenia: the choice between splenectomy or a medical therapy as a second-line treatment. *Blood* 2012;120(5):960–9. doi:10.1182/blood-2011-12-309153.
6. Stevens W, Koene H, Zwaginga JJ, Vreugdenhil G. Chronic idiopathic thrombocytopenic purpura: present strategy, guidelines and new insights. *Neth J Med* 2006;64(10):356–63. PMID 17122451.

38 Hematologic Emergencies: Sickle Cell Disease

Kevin Baumgartner and Christopher Brooks

GENERAL PRINCIPLES

Classification

- Sickle cell disease (SCD) is classified by the mutant alleles involved: HgbSS, HgbSC, and HgbS-β-thalassemia.
- Patients with HgbSS are severely affected and patients with HgbSC are moderately affected. Severity of disease in HgbS-β-thalassemia varies from mild to severe based on subtype.[1]
- People who are heterozygous for the sickle allele are said to have sickle cell trait. In general, they do not suffer the complications of SCD.

Epidemiology/Etiology

- SCD is common in African Americans but can also be found in people of African, Mediterranean, Middle Eastern, and Indian descent.[1]

Pathophysiology

- A mutation of the hemoglobin molecule alters its structure when deoxygenated, leading to characteristic "sickle" deformity of red blood cells (RBCs).
- Even when "sickle" RBCs are not present, the blood and vascular endothelium of SCD patients are abnormal; cell adhesion molecules, platelet adhesion, endothelial adhesion and activation, and acute-phase reactant activation are all abnormal in SCD and contribute to microvascular occlusion.[1,2]
- The most common complication of SCD in patients presenting to the ED is acute vasoocclusive episode (VOE). These episodes are painful, resulting from localized vasoocclusion with resulting hypoxia and tissue ischemia.
  - Acute chest syndrome is a potentially life-threatening syndrome of pulmonary hypoxia and vasoocclusion, which can progress to complete respiratory failure if untreated. It may be caused by infection, infarction of the pulmonary vasculature, pulmonary edema, or fat emboli from bone marrow infarction.[1] Acute chest syndrome is clinically indistinguishable from pneumonia.
  - Fever in a patient with SCD is a medical emergency, as patients are typically functionally asplenic.
  - Patients with SCD are at increased risk of cerebrovascular accident (CVA), intracranial hemorrhage (ICH), and sinus venous thrombosis.[3]
  - Splenic sequestration can occur in SCD patients who have not yet become functionally asplenic due to splenic infarcts, leading to sepsis, acute anemia, and hypovolemia.
  - Osteomyelitis is common in SCD due to infection of infarcted bone tissue.
  - Ischemic priapism due to obstruction of venous outflow is common.[1]
  - SCD patients are at high risk for cholelithiasis and choledocholithiasis due to increased formation of bilirubin stones.[4] Acute hepatic crisis is a variant of VOE involving the hepatic circulation, which causes painful infarction and inflammation of the liver.
  - In addition to chronic renal failure due to medullary infarcts, patients with SCD are at risk of papillary necrosis due to renal infarction. The sloughed papillae can obstruct the ureter, mimicking renal colic and requiring urologic intervention.[6]
  - Patients with SCD who suffer eye trauma are at high risk of developing a traumatic hyphema that can cause acute angle-closure glaucoma, ocular rebleeding, and vision loss.

DIAGNOSIS

Clinical Presentation

History
- All patients with SCD should be asked about their history of complications of SCD (especially acute chest and stroke), their home medication regimen and frequency of crises, their transfusion history, and the characteristics of their typical sickle crises.[1]
- Symptoms to inquire about: fever, chest pain, dyspnea, cough, abdominal pain, myalgias, arthralgias, headache, focal neurologic symptoms, and persistent painful erections.

Physical Examination
- Hypoxia is a sign of acute chest syndrome.
- Fever should prompt assessment for serious bacterial infections.
- Abdominal exam may demonstrate generalized tenderness, which can be suggestive of uncomplicated VOE (or in rare cases mesenteric ischemia), liver, or biliary pathology.
- Any focal neurologic deficit should prompt immediate evaluation for CVA.
- The extremities are frequently tender to palpation in uncomplicated VOE. However, focal tenderness to palpation is concerning for osteomyelitis or avascular necrosis (AVN). Swollen, erythematous, painful digits are a sign of dactylitis.
- Focal midline spinal tenderness should prompt consideration of vertebral osteomyelitis or epidural abscess.
- A careful ocular exam in patients who have suffered eye or head trauma is essential to screen for traumatic hyphema.[1]

Differential Diagnosis
- Sickle cell disease has multiple different presentations that have a wide range of diagnoses consistent with abnormalities in the effected organ system.

Diagnostic Testing
Laboratories
- No laboratory test is reliably diagnostic of VOE.[1]
- CBC: hemoglobin level assists in determining the necessity of transfusion and should be compared to the patient's baseline if known
- Reticulocyte count: can help differentiate aplastic (retic low) from hemolytic or sequestration-related (retic normal or high) anemia.
- Basic metabolic panel (BMP): serum creatinine may overestimate true renal function in SCD patients, due to renal infarction.[1,6]
- Type and screen: send on any patient who may require exchange or simple transfusion

Imaging
- Chest radiography is indicated to screen for the pulmonary infiltrates that are typical of acute chest syndrome. Any new pulmonary infiltrate in conjunction with fever, chest pain, hypoxia, or respiratory symptoms should be treated as acute chest syndrome.
- Plain films may be used to assess for the presence of osteomyelitis or AVN.

TREATMENT

- VOE requires prompt treatment with analgesics. Parenteral opioids are the recommended first-line agents.[2] Home NSAIDs have not been shown to decrease pain or "spare" opioids in the ED.[1]
- Patients with VOE are frequently dehydrated and may benefit from gentle hypotonic maintenance fluids but should not receive boluses of isotonic fluids unless they are clinically hypovolemic. Overuse of normal saline boluses can lead to a nongap metabolic acidosis, which worsens RBC sickling.[1]
- Transfusion has no role in the treatment of uncomplicated VOE.[2]
- Supplementary oxygen should be used only if the patient is hypoxic and then only to maintain oxygen saturations >92% on pulse oximetry.
- Treatment of acute chest syndrome must include supplemental oxygen (as needed to maintain oxygen saturations >95%), incentive spirometry, analgesia and fluids as in uncomplicated VOE, and broad-spectrum antibiotics, typically a parenteral third-generation cephalosporin an oral macrolide and (e.g., ceftaroline 1–2 g and

azithromycin 500 mg).[2] Simple transfusion should be considered if the patient's Hgb is <9 mg/dL and is at least 1 mg/dL below the patient's baseline.[2] Noninvasive positive pressure ventilation has not been shown to be helpful.[1]

- Patients with acute chest syndrome who have refractory hypoxia, progressively worsening respiratory distress, anemia refractory to simple transfusion, or respiratory failure should undergo urgent exchange transfusion, in consultation with a hematologist.[2]
- CVA in a patient with SCD should be treated with emergent exchange transfusion in consultation with a hematologist.[2] Typical treatments for ischemic stroke such as thrombolytics and clot retrieval may be considered in consultation with a neurologist and hematologist in adults with SCD, who are at risk of "typical" atherothrombotic ischemic CVA.[1]
- Aplastic crisis should be treated with urgent simple transfusion. It is also very important to isolate these patients from all pregnant women (whether health care workers, visitors, or other patients) as parvovirus B19 can cause fatal hydrops fetalis in unborn children.[1]
- Patients with renal colic with significant ureteral obstruction or infection may require urgent surgical or cystoscopic decompression of the urinary tract. These patients warrant urgent urologic consultation.
- Priapism lasting <2 hours should first be treated with IV hydration and analgesia as in uncomplicated VOE. Priapism lasting longer than 2 hours requires urgent treatment with aspiration and phenylephrine injection into the corpora cavernosa. If this fails, they must undergo immediate surgical shunting.[6]
- Traumatic hyphema in patients with SCD or sickle cell trait (SCT) should prompt immediate ophthalmologic consultation. The head of the patient's bed should be elevated >30 degrees and they should be treated with topical timolol eyedrops.[1]

SPECIAL CONSIDERATIONS

Disposition

- Patients with a minor VOE whose pain can be successfully controlled in the ED may be discharged with outpatient hematology follow-up.
- Patients with severe VOE requiring repeated or continuous IV analgesia or with any of the major acute complications of SCD should be admitted to the hospital.[1]
- Acute chest syndrome should be admitted to an ICU.

Complications

- Chronic complications of SCD include hemochromatosis (due to increased RBC turnover and frequent transfusions); severe arthritis due to AVN, which may require arthroplasty; chronic pain syndromes and opiate hyperalgesia; and end-stage renal disease.

REFERENCES

1. Gebreselassie S, Simmons MN, Montague DK, et al. Genitourinary manifestations of sickle cell disease. *Clev Clin J Med* 2015 Oct;82(10):679–83.
2. Yawn BP, Buchanan GR, Afenyi-Annan AN, et al. Management of sickle cell disease: summary of the 2014 evidence-based report by panel members. *JAMA* 2014;312(10):1033–48.
3. Uprety D, Baber A, Foy M, et al. Ketamine infusion for sickle cell pain crisis refractory to opioids: a case report and review of literature. *Ann Hematol* 2014;93:769–71.
4. Glassberg J. Evidence-based management of sickle cell disease in the emergency department. *Emerg Med Pract* 2011;13(8):1–20.

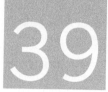

39 Hematologic Emergencies: Transfusion Reactions and Complications

Aimee Wendelsdorf

GENERAL PRINCIPLES

Definition

- Acute/immediate transfusion reactions
  - Transfusion-associated sepsis/bacterial infection
    - Infectious symptoms after the transfusion of contaminated blood products, more common with platelet transfusions
  - Acute hemolytic reaction
    - A medical emergency resulting from transfusion of ABO incompatible blood products resulting in massive hemolysis of erythrocytes leading to DIC, shock, and acute renal failure
  - Febrile nonhemolytic reaction (FNHR)
    - Acute, nonlife-threatening rise in a patient's temperature after transfusion of at least 1°C and is a result of antibodies in the recipient's serum reacting against white blood cells in the donor product.[3]
  - Urticaria/anaphylactic reactions
    - A reaction to allergens present in donor blood
  - Transfusion-related acute lung injury (TRALI)
    - A new acute lung injury that occurs during or within 6 hours after a transfusion of blood products that results in onset of respiratory distress.[4]
  - Transfusion-associated circulatory overload (TACO)
    - Hydrostatic pulmonary edema resulting from the transfusion of excess blood product volume[5]
  - Metabolic reactions (citrate toxicity,[6] hyperkalemia, hypocalcemia, respiratory alkalosis)
  - Hypothermia
- Delayed transfusion reactions
  - Delayed hemolytic transfusion reactions (DHTR)
    - A milder reaction than acute hemolysis
    - Asymptomatic hemolysis and decrease in hemoglobin
  - Transfusion-associated graft versus host disease (GVHD)
    - Rare but fatal
    - Immunocompetent donor lymphocytes attack and destroy the organs and tissues of an immunosuppressed recipient leading to multiorgan failure and death.[5]
  - Alloimmunization to red cell antigens and/or leukocyte antigens
  - Posttransfusion purpura (PTP)
    - A rare transfusion reaction caused by platelet-specific alloantibodies, which results in thrombocytopenia < 20,000.

Epidemiology/Etiology

- An estimated 20% of patients who receive a blood transfusion will experience some form of a transfusion reaction.[1]
- Plasma-related transfusion reactions may occur in as many as 1 out of 360 plasma transfusions.[7]
- Acute hemolytic reactions now only occur anywhere from 1 in 10,000 to 1 in 50,000 transfusions. Mortality increases as the volume of incompatible blood transfused increases and can be as high as 44% if >1 L of blood is administered.[7]
- The highest rate of bacterial infection is associated with platelet transfusion despite mitigating strategies (1 out of 3,000 transfused units).
- FNHRs occur in <1% of all transfusions.[3]
- TRALI accounts for ~65% of blood transfusion–related deaths.[2,8]
- TACO is estimated to occur in up to 11% of transfusions.[5]
- PTP is five times more likely to occur in women than men and primarily affects women who have developed antibodies against platelets from prior pregnancies.[5]
- Patients who receive frequent and numerous blood transfusions are more likely to have transfusion reactions due to alloimmunization.[3]
- The risk of developing TRALI has been shown to increase as the volume of transfused product increases; however, as little as 10–20 mL of plasma-rich blood product has been known to lead to lung injury.[8]
  - Risk for TRALI includes patients with sepsis, recent surgery, congestive heart failure, shock, and on mechanical ventilation or that are at extremes of age, are chronic tobacco users, or have chronic alcohol abuse.[2,8]
- Transfusion-associated circulatory overload
  - Any risk factor that predisposes a patient to hypervolemia such as extremes of age and pre-existing cardiac or renal failure can predispose recipients to circulatory overload secondary to transfusion.[2,7]

Pathophysiology

- Transfusion reactions are caused by either acute immune reactions or hemolysis and its sequelae.
- Nonhemolytic transfusion reactions—cytokine mediated and antibody production leading to prostaglandin E2 production in the hypothalamus causing fever[9]
- Allergic reactions—allergens in the donor plasma react to IgE bound to recipient mast cells causing a histamine release[6]
- Acute hemolytic reactions—hemolysis and the release of cytokines and interleukins causing vasodilation, hypotension, microthrombi/procoagulants state, and renal failure[7]
- DHTRs—previously immunization to blood components via prior transfusions or pregnancies.[10]
- TRALI—a prior inflammatory process (sepsis/surgery) prime neutrophils in the lung endothelium resulting in protease release, capillary leakage, and pulmonary edema.

DIAGNOSIS

Clinical Presentation

History
- The onset of symptoms in acute hemolytic transfusion reactions is rapid and usually begins with fever and chills. The classic triad of fever, flank pain, and hemoglobinuria is rare.

Physical Examination

- Patients presenting with TRALI and TACO are clinically indistinguishable. They present with similar signs and symptoms of increased pulmonary congestion and progressive respiratory distress including dyspnea, cyanosis, hypoxemia, and tachypnea, copious pink, frothy sputum, fever, or hypotension may be present. They may also have evidence of an S3 on cardiac exam or elevated jugular venous pressures.[7,8]
- Symptoms of sepsis related to contaminated blood products typically develop rapidly and often within minutes of transfusion.[11]
- Transfusion-associated GVHD typically develops anywhere between 4 and 30 days after blood transfusion. Patients may present with a generalized erythematous, maculopapular rash or right upper quadrant abdominal pain, fever, vomiting, and diarrhea.[11]
- PTP may present as mild manifestations of thrombocytopenia such as epistaxis and hematuria or can lead to life-threatening gastrointestinal hemorrhage.[5]
- Flushing, pruritus, urticarial rash, wheezing, and hypotension are all potential symptoms associated with allergic reactions and anaphylaxis.

Differential Diagnosis

- Cardiogenic pulmonary edema secondary to heart failure and other causes of acute lung injury/acute respiratory distress syndrome must be excluded prior to making a diagnosis of TRALI.[8]

Diagnostic Criteria and Testing

- Suspected TRALI requires all of the following:
  - Acute onset of respiratory distress within 6 hours of blood transfusion
  - PaO_2/FiO_2 < 300 mm Hg or worsening PaO_2 to FiO_2 ratio
  - Bilateral infiltrative changes on chest radiograph
  - No sign of hydrostatic pulmonary edema (pulmonary artery occlusion pressure < 18 mm Hg or central venous pressure [CVP] < 15 mm Hg)
  - No other risk factor for acute lung injury
- Delayed TRALI
  - Same as for suspected TRALI, but criteria and symptoms develop 6–72 hours after blood transfusion.
- Suspected TACO requires the following[9]:
  - Acute respiratory distress (dyspnea, orthopnea, cough)
  - Evidence of positive fluid balance
  - Increased B-type natriuretic protein (BNP)
  - Radiographic evidence of pulmonary edema
  - Evidence of left heart failure
  - An increase in CVP

Laboratories

- Direct antiglobulin (Coombs test): positive in acute hemolysis.[11]
- CBC: neutropenia may develop in 5–35% of TRALI patients.
- Platelets: <20,000 is required for the diagnosis of PTP.
- BNP: elevated in TACO.[12]
- Bilirubin and alkaline phosphatase: elevated in GVHD.[11]
- Blood cultures should be drawn in transfusion patients with a fever, especially if the rise in temperature is more than 2°C.
- Urinalysis: hemoglobinuria.

Imaging
- Chest radiography (CXR) is helpful for differentiating allergic reaction from acute lung injury when respiratory distress develops after blood transfusion. The CXR in TRALI and TACO, however, are nonspecific showing interstitial opacities and diffuse lung haziness that may obscure the pulmonary vasculature.
- Echocardiography demonstrating decrease left-ventricular function may be useful in distinguishing TACO from other blood transfusion–related reactions.[2]

TREATMENT

- Management of most blood transfusion reactions is supportive care.[2]
- Stop the transfusion and immediately notify the blood bank.
- A new type and screen should be collected from any patient who is believed to have received mismatched or infected blood.
- Acute hemolytic transfusion reactions should be managed with aggressive IV crystalloid hydration to avoid the negative effects of hemoglobinuria. IV hydration therapy should be titrated to achieve a urine output of 100 to 200 mL/h.
- By definition, all TRALI and TACO patients require supplemental oxygen.[2,13] A low-tidal volume lung protective strategy is recommended to prevent further lung injury.[13]
- The use of steroids, antipyretics, or diphenhydramine to prevent allergic transfusion is currently not recommended.[14]

Medications
- Oral antipyretics may be used to treat symptomatic fever.
- Diphenhydramine 25 to 50 mg may be given either for pruritus or urticaria.
- Epinephrine 0.5 mg IM of a 1:1000 solution or 0.1 mg of a 1:10,000 solution may be given either intramuscularly or intravenously for anaphylaxis.
- Corticosteroid administration is not recommended for management of suspected TRALI.[15]
- Diuretics are not recommended for the treatment of chest plain radiograph infiltrates seen in TRALI.[13] IVIG has been used to treat severe delayed hemolytic reactions and is now considered the first-line therapy for treatment of symptomatic posttransfusion purpura.[10]

SPECIAL CONSIDERATIONS

- Plasma from female donors with past pregnancies has a higher likelihood of containing leukocyte antibodies so some centers have restricted the use of female donors with past pregnancies and donors with multiple prior transfusions in an attempt to limit the incidence of TRALI.[7]
- PTP may develop 5 to 10 days after transfusion of any platelet containing blood product and carries a mortality related to bleeding complications of 5–10%.[5]
- Immunocompromised patients should receive only blood products that are both irradiated and leukoreduced.

Disposition
- Minor febrile and cutaneous reactions do not require prolonged monitoring and patients may be discharged if there are no other concerns regarding acute blood loss or the need for further resuscitation or transfusion.

TABLE 39.1	Risk of Transfusion-Transmitted Viral Infection
Virus	Risk of transmission per unit transfused
Human immunodeficiency virus	1 in 1.4 million
Hepatitis C virus	1 in 1.1 million
Hepatitis B virus	1 in 280,000
West Nile virus	1 in 350,000
Human T-cell lymphotropic virus II	1 in 2.9 million

Adapted from Bihl F, Castelli D, Marincola F, et al. Transfusion-transmitted infections. *J Transl Med* 2003;14:5–25 and Pandey S, Vyas GN. Adverse effects of plasma transfusion. *Transfusion* 2012;52:655–79.

• Patients with suspected acute hemolysis or respiratory distress from either TRALI or TACO should be admitted to the hospital for monitoring and supportive care. Patients requiring vasopressor support, supplemental oxygen, and those with the potential for developing acute renal failure should be admitted to the intensive care unit for close monitoring.

Complications

• Viral infection from receiving blood products (Table 39.1)

REFERENCES

1. Coil CJ, Santen SA. Transfusion Therapy. In: Tintinalli JE, ed. *Emergency Medicine: A Comprehensive Study Guide.* 7th ed. New York: McGraw-Hill, 2011:1493–500.
2. Carcano C, Okafor N, Martinez F, et al. Radiographic manifestations of transfusion-related acute lung injury. *Clin Imaging* 2013;37:1020–23.
3. Mosley JC, Blinder MA. Transfusion Practices. In: Kollef M, ed. *The Washington Manual of Critical Care.* 2nd ed. Philadelphia: Lippincott Williams & Wilkins, 2012:505–10.
4. Alam A, Lin Y, Lima A, et al. The prevention of transfusion-associated circulatory overload. *Transfus Med Rev* 2013;27:105:12.
5. Klein HG, Anstee DJ. Some Unfavourable Effects of Transfusion. In: *Mollison's Blood Transfusion in Clinical Medicine.* Somerset, GB: Wiley-Blackwell, 2013:660–95.
6. Heddle N, Webert KE. Febrile, Allergic, and Other Noninfectious Transfusion Reactions. In: *Hillyer's Blood Banking and Transfusion Medicine.* 2nd ed. Philadelphia: Churchill Livingstone, 2007:677–90.
7. Pandey S, Vyas GN. Adverse effects of plasma transfusion. *Transfusion* 2012;52:655–79.
8. Sayah DM, Looney MR, Toy P. Transfusion reactions: new concepts of the pathophysiology, incidence, treatment and prevention of transfusion-related acute lung injury. *Crit Care Clin* 2012;28:363–72.
9. Shanwell A, Kristiansson M, Remberger M, Ringden O. Generation of cytokines in red cell concentrates during storage is prevented by prestorage white cell reduction. *Transfusion* 1997;37:678–84.
10. Klein HG, Anstee DJ. Haemolytic Transfusion Reactions. In: *Mollison's Blood Transfusion in Clinical Medicine.* Somerset, GB: Wiley-Blackwell, 2013:458–98.
11. Kopko PM, Holland PV. Mechanisms of severe transfusion reactions. *Transfus Clin Biol* 2001;8:278–81.
12. Zhou L, Giacherio D, Cooling L, Davenport RD. Use of B-natriuretic peptide as a diagnostic marker in the differential diagnosis of transfusion-associated circulatory overload. *Transfusion* 2005;45:1056–63.

13. Jawa RS, Anillo S, Kulaylat MN. Transfusion-related acute lung injury. *J Intensive Care Med* 2008;23(2):109–21.
14. Sarai M, Tejani AM. Loop diuretics for patients receiving blood transfusions. *Cochrane Database Syst Rev* 2015;(2). Art. No.: CD010138. doi:10.1002/14651858.CD010138.pub2.
15. Goldberg AD, Kor DJ. State of the art management of transfusion-related acute lung injury (TRALI). *Curr Pharm Des* 2012;18:3273–84.

Hematologic Emergencies: Thrombotic Thrombocytopenic Purpura (TTP)

Jordan Maryfield

GENERAL PRINCIPLES

Definition

- Thrombotic thrombocytopenic purpura (TTP) is a thrombotic microangiopathy (TMA) characterized by severe ADAMTS13 deficiency resulting in large platelet von Willebrand factor (vWF) aggregates that causes microangiopathic hemolytic anemia (MAHA) and thrombocytopenia.[1]

Epidemiology/Etiology

- The median age at diagnosis is 41 years with a 3:1 female-to-male ratio.[2]
- One-third of cases occur in African American patients with a sevenfold increased risk of TTP.[2]

Pathophysiology

- The key pathologic mechanism causing TTP is a severely decreased activity of the serine metalloproteinase ADAMTS13 (most often secondary to an autoantibody), leading to the inability to cleave ultra large von Willebrand factor (ULvWF) multimers resulting in platelet aggregation, followed by organ ischemia due to occlusion of vessels by platelet-rich thrombi.[3]

DIAGNOSIS

- The diagnosis is initially based on the clinical history, exam, and the presence of thrombocytopenia and MAHA with schistocytes on peripheral blood smear.

Clinical Presentation

- The classic pentad of TTP includes thrombocytopenia, MAHA, renal failure, fever, and neurologic deficits; however, this is only seen in 5% of presentations.

- TTP must be considered strongly even when only thrombocytopenia and MAHA are present.

History
- A comprehensive history is essential considering the broad differential diagnosis in patients with MAHA and thrombocytopenia.

Physical Examination
- There are no physical exam findings that are specific to TTP.
  - Patients may have petechiae, purpura, or bleeding depending on the severity of thrombocytopenia. Pallor of the skin and conjunctiva can be manifestations of anemia. Neurologic findings such as confusion or focal deficits may occur.

Differential Diagnosis

- Autoimmune hemolysis, autoimmune disease (lupus), disseminated intravascular coagulation (DIC), vasculitis, and hemolytic uremic syndrome
- Pregnancy-associated hemolysis, elevated liver enzymes, and low platelets (HELLP)
- Infection: viral (cytomegalovirus, adenovirus, herpes simplex, etc.) or severe bacterial or fungal infection
- Drug induced: quinine, calcineurin inhibitors, interferon, and simvastatin[4]

Diagnostic Testing

Laboratories
- Complete blood count (CBC) with peripheral smear: assess for anemia, thrombocytopenia, and schistocytes.
- Reticulocyte count and lactase dehydrogenase (LDH) may be elevated in TTP.
- Haptoglobin may be low in TTP.
- Direct Coombs test, fibrinogen, and liver enzyme are usually negative in TTP.
- Blood type and screen.
- ADAMTS13 activity and antibody testing: ideally obtain prior to treatment.

TREATMENT

- Hematology consult should be obtained.
- Plasma exchange (PEX) is the key therapy for TTP and should be instituted urgently.
  - PEX is the preferred treatment, but if not available, consider fresh frozen plasma in conjunction with steroids and consider urgent transfer to a center with PEX capabilities.[5]
  - Try to obtain laboratory tests prior to PEX; however, treatment should not be delayed while waiting for ADAMTS13 testing to result.
- Central venous access (specifically an exchange catheter) is preferred for PEX, regardless of platelet count, especially in setting of neurologic impairment.
- Immediately after starting PEX, administer steroids, either oral prednisolone 1 mg/kg/d or IV methylprednisolone 1 g/d for 3 days.
- When the platelet count is >50,000, start aspirin and prophylactic dose heparin to prevent thrombosis.

- Platelet transfusion is strictly contraindicated.
- Red blood cell transfusion is recommended to maintain hemoglobin > 7.

SPECIAL CONSIDERATIONS

- Hemolytic uremic syndrome (HUS)
  - Diarrhea-positive HUS is associated with bloody diarrhea in addition to MAHA and thrombocytopenia and is treated with supportive care.
  - Diarrhea-negative (atypical) HUS can present very similar to acquired TTP (though is more commonly associated with renal failure than TTP), and thus, with such diagnostic overlap, it is appropriate to treat with urgent PEX.[4,5]
- HIV-related TTP
  - Infectious disease should be consulted, and highly active antiretroviral therapy (HAART) should be started immediately after PEX to allow time for maximal absorption.
- TTP in pregnancy
  - If TMA is not fully explained by a non-TTP thrombotic microangiopathy, PEX should be started and maternal fetal medicine consulted.
- Drug-associated TTP
  - Medicines associated with TTP should be avoided in the future to prevent relapse.

Disposition

- Once the patient is stabilized, consider transfer to an institution experienced in the complex management of TTP. Most of these patients are best suited in an ICU setting given the need for central line placement, plasma exchange, the resuscitation required, and clinical instability, especially in the first 72 hours.

Complications

- Major complications of PEX include sepsis, venous thrombosis, and hypotension requiring pressors. About one in four patients will have one of these complications.[4]

REFERENCES

1. Reese JA, Muthurajah DS, Kremer Hovinga JA, et al. Children and adults with thrombotic thrombocytopenic purpura associated with severe, acquired ADAMTS13 deficiency: comparison of incidence, demographic and clinical features. *Pediatr Blood Cancer* 2013;60:1676.
2. Terrell DR, Vesely SK, Kremer Hovinga JA, et al. Different disparities of gender and race among the thrombotic thrombocytopenia purpura and hemolytic uremic syndromes. *Am J Hematol* 2010;85:844.
3. Blombery P, Scully M. Management of thrombotic thrombocytopenic purpura: current perspectives. *J Blood Med* 2014;5:15–23.
4. Mcdonald V, Laffan M, Benjamin S, et al. Thrombotic thrombocytopenic purpura precipitated by acute pancreatitis: a report of seven cases from a regional UK TTP registry. *Br J Haematol* 2009;144:430–3.
5. Rock GA, Shumak KH, Buskard NA, et al. Comparison of plasma exchange with plasma infusion in the treatment of thrombotic thrombocytopenic purpura. Canadian Apheresis Group. *N Engl J Med* 1991;325:393–7.
6. Scully M, Hunt BJ, Benjamin S, et al.; On behalf of British Committee for Standards in Haematology. Guidelines on the diagnosis and management of thrombotic thrombocytopenic purpura and other thrombotic microangiopathies. *Br J Haematol* 2012;158:323–35. doi:10.1111/j.1365-2141.2012.09167.x.

41 Allergic Reactions and Anaphylaxis

W. Scott Gilmore

GENERAL PRINCIPLES

Definition

- Allergic rhinitis is defined as an IgE-mediated inflammation of the mucous membranes of the nasal cavity.
- Acute urticaria is defined as hives that have been present for <6-week duration.
- Angioedema is defined as localized subcutaneous or submucosal swelling.
- Anaphylaxis is an acute, life-threatening, multisystem syndrome.

Epidemiology/Etiology

- Allergies are the sixth leading cause of chronic illness in the United States.
- Common causes of acute urticaria include infections, foods, and medications.
- Common cause of chronic urticaria include autoimmune forms, physical urticarias (cholinergic, aquagenic, pressure, cold, solar, heat, dermatographism, and exercise induced), and idiopathic urticaria, which is a diagnosis of exclusion.
- Food allergens are the main triggers for anaphylaxis.
  ○ Most common foods that trigger anaphylaxis include peanuts, tree nuts, fish, and shellfish.
- Other causes of anaphylaxis include medications (β-lactam antibiotics, NSAIDs, biologics, and monoclonal antibodies), insect stings, seminal fluid, vaccines or vaccine components, exercise, and latex.

Pathophysiology

- Allergic reactions occur when hypersensitivity to a foreign protein or antigen that normally would not be deleterious is acquired.
- Angioedema results from extravasation of fluid into interstitial tissues that will often affect the face, lips, mouth, throat, larynx, extremities, and genitalia. Bradykinin is the primary mediator in the compliment-mediated form of angioedema and is typically slower in onset and more severe than mast cell forms of angioedema.
- Anaphylaxis results from the sudden release of mediators derived from mast cells and basophils.
  ○ Augmenting factors include exercise, NSAIDs, angiotensin-converting enzyme (ACE) inhibitors, β-blockers, estrogens, lipid-lowering drugs, and alcohol.

DIAGNOSIS

Clinical Presentation

- Anaphylaxis, which is underdiagnosed, will present in one of the following manners:
  ○ In the absence of an allergen, anaphylaxis is diagnosed by a rapid onset (minutes to hours) of a reaction that involves the skin, mucosal tissue, or both, alongside

at least one of the following symptoms: respiratory compromise, reduced blood pressure, or symptoms of end-organ dysfunction.
- ○ After a likely allergen exposure, two or more of the following occur: involvement of the skin or mucosal tissue, respiratory symptoms, decreased blood pressure, and/or gastrointestinal involvement.
- ○ In the case of a known allergen, reduced blood pressure alone is sufficient for the diagnosis of anaphylaxis.

History
- The patient can present with a myriad of complaints depending upon the severity of the allergic reaction.
- Review the patient's medications, paying particular attention to the following: NSAIDs, ACE inhibitors or angiotensin receptor blockers (ARBs), estrogen, any new medications, or significant increases in doses of medications.
- Inquire about exposure to potential allergens including stinging or biting insects, latex, foods, and food additives.
- Allergic rhinitis will present with sneezing, watery rhinorrhea, nasal itching, nasal congestion, and nasal obstruction. Allergic rhinitis is often accompanied by atopic ocular disease, ear complaints, or laryngeal complaints.
- Urticaria will report pruritic skin lesions after exposure to a trigger.

Physical Examination
- A thorough physical examination should be undertaken paying attention to the airway, lungs, abdomen, and skin in addition to any other body system that the patient complains about.
- Urticarial lesions are circumscribed, raised, erythematous plaques, often with central pallor. Lesions may be round, oval, or serpiginous in shape and vary in size from one to several centimeters in diameter.
- Angioedema is localized swelling of the skin or of the mucous membranes of the upper respiratory or gastrointestinal tracts. It is not gravitationally dependent, and it is usually asymmetrical and nonpitting.

Differential Diagnosis
- The differential for allergic rhinitis includes nonallergic rhinitis, nonallergic rhinitis with eosinophilia, gustatory rhinitis, medication-induced rhinitis, infectious rhinitis, and atrophic rhinitis.
- The differential for urticaria includes viral exanthems, Sweet syndrome, atopic dermatitis, contact dermatitis, drug eruptions, insect bites, bullous pemphigoid, erythema multiforme, and plant-induced reactions.
- The differential for angioedema includes contact dermatitis, cellulitis, erysipelas, facial lymphedema, autoimmune conditions, eyelid edema, parasitic infections, hypothyroidism, superior vena cava syndrome and tumors, cheilitis granulomatosa, Melkersson-Rosenthal syndrome, idiopathic edema, tonsillitis, peritonsillar abscess, and pharyngeal foreign body.
- The differential diagnosis for anaphylaxis includes myocardial infarction, arrhythmia, pulmonary embolism, asthma, scombroid, septic shock, hemorrhagic shock, anxiety, cerebrovascular accident (CVA), seizure, ACE angioedema, pheochromocytoma.

Diagnostic Criteria and Testing
- The diagnosis of allergic reactions in the emergency department is based on clinical findings.

Laboratories
- There are no specific laboratory tests that are diagnostic for allergic reactions.

Imaging
- There are no specific radiographic studies that are diagnostic for allergic reactions.

TREATMENT

- In patient presenting with angioedema affecting the airway, airway protection must be given priority over a comprehensive diagnostic evaluation.

Medications

- For the treatment of allergic rhinitis:
  - Oral antihistamines are first-line therapy for mild to moderate allergic disease and specifically for allergic rhinitis.
    - Second-generation H1 antihistamines (loratadine, fexofenadine, cetirizine, levocetirizine, and desloratadine) are preferred.
    - Oral antihistamines control the symptoms of nasal itching, rhinorrhea, sneezing, and ocular irritation but have not been shown to be as effective at relieving nasal congestion.
  - Combination therapy using an oral antihistamine and an oral decongestant has developed to target the full spectrum of allergic symptoms.
  - Intranasal corticosteroids can also provide effective first-line treatment.
    - Intranasal corticosteroids (beclomethasone, budesonide, ciclesonide, flunisolide, fluticasone furoate, fluticasone propionate, mometasone, and triamcinolone) can be used.
    - Intranasal corticosteroids are successful in ameliorating the inflammatory effects of allergic process and are therefore effective in relieving nasal congestion in allergic rhinitis, as well as rhinorrhea, sneezing, and itching.
- For the treatment of urticaria:
  - First- and second-generation H1 antihistamines can be used in both acute and chronic urticaria and are effective in most patients. Although first-generation H1 antihistamines are frequently used for urticaria, second-generation H1 antihistamines are often just as efficacious, and the dose can be advanced further given the lower side effect profile of the second-generation H1 antihistamines. It has been shown that a two- to fourfold increase in the Food and Drug Administration (FDA)-approved dose of second-generation antihistamines can be effective for achieving control in some patients.
  - H2 antihistamines (ranitidine, nizatidine, famotidine, and cimetidine) can be used in conjunction with H1 antihistamines.
- For the treatment of allergic angioedema that is less severe than anaphylaxis use the following:
  - H1 and H2 antihistamines at standard doses
  - Glucocorticoids (methylprednisolone or prednisone)
- For the treatment of ACE inhibitor–induced angioedema:
  - There is no specific medication given in the treatment of ACE inhibitor–induced angioedema. Management involves discontinuing the drug and monitoring for resolution.
- For the treatment of anaphylaxis, epinephrine 1:1000 (1 mg/mL) at a dose of 0.3–0.5 mg every 5 minutes is the first-line treatment. Injection in a large muscle, usually the lateral thigh, results in better absorption of the medication.

- In patients who take oral or use ophthalmic β-blockers and who do not respond to epinephrine, intravenous glucagon should be given at a dose of 1–5 mg in adults, followed by an infusion at a rate of 5–15 μg/min titrated to clinical response.
- Intravenous fluids should be initiated to maintain adequate perfusion.
- Other supportive measures could be considered as second-line therapy. These include oxygen use, H1 and H2 antihistamines for the treatment of hives, and albuterol for the treatment of bronchospasm.
- Corticosteroids are not useful for the acute treatment of anaphylaxis but may be effective in preventing biphasic or protracted anaphylaxis.

SPECIAL CONSIDERATIONS

- Disposition is based on the patient's clinical condition. Patients with anaphylaxis should be observed in the emergency department for at least 6 hours after stabilization. Patients with angioedema requiring intubation should be admitted to the intensive care unit. All patients with angioedema should be observed for a period of time to ensure that the airway is not being compromised. Patients with rhinitis or isolated urticaria can be discharged home with follow-up with a primary care physician.

SUGGESTED READINGS

Ayars AG, Altman MC. Pharmacologic therapies in pulmonology and allergy. *Med Clin North Am* 2016;100(4):851–68. doi:10.1016/j.mcna.2016.03.010.

Franzese CB, Burkhalter NW. The patient with allergies. *Med Clin North Am* 2010;94(5):891–902. doi:10.1016/j.mcna.2010.05.006.

Sampson HA, Muñoz-Furlong A, Campbell RL, et al. Second symposium on the definition and management of anaphylaxis: summary report—second National Institute of Allergy and Infectious Disease/Food Allergy and Anaphylaxis Network symposium. *Ann Emerg Med* 2006;47(4):373–80.

Simons FE, Ebisawa M, Sanchez-Borges M, et al. 2015 update of the evidence base: World Allergy Organization anaphylaxis guidelines. *World Allergy Organ J* 2015;8(1):32. doi:10.1186/s40413-015-0080-1. eCollection 2015.

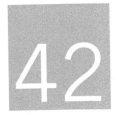

Antimicrobial Selection and Stewardship in the Emergency Department

Diana Zhong and Stephen Y. Liang

Antimicrobial Therapy

GENERAL PRINCIPLES

- Appropriate and timely initiation of antimicrobial therapy in the ED reduces morbidity and mortality.
- Optimizing the use of existing antimicrobials in the ED not only maximizes their intended effect but can safeguard against the development of antimicrobial resistance.

Approach to Infection in the Emergency Department

- A reasonable clinical suspicion for infection should drive any decision to start antimicrobial therapy.
- Rapid diagnostic tests for viral pathogens (e.g., influenza) can aid in identifying common respiratory infections unlikely to benefit from antibacterial agents.
- Whenever feasible, microbiologic cultures should be obtained from the suspected site(s) of infection (e.g., urine, blood, wound) before antimicrobials are administered, particularly in patients with moderate to severe disease requiring hospital admission.[1]

Antimicrobial Therapy in Emergency Care

- Antibiotic usage should take into account the following:
  - Spectrum of antimicrobial coverage
    - For mild-to-moderate infections, narrow-spectrum antibiotic coverage targeting the most likely causative microorganism is recommended (e.g., *Escherichia coli* for urinary tract infection).
    - For severe infection or in critically ill patients, broad-spectrum antimicrobial therapy is warranted and should cover both gram-positive and gram-negative bacteria (including *Pseudomonas aeruginosa*).
      - In the setting of chronic comorbid diseases (e.g., diabetes mellitus, chronic kidney disease), immunosuppression, or suspected health care–associated infection, empiric coverage should also include multidrug-resistant organisms (e.g., methicillin-resistant *Staphylococcus aureus*, vancomycin-resistant *Enterococcus*, multidrug-resistant gram-negative bacilli).
      - Empiric antifungal coverage may be considered in patients with significant risk factors for invasive candidiasis (e.g., central venous catheter, total parenteral nutrition, hemodialysis, prior broad-spectrum antibiotics, gastrointestinal procedures, and immunocompromised state).
    - Institutional and/or ED-specific antibiograms can aid empiric antimicrobial selection, particularly when common organisms are suspected (e.g., *S. aureus*, *E. coli*, *P. aeruginosa*).
    - Prior microbiologic culture data in patients with recurrent infections including antibiotic resistance profiles can also inform antimicrobial selection.
  - Adequate dosing to achieve and sustain activity
    - For mild-to-moderate infection, oral antimicrobial therapy is acceptable.
    - In critically ill patients or other patients where gastrointestinal absorption may be compromised, intravenous therapy is preferred to achieve adequate serum drug concentrations.
    - Dose adjustment may be necessary in patients presenting with impaired renal and/or hepatic function.[2]
  - Potential drug toxicity
    - Be aware of potential drug–drug interactions with the patient's home medications or other medications administered in the ED.
    - In the setting of acute kidney injury, avoid potentially nephrotoxic agents.
    - In women, antimicrobial selection should factor in pregnancy and active breastfeeding.
      - Category B antimicrobials are considered safe in most instances (penicillins, cephalosporins, macrolides).
        - Metronidazole is generally considered safe to use in pregnancy. There is a theoretical risk in the first trimester because it crosses the placenta, but it can be given in all trimesters.[3]

- Categories C (trimethoprim–sulfamethoxazole [TMP–SMX], fluoroquinolones, aminoglycosides) and D antimicrobials (tetracyclines) are generally not recommended in pregnancy.
  - Generally, penicillins and cephalosporins are always safe. Cephalexin should be dosed qid in pregnant women.
  - Avoid oral fluconazole in early pregnancy due to reports of first trimester miscarriage. Instead, use topical agents such as topical metronidazole.
  - Avoid TMP/SMX in the first trimester and near term. TMP/SMX causes inhibition of the folate pathway, which is associated with spina bifida.
  - Avoid nitrofurantoin near term due to G6PD-related hemolytic anemia and therefore hyperbilirubinemia.
  - Obstetrics consultation should be considered to weigh risks and benefits of antimicrobial use in situations where no safe options are available.[3] Sulfonamides and nitrofurantoins should still be used as first-line therapy during third-trimester infections when appropriate.
- Early administration
  - For severe infection or in patients who are critically ill, antimicrobial therapy should be started after microbiologic cultures have been obtained. However, if the patient is clinically or hemodynamically unstable, cultures should not significantly delay therapy.
- Shortest treatment duration clinically acceptable
  - For most uncomplicated infections treated on an outpatient basis, the shortest duration of antimicrobial therapy indicated to treat the infection is preferred.
  - Decisions to treat for longer durations should be made in collaboration with the patient's primary care provider or an infectious disease specialist.

Antimicrobial Stewardship

GENERAL PRINCIPLES

- Antimicrobial stewardship seeks to optimize clinical outcomes, minimize antimicrobial-associated adverse events (e.g., medication toxicity, *Clostridium difficile* infection), and reduce selection pressure for antimicrobial resistance.[4]
- The Centers for Disease Control and Prevention (CDC) estimates that anywhere from 20% to 50% of all antibiotics prescribed in US acute care hospitals are either unnecessary or inappropriate.[5]
- Antimicrobial stewardship may also reduce health care costs by decreasing drug utilization and preventing antimicrobial-resistant infections and other complications of antimicrobial use.
- Antimicrobial therapy is frequently initiated or prescribed in the ED for a range of diseases based on varying degrees of suspicion for infection, and empiric therapy started in the ED often continues well into the course of a hospital admission.[6,7]
- On a day-to-day basis, a rational approach to antimicrobial stewardship in the ED at the bedside should take into consideration the following:
  - Acute respiratory tract infections
    - Avoid prescribing antibiotics for the common cold, nasopharyngitis, acute rhinosinusitis, otitis media, acute uncomplicated bronchitis or bronchiolitis, viral pneumonia, or influenza.[2]
    - Studies show that patients respond positively to education and guidance about managing viral illness without the prescription of antibiotics.[8]

- Recognize that the majority of pharyngitis cases are caused by viruses.
  - Apply the Centor score (one point each for fever, absence of cough, tonsillar exudates, swollen or tender anterior cervical lymph nodes) or the modified Centor score (add one point for ages 3–14, subtract one point for age > 45). Avoid Rapid Antigen Detection Test (RADT) testing for group A *Streptococcus* or prescribing antibiotics for scores of 0 and 1. Treat only positive RADTs for scores of 2 or greater.[9,10]
- In sinusitis, bacterial infections should generally be considered only if the patient has a high fever (≥39°C), persistent symptoms (>10 days), or worsening of symptoms.[11]
- Skin and soft tissue infections
  - Uncomplicated skin abscesses do not require antibiotic treatment after successful bedside incision and drainage.[12]
  - Utilize oral antibiotics for mild uncomplicated cellulitis and reserve parenteral antibiotics for patients with signs of systemic toxicity and rapid progression of erythema, patients who are immunocompromised, or patients who have progression of symptoms despite 48–72 hours of oral therapy.[12]
- Urinary tract infections (UTIs)
  - Avoid treatment of asymptomatic bacteriuria except in pregnant women or those undergoing a urologic procedure where mucosal bleeding is anticipated.
  - Consider alternative causes of asymptomatic bacteriuria (sexually transmitted illnesses).[13]

REFERENCES

1. Dellinger RP, Levy MM, Rhodes A, et al. Surviving sepsis campaign: international guidelines for management of severe sepsis and septic shock, 2012. *Intensive Care Med* 2013;39(2):165–228.
2. Trinh T, Klinker K. Antimicrobial Stewardship in the Emergency Department. *Infect Dis Ther* 2015;4(Suppl 1):39–50.
3. American College of Obstetricians and Gynecologists Committee on Obstetric Practice. ACOG Committee Opinion No. 494: Sulfonamides, nitrofurantoin, and risk of birth defects. *Obstet Gynecol* 2011;117(6):1484–85.
4. Dellit TH, Owens RC, McGowan JE Jr, et al. Infectious Diseases Society of America and the Society for Healthcare Epidemiology of America guidelines for developing an institutional program to enhance antimicrobial stewardship. *Clin Infect Dis* 2007;44(2):159–77.
5. CDC. Core Elements of Hospital Antibiotic Stewardship Programs. 2015. Available at: http://www.cdc.gov/getsmart/healthcare/implementation/core-elements.html
6. Percival KM, Valenti KM, Schmittling SE, et al. Impact of an antimicrobial stewardship intervention on urinary tract infection treatment in the ED. *Am J Emerg Med* 2015;33(9):1129–33.
7. Borde JP, Kern WV, Hug M, et al. Implementation of an intensified antibiotic stewardship programme targeting third-generation cephalosporin and fluoroquinolone use in an emergency medicine department. *Emerg Med J* 2015;32(7):509–15.
8. Ong S, Nakase J, Moran GJ, et al. Antibiotic use for emergency department patients with upper respiratory infections: prescribing practices, patient expectations, and patient satisfaction. *Ann Emerg Med* 2007;50(3):213–20.
9. Centor RM, Witherspoon JM, Dalton HP, et al. The diagnosis of strep throat in adults in the emergency room. *Med Decis Making* 1981;1(3):239–46.
10. Fine AM, Nizet V, Mandl KD. Large-scale validation of the Centor and McIsaac scores to predict group A streptococcal pharyngitis. *Arch Intern Med* 2012;172(11):847–52.

11. Chow AW, Benninger MS, Brook I, et al. IDSA clinical practice guideline for acute bacterial rhinosinusitis in children and adults. *Clin Infect Dis* 2012;54(8):e72–112.
12. Stevens DL, Bisno AL, Chambers HF, et al. Practice guidelines for the diagnosis and management of skin and soft tissue infections: 2014 update by the Infectious Diseases Society of America. *Clin Infect Dis* 2014;59(2):e10–52.
13. Hecker MT, Fox CJ, Son AH, et al. Effect of a stewardship intervention on adherence to uncomplicated cystitis and pyelonephritis guidelines in an emergency department setting. *PLoS One* 2014;9(2):e87899.
14. Nicolle LE, Bradley S, Colgan R, et al. Infectious Diseases Society of America guidelines for the diagnosis and treatment of asymptomatic bacteriuria in adults. *Clin Infect Dis* 2005;40(5):643–54.

Infectious Emergencies: Emerging Infectious Diseases

Diana Zhong and Stephen Y. Liang

GENERAL PRINCIPLES

- Several factors contribute to the emergence of new infectious diseases:
  - Changes in demographics and behavior (e.g., changes in host susceptibility, risky behavior, environmental exposures)
  - Environmental and land use change (e.g., climate, ecosystem)
  - Breakdown of public health measures (e.g., social upheaval, social inequality, poverty, famine)
  - Microbial adaptation (e.g., increased virulence, microbial resistance)
  - International travel and commerce
  - Changes in technology and industry (e.g., food storage)
- Maintain awareness and high clinical suspicion for emerging infectious diseases.
- Solicit travel history when appropriate.
- Contact local/state health department when clinical suspicion is high for an emerging infection.

EMERGING VIRAL INFECTIONS

Zika Virus

GENERAL PRINCIPLES

- *Flavivirus* genus (same as dengue, yellow fever, and West Nile virus)[1]

- Transmission:
  - Vector-borne: *Aedes aegypti* (tropics, subtropics), *Aedes albopictus* (temperate)[1]
  - Nonvector-borne: vertical transmission during pregnancy, less commonly through blood transfusion and sexual intercourse[1]

Epidemiology

- Currently prevalent in South and Central America. Refer to the CDC Web site for updated territories of active Zika transmission.[2,3]

Clinical Presentation

- Most common symptoms: macular and/or papular rash, low-grade fever, arthralgia and arthritis, nonpurulent conjunctivitis, myalgia, headache, edema, and vomiting.[4]
- Usually mild, self-limited illness lasting 2–7 days. Rash or arthralgias can persist for over 2 weeks. Severe or fatal disease is uncommon.[4]

Complications

- Fetal microcephaly and/or ophthalmic abnormalities. Highest risk if infection occurs during first trimester of pregnancy
- Association with Guillain–Barré syndrome.[5]

Diagnosis and Testing

- Testing can be performed with RT-PCR or ELISA for Zika IgM antibody.[6]
- Guidelines are dynamic, and all suspected cases warrant CDC consultation.
- Differential diagnosis should include dengue, chikungunya, and malaria, which have overlapping clinical presentations, modes of transmission, endemic areas.

Management

- Supportive care including hydration and rest. Acetaminophen can be used as an analgesic and antipyretic. Aspirin and nonsteroidal anti-inflammatory drugs (NSAIDs) should be avoided until dengue or other hemorrhagic fevers are ruled out.[7]

Chikungunya

GENERAL PRINCIPLES

- *Togaviridae* family, *Alphavirus* genus[8]
- Transmission: *A. aegypti* and *A. albopictus*[8]

Epidemiology

- Most prevalent in the Caribbean and Central America; however, cases have been reported throughout the world.[9,10]

Clinical Presentation

- The mean incubation period is 3 days, and acute infection lasts 1 week.[8,11]
- The presentation typically begins with high-grade fevers (over 39°C) followed by severe myalgias and polyarthralgias. Fevers typically last 1 week. Other symptoms include rash (usually maculopapular), headache, and asthenia.[8]
- Arthralgias are usually polyarticular and symmetric. Frequently involves distal joints including the interphalangeal joints, wrists, and ankles.[8]

Complications
- Many patients develop persistent and debilitating polyarthritis and tenosynovitis.[12]
- Severe cases can result in encephalopathy and encephalitis, myocarditis, hepatitis, and multiorgan failure.[8]

Diagnosis
- IgM antibodies are usually detectable 3–8 days after symptom onset and can persist for weeks to months. IgG antibodies usually appear 4–10 days after symptom onset and can persist for years. Acute illness can also be detected by viral culture after 3 days and RT-PCR.[8,13]

Management
- Supportive care for acute infection[14]

EBOLA AND OTHER VIRAL HEMORRHAGIC FEVERS (VHF)

Ebola Virus Disease

GENERAL PRINCIPLES[15]

- *Filoviridae* family
- Transmission
  - The main animal reservoir is the fruit bat. Other potential reservoirs include pigs and rodents. Transmission to human occurs after direct contact with infected tissues or bodily fluids.
  - Human-to-human transmission occurs through direct contact with infected tissues or bodily fluids.

Epidemiology
- Most prominent in West Africa, though cases have been reported worldwide.

Clinical Presentation
- Incubation period typically 5–7 days.
- There is an early febrile phase, usually in the first 3 days of symptoms. This includes nonspecific symptoms such as fever, malaise, fatigue, and body aches.
- There is a subsequent gastrointestinal phase in the first 3–10 days, comprised of epigastric pain, nausea, vomiting, and diarrhea. This can also be associated with other nonspecific symptoms such as persistent fever, asthenia, headache, conjunctivitis, chest pain, abdominal pain, arthralgias, myalgias, hiccups, and delirium.
- During days 7–12, the patient will either worsen and develop shock or mount a clinical recovery.
  - The shock phase includes diminished consciousness or coma, tachycardia, hypotension, tachypnea, and oliguria or anuria.
- After 10 days, if there is no recovery, complications can include gastrointestinal hemorrhage, secondary infections, meningoencephalitis, and neurocognitive abnormalities.[15]

Diagnosis

- RT-PCR is the standard diagnostic test.[15,16]

Management

- Supportive care
- Limited research on the benefit of existing antivirals and vaccines or blood product transfusion
- Prevent further transmission by isolating patients and monitoring contacts

Other Viral Hemorrhagic Fevers

GENERAL PRINCIPLES

- *Arenaviridae* (Lassa, Argentine, Bolivian, Venezuelan)
- *Bunyaviridae* (hantavirus—hemorrhagic fever with renal syndrome—HFRS, Congo-Crimean, Rift Valley)
- *Filoviridae* (Ebola, Marburg)
- *Flaviviridae* (dengue, yellow fever, Omsk hemorrhagic fever, Kyasanur Forest disease)

DIAGNOSIS

- Laboratory assays vary and require biosafety level 4 containment capability.

TREATMENT

- Antiviral treatments only as investigational drugs. IV ribavirin can be helpful in some cases (*Bunyaviridae, Arenaviridae*—Lassa, Crimean-Congo, Old World hantavirus), convalescent plasma—Argentine or Bolivia.

Prevention

- Only licensed vaccine is 17D yellow fever vaccine.

Clinical Presentation

- Fever, flushing of face and chest, petechiae, frank bleeding, edema, hypotension, shock, malaise, myalgias, headache, vomiting, diarrhea

MERS-CoV

Presentation

- Fevers, chills, cough, shortness of breath, myalgias, diarrhea, vomiting, hemoptysis, sore throat.[17] Many patients experience severe illness including pneumonia, ARDS, AKI, GI symptoms, pericarditis, and DIC.
- Suspect in patients with fever and pneumonia or ARDS and travel from countries in or near the Arabian peninsula (or other confirmed MERS-CoV area) within 14 days before symptom onset, or close contact with such individuals.[18]

Diagnosis and Testing

- Abnormalities on chest radiography are variable but nearly always present.[19]
- Collect all of the following: lower respiratory tract specimens (sputum, endotracheal aspirate, bronchoalveolar lavage), upper respiratory tract specimens, serum

specimens for rRT-PCR, a serum serology sample if symptom onset was 14 or more days ago.[20]

Pandemic, Swine, and Avian Flu

Avian flu[17,21]

- Novel influenza A viruses with the potential to cause severe illness in humans, including strains of Asian-lineage avian influenza A (H5N2), (H5N8), and (H5N1)
- Consider the diagnosis in patients with influenzalike illness and acute respiratory infection who have had recent contact with sick or dead birds.
- Highly pathogenic avian influenza (HPAI) H5 infection can begin with signs and symptoms of uncomplicated seasonal influenza such as fever, upper respiratory tract symptoms, and myalgias. It can progress to pneumonia and more severe illness including multiorgan failure, encephalitis, and septic shock.
- To date, no human infections with HPAI H5 viruses have been identified in the United States.

Swine flu[22]

- Variant strains of swine flu have been known to cause disease in humans, including H1N1v, H3N2v, and H1N2v. Such strains have been detected in the United States.
- Suspect in individuals with exposure to infected pigs, such as pigs at a fair or workers in the swine industry.
- The vast majority of strains do not result in person-to-person spread but warrant further CDC investigation.

ANTIMICROBIAL RESISTANCE

MRSA

- Suspect methicillin-resistant *Staphylococcus aureus* (MRSA) in skin and soft tissue infections when there is an abscess or pus.[23]
- Treat symptomatic infections, not colonization.
- Common oral agents for MRSA include trimethoprim-sulfamethoxazole (TMP-SMX), clindamycin, and doxycycline. These agents are commonly used to empirically treat skin and soft tissue infections.

Vancomycin-Resistant *Enterococcus* (VRE)

- Treat symptomatic infections, not colonization.
- Symptomatic and severe infections will require agents such as linezolid, daptomycin, tigecycline, telavancin, and quinupristin–dalfopristin.[24]

REFERENCES

1. Waggoner JJ, Pinsky BA. Zika Virus: diagnostics for an emerging pandemic threat. *J Clin Microbiol* 2016;54(4):860–7.
2. CDC. All Countries and Territories with Active Zika Virus Transmission. 2016. Available at: http://www.cdc.gov/zika/geo/active-countries.html
3. CDC. Areas with Zika. 2016. Available at: http://www.cdc.gov/zika/geo/index.html
4. Duffy MR, Chen TH, Hancock WT, et al. Zika virus outbreak on Yap Island, Federated States of Micronesia. *N Engl J Med* 2009;360(24):2536–43.

5. Bautista LE, Sethi AK. Association between Guillain-Barre syndrome and Zika virus infection. *Lancet* 2016;387(10038):2599–600.
6. CDC. Zika Virus—Diagnostic Testing. 2016. Available at: http://www.cdc.gov/zika/hc-providers/diagnostic.html
7. Zika Virus—Treatment. 2016. Available at: http://www.cdc.gov/zika/symptoms/treatment.html
8. Weaver SC, Lecuit M. Chikungunya virus and the global spread of a mosquito-borne disease. *N Engl J Med* 2015;372(13):1231–9.
9. CDC. Chikungunya Virus—Geographic Distribution. 2016. Available at: http://www.cdc.gov/chikungunya/geo/index.html
10. Gibney KB, Fischer M, Prince HE, et al. Chikungunya fever in the United States: a fifteen year review of cases. *Clin Infect Dis* 2011;52(5):e121–6.
11. Rudolph KE, Lessler J, Moloney RM, et al. Incubation periods of mosquito-borne viral infections: a systematic review. *Am J Trop Med Hyg* 2014;90(5):882–91.
12. Assiri A, Al-Tawfiq JA, Al-Rabeeah AA, et al. Epidemiological, demographic, and clinical characteristics of 47 cases of Middle East respiratory syndrome coronavirus disease from Saudi Arabia: a descriptive study. *Lancet Infect Dis* 2013;13(9):752–61.
13. CDC. Chikungunya Virus—Diagnostic Testing. 2016. Available at: http://www.cdc.gov/chikungunya/hc/diagnostic.html
14. CDC. *Chikungunya Virus—Clinical Evaluation & Disease.* Atlanta, 2015.
15. Kanapathipillai R. Ebola virus disease—current knowledge. *N Engl J Med* 2014;371(13):e18.
16. Chertow DS, Kleine C, Edwards JK, et al. Ebola virus disease in West Africa—clinical manifestations and management. *N Engl J Med* 2014;371(22):2054–7.
17. CDC. Interim Guidance on Testing, Specimen Collection, and Processing for Patients with Suspected Infection with Novel Influenza A Viruses with the Potential to Cause Severe Disease in Humans. 2016. Available at: http://www.cdc.gov/flu/avianflu/severe-potential.htm
18. CDC. Middle East Respiratory Syndrome (MERS)—Interim Guidance for Healthcare Professionals. 2015. Available at: http://www.cdc.gov/coronavirus/mers/interim-guidance.html
19. Chan JF, Lau SK, To KK, et al. Middle East respiratory syndrome coronavirus: another zoonotic betacoronavirus causing SARS-like disease. *Clin Microbiol Rev* 2015;28(2):465–522.
20. CDC. Interim Guidelines for Collecting, Handling, and Testing Clinical Specimens from Patients Under Investigation (PUIs) for Middle East Respiratory Syndrome Coronavirus (MERS-CoV) 2015. Available at: http://www.cdc.gov/coronavirus/mers/guidelines-clinical-specimens.html
21. CDC. HPAI A H5 Virus Background and Clinical Illness. 2015. Available at: http://www.cdc.gov/flu/avianflu/hpai/hpai-background-clinical-illness.htm
22. CDC. *Variant (Swine Origin) Influenza Viruses in Humans.* Atlanta, 2014.
23. Dellit TH, Owens RC, McGowan JE Jr, et al. Infectious Diseases Society of America and the Society for Healthcare Epidemiology of America guidelines for developing an institutional program to enhance antimicrobial stewardship. *Clin Infect Dis* 2007;44(2):159–77.
24. O'Driscoll T, Crank CW. Vancomycin-resistant enterococcal infections: epidemiology, clinical manifestations, and optimal management. *Infect Drug Resist* 2015;8:217–30.
25. Zeana C, Kelly P, Heredia W, et al. Post-chikungunya rheumatic disorders in travelers after return from the Caribbean. *Travel Med Infect Dis* 2016;14(1):21–5.

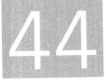

44 Infectious Emergencies: Infections in the Immunocompromised Patient

Julianne S. Dean and Stephen Y. Liang

GENERAL PRINCIPLES

Neutropenic Fever

- Neutropenia is common in patients undergoing chemotherapy or presenting with a primary hematologic malignancy.
- Neutropenic fever is defined as an absolute neutrophil count (ANC) of <500 cells/mm³ or <1000 cells/mm³ and the presence of a single temperature of ≥38.3°C (101°F) or a persistent temperature of ≥38.0°C (100.4°F) for ≥1 hour.
- Infection should always be considered high on the differential diagnosis.
- Early empiric antimicrobial therapy is critical to reduce mortality, preferentially after appropriate microbiologic cultures (e.g., blood, urine) have been obtained.
  - Depending on local antimicrobial resistance patterns, monotherapy with an antipseudomonal cephalosporin (cefepime), beta-lactam (piperacillin–tazobactam), or carbapenem (meropenem, imipenem/cilastatin) for broad gram-negative coverage is recommended.
  - Gram-positive coverage (commonly achieved with the addition of vancomycin) should be considered in the setting of sepsis or other hemodynamic instability, pneumonia, skin or soft tissue infection, gram-positive bacteremia, or suspected central line–associated bloodstream infection (CLABSI).
  - Antifungal therapy is not recommended in the emergency department.
  - Empiric antiviral therapy is not recommended unless characteristic skin or cutaneous lesions suggestive of herpes simplex virus (HSV) or varicella zoster virus (VZV) infection are identified or active influenza is known to be circulating in the community.

SOLID ORGAN TRANSPLANTATION

- The risk for different types of infection after solid organ transplantation can be broken into three phases of immunosuppression based on time since transplant.
  - First month: surgical and health care–associated infections
  - 1 to 6 months: opportunistic infections with bacterial or fungal superinfection
  - Greater than 6 months: community-acquired infections; opportunistic infections if high-level immunosuppression persists

HEMATOPOIETIC STEM CELL TRANSPLANTATION

- Infections following hematopoietic stem cell transplantation (HSCT) can also be divided into three phases of immunosuppression based on time since transplant.
  - Less than 3 weeks: bacterial and fungal infections
  - Three weeks to three months: opportunistic infections (particularly in the setting of acute graft versus host disease requiring profound immunosuppression)
  - Greater than 6 months: community-acquired infections; opportunistic infections in patients with chronic graft versus host disease

ASPLENIA

- Patients with functional asplenia (e.g., sickle cell disease, splenic artery thrombosis, parasitic infection) or who have undergone splenectomy or splenic embolization due to trauma are at increased risk for severe infection due to encapsulated organisms including *Streptococcus pneumoniae*, *Neisseria meningitidis*, and *Haemophilus influenzae*.

BIOLOGIC AGENTS

- Standard and high-dose biologic agents with or without disease-modifying antirheumatic drugs (DMARD) increase the risk of infection.
- Patients with untreated latent *Mycobacterium tuberculosis* infection are susceptible to developing active disease after initiation of a TNF antagonist.
- Infections due to opportunistic organisms (*Toxoplasma gondii*, endemic fungi, *Pneumocystis jirovecii*), *Legionella pneumophila*, *Listeria monocytogenes*, *Nocardia*, and *Actinomyces* as well as nontuberculous mycobacteria should be considered.

HUMAN IMMUNODEFICIENCY VIRUS

- The risk for opportunistic infections in patients with human immunodeficiency virus (HIV) can stratified by CD4+ lymphocyte cell count, when available.
  - CD4+ < 200 cells/mm^3: *P. jirovecii*, *Histoplasma capsulatum*
  - CD4+ < 100 cells/mm^3: *T. gondii*, *Cryptococcus neoformans*
  - CD4+ < 50 cells/mm^3: *Mycobacterium avium complex* (MAC), CMV, EBV, VZV, JC polyomavirus (progressive multifocal leukoencephalopathy)
- Infections due to common community-acquired bacteria and *M. tuberculosis* can occur at any CD4+ count.
- As high as 15% of patients recently started on antiretroviral therapy (ART) for HIV may develop immune reconstitution inflammatory syndrome (IRIS), characterized by worsening or reactivation of opportunistic infections (e.g., *P. jirovecii*, *C. neoformans*, JC polyomavirus, mycobacteria).
  - Risk factors include ART following treatment for an opportunistic infection, lower CD4+ count at time of initiation of ART (CD4+ < 100), rapid reduction in HIV viral load following initiation, and use of ritonavir-boosted protease inhibitors or integrase inhibitors.

SUGGESTED READINGS

Akgun K, Miller R. Critical care in human immunodeficiency virus infected patients. *Semin Respir Crit Care Med* 2016;37:303–17.

Corona A, Raimondi F. Caring for HIV-infected patients in the ICU in the highly active antiretroviral therapy era. *Curr HIV Res* 2009;7:569–79.

Fishman JA. Infection in solid-organ transplant recipients. *N Engl J Med* 2007;357:2601–14.

Frefield AG, Bow EJ, Sepkowitz KA, et al. Clinical practice guideline for the use of antimicrobial agents in neutropenic patients with cancer: 2010 update by the Infectious Diseases Society of America. *Clin Infect Dis* 2011;52(4):e56–93.

Hiemenz JW. Management of infections complicating allogeneic hematopoietic stem cell transplantation. *Semin Hematol* 2009;46:289–312.

Linden PK. Approach to the immunocompromised host with infection in the intensive care unit. *Infect Dis Clin North Am* 2009;23:535–56.

45 Infectious Emergencies: Sepsis

Christopher Holthaus and Stephen Y. Liang

GENERAL PRINCIPLES

Definition and Classification

- Several important definitions have evolved over time, with the 3rd International Consensus Definitions for Sepsis and Septic Shock representing the most recent iteration.
- *Sepsis*:
  - "Life-threatening organ dysfunction due to a dysregulated host response to an infection."[1]
    - Evolving recommendations suggest quantifying severity of organ dysfunction using the SOFA score (sequential [sepsis-related] organ failure assessment). If SOFA score ≥2 points from baseline, the criteria for sepsis are met (Table 45.1).
    - A quick SOFA score (1 point is assigned for each of the following: altered mental status, systolic blood pressure (SBP) ≤ 100 mm Hg, respiratory rate (RR) ≥ 22 breaths/min) ≥2 points is associated with a mortality risk of 10% and should prompt evaluation for sepsis and organ dysfunction.[1]
- *Severe Sepsis*:
  - No severe sepsis definition as the most current sepsis definition is already inclusive of organ dysfunction.
- *Septic Shock*:
  - "Persisting hypotension requiring vasopressors to maintain mean arterial pressure (MAP) ≥ 65 mm Hg and having a serum lactate level >2 mmol/L despite adequate volume resuscitation"[1]

Epidemiology/Etiology

- Significant risk factors for sepsis include previous hospitalization, bacteremia, age ≥ 65, immunosuppression, diabetes, and cancer.[2]
- Patients ≥65 years of age account for the majority of sepsis patients (60–85%) with the greatest incidence during the winter.[1,2]
- The most common severe organ dysfunctions are acute respiratory distress syndrome (ARDS), acute renal failure, and disseminated intravascular coagulation (DIC).[2]

TABLE 45.1 SOFA (Sequential [Sepsis-related] Organ Failure Assessment) Score[a]

System		Score			
	0	1	2	3	4
Respiration					
PaO₂/FIO₂, mm Hg (kPa)	≥400 (53.3)	<400 (53.3)	<300 (40)	<200 (26.7) with respiratory support	<100 (13.3) with respiratory support
Coagulation					
Platelets, × 10³/μL	≥150	<150	<100	<50	<20
Liver					
Bilirubin, mg/dL (μmol/L)	<1.2 (20)	1.2–1.9 (20–32)	2.0–5.9 (33–101)	6.0–11.9 (102–204)	>12.0 (204)
Cardiovascular	MAP ≥ 70 mm Hg	MAP < 70 mm Hg	Dopamine < 5 or dobutamine (any dose)[b]	Dopamine 5.1–15 or epinephrine ≤ 0.1 or norepinephrine ≤ 0.1[b]	Dopamine > 15 or epinephrine > 0.1 or norepinephrine > 0.1[b]
Central nervous system					
Glasgow Coma Scale score[c]	15	13–14	10–12	6–9	<6
Renal					
Creatinine, mg/dL (μmol/L)	<1.2 (110)	1.2–1.9 (110–170)	2.0–3.4 (171–299)	3.5–4.9 (300–440)	>5.0 (440)
Urine output, mL/d				<500	<200

[a]Adapted from Vincent et al.[27]
[b]Catecholamine doses are given as μg/kg/min for at least 1 hour.
[c]Glasgow Coma Scale scores range from 3-15; higher score indicates better neurologic function.
FIO₂, fraction of inspired oxygen; MAP, mean arterial pressure; PaO₂, partial pressure of oxygen.

Pathophysiology

- The most current understanding of "sepsis" is that it is "life-threatening organ dysfunction due to a dysregulated host response to an infection."[1]
- Severity of infection can exist on a continuum ranging from infection without organ dysfunction to bacteremia, organ dysfunction, shock, and death.[2]
- The most frequent pathogens are gram-positive bacteria followed by gram-negative bacteria and fungi.[2]

DIAGNOSIS

Clinical Presentation

History
- Tachycardia, tachypnea, fever, hypotension, and leukocytosis are frequently present in sepsis. However, patients may also have occult presentations accompanied by varying degrees of vital signs, physical examination, and laboratory abnormalities.
- Clinical manifestations may reflect localized infection and/or subsequent organ dysfunction with progressive disease.

Physical Examination
- A thorough examination may yield findings characteristic of organ-specific infection (i.e., pneumonia, skin, and soft tissue infection).
- Evidence of significant hypoperfusion and normotensive shock ("cryptic" or occult shock) may include delayed capillary refill, cyanosis, mottling of the extremities, acute oliguria (<0.5 mL/kg/h), or absent bowel sounds (ileus).

Differential Diagnosis

- Systemic inflammatory response syndrome due to noninfectious etiologies
- Other types of shock
- Endocrinopathies (i.e., thyroid, adrenal)
- Overdose, toxic, and withdrawal syndromes
- Environmental exposure

Diagnostic Criteria and Testing

Laboratories
- A complete blood cell count may be notable for leukocytosis (WBC > 12,000/μL), leukopenia (WBC < 4000/μL), or a normal WBC with bandemia (>10%). Thrombocytopenia (platelet count < 100,000/μL) may be present.
- Laboratory evidence of organ dysfunction may include elevated creatinine (Cr > 2.0 mg/dL), hyperglycemia (plasma glucose > 110 mg/dL), coagulopathy (INR > 1.5), and hyperbilirubinemia (total bilirubin > 4 mg/dL).
- Elevated serum lactate and lactic acidosis are indications of significant tissue hypoperfusion.
- Obtain microbiologic culture from suspected site(s) of infection.

Imaging
- Chest radiography can help identify pulmonary infections and alternate etiologies for hypoxia.
- Bedside echocardiography can help to evaluate cardiac function and assist in gauging the likelihood of volume tolerance during fluid resuscitation.
- Computed tomography and ultrasound can aid with the identification of infection.

TREATMENT

- Resuscitation
  - Fluid resuscitation should consist initially of crystalloid (≥30 mL/kg bolus in the setting of hypoperfusion with suspicion for hypovolemia). Albumin may be considered if substantial volumes of crystalloid have been administered; avoid hydroxyethyl starch. Continue fluid challenges as long as there is hemodynamic improvement.[3]
  - Resuscitation should be centered on optimization of oxygen delivery and utilization. This is accomplished through adequate preload, afterload, cardiac contractility, hemoglobin, and reduced demand (source control, pain, agitation, fever, shivering, work of breathing).
  - Commonly used quantitative markers of organ perfusion include vital signs (MAP > 65 mm Hg, improvements in heart rate and respiratory rate), physical examination (capillary refill <2 seconds, improved pulses, decreased pallor), lactate clearance (≥10%), $ScvO_2$ (≥70%), and urine output (≥0.5 mL/kg/h).[6]
- Source Control
  - Incision and drainage, surgical debridement, removal of infected hardware (i.e., vascular catheters, urinary catheters, other medical devices) within 12 hours.

Medications

- Antibiotics
  - Early administration of antimicrobials (generally <3 hours, <1 hour if shock) is paramount.
  - Tailor antimicrobial selection to the most likely pathogen(s) and affected organ(s). Modify based on medical comorbidities and risk factors for health care–associated infection.
- Vasopressors[3]
  - Norepinephrine (5–20 μg/min)[4]: first-choice vasopressor.
  - Epinephrine (5–20 μg/min)[4]: can be added to or potentially substituted for norepinephrine when another agent is needed to maintain adequate MAP.
  - Vasopressin (up to 0.03 U/min): can be added to norepinephrine with the intent of raising MAP to target or decreasing norepinephrine dosage but should not be used alone
  - Dopamine (2–20 μg/kg/min)[4]: should only be used as an alternative to norepinephrine in highly select patients (i.e., low risk of tachyarrhythmias and absolute or relative bradycardia)
  - Phenylephrine (2–20 μg/min)[4]: not recommended except when (a) norepinephrine is associated with serious arrhythmias, (b) cardiac output is known to be high and blood pressure persistently low, or (c) salvage therapy when combined inotrope/vasopressors and low-dose vasopressin has failed to achieve target MAP
- Inotropes[3]
  - A trial of dobutamine (maximum 20 μg/kg/min) can be considered in the presence of (a) myocardial dysfunction or (b) ongoing signs of hypoperfusion despite adequate intravascular volume and adequate MAP.
- Steroids[3]
  - Consider adding intravenous hydrocortisone (200 mg/d continuous flow) if adequate fluid resuscitation and vasopressor therapy are not able to restore hemodynamic stability. Do not use the (adrenocorticotropic hormone) ACTH stimulation test to identify who should receive hydrocortisone.

Other Nonpharmacologic Therapies[3]

- Blood product administration
  - Transfuse packed red blood cells if hemoglobin < 7 g/dL to a target of 7–9 g/dL unless myocardial ischemia, severe hypoxemia, acute hemorrhage, or ischemic heart disease.
  - Transfuse platelets if (a) platelets < 10,000/μL, (b) <20,000/μL and risk for bleeding, or (c) <50,000/μL and active bleeding, surgery, or invasive procedures.
- Mechanical ventilation of sepsis-induced ARDS
  - A target tidal volume of 6 mL/kg of predicted body weight and goal plateau pressure ≤30 cm H_2O are recommended.
  - Favor higher positive end expiratory pressures (PEEP) with moderate to severe ARDS.
  - Elevate head of bed to 30–45 degrees to reduce the risk of aspiration.
  - Conservative rather than liberal fluid strategy with ARDS who do not have tissue hypoperfusion.
- Sedation, Analgesia, Neuromuscular Blockade Agents (NMBA) in Intubated Patients
  - Minimize sedation targeting specific titration endpoints.
  - Avoid NMBAs whenever possible.
- Glucose Control
  - If two consecutive levels are >180 mg/dL, target goal to 110–180 mg/dL.
  - Monitor levels every 1–2 hours until stable then recheck every 4 hours.

SPECIAL CONSIDERATIONS

Disposition
- Patients with shock and/or poor functional reserve should be admitted to the ICU.

REFERENCES

1. Singer M, Deutschman CS, Seymour C, et al. The third international consensus definitions for sepsis and septic shock (sepsis-3). *JAMA* 2016;315(8):801–10.
2. Remi Neviere MD. Sepsis syndromes in adults: epidemiology, definitions, clinical presentation, diagnosis, and prognosis. *UpToDate* 2016. (last accessed 07/15/16).
3. Dellinger RP, Levy MM, Rhodes A, et al. Surviving sepsis campaign: international guidelines for management of severe sepsis and septic shock: 2012. *Crit Care Med* 2013;41(2): 580–637.
4. Shapiro NI, Zimmer GD, Barkin AZ. Sepsis Syndromes. *Rosen's Emergency Medicine—Concepts and Clinical Practice*. Philadelphia: Elsevier, 2014:1864–73.
5. Jones AE, Brown MD, Trzeciak S, et al. The effect of a quantitative resuscitation strategy on mortality in patients with sepsis: a meta-analysis. *Crit Care Med* 2008;36(10):2734–9.
6. Rivers E, Nguyen B, Havstad S, et al. Early goal-directed therapy in the treatment of severe sepsis and septic shock. *N Engl J Med* 2001;345(19):1368–77.

46

Infectious Emergencies: Sexually Transmitted Diseases (STDs)

SueLin M. Hilbert

GENERAL PRINCIPLES

- Workup for patients presenting with pelvic or genitourinary (GU) complaints may include the following:
  - A complete genital exam, urinalysis, screening for HIV, gonorrhea, and syphilis
  - For women: wet prep microscopy and urine hCG

Epidemiology/Etiology

- Estimated 20 million new sexually transmitted infections in the United States each year
  - Half occur in young people 15–24 years old.
- Risk factors include multiple partners or a new partner, previous or coexisting sexually transmitted diseases (STD), and community prevalence of particular infections.

Differential Diagnoses

- Females: bacterial vaginosis, candidiasis, physiologic discharge, gonorrhea, or chlamydia
- Males: urethritis, prostatitis, gonorrhea, or chlamydia

SPECIAL CONSIDERATIONS

- Expedited Partner Therapy (EPT) or Patient-Delivered Partner Therapy (PDPT)
  - Refers to the practice of prescribing medications to treat the sexual partners of patients diagnosed with an STD—specifically gonorrhea or chlamydia—without examining them
  - Also referred to as "Patient-Delivered Partner Therapy" (PDPT)

Disposition

- Most patients can be discharged.

Complications

- Undiagnosed STDs lead to an estimated 20,000 cases of infertility among women each year as well as an increased risk of ectopic pregnancy, congenital infections and pelvic inflammatory disease (PID), Fitz-Hugh-Curtis syndrome, epididymitis, and orchitis.

Human Papillomavirus (HPV)

GENERAL PRINCIPLES

Epidemiology

- Most common cause of anogenital warts
  - Most sexually active people will become infected with HPV at least once in their lifetime and most will be asymptomatic.

- Risk factors include unprotected vaginal, anal, or oral intercourse.
  - It is possible to transmit during genital contact without penetration.

DIAGNOSIS

Clinical Presentation

History
- Typically asymptomatic but may report pruritic or painful lesions anywhere along the anogenital tract

Physical Examination
- Flat, papular, or pedunculated lesions most commonly found around vaginal introitus mucosa
  - Can also be located anywhere along the anogenital tract epithelium or mucosa

TREATMENT

- No treatment indicated in the ED

Trichomoniasis

GENERAL PRINCIPLES

Epidemiology/Etiology
- Transmitted by the protozoan *T. vaginalis.*
- Most prevalent nonviral STD in the United States.
- Infected persons are often asymptomatic.

DIAGNOSIS

Clinical Presentation

History
- Patients may report a malodorous vaginal discharge, vaginal irritation or itching, dysuria, lower abdominal pain, or dyspareunia.

Physical Examination
- Vaginal discharge (70% of patients): frothy and gray or yellow/green.
- The patient may have a "strawberry" cervix.

Diagnostic Testing

Laboratories
- Visualization of motile protozoa on wet prep microscopy

TREATMENT

- All sexual partners in the past 60 days should be evaluated, tested, and treated to prevent reinfection.

Medication
- Metronidazole 2 g PO in a single dose or 500 mg PO bid × 7 days
  - Intravaginal preparation is less efficacious and not recommended.
  - In order to avoid a disulfiram-like reaction, patients should be counseled to abstain from alcohol during and for 24 hours after completion of treatment.

SPECIAL CONSIDERATIONS

- Women who are pregnant can still be treated safely at any stage of pregnancy.
- Women who are lactating should defer breast-feeding for 12–24 hours if they receive the single-dose regimen.
- Women who are HIV+ should received the extended, 7 days, treatment.
- In pregnant women, *Trichomonas* is associated with premature rupture of membranes, preterm delivery, and delivery of low-birth-weight infants, regardless of treatment.

Gonorrhea

GENERAL PRINCIPLES

Epidemiology/Etiology
Gonorrhea is the second most commonly reported infectious disease in the United States.

DIAGNOSIS

Clinical Presentation
History
- Men may report dysuria or penile discharge.
- Women often asymptomatic or may not present until complications (i.e., PID) occur but may report vaginal discharge, dysuria, dyspareunia, abnormal vaginal bleeding, or lower abdominal pain.
- Nongenital/nonurinary symptoms include the following:
  ○ Oropharyngeal symptoms (e.g., sore throat, tonsillar swelling)
  ○ Anorectal symptoms (e.g., rectal pain or discomfort, tenesmus, purulent or mucoid anal discharge or bleeding)
  ○ Disseminated gonococcal infection (DGI) symptoms (e.g., petechial or pustular rash, mono- or polyarticular arthritis)

Physical Examination
- Urethritis/cervicitis
  ○ Men: purulent urethral discharge, meatal erythema
  ○ Women: purulent vaginal discharge
    ▪ If cervical motion and uterine or adnexal tenderness, consider PID.
- Disseminated gonococcal infection
  ○ Tender, peripheral rash comprised of necrotic pustules on an erythematous base.
  ○ Erythema, swelling, and painful range of motion (ROM) of one or more joints—most commonly knees, then elbows, ankles, wrists, and hands.

Diagnostic Testing
Laboratories
- Swab for Gram stain and culture (e.g., urethra, cervix, oropharynx, synovium, etc.)
- Nucleic acid amplification testing (NAAT) can be used for cervical, urethral, and urine samples only.

TREATMENT

- All sexual partners in the past 60 days should be evaluated, tested, and treated to prevent reinfection.
  ○ Consider EPT where permissible by law.

Medication

For patients where there is a high clinical suspicion, treat empirically.

- Coverage with azithromycin is recommended. This covers likely chlamydia coinfection.
- Uncomplicated infection (e.g., urethritis/cervicitis, prostatitis, etc.)
  - Ceftriaxone 250 mg IM as a single dose plus azithromycin 1 g PO in a single dose
    - If ceftriaxone is not available, may use cefixime 400 mg PO in a single dose.
    - If patient has a severe penicillin allergy (i.e., anaphylaxis, Stevens-Johnson syndrome, or toxic epidermal necrolysis), consult infectious disease.
- Disseminated gonococcal infection
  - Ceftriaxone 250 mg IM or IV q day plus azithromycin 1 g PO in a single dose
  - Cefotaxime 1 g IV q8 hours or ceftizoxime 1 g IV q8 hours plus azithromycin 1 g PO in a single dose

SPECIAL CONSIDERATIONS

Complications

- Pelvic inflammatory disease, epdidymitis, prostatitis, or disseminated gonococcal infection

Disposition

- Instruct patients who receive treatment in the ED to abstain from sexual activity for 7 days and until all partners are adequately treated.
- All patients with suspected DGI should be admitted to the hospital.

Chlamydia

GENERAL PRINCIPLES

Epidemiology

- Most commonly reported infectious disease in the United States
- Highest prevalence in persons <24 years

DIAGNOSIS

Clinical Presentation

History
- 50% of men and 75% of infected women are asymptomatic.
- Patients may report penile or vaginal discharge, dysuria, dyspareunia, abnormal vaginal bleeding, pelvic or lower abdominal pain, or unilateral testicular pain.

Physical Examination
- Men: mucoid or watery urethral discharge and unilateral testicular tenderness or swelling
- Women: mucoid endocervical discharge or easily induced endocervical bleeding
  - If cervical motion and uterine or adnexal tenderness is present, consider PID.

Diagnostic Testing

Laboratories
- Nucleic acid amplification testing (NAAT) of urethral/endocervical swab or first-catch urine specimens

TREATMENT

- All sexual partners in the past 60 days should be evaluated, tested, and treated to prevent reinfection.
  ○ Consider EPT where permissible by law.

Medical Management

- Azithromycin 1 g PO in a single dose or doxycycline 100 mg PO bid × 7 days
  ○ Doxycycline is contraindicated in the second and third trimesters of pregnancy.
    ▪ Alternative regimen: amoxicillin 500 mg PO tid × 7 days
- For patients where there is a high clinical suspicion, treat empirically.
- Due to high rates of gonorrheal coinfection, consider adding ceftriaxone 250 mg IM as a single dose.

Syphilis

GENERAL PRINCIPLES

Epidemiology

- Syphilis cases continue to rise particularly among women and men who have sex with men.

DIAGNOSIS

Clinical Presentation

- Divided into stages based on history and clinical findings:
  ○ Primary: presence of a painless chancre at the site of inoculation
    ▪ Lasts 2–4 weeks and then resolves spontaneously
  ○ Secondary: development of a fine, macular rash that starts on the trunk and spreads outward to include the palms and soles
    ▪ Over time, becomes more papulosquamous and resembles pityriasis rosea.
    ▪ Constitutional signs and symptoms: fever, malaise, fatigue, and generalized lymphadenopathy.
    ▪ Symptoms resolve spontaneously if not treated.
  ○ Tertiary: end-organ manifestations (e.g., thoracic aortic aneurysm, tabes dorsalis, gummas)
    ▪ Typically cardiac and neurologic
  ○ Latent: seroreactive but no clinical signs or symptoms
    ▪ "Early" if infection acquired in the last year, otherwise considered "late."

Differential Diagnoses

- Depends on stage of disease at time of diagnosis:
  ○ Primary: herpes simplex virus (HSV) and chancroid
  ○ Secondary: pityriasis rosea, Rocky Mountain spotted fever, and coxsackievirus
  ○ Tertiary: B_{12} deficiency, stroke, and malignancy

Diagnostic Testing

Laboratories

- Nontreponemal screening test: the Venereal Disease Research Laboratory (VDRL) and rapid plasma reagin (RPR)
  ○ Most commonly performed in the ED

- Definitive diagnosis requires close follow-up for confirmatory testing.
- If there are concerns for neurosyphilis, send CSF for VDRL testing.

TREATMENT

Medications
- Benzathine penicillin G 2.4 million units IM in a single dose

SPECIAL CONSIDERATIONS

Disposition
- Patients with suspected tertiary syphilis will likely need admission for further evaluation and likely neurology, ophthalmology, and/or infectious disease consultation.

Complications
- Neurosyphilis
  - Early: cranial nerve dysfunction, stroke, meningitis, and acute altered mental status
  - Late: tabes dorsalis and paresis

Pelvic Inflammatory Disease (PID)

GENERAL PRINCIPLES

- Refers to a spectrum of infection of the upper female genital tract from endometritis, salpingitis, tuboovarian abscess (TOA), and pelvic peritonitis

Epidemiology
- Sexually transmitted organisms—particularly gonorrhea and chlamydia—have been frequently implicated but can also be caused by species of normal vaginal flora, *Mycoplasma* sp. and CMV.
- Risk factors include a prior history of STD or PID and may occur in the first 3 weeks after insertion of an IUD.

DIAGNOSIS

Clinical Presentation
- PID is a clinical diagnosis.

History
- The patient may have nonspecific symptoms of abdominal or pelvic pain, fever, or pain with intercourse.

Physical Examination
- Cervical motion tenderness, uterine tenderness, or adnexal tenderness may be present on pelvic exam.
- Other findings may include fever, abnormal cervical discharge, or cervical friability.

Differential Diagnoses
- Ectopic pregnancy, ovarian cyst rupture, and ovarian torsion
- Other nongynecologic causes of abdominal pain (e.g., appendicitis, renal stone, cystitis/pyelonephritis)

Diagnostic Testing

Laboratories
- Consider CBC, CMP, and other studies as needed by consultant.

Imaging
- Transvaginal ultrasound may show tubal thickening or pelvic free fluid.
  - Similar findings may also be seen on abdominal/pelvic CT, but ultrasound is the modality of choice.

TREATMENT

Medications

- For mild to moderate cases (e.g., tolerating PO, hemodynamically stable, etc.):
  - Ceftriaxone 250 mg IM in a single dose plus doxycycline 100 mg orally twice a day for 14 days with or without metronidazole 500 mg orally twice a day for 14 days
- For moderate to severe cases (e.g., unable to tolerate PO, hemodynamically unstable, signs of peritonitis or TOA, etc.):
  - Cefotetan 2 g IV every 12 hours plus doxycycline 100 mg orally or IV every 12 hours
  - Clindamycin 900 mg IV every 8 hours plus gentamicin loading dose IV or IM (2 mg/kg), followed by a maintenance dose (1.5 mg/kg) every 8 hours

Surgical Management

- TOAs require surgical intervention.

SPECIAL CONSIDERATIONS

Disposition

- Patients should abstain from sexual activity until treatment is completed, symptoms have resolved, and partners have been adequately treated.
- Mild to moderate cases: discharge home with OB/GYN follow-up in 3 days if symptoms are not improving.
- Moderate to severe cases, pregnant patients, or patients who fail outpatient therapy should receive gynecology consultation and admission to the hospital.

SUGGESTED READINGS

http://www.cdc.gov/std/ept

Birnbaumer DM. Chapter 98: Sexually Transmitted Diseases. In: *Rosen's Emergency Medicine-Concepts and Clinical Practice.* 8th ed. Philadelphia: Elsevier, 2014:1312–25.e1.

Centers for Disease Control and Prevention. *Sexually Transmitted Disease Surveillance 2014.* Atlanta: U.S. Department of Health and Human Services, 2015.

Markowitz LE, Liu G, Hariri S, et al. Prevalence of HPV after introduction of the vaccination program in the United States. *Pediatrics* 2016 Mar; 137(3). doi:org/10.1542/peds.2015-1968.

Pelvic Inflammatory Disease—CDC Fact Sheet (Detailed). Available at: www.cdc.gov/std/pid/stdfact-pid-detailed.htm. Page last reviewed: January 24, 2014; Page last updated: May 4, 2015.

Syphilis—CDC Fact Sheet (Detailed). Available at: http://www.cdc.gov/std/syphilis/stdfact-syphilis-detailed.htm. Page last reviewed: September 24, 2015; Page last updated: July 19, 2016.

Workowski KA, Bolan GA. Sexually transmitted diseases treatment guidelines. *MMWR Recomm Rep* 2015;64(RR-03):1–137.

47

Infectious Emergencies: Tick Borne Diseases

Steven Hung and Stephen Y. Liang

GENERAL PRINCIPLES

- Tick borne infections are seasonal, peaking during the summer months when tick vectors, animal reservoirs, and humans are likely to come in close contact outdoors.
- Tick bites often go unnoticed and may not be a reliable marker of tick exposure. Compatible symptoms following recent outdoor activity in an endemic area during the appropriate season should prompt consideration of tick borne infection.
- Coinfection with more than one tick borne infection is possible.

Lyme Borreliosis (Lyme Disease)

Epidemiology/Etiology
- Lyme disease is the most common vector-borne infection in the United States.
  - Endemic to northeastern United States (from Maine to Maryland) and parts of the midwest (Minnesota, Wisconsin) and western coast (northern California and Oregon)
- The causative spirochete for Lyme disease, *Borrelia burgdorferi*, is transmitted by ticks of the *Ixodes* family.

DIAGNOSIS

Clinical Presentation
History
- An incubation period of 7–10 days follows the initial tick bite, with clinical disease presenting in the following progressive stages (when untreated):
  - Stage 1 (erythema migrans): follows incubation period after bite
    - A localized, slowly expanding, erythematous rash with central clearing may appear at the site of the tick bite.
    - Fever, malaise, fatigue, headache, arthralgias, and myalgias may accompany the rash.
  - Stage 2 (disseminated infection): days to weeks after initial infection
    - Arthralgias and muscular complaints
    - Neurologic disease (10–15%): visual complaints and dizziness
  - Stage 3 (persistent infection): weeks to months after initial infection
    - Intermittent versus persistent arthritis (60%), primarily involving large joints (e.g., knee)
    - Chronic neurologic disease: polyneuropathy and encephalopathy

Physical Examination
- Stage 1 (erythema migrans): follows incubation period after bite
  - A localized, slowly expanding, erythematous rash with central clearing may appear at the site of the tick bite.

215

- Stage 2:
  - Multiple erythema migrans lesions may appear.
  - Neurologic disease (10–15%): lymphocytic meningitis and/or encephalitis, unilateral/bilateral facial nerve palsy, cerebellar ataxia, myelitis, and mononeuritis multiplex.
- Stage 3:
  - Intermittent versus persistent arthritis (60%), primarily involving large joints (e.g., knee)

Differential Diagnosis

- *Borrelia mayonii* and *Borrelia miyamotoi*
  - Transmitted by the tick *Ixodes scapularis*—causes illness similar to Lyme disease
- Southern tick–associated rash illness (STARI)
  - Transmitted by the Lone Star tick (*Amblyomma americanum*) in Alabama, Missouri, New Jersey, North Carolina, Oklahoma, and Texas—illness similar to Lyme

Diagnostic Testing

Laboratories
- Lyme serologies may be falsely negative early on during infection.
- During later-stage disease, an ELISA and Western blot can aid in diagnosis.
- Serologic testing should not be ordered for screening purposes.
- Serologies may remain positive after successful treatment of Lyme disease.

Electrocardiography
- Atrioventricular blocks may commonly be seen in stage 2.

TREATMENT

Medications

- Prophylaxis with a single dose of doxycycline 200 mg may prevent Lyme disease if given within 72 hours of a tick bite.
- For Lyme disease without neurologic or cardiac involvement, oral antibiotic therapy with one of the following agents for 10–21 days is recommended:
  - Doxycycline 100 mg PO bid (first line)
  - Amoxicillin 500 mg PO tid (for children under 8 or pregnant women)
  - Cefuroxime axetil 500 mg PO bid
- For severe neurologic or cardiac disease, parenteral therapy with one of the following agents for 14–28 days is recommended:
  - Ceftriaxone 2 g IV daily (preferred)
  - Cefotaxime 2 g IV q8h
  - Penicillin G 3–4 million units IV q4h

SPECIAL CONSIDERATIONS

- Tick removal within 24 hours renders Lyme disease unlikely.

Disposition

- Patients may be discharged home with oral antibiotics. If neurologic or cardiac involvement is considered, the patient will need to be admitted for IV antibiotics.

Rocky Mounted Spotted Fever

EPIDEMIOLOGY/ETIOLOGY

- Prevalent in southeastern and south central United States.
- Rocky Mountain spotted fever (RMSF) is caused by *Rickettsia rickettsii*, a gram-negative obligate intracellular organism, and transmitted by *Dermacentor variabilis* (American dog tick), *Dermacentor andersoni* (Rocky Mountain wood tick), and *Rhipicephalus sanguineus* (common brown dog tick).
- Individuals with exposure to dogs residing near wooded or tall grass areas may be at greater risk for infection.

PATHOPHYSIOLOGY

- *Rickettsia rickettsii* infects vascular endothelial cells, resulting in vascular injury.
- Transmission of disease can occur in as little as 6–10 hours after the tick bite but may be delayed up to 24 hours.

DIAGNOSIS

Clinical Presentation

History
- A febrile illness usually precedes a rash, and other symptoms can include headache, nausea, vomiting, abdominal pain, myalgias, or anorexia.

Physical Examination
- A macular nonpruritic rash within 2–5 days involving the extremities (including palms and soles) and progressing to the trunk. Later, this transitions to a petechial rash heralding severe disease. Conjunctival injection may be seen.

Differential Diagnosis

- Thrombotic thrombocytopenic purpura, vasculitis, other rickettsial infection, leptospirosis, infectious mononucleosis, bacterial sepsis, and meningitis.
- *Rickettsia parkeri* and 364D rickettsiosis can have a similar presentation as RMSF.

Diagnostic Testing

Laboratories
- Culture, PCR, or staining of skin biopsy helps confirm the diagnosis.
- Serologic testing may be negative early on during infection.

TREATMENT

- Treatment should not be delayed pending definitive testing.

Medications

- Antibiotic therapy should consist of one of the following:
  - Doxycycline 100 mg q12h IV or PO for 7 days
  - Chloramphenicol (alternative)

SPECIAL CONSIDERATIONS

Disposition
- Admission to the hospital is usually indicated.

Complications

- Complications result from the vasculitis and includes encephalitis, noncardiogenic pulmonary edema, acute respiratory distress syndrome, cardiac arrhythmia, coagulopathy, gastrointestinal bleeding, and skin necrosis.
- Death occurs 8–15 days after onset of symptoms in untreated patients.
- Patients with G6PD deficiency may experience a more rapid progression to death.

Ehrlichiosis and Anaplasmosis

Epidemiology/Etiology

- Human monocytic ehrlichiosis (HME) is caused by *Ehrlichia chaffeensis*, is transmitted by the lone star tick (*A. americanum*), and is endemic to south and south central United States.
- Human granulocytic anaplasmosis (HGA) is caused by *Anaplasma phagocytophilum*, is transmitted by *I. scapularis*, and shares the same geographical distribution as Lyme disease due to a common tick vector.

Pathophysiology

- The parasite infects RBCs and causes hemolysis, leading to anemia and microvascular stasis.

DIAGNOSIS

Clinical Presentation

History
- HME and HGA present similarly with illness onset usually up to a week after tick exposure.
- Nonspecific symptoms including fever, chills, malaise, myalgia, and headache are common in most patients. Some may also have nausea, vomiting, arthralgias, or cough.

Physical Examination
- Some patients may develop rash that can be macular, maculopapular, or petechial.
- Mental status changes, stiff neck, and clonus can also be seen.

Differential Diagnosis

- RMSF, thrombotic thrombocytopenic purpura, cholangitis, hepatitis, Lyme disease (a common coinfection with HGA), or other viral infection (e.g., mononucleosis)

Diagnostic Testing

Laboratories
- Blood work including a CBC, basic metabolic panel, and liver function tests may show leukopenia with a left shift, anemia, thrombocytopenia, renal insufficiency, elevated transaminases, elevated lactate dehydrogenase, and elevated alkaline phosphatase.
- In patients with neurologic symptoms, cerebrospinal fluid analysis usually demonstrates a lymphocytic pleocytosis and elevated protein.
- PCR of the blood is preferred for definitive testing.

TREATMENT

Medications

- Antibiotic therapy should consist of one of the following:
  - Doxycycline 100 mg PO or IV q12h

- ○ Tetracycline 25 mg/kg/d PO divided qid for 7–14 days
- ○ Rifampin 300 mg PO q12h for 7–10 days

SPECIAL CONSIDERATIONS

Disposition
- Most patients can be admitted to the hospital floor.

Complications
- Seizures, coma, renal failure, and respiratory failure.
- HGA infection can be complicated by opportunistic infections.

Tularemia

Epidemiology/Etiology
- Caused by gram-negative bacteria, *Francisella tularensis*, that is endemic to south central United States and transmitted by tick bite, exposure to infected animals, or exposure by infectious aerosol.
- Tularemia is not transmitted from person to person.

Pathophysiology
- Tularemia is an intracellular parasite that infects macrophages.

DIAGNOSIS

Clinical Presentation
History
- Fever and malaise develop 2–5 days after exposure.

Physical Examination
- Ulceroglandular disease (most common presentation)
  - ○ A single erythematous papuloulcerative lesion with central eschar at the site of tick bite accompanied by tender regional lymphadenopathy
- Glandular disease (common in children)
  - ○ Tender regional lymphadenopathy in absence of a skin lesion at the site of the tick bite. Some lymph nodes may become suppurative.
- Oculoglandular disease
  - ○ Results from exposure to conjunctiva.
  - ○ Eye pain, photophobia, conjunctival erythema edema and vascular engorgement, and increased tearing are present. Unilateral conjunctivitis with associated preauricular lymphadenopathy may be seen.
  - ○ Complications may include corneal ulceration and dacryocystitis.
- Typhoidal disease (systemic disease)
  - ○ Nonspecific symptoms dominate including fever, chills, headache, myalgias, sore throat, diarrhea, and anorexia.
- Pneumonic disease
  - ○ Primary disease results from direct inhalation of infectious aerosol. Secondary disease may stem from either typhoidal or ulceroglandular disease, although other forms can also cause this.
  - ○ Early symptoms include fever, cough, and pleuritic chest pain and may progress to respiratory failure.

Differential Diagnosis

- Cat scratch disease, bacterial lymphadenitis, toxoplasmosis, rat-bite fever, anthrax, plague, typhoid, salmonella, Q fever, mycobacterial infection, or malignancy

Diagnostic Testing

Laboratories

- Laboratory personnel must be made aware of any suspicion for tularemia in order to assure appropriate use of biosafety precautions when handling clinical specimens.
- Tularemia is diagnosed through serology or culture of suspected infected fluid (blood, sputum, pleural fluid).

Imaging

- Chest radiography should be obtained if pneumonic disease is suspected.

TREATMENT

Medications

- Antibiotic therapy should include one of the following:
  - Streptomycin 1 g IM q12h for 10 days (treatment of choice)
  - Gentamicin 5 mg/kg IV divided q8h
  - Doxycycline 100 mg PO or IV q12h for 14–21 days
  - Ciprofloxacin 500–750 mg PO bid for 14–21 days may also be effective

SPECIAL CONSIDERATIONS

Disposition

- Patients should be discharged to home, as person–person transmission does not occur.

Complications

- Lymph node suppuration, sepsis, renal failure, rhabdomyolysis, hepatitis, pericarditis, meningitis, endocarditis, osteomyelitis

Babesiosis

EPIDEMIOLOGY/ETIOLOGY

- Found in northeastern and midwestern United States (including Connecticut, Massachusetts, Minnesota, New Jersey, New York, Rhode Island, and Wisconsin)
- Caused by the intraerythrocytic parasite *Babesia microti* and transmitted by the *I. scapularis* tick

PATHOPHYSIOLOGY

- Infection causes lysis of red blood cells.

DIAGNOSIS

Clinical Presentation

- Babesiosis resembles malaria and can range from asymptomatic to fatal disease.

History
- Symptoms develop 1–6 weeks after the bite of an infected tick.
- Mild illness includes gradual onset of fatigue, malaise, and weakness accompanied by intermittent fever, chills, and sweats. Headache, myalgias, and arthralgias are less common.

Physical Examination
- Patients may have splenomegaly and/or hepatomegaly on examination.

Laboratories
- Anemia with elevated lactate dehydrogenase, total bilirubin, and reticulocyte count and low haptoglobin is indicative of hemolytic anemia. Thrombocytopenia may also be present.
- Liver enzymes (AST, ALT, and alkaline phosphatase) can be elevated.
- Diagnosis is made through examination of thin blood smears to identify intraerythrocytic parasite. Serology and PCR may also be available.

Differential Diagnosis
- Malaria, leptospirosis, hepatitis, hemolytic anemia, or bacteremia

TREATMENT

Medications
- Antibiotic therapy should consist of one of the following regimens:
  ○ Azithromycin 500 mg PO on day 1 and then 250 mg daily for 7–10 days, in combination with atovaquone 750 mg PO bid
  ○ Life-threatening disease: clindamycin 600 mg IV q8 plus quinine 650 mg PO q8h for 7–10 days

Other Nonpharmacologic Therapies
- Exchange transfusion may be considered in the setting of severe anemia and high parasitemia.

SPECIAL CONSIDERATIONS

Disposition
- Patients may be discharged or admitted to the hospital based on degree of illness.

Prognosis
- Severe illness, including hemolytic anemia, can lead to prolonged hospitalization or death, particularly in those aged 50 years and over, who have undergone splenectomy, or who are immunosuppressed.

Other Tick Borne Infections (Table 47.1)

Colorado Tick Fever
- Caused by virus transmitted by Rocky Mountain wood tick (*D. andersoni*) in the Rocky Mountains.
- Symptoms include fever, chills, headache, body aches, and malaise.
- There is no specific treatment.

TABLE 47.1	Other Tick-Borne Infections Encountered in the United States		
	Tick vector	Geographic distribution	Clinical presentation
Colorado tick fever	Rocky Mountain wood tick (Dermacentor andersoni)	Colorado	Fever, chills, headache, body aches, malaise
Heartland virus	Lone star tick	Missouri, Tennessee	Fever, malaise, headache, myalgias, diarrhea, anorexia, nausea
Powassan disease	Ixodes scapularis tick	Northeast United States and Great Lakes region	Fever, headache, vomiting, weakness, confusion, seizures, memory loss. Long-term neurologic sequelae possible
Southern tick–associated rash illness (STARI)	Lone star tick (Amblyomma americanum)	Alabama, Missouri, New Jersey, North Carolina, Oklahoma, and Texas	Rash resembling erythema migrans (Lyme disease) with associated flu-like symptoms
Spotted fever group Rickettsii (other than RMSF):			
Rickettsia parkeri	Gulf Coast tick (Amblyomma maculatum)	Eastern and southern United States	Fever, headache, eschar, rash
Rickettsia species 364D	Pacific Coast tick (Dermacentor occidentalis)	Northern California and Pacific coast	Fever, eschar
Tick-borne relapsing fever (Borrelia species)	Soft tick, body louse	Western United States	Fever, headache, muscle and joint aches, and nausea

Data from: U.S. Centers for Disease Control and Prevention; http://www.cdc.gov/ticks/diseases; http://www.cdc.gov/otherspottedfever.

Tick Borne Relapsing Fever (TBRF)

• Bacterial infection (*Borrelia* spirochetes) found in western United States transmitted by both tick and louse.
• Symptoms include fever, headache, muscle and joint aches, and nausea.
• Can be treated with penicillin, beta-lactam antibiotics, tetracyclines, macrolides, and possibly fluoroquinolones.

SUGGESTED READINGS

http://www.cdc.gov/ticks/diseases/

Dantas-Torres F. Rocky Mountain spotted fever. *Lancet Infect Dis* 2007;7(11):724–32.

Dennis DT, Inglesby TV, Henderson DA, et al.; Working Group on Civilian Biodefense. Tularemia as a biological weapon: medical and public health management. *JAMA* 2001;285(21):2763–73.

Dumler JS, Madigan JE, Pusterla N, Bakken JS. Ehrlichioses in humans: epidemiology, clinical presentation, diagnosis, and treatment. *Clin Infect Dis* 2007;45(Suppl 1):S45–51.

Hamburg BJ, Storch GA, Micek ST, Kollef MH. The importance of early treatment with doxycycline in human ehrlichiosis. *Medicine (Baltimore)* 2008;87(2):53.

Steere AC. Lyme disease. *N Engl J Med* 2001;345(2):115–25.

Thorner AR, Walker DH, Petri WA Jr. Rocky mountain spotted fever. *Clin Infect Dis* 1998;27(6):1353–9

Vannier E, Krause PJ. Human babesiosis. *N Engl J Med* 2012;366(25):2397–407.

Weber IB, Turabelidze G, Patrick S, et al. Clinical recognition and management of tularemia in Missouri: a retrospective records review of 121 cases. *Clin Infect Dis* 2012;55(10):1283–90.

Wormser GP, Dattwyler RJ, Shapiro ED, et al. The clinical assessment, treatment, and prevention of lyme disease, human granulocytic anaplasmosis, and babesiosis: clinical practice guidelines by the Infectious Diseases Society of America. *Clin Infect Dis* 2006;43(9):1089–134.

48 Infectious Emergencies: Tropical Infectious Diseases

Steven Hung and Stephen Y. Liang

Malaria

GENERAL PRINCIPLES

Epidemiology/Etiology

- Caused by parasitic protozoan including *Plasmodium falciparum*, *P. ovale*, *P. vivax*, *P. malariae*, and *P. knowlesi*.
- *Plasmodium falciparum* malaria is the most severe form.

DIAGNOSIS

Clinical Presentation

History

- Onset of illness may occur within weeks or up to 12 months after infection.
- Symptoms usually include headache, myalgias, and fatigue.
- Characterized by periodic paroxysms of rigors and fevers with headache, cough, and nausea culminating in profuse sweating.

Physical Examination
- The examination is relatively unremarkable apart from episodes of fever, rigors, sweats, and nausea.

Diagnostic Criteria and Testing
Laboratories
- Diagnosis is made by the visualization of parasites on blood smear; these should be obtained during febrile episodes to maximize yield.

TREATMENT

- Treatment depends on type and severity as well as resistance patterns to chloroquine.

Medications

- Uncomplicated malaria (*P. falciparum, P. ovale, P. vivax, P. malariae*, and *P. knowlesi*) can be treated with chloroquine if the patient reports travel to a chloroquine-sensitive area.
- Uncomplicated *P. falciparum* from chloroquine-resistant areas and *P. vivax* from Australia, Indonesia, or South America can be treated with quinine and doxycycline; an alternative is atovaquone–proguanil.
- For *P. ovale* or *P. vivax*, add primaquine to above regimens to prevent relapse.
- For complicated severe malaria (most commonly by *P. falciparum*), treat with intravenous quinidine and doxycycline.

SPECIAL CONSIDERATIONS

Disposition
- Patients should be admitted to the hospital for further diagnosis and treatment.

Complications
- Complications include cerebral malaria, hypoglycemia, lactic acidosis, renal failure, acute respiratory distress syndrome, and coagulopathy.

Chagas Disease

GENERAL PRINCIPLES

Epidemiology/Etiology
- Chagas disease is a disease mainly affecting the lymph nodes, heart, and esophagus caused by the protozoan *Trypanosoma cruzi*, found mainly in Latin America.
- Spread by Triatominae or the "kissing bug"; bites often occur on the face.

DIAGNOSIS

Clinical Presentation
History
- The patient may complain of a febrile illness, headache, or body aches in the early stage.
- After 8–12 weeks, the disease enters the chronic phase; 60–70% of patients are asymptomatic.

Physical Examination
- In the early stage of the illness, findings can include swollen lymph nodes, a rash, and/or a local swelling at site of bite.
- Romana sign is characterized by swelling of the eyelids on the side of the face near the insect bite.

Diagnostic Testing

Laboratories
- Diagnosis of early disease is made by identification of the parasite in the blood.
- Chronic disease is diagnosed by detection of serum antibodies against *T. cruzi.*

TREATMENT

- Benznidazole or nifurtimox may be used.
- Cure rates decline the longer the patient has been infected.

SPECIAL CONSIDERATIONS

Disposition
- Patients should be admitted to the hospital for further diagnosis and treatment.

African Trypanosomiasis (Sleeping Sickness)

GENERAL PRINCIPLES

- African trypanosomiasis is a parasitic protozoa that causes "sleeping sickness."

Epidemiology/Etiology
- Endemic to sub-Saharan Africa
- Caused by protozoa *Trypanosoma brucei* and is transmitted by the bite of the tsetse fly
  - *Trypanosoma brucei gambiense* (T.b.g.) is the most common, causing ~98% of infections.
  - *Trypanosoma brucei rhodesiense* (T.b.r.).

DIAGNOSIS

Clinical Presentation
History
- In the first 1–3 weeks after the bite (first stage), the patient usually complains of fever, headache, itchiness, and joint pains.
- The second stage begins weeks to months later and consists of confusion, poor coordination, numbness, irritability, psychosis, aggressive behavior, apathy, and trouble sleeping.
- There may be a fragmented 24-hour rhythm of sleep, daytime sleep episodes, and nighttime wakefulness.

Physical Examination
- There may be swelling of lymph nodes along the back of neck (Winterbottom sign).

Diagnostic Criteria and Testing
Laboratories
- Identification of the parasite in blood smear or from lymph node biopsy is pathognomonic.

TREATMENT

- Without treatment, the disease is fatal.
- Treatment is pentamidine for *T.b.g.* or suramin for *T.b.r.* in first stage.
- Treatment of the second stage is with eflornithine or combination of nifurtimox and eflornithine for *T.b.g.*

SPECIAL CONSIDERATIONS

Disposition

- Patients should be admitted to the hospital for further diagnosis and treatment.

Leishmaniasis

GENERAL PRINCIPLES

Epidemiology/Etiology

- Leishmaniasis is a disfiguring infection caused by protozoan parasites of the genus *Leishmania* found in Central and South America, Asia, the Middle East, and Africa.
- It is spread by bite of certain sandflies.

DIAGNOSIS

Clinical Presentation

History
- The patient may complain of ulcerations to the skin, scars, and pain with ulcers in the mouth and nose.

Physical Examination
- Cutaneous
  - Skin ulcers at bite site
  - Last for months to a year and a half, heals as a scar
- Mucocutaneous
  - Ulcers of the skin, mouth, and nose
- Visceral leishmaniasis—kala-azar ("black fever")
  - Begins with skin ulcers and progresses to fever and hepatosplenomegaly.

Diagnostic Testing

Laboratories
- Leishmaniasis is diagnosed in hematology lab by direct visualization of the amastigotes (Leishman-Donovan bodies) in blood smear.

TREATMENT

Medications

- Miltefosine
- Liposomal amphotericin B (visceral)
- Pentavalent antimonials and paromomycin

SPECIAL CONSIDERATIONS

Disposition
- Patients should be admitted to the hospital for further diagnosis and treatment.

Schistosomiasis

GENERAL PRINCIPLES

Epidemiology/Etiology
- Schistosomiasis is a disease caused by a parasitic flatworm that infects either the urinary tract or intestine.
- Most human infections are caused by *Schistosoma mansoni, S. haematobium,* and *S. japonicum,* which are found throughout Africa, South America, Indonesia, and China.

DIAGNOSIS

Clinical Presentation
History
- Incubation is 14–84 days; however, many people are asymptomatic.
- Patients with acute infection (Katayama syndrome) may present with rash, fever, headache, myalgia, and respiratory symptoms.
- Chronic infection may lead to complaints of dysuria, diarrhea, constipation, and blood in stool.

Physical Examination
- *S. mansoni and S. japonicum* infection can lead to ascites.
- *S. haematobium* infection can cause hematuria.

Diagnostic Testing
Laboratories
- A complete blood count (CBC) may assist in the diagnosis, as eosinophilia is frequently present.
- Stool samples should be sent for ova and parasites.
- Parasite eggs can be seen in stool (*S. mansoni, S. japonicum*) or urine (*S. haematobium*).

TREATMENT

Medications
- Praziquantel

SPECIAL CONSIDERATIONS

Disposition
- Patients should be admitted to the hospital for further diagnosis and treatment.

Complications
- Severe chronic inflammation can lead to bowel wall ulceration, liver fibrosis, and portal hypertension. There is also an increased risk of bladder cancer.

Onchocerciasis (River Blindness)

GENERAL PRINCIPLES

Epidemiology/Etiology
- Onchocerciasis is caused by the parasitic worm *Onchocerciasis volvulus*.
- Transmitted by repeated bites by blackflies, found mostly in sub-Saharan Africa.
- Flies that transmit the disease live and breed near fast-flowing streams and rivers and are normally active during the day.

Pathophysiology
- Incubation time is 3 months to 1 year.
- Fibrous nodules form under the skin, where they are protected from the immune system.
- Inflammation by larvae in the eye causes permanent clouding of the cornea and can cause direct inflammation of the optic nerve.

DIAGNOSIS

Clinical Presentation
History
- The patient may present with complaints of nonpainful swelling of the lymph nodes.

Physical Examination
- Can cause a "leopard skin" appearance with thinning of the skin and loss of elastic tissue ("cigarette paper" consistency)

Diagnostic Testing
Laboratories
- Skin snip—taking skin shaving or biopsy to examine for worms

Diagnostic Procedures
- Infections of eye can be diagnosed with slit-lamp exam where larvae can be seen.

TREATMENT

Medications
- Ivermectin, given every 6 months for the life span of the adult worms since the medication only kills the larva

SPECIAL CONSIDERATIONS

Disposition
- Patients should be admitted to the hospital for further diagnosis and treatment.

Lymphatic Filariasis

GENERAL PRINCIPLES

Epidemiology/Etiology
- Lymphatic filariasis is caused by a parasitic, microscopic, thread-like worm that lives in the lymphatic system commonly found in tropic and subtropic areas of Asia and Africa, the Caribbean, and South America.

- Most infections are caused by *Wuchereria bancrofti, Brugia malayi,* and *Brugia timori.*
- Spread from person to person by mosquitoes but requires multiple exposures over months to years. Short-term tourists are at lower risk for acquiring the disease.

DIAGNOSIS

Clinical Presentation

History
- Most infected people have no symptoms.

Physical Examination
- A small percentage of patients will develop lymphedema and elephantiasis.
- *W. bancrofti* can cause swelling of the scrotum.

Diagnostic Testing

Laboratories
- A blood smear should be sent to the lab, as microfilariae will be seen.
- Blood should be drawn at night when the parasite circulates throughout the body.

TREATMENT

Medications
- Diethylcarbamazine (DEC)
  - DEC should not be given to patients who have onchocerciasis as it can worsen eye disease.
- Ivermectin kills only microfilariae, but not the adult worms.

SPECIAL CONSIDERATIONS

Disposition
- Patients should be admitted to the hospital for further diagnosis and treatment.

Leprosy

GENERAL PRINCIPLES

Epidemiology/ Etiology
- Leprosy, also known as Hansen disease, is an infection caused by the bacteria *Mycobacterium leprae* and *Mycobacterium lepromatosis.*
- Spread between humans via droplet transmission but up to 95% of adults are naturally immune to the disease.
- Found in India, Brazil, Indonesia, and parts of Africa.

DIAGNOSIS

Clinical Presentation

History
- The patient may report dermatologic findings, particularly of the nasal mucosa, weakness, and decreased sensation of the limbs.

Physical Examination
- Paucibacillary—hypopigmented skin macules that are asymmetrically distributed.
- Multibacillary—symmetric skin lesions, nodules, plaques, thickened dermis, and frequent involvement of the nasal mucosa.
- Can progress to numbness of affected areas and muscle weakness/paralysis.
- Loss of sensation leads to repeated trauma of affected limbs and loss of tissue.

Diagnostic Testing
- Skin smears

TREATMENT

- Paucibacillary—treated with daily dapsone and daily or monthly rifampin for 6 months
- Multibacillary—daily dapsone and clofazimine along with daily or monthly rifampicin for 12 months

SPECIAL CONSIDERATIONS

Disposition
- Patients should be admitted to the hospital for further diagnosis and treatment.

Dengue Fever (Breakbone Fever)

GENERAL PRINCIPLES

Epidemiology/Etiology
- Dengue fever is a hemorrhagic fever disease caused by the dengue virus and is also known as "breakbone fever."
- It is transmitted by mosquitoes and is more common in countries around the equator.
- There are five different types of virus that cause dengue; infection with one provides lifelong immunity after first infection and transient immunity to other types.

DIAGNOSIS

Clinical Presentation
History
- Incubation time is usually between 3 and 14 days.
- Patients will have high fever, headache, vomiting, and muscle and joint pains.

Physical Examination
- Fever is biphasic, breaking then returning for 1–2 days.
- Some patients may develop a blanching, flushed skin rash with petechiae.
- May progress to dengue hemorrhagic fever, resulting in bleeding and low platelets.

Diagnostic Testing
- Serologic, PCR, or viral antigen testing.
- A full set of laboratories should be obtained, as patients with dengue fever may have thrombocytopenia, metabolic acidosis, or elevated liver enzymes.

TREATMENT

- Supportive care and intravenous fluids.
- Recommend avoiding NSAIDs due to risk of increased bleeding.

SPECIAL CONSIDERATIONS

Disposition

• Patients should be admitted to the hospital for further diagnosis and treatment.

SUGGESTED READINGS

Barrett MP, Croft SL. Management of trypanosomiasis and leishmaniasis. *Br Med Bull* 2012;104(1):175–196. doi:10.1093/bmb/lds031.

Basáñez MG, Pion SD, Churcher TS, et al. River blindness: a success story under threat? *PLoS Med* 2006;3(9):e371.

Freerksen E, Rosenfeld M, Depasquale G, et al. The Malta Project—a country freed itself of leprosy. A 27-year progress study (1972–1999) of the first successful eradication of leprosy. *Chemotherapy* 2001;47(5):309.

Griffith KS, Lewis LS, Mali S, Parise ME. Treatment of malaria in the United States: a systematic review. *JAMA* 2007;297(20):2264–77.

Gubler DJ. Dengue and dengue hemorrhagic fever. *Clin Microbiol Rev* 1998;11(3):480.

Kramer CV, Zhang F, Sinclair D, Olliaro PL. Drugs for treating urinary schistosomiasis. *Cochrane Database Syst Rev* 2014;(8):CD000053.

Malvy D, Chappuis F. Sleeping sickness. *Clin Microbiol Infect* 2011;17(7):986–95.

Rassi A Jr, Rassi A, Marin-Neto JA. Chagas disease. *Lancet* 2010;375(9723):1388–402.

Ross AG, Bartley PB, Sleigh AC, et al. Schistosomiasis. *N Engl J Med* 2002;346(16):1212–20.

Schwartz E, Mendelson E, Sidi Y. Dengue fever among travelers. *Am J Med* 1996;101(5):516.

Tisch DJ, Michael E, Kazura JW. Mass chemotherapy options to control lymphatic filariasis: a systematic review. *Lancet Infect Dis* 2005;5(8):514.

Additional resources can be found at www.cdc.gov.

49 Electrolyte Emergencies: Calcium

Mark D. Levine

GENERAL PRINCIPLES

Definition

• Calcium disorders occur from malignancy or parathyroid disorders.
• Approximately 50% of calcium is ionized, 40% is bound to proteins, and 10% is bound to anions.

Pathophysiology

• Tumors may secrete humoral factor (parathyroid hormone-related protein [PTHrP]) leading to metastases and osteolysis.
• Other causes of hypercalcemia include milk-alkali syndrome, alkalosis with renal insufficiency, and medication-induced hypercalcemia.

- Hypocalcemia causes neuromuscular irritability and tetany. It may also lead to decreased myocardial contractility, which can lead to heart failure or hypotension.

Hypercalcemia

GENERAL PRINCIPLES

Epidemiology/Etiology

- Common causes of hypercalcemia are usually secondary to malignancy and hyperparathyroidism.
- Other causes may be due to increased intake, thiazide diuretic use, immobilization, and granulomatous disease.
- 20–40% of patients with cancer may develop hypercalcemia during their disease process.
- Women and the elderly have increased rates of non–cancer-related hypercalcemia.
- The incidence of primary hyperparathyroidism increases with age.

DIAGNOSIS

Clinical Presentation

History

- Symptoms of hypercalcemia depend on the cause of the disease and the time period of the disease development.
- Mild elevations are usually asymptomatic and discovered incidentally.
- Patients with clinically significant hypercalcemia may report nausea, vomiting, abdominal or flank pain, constipation, lethargy, vague myalgias, polyuria, polydipsia, or mental status changes.

Physical Examination

- The examination of patients with hypercalcemia will usually be nonspecific or may be consistent with other medical issues.
- Hyperreflexia and tongue fasciculations may be seen.
- Weakness in the proximal lower extremities may be present, and abdominal discomfort may also be present.

Differential Diagnosis

- Intoxication, medication overdose, tumor, pancreatitis, renal colic, MS, ulcer disease, or musculoskeletal pain

Diagnostic Criteria and Testing

Laboratories

- Calcium levels and ionized calcium levels should be checked, and if abnormal, the corrected calcium should be calculated (measured total calcium mg/dL + [0.8 for every decrease in serum albumin of 1 g/dL below the reference level]).
  - (Subtract 0.8 for every increment of 1 g/dL above the reference level of albumin.)
- PTH and serum phosphate levels should be measured.

Electrocardiography

- QT shortening is common and PR intervals are frequently prolonged.
- At high calcium levels, the QRS may widen, T waves may flatten or invert, and heart block may occur.

Imaging
- No imaging studies are specifically diagnostic for hypercalcemia.

TREATMENT

Medications
- Hydration should occur with normal saline, as these patients are very dehydrated, and this will help dilute the calcium level and increase renal clearance.
- Loop diuretics (furosemide) will help increase calcium excretion.
- Thiazide diuretics will increase reabsorption of calcium.
- In severe cases of hypercalcemia, calcitonin may be administered in consultation with endocrinology.

Other Nonpharmacologic Therapies
- Dialysis is indicated in anuric patients, as no diuresis occurs.

SPECIAL CONSIDERATIONS

Disposition
- All patients with hypercalcemia should be admitted to the hospital.

Hypocalcemia

GENERAL PRINCIPLES

Epidemiology/Etiology
- Causes of hypocalcemia include low albumin states, hypomagnesemia, medication or surgical effects, and PTH or vitamin D deficiency.
- Patients who have large burns, have received massive transfusions, have been exposed to hydrofluoric acid, have rhabdomyolysis, or have pancreatitis or septic shock frequently are hypocalcemic.
- Age and nutritional status affect the prevalence of hypocalcemia in patients.

DIAGNOSIS

Clinical Presentation
History
- Patients may report numbness or tingling periorally and in the extremities.
- They may complain of muscle cramps or carpopedal spasm.
- Wheezing, dysphagia, or vocal changes may be reported, as well as altered mentation, personality changes, fatigues, or new seizures may be present.

Physical Examination
- In addition to findings per the history, patients with chronic hypocalcemia may have coarse hair, brittle nails, psoriasis, dry skin, poor dentition, or cataracts.
- Chvostek and Trousseau signs may be present.
- Patients may have abnormal movements as well.

Differential Diagnosis
- Renal injury, pancreatitis, hypomagnesemia, malnutrition, metabolic alkalosis, hydrofluoric acid burn, or hypoparathyroidism

Diagnostic Criteria and Testing
Laboratories
- Calcium levels and ionized calcium levels should be checked, and if abnormal, the corrected calcium should be calculated (see calculation in hypercalcemia).
  - (Subtract 0.8 for every increment of 1 g/dL above the reference level of albumin.)
- PTH and serum phosphate levels should be measured.

Electrocardiography
- A prolongation of the QT interval may be seen.

Imaging
- No imaging studies are specifically diagnostic for hypocalcemia.

TREATMENT
Medications
- Mild hypocalcemia (no clinical symptoms) can be treated with oral replacement therapy.
- Patients with symptomatic hypocalcemia should receive 100–300 mg of calcium gulconate IV. Calcium chloride has three times the available elemental calcium but should be given via central access if needed for rapid correction.
- If the patient is on digitalis, there should be continuous ECG monitoring, as calcium will potentiate the effects of digitalis.

SPECIAL CONSIDERATIONS
Disposition
- Symptomatic patients should be admitted to the hospital.

50 Electrolyte Emergencies: Potassium

Lauren O'Grady

Hypokalemia

GENERAL PRINCIPLES
Definition
- A serum potassium level <3.5 mEq/L (reference ranges vary between institutions).
- Patients usually become symptomatic at levels <2.5 mEq/L.

Epidemiology/Etiology
- Decreased potassium intake, renal losses by acidosis, hemolytic uremic syndrome (HUS), chronic kidney disease (CKD), loop diuretics, and other illnesses may lead to hypokalemia.
- Large bowel adenomas, diarrhea/chronic laxative abuse, drug-induced causes such as penicillin, lithium, levodopa, or theophylline, and ingestion of clay may also lead to hypokalemia.

Pathophysiology
- Increased loss or increased shifting of potassium into the cells causes hypokalemia.

DIAGNOSIS

Clinical Presentation
History
- The patient may report weakness, muscle cramps, constipation, or paresthesias.

Physical Examination
- A full neurologic exam should be done looking for hyporeflexia, alterations in blood pressure, or reentrant or ventricular dysrhythmias.

Differential Diagnosis
- Hyperthyroidism, hypocalcemia, hypomagnesemia, Cushing syndrome, or metabolic alkalosis

Diagnostic Criteria and Testing
Laboratories
- A basic metabolic panel and magnesium should be drawn.

Electrocardiography
- U waves, prolonged QT intervals, and ST segment depression may be seen.

Imaging
- There are no imaging studies that will diagnose potassium abnormalities.

TREATMENT

Medications
- Potassium supplementation of 20 mEq will raise the serum K by 0.25 mEq/L.
- Oral supplementation is adequate for stable patients without ECG changes.
- IV supplementation should be used for unstable patents, but faster repletion should be administered through central access.

SPECIAL CONSIDERATIONS

- Patients with heart failure and myocardial infarction should have a potassium goal closer to 4.5 mEq to decrease incidence of ventricular dysrhythmias.
- Patients should be on a cardiac monitor while they have uncorrected electrolyte imbalance or are receiving potassium supplementation.

Disposition
- Patients with symptomatic hypokalemia need to be admitted.

Hyperkalemia

GENERAL PRINCIPLES

Definition
• A serum potassium level >5.5 mEq/L (reference ranges vary between institutions)

Epidemiology/Etiology
• Patients may have hyperkalemia if they have acute or chronic kidney failure, rhabdomyolysis, trauma or burns resulting in substantial tissue damage, Addison disease, DKA, or ingestions (including but not limited to American society of Anesthesiologist (ASA), ethylene glycol, methanol, digitalis, and potassium supplements).

Pathophysiology
• An elevation of the extracellular potassium concentration partially depolarizes the cell membrane and increases membrane excitability, inactivating sodium channels causing impaired cardiac conduction and neuromuscular weakness.

DIAGNOSIS

Clinical Presentation
History
• Patients may experience weakness, vomiting, colic, diarrhea, and paralysis but may also present in cardiac arrest.

Physical Examination
• A full neurologic exam is necessary with evaluation for weakness and movement issues. Ascending muscle weakness leads to flaccid paralysis.

Differential Diagnosis
• Acute tubular necrosis (ATN), digitalis toxicity, adrenal hyperplasia, head trauma, burn injuries, hypocalcemia, metabolic acidosis, rhabdomyolysis, or tumor lysis syndrome

Diagnostic Criteria and Testing
Laboratories
• A basic metabolic panel and magnesium should be drawn.

Electrocardiography
• Patients usually show ECG changes at levels >6.5 mEq/L
  ○ Peaked T waves, prolonged PR, and shortened QT interval at levels of 6.5–7.5 mEq/L
  ○ QRS widening and P-wave flattening at levels of 7.5–8 mEq/L
  ○ Sine-wave pattern, VF, and heart block at levels >8 mEq/L

Imaging
• There is no imaging modality that will diagnosis potassium disorders.

TREATMENT

Medications
• Three different treatment strategies should be employed simultaneously:

- Membrane stabilization
  - Calcium gluconate (4.65 mEq Ca/g) or calcium chloride (13.6 mEq Ca/g)—1 g over 10 minutes
    - Immediate onset
    - Duration of action 30–60 minutes
    - Consider calcium drip if ECG changes and potential delay in definitive management
- Cellular shift
  - Fast-acting insulin (10 units) with dextrose supplementation (D50 bolus and drip)
    - Onset of action at 20 minutes
    - Duration of action 4–6 hours
    - Requires frequent blood glucose monitoring
  - Albuterol (10–20 mg in 4 mL NS given over 10 minutes)
    - Onset of action within 30 minutes
    - Duration of action about 2 hours
- Potassium excretion
  - Furosemide (40–80 mg IV)
    - Contraindicated in anuric patients
    - Onset of action within 15 minutes
    - Duration of action 2–3 hours
  - Sodium bicarbonate (150 mEql/L IV at 1 mL/kg/h of ideal body weight)
    - Onset of action is hours
  - Sodium polystyrene sulfonate (15–30 g in 15–30 mL)
    - Less commonly used and not widely recommended due to concern for bowel wall necrosis and electrolyte disturbances
    - Onset of action anywhere from hours to days

Other Nonpharmacologic Therapies

- Clinically significant hyperkalemia is an indication for initiating dialysis.

SPECIAL CONSIDERATIONS

- Always check a potassium level on DKA patients before starting insulin. Supplement potassium if <4.0 mEq/L as true total body potassium is generally low in these patients even is serum potassium is normal or slightly elevated.
- ASA overdoses will always require aggressive potassium supplementation, even if serum potassium is normal or slightly elevated, due to substantial renal losses due to acidosis and cellular shifts.

Disposition

- These patients should be admitted to the hospital, with unstable patients admitted to the ICU.

SUGGESTED READINGS

Bruder Stapleton F, MD reviewing Sterns RH, et al. Is kayexalate effective for hyperkalemia, and is it safe? *J Am Soc Nephrol* 2010.

Tintinalli J, Stapczynski O, John Ma. *Tintinalli's Emergency Medicine: A Comprehensive Study Guide.* 7th ed. (Book and DVD) (Emergency Medicine (Tintinalli)).

Krogager ML, Eggers-Kaas L, Aasbjerg K, et al. Short-term mortality risk of serum potassium levels in acute heart failure following myocardial infarction. *Eur Heart J Cardiovasc Pharmacother* 2015;1(4):245–51.

51 Electrolyte Emergencies: Sodium

Emily Harkins and Lauren O'Grady

Hyponatremia

GENERAL PRINCIPLES

Definition
- Refers to a sodium level <135 mmol/L.
- Symptoms generally start at levels <120 mmol/L.

Epidemiology/Etiology

Hyponatremia can be divided into hypotonic hyponatremia (true hyponatremia), isotonic hyponatremia, or hypertonic hyponatremia (pseudohyponatremia).

Hypertonic Hyponatremia
- Pseudohyponatremia is generally due to abnormalities of other osmotically active solutes such as protein, lipids, or glucose.

Hypotonic Hyponatremia
- Hypovolemic
  - Salt loss (sweating, vomiting, diarrhea, and fistulas that lead to fluid and sodium losses)
  - Third spacing (pancreatitis, burns, sepsis)
  - Iatrogenic (fluid replacement with hyponatremic IV fluids)
- Euvolemic
  - Syndrome of inappropriate antidiuretic hormone (SIADH)
  - Water intoxication (psychogenic polydipsia)
- Hypervolemic
  - Renal failure
  - Nephrotic syndrome
  - Cirrhosis
  - Congestive heart failure (CHF)

Pathophysiology
- Acute hyponatremia results in a release of glutamate. Excess glutamate causes seizures. Severe hyponatremia leads to osmotic movement of water, resulting in brain swelling, increased intracranial pressure (ICP), and herniation.

DIAGNOSIS

Clinical Presentation
History
- The majority of patients will be asymptomatic.
- Patients may report vague symptoms such as confusion, muscle weakness, muscle spasm, decreased appetite, vomiting, lethargy, fatigue, somnolence, coma, and seizures.

Physical Examination
- A full neurologic exam should be performed, as the patient may present with a seizure, have an altered mentation, or have movement disorders.

Differential Diagnosis
- Adrenal crisis, cardiogenic pulmonary edema, cirrhosis, or hypothyroidism

Diagnostic Criteria and Testing
Laboratories
- Basic metabolic panel, urine osmolality, and urine electrolytes

Imaging
- There are no specific imaging studies that will diagnose hyponatremia.

TREATMENT

Medications
- Severe hyponatremia of <120 mEq/L with symptoms of central nervous system (CNS) abnormalities or seizures should receive hypertonic saline.
  - For hyponatremic seizure, push 100 mL of 3% saline up to three times for a max correction of 4–6 mEq/L. Avoid increasing serum sodium by more than 8 mmol/d if hyponatremia is of unknown duration.
- Patients with symptoms such as dizziness, nausea, vomiting, confusion, or lethargy can be treated with hypertonic saline at 15–30 mL/h and desmopressin 1–2 μg IV every 8 hours for 24–48 hours along with free water restriction.
- Patients who are asymptomatic may receive normal saline unless they are fluid overloaded or have SAIDH.

Other Nonpharmacologic Therapies
- If the patient is euvolemic or hypervolemic and does not have significant symptoms, implement fluid restriction to 500–1500 mL daily.

SPECIAL CONSIDERATIONS

- Hyperlipidemia and other osmotically active solutes can cause falsely lower sodium.
- Hyperglycemia is a common cause of pseudohyponatremia.
  - The corrective factor is 1.6 mEq/L Na for every 100 mg/dL glucose over 100.
- Rapid sodium correction has been associated with central pontine myelinolysis.
- Do not treat hyponatremia secondary to SIADH with isotonic solutions.

Disposition
- Patients should be admitted to the hospital.

Hypernatremia

GENERAL PRINCIPLES

Definition
- Refers to a sodium level >145 mmol/L.
- Symptoms usually manifest at levels >158 mmol/L.

Epidemiology/Etiology

- Hypovolemic
  - Poor fluid intake (immobile, (elderly at high risk))
  - Osmotic diuresis (hyperglycemia or medications)
  - Excessive sweating (endurance athletes, thyrotoxicosis)
  - Severe diarrhea
- Euvolemic
  - Diabetes insipidus
  - Drug induced (lithium, phenytoin)
- Hypervolemic
  - Iatrogenic due to hypertonic infusions
  - Excess mineralocorticoid release
  - Intentional salt ingestion
    - Drinking salt water and excessive dietary ingestion
    - Munchausen and Munchausen by proxy

Pathophysiology

- Rapidly developing hypernatremia can cause shrinking of the brain, followed by damage of the brain vasculature or intracranial hemorrhage.

DIAGNOSIS

Clinical Presentation

History
- Thirst is the first clinical response to hypernatremia.
- Patients may have vague complaints of weakness, irritability, twitching, muscle spasm, seizure, or coma.

Physical Examination
- A full neurologic exam should be performed, as the patient may present with a seizure, have an altered mentation, or have movement disorders.

Differential Diagnosis

- Cirrhosis, hypocalcemia, hyponatremia, or diabetes mellitus

Diagnostic Criteria and Testing

Laboratories
- Basic metabolic panel, urine osmolality, urine electrolytes

Imaging
- There are no imaging studies that will diagnose hypernatremia.

TREATMENT

Medications

- Administer free water or ½NS and consider emergent dialysis.
- Furosemide may be used if there is inadequate urine output after fluid administration.
- If the onset of hypernatremia is over the course of 1–2 days, decrease the plasma sodium by 2 mEq/L/h until the serum concentration reaches 145 mEq/L.
- If the onset of hypernatremia is over longer than 2 days, decrease the plasma sodium by 10 mEq/L/d.
- Calculate free water deficit (L) = (measured [Na]/desired [Na]) + 1.

SPECIAL CONSIDERATIONS

- Diabetes insipidus should be treated with desmopressin with monitoring of urinary output and electrolytes.

Disposition

- Patients should be admitted to the hospital.

Complications

- Osmotic demyelination may be a results of rapid correction of hyponatremia followed by onset of new neurologic changes.
- Locked-in syndrome may be a result of osmotic demyelination.

SUGGESTED READINGS

Leroy C, Karrouz W, Douillard C, et al. Diabetes insipidus. *Ann Endocrinol (Paris)* 2013;74(5–6): 496–507. doi: 10.1016/j.ando.2013.10.002. PMID 24286605.

Muhsin SA, Mount DB. Diagnosis and treatment of hypernatremia. *Best Pract Res Clin Endocrinol Metab* 2016;30(2):189–203. doi: 10.1016/j.beem.2016.02.014. PMID 27156758.

Reynolds RM, Padfield PL, Seckl JR. Disorders of sodium balance. *BMJ* 2006;332(7543):702–5. doi: 10.1136/bmj.332.7543.702. PMC 1410848. PMID 16565125.

Rosenson J, Smollin C, Sporer KA, et al. Patterns of ecstasy-associated hyponatremia in California. *Ann Emerg Med* 2007;49(2):164–71.e1.

Sterns RH. Disorders of plasma sodium—causes, consequences, and correction. *N Engl J Med* 2015;2015(372):55–65.

Sterns RH, Emmett M, Forman JP. General principles of disorders of water balance (hyponatremia and hypernatremia) and sodium balance (hypovolemia and edema). *Basow DS, Waltham MA.* 2012.

Petrino R, Marino R. Fluids and Electrolytes. In: Tintinalli J, Stapczynski J, John Ma O, eds. *Tintinalli's Emergency Medicine: A Comprehensive Study Guide.* 8th ed. New York: McGraw-Hill Education, 2016.

52 Musculoskeletal Emergencies: Ankylosing Spondylitis

Al Lulla

GENERAL PRINCIPLES

Definition

- Ankylosing spondylitis (AS) is a rheumatic disease and type of spondyloarthritis characterized by chronic inflammation of the axial skeleton. Over time, this inflammation leads to significant rigidity of the spine and inability to accommodate stress.[1–3]

Epidemiology/Etiology

- Males have a greater predilection for AS than females, with the frequency of the disease in males being two to three times higher than in females.[1,4,5]
- The disease most often manifests itself in the second and third decades of life.[4]
- HLA-B27 seropositivity and a family history have a very strong association with AS.[1,6,9]

Pathophysiology

- AS is thought to be driven by chronic inflammation, bone erosion, and bone formation.[6]
- In addition to inflammatory back pain and stiffness of the spine, other manifestations of the spondyloarthritis include peripheral oligoarthritis, enthesitis, anterior uveitis, psoriasis, and inflammatory bowel disease.[1,4]

DIAGNOSIS

Clinical Presentation

History

- Patients with AS typically present with inflammatory low back pain that is insidious in onset and has a dull quality. Patients often have morning stiffness that improves with activity and returns with inactivity. Often times, the pain is worse at night.[1,4]
- Arthritis of the hips and shoulders can also occur. Some patients may have asymmetric arthritis of the lower extremities. Neck pain and stiffness are seen in advanced stages of the disease.[1,4]
- Anterior uveitis is the most common extra-articular manifestation of AS. Patients present with lacrimation, photophobia, and unilateral eye pain. Inflammatory bowel disease can also be seen in a subset of patients.[4]
- Red flag symptoms such as saddle anesthesia or loss of bowel and bladder function should be addressed.

Physical Examination

- Patients with low back pain and a history of AS should undergo a thorough neurologic examination, with an emphasis on identifying any possible spinal fracture. Patients with AS typically have many important physical exam findings, including loss of flexion and extension of the spine and pain in the sacroiliac joints when pressure is applied. Extra-articular manifestations of the disease (i.e., anterior uveitis, inflammatory bowel disease) should be assessed as well.[4]

Differential Diagnosis

- The differential diagnosis for AS is extremely broad given the numerous etiologies for lower back pain.

Diagnostic Criteria and Testing

- Inflammatory back pain should be considered in patients who have four of the following five features: age <40, back pain lasting >3 months, insidious onset, pain associated with morning stiffness, and improvement in symptoms with exercise.[7]

Laboratories

- There is no specific laboratory test in the ED that is diagnostic for AS.

Imaging

- Pelvis radiographs can demonstrate presence of sacroiliitis, which is the radiologic hallmark of AS. Sacroiliitis is the earliest manifestation of AS and appears as bony erosions and sclerosis at the level of the sacroiliac joints. Over time, these changes can progress to bony ankylosis and calcification and give the classic "bamboo spine" appearance of AS on imaging.[1,4]

TREATMENT

- There is currently no cure for AS. Current treatment guidelines are centered around management of symptoms and exercise programs.[1]

Medications

- NSAIDs are the mainstay of medical therapy for patients with AS.[1]
- Other medications may be initiated after consultation with a rheumatologist.

Other Nonpharmacologic Therapies

- Physical therapy as an outpatient is largely recommended by many experts and may offer some benefit to patients with AS.[8]

SPECIAL CONSIDERATIONS

Disposition

- Patients with AS should be referred to their PMD or rheumatologist for further care.
- Patients with AS should be educated to avoid strenuous activities that may increase risk of trauma and subsequent fracture.

Complication

- Providers in the ED should be aware of the risk of spinal fracture in patients who have a history of AS.[3]

REFERENCES

1. Braun J, Sieper J. Ankylosing spondylitis. *Lancet* 2007;369:1379–90.
2. Vosse D, Feldtkeller E, Erlendsson J, et al. Clinical vertebral fractures in patients with ankylosing spondylitis. *J Rheumatol* 2004;31:1981–5.
3. Waldman SK, Brown C, Lopez De Heredia L, Hughes RJ. Diagnosing and managing spinal injury in patients with ankylosing spondylitis. *J Emerg Med* 2013;44:e315–19.
4. Sieper J, Braun J, Rudwaleit M, et al. Ankylosing spondylitis: an overview. *Ann Rheum Dis* 2002;61:iii8–18.
5. Wang H, Ramakrishnan A, Fletcher S, et al. Epidemiology of Spondyloarthritis. *Rheum Dis Clin North Am* 2012;38:441–76.
6. Tam L, Gu J, Yu D. Pathogenesis of ankylosing spondylitis. *Nat Rev Rheumatol* 2010;6:399–405.
7. Calin A, Porta J, Fries JF, Schurman DJ. Clinical history as a screening test for ankylosing spondylitis. *JAMA* 1977;237:2613–14.
8. Dagfinrud H, Kvien TK, Hagen KB. The Cochrane review of physiotherapy interventions for ankylosing spondylitis. *J Rheumatol* 2005;32:1899–1906.
9. Feldtkeller E, Vosse D, Geusens P, Van Der Linden S. Prevalence and annual incidence of vertebral fractures in patients with ankylosing spondylitis. *Rheumatol Int* 2006;26:234–9.

Musculoskeletal Emergencies: Arthropathies

Mark D. Levine

Osteoarthritis (OA)

GENERAL PRINCIPLES

Definition
- A generalized inflammatory process of joint tissues and synovial fluid that leads to joint space narrowing, cartilage loss, and bony changes

Epidemiology/Etiology
- It is present in over 97% of patients over the age of 65.
- Risk factors for OA include female sex, obesity, previous injury, and genetic predisposition. Osteoporosis is thought to be protective against OA.

Pathophysiology
- Meniscal and ligament damage along with synovitis lead to the influx of inflammatory markers that affect articular cartilage and subchondral bone.

DIAGNOSIS

Clinical Presentation
History
- Patients usually complain of pain and stiffness that has increased over a period of time and may cause restriction of daily activities.
- Pain is usually increased in the late afternoon/evening or within the first 30 minutes of wakening.

Physical Examination
- The examination should be focused on the joints, looking for joint line tenderness, bony swelling/deformity, joint instability, and limited range of motion. There may be periarticular soft tissue lesions. OA has a predilection for the knees, hips, hand/fingers, and lower cervical and lumbar spine.

Differential Diagnosis
- Rheumatoid arthritis, septic arthritis, crystal arthropathy, or soft tissue trauma

Diagnostic Criteria and Testing
Laboratories
- Synovial fluid in noninflammatory OA will have <2000 wbc/mm^3 and may show calcium pyrophosphate crystals.

Imaging
- Plain radiography is used for evaluation of joint spaces and bony deformities and to rule out fractures.

TREATMENT

Medications
- Acetaminophen for noninflammatory OA
- NSAIDs for failure of acetaminophen or for inflammatory OA
  - Topical NSAIDs or capsaicin may be used as an alternate to oral NSAIDs or acetaminophen.

SPECIAL CONSIDERATIONS

Disposition
- Patients can usually be safely discharged home to follow-up with their primary physician.

Rheumatoid Arthritis (RA)

GENERAL PRINCIPLES

Definition
- A symmetric, inflammatory, or peripheral polyarthritis

Epidemiology/Etiology
- Age of onset is between 50 and 65 and is more common in females.
- Genetic components and cigarette smoking are implicated in the development of RA.

Pathophysiology
- Autoimmune breakdown of the synovium causing destruction of bone and cartilage

DIAGNOSIS

Clinical Presentation
History
- Patients will report peripheral joint pain, swelling, and more than 30 minutes of stiffness upon wakening, usually lasting for >6 weeks.
- Systemic complaints such as myalgias, fever, fatigue, weight loss, and depression may be present.
- RA usually improves over the course of the day.

Physical Examination
- The examination should be focused on joints, looking for joint line tenderness, bony swelling/deformity, joint instability, and limited range of motion. Erythema and warmth are not features of RA.
- Pathognomonic findings include ulnar deviation, boutonniere, and swan-neck deformities, hammer toes, and joint ankylosis.

Differential Diagnosis
- Gout, pseudogout, Reiter syndrome, systemic lupus erythematosus (SLE), scleroderma, polymyositis, polymyalgia rheumatica (PMR), viral polyarthritis, or systemic rheumatic diseases

Diagnostic Criteria and Testing

The diagnosis or RA can be made when the following criteria are present:

- Inflammatory arthritis involving three or more joints
- Positive rheumatoid factor (RF)
- Elevated CRP or erythrocyte sedimentation rate (ESR)
- Exclusion of other diseases on the differential diagnosis
- Duration of symptoms >6 weeks

Laboratories

- CBC, antinuclear antibody (ANA), C-reactive protein (CRP), erythrocyte sedimentation rate (ESR), and rheumatoid factor (RF) should be drawn.
- Synovial fluid with a cell count between 1500 and 25,000 cells/mm^3 is frequently present. The fluid will also have low glucose levels and protein levels near serum protein levels.

Imaging

- Plain radiographs of joints may show characteristic joint erosion.

TREATMENT

Medications

- NSAIDs are the primary initial medication in the emergency department (ED).
- Glucocorticoids or methotrexate may be started in consultation with a rheumatologist.

SPECIAL CONSIDERATIONS

Disposition

- Most patients may be discharged home with rheumatology follow-up.

Septic Arthritis

GENERAL PRINCIPLES

Definition

- Infection of a joint

Epidemiology/Etiology

- Usually bacterial, but may be viral or fungal, spread from a hematogenous source or from violation of the joint space iatrogenically or from trauma.
- Risk factors include older age (>80 years), diabetes, RA, presence of a prosthetic joint, recent joint surgery, cellulitis, IV drug use, or prior violation of the joint space.

Pathophysiology

- Bacteria in the joint space cause an acute inflammatory response, with bacteria entering the synovial fluid, leading to inflammation and purulence. This causes cartilage and bone destruction.

DIAGNOSIS

Clinical Presentation

History
- Patients usually complain of joint pain, swelling, warmth, and difficulty moving the joint. Some patients report fever.

Physical Examination
- Swelling and warmth are usually found in the affected joint. Most of the time, only one joint is affected but all joints should be examined. Range of motion is limited by pain. The patient may be febrile.

Differential Diagnosis
- Crystal arthropathy, hemarthrosis, tumor, systemic rheumatic disease, OA, or trauma

Diagnostic Criteria and Testing

Laboratories
- WBC may be drawn along with ESR or CRP and may all be elevated.
- Synovial fluid should be sent for cell count, Gram stain/culture, and crystal analysis (Table 53.1).

TABLE 53.1	Categories of Synovial Fluid Based on Clinical and Laboratory Findings			
Measure	Normal	Noninflammatory	Inflammatory	Septic	Hemorrhagic
Volume, mL (knee)	<3.5	Often >3.5	Often >3.5	Often >3.5	Usually >3.5
Clarity	Transparent	Transparent	Translucent–opaque	Opaque	Bloody
Color	Clear	Yellow	Yellow to opalescent	Yellow to green	Red
Viscosity	High	High	Low	Variable	Variable
WBC, per mm³	<200	200–2000	2000–100,000	15,000 to >100,000[a]	200–2000
PMNs, percent	<25	<25	≥50	≥75	50–75
Culture	Negative	Negative	Negative	Often positive	Negative
Total protein, g/dL	1–2	1–3	3–5	3–5	4–6
Glucose, mg/dL	Nearly equal to blood	Nearly equal to blood	>25, lower than blood	<25, much lower than blood	Nearly equal to blood

[a]Lower part of range with infections caused by partially treated or low virulence organisms.

PMN, polymorphonuclear leukocyte. Source: Sholter DE, Russell AS. Synovial Fluid Analysis: Septic Arthritis in Adults. In: Curtis MR, ed. *UpToDate*. Waltham: UpToDate (last accessed 4/6/17).

Imaging
- There are no imaging studies that are diagnostic for septic arthritis, but concurrent osteomyelitis may be present.

Diagnostic Procedures
- Arthrocentesis will help differentiate a septic joint from other causes, but care should be taken not to tap the joint over cellulitic skin.

TREATMENT

Medications

- Initial choice of antibiotics should be based on likely organisms and Gram stain results.
- Gram-positive cocci:
  - Vancomycin 30 mg/kg IV q24 hours is divided into two doses (2 g max q24h).
  - If vancomycin allergic, daptomycin, clindamycin, or linezolid may be substituted.
- Gram-negative bacilli:
  - Ceftriaxone 2 g IV qD
  - Cefotaxime 2 g IV q8 hours
  - Ceftazidime 1–2 g IV q8 hours
- If clinical suspicion for *Pseudomonas aeruginosa* exists (IV drug users):
  - Add gentamicin 3–5 mg/kg/d in 2–3 divided doses.
- If negative Gram stain, vancomycin should still be used. If the patient is immunocompromised, treatment with vancomycin and an aminoglycoside is recommended.

SPECIAL CONSIDERATIONS

Disposition
- These patients should be admitted to the hospital.

Complications
- Endocarditis, osteomyelitis, or sepsis

Gout

GENERAL PRINCIPLES

Definition
- Gout—monosodium urate crystal arthropathy

Epidemiology/Etiology
- The disease presents in later years with a slight male predominance.
- Risk factors include obesity, trauma, surgery, starvation, alcohol consumption, dehydration, fatty food consumption, or consumption of high-fructose corn syrup–containing foods.
- Gout attacks occur more frequently overnight or in the early morning.

Pathophysiology
- Monosodium urate crystals in the joint space cause an inflammatory response, arthritis, and potential tophus formation. The inflammatory response usually resolves within a few weeks, even without treatment.

DIAGNOSIS

Clinical Presentation

History
- The patient will frequently report a painful swollen monoarticular joint, usually in the extremities (usually spares axial joints). Polyarticular involvement is less common.

Physical Examination
- The affected joint may be warm, have pain with range of motion, and have swelling that extends beyond the primary joint.
- The majority of initial attacks are monoarticular (knee or base of the great toe).

Differential Diagnosis
- Septic arthritis, trauma, pseudogout, cellulitis, or rheumatic disease

Diagnostic Criteria and Testing

Laboratories
- There are no specific serum laboratory values that will diagnose gout, but serum uric acid levels may be falsely decreased as the uric acid crystals are being deposited into the joint early in a gouty attack.
- Synovial fluid will show intracellular monosodium urate crystals. The white cell count in the aspirate ranges between 10,000 and 100,000 with neurophilic predominance.

Imaging
- Plain imaging may show gouty tophi or erosions but are not usually seen in initial attacks.

Diagnostic Procedures
- Arthrocentesis

TREATMENT

Medications
- Initial therapy is with naproxen 500 mg PO bid or indomethacin 50 mg PO tid.
  - Indomethacin should be avoided in older adults.
- Colchicine may be used in patients who have contraindications to NSAIDs.
  - Initial dose is 1.2 mg PO followed an hour later by 0.6 mg.
  - 0.6 mg once or twice daily is prescribed until response or resolution is achieved.
  - Colchicine is contraindicated with severe renal (CrCl < 30 mL/min) or hepatic impairment or if the patient is on medication that inhibits P-glycoprotein and/or CYP3A4.
- Corticosteroids may also be administered if the patient cannot tolerate NSAIDs or colchicine, but this should be done in consultation with a rheumatologist.

SPECIAL CONSIDERATIONS

Disposition
- Patients may be discharged home with follow-up with their primary physician or rheumatologist.

Bursitis

GENERAL PRINCIPLES

Definition
• Inflammation of the lining of the synovial membranes

Epidemiology/Etiology
• Causes may include trauma, prolonged pressure on a joint, overuse, crystal-induced arthropathy, inflammatory arthritis, or infection.
• *Staphylococcus aureus* is the most common causative organism in septic bursitis cases.

Pathophysiology
• Local trauma leads to a release in inflammatory cells, causing effusion and pain with range of motion. Infectious bursitis can be caused by local, traumatic, or hematologic spread of bacteria.

DIAGNOSIS

Clinical Presentation
History
• Patients may complain of swelling and tenderness in the affected joint.

Physical Examination
• Evaluate the joint for tenderness directly over the bursa with pain elicited on active motion of the bursa/joint. Passive motion is usually painless.
• Evaluate for evidence of penetrating trauma, cellulitis, abrasion, or signs of systemic polyarthropathy.

Differential Diagnosis
• Deep bursitis, cellulitis, OA, RA, trauma, crystal-induced bursitis, or osteomyelitis

Diagnostic Criteria and Testing
Laboratories
• In noncomplicated bursitis, the bursal fluid should have a cell count of <500 cells/mm^3 and be nonbloody.
• WBC over 2000 cells/mm^3 from aspirated fluid may be indicative for septic bursitis.
• Gram stain of the bursal fluid is indicated if septic bursitis is considered.
  ○ Bacteria may not be present in one-third of cases.

Diagnostic Procedures
• Aspiration of the bursal fluid is warranted to evaluate for septic bursitis and for symptomatic control.

TREATMENT

Medications
• NSAIDs are the first-line therapy for an uncomplicated superficial bursitis.
• Septic bursitis with mild inflammation.
  ○ Dicloxacillin 500 mg PO qid. If penicillin allergic,
    ▪ Clindamycin, doxycycline, or trimethoprim–sulfamethoxazole may be used.

- Septic bursitis with severe inflammation or immunocompromise.
  - Vancomycin 15–20 mg/kg/dose q8–12 hours (not exceeding 2 g daily).
  - Antipseudomonal coverage should be added for immunocompromised patients.

Other Nonpharmacologic Therapies

- Short-term ice pack use for superficial bursitis, heating pad for deeper bursitis, and joint padding to prevent recurrence should be discussed with the patient.
- Surgical intervention may be necessary for deep aspiration, failed aspiration, foreign body presence, or adjacent skin/soft tissue infection needing debridement.

SPECIAL CONSIDERATIONS

Disposition

- Patients with uncomplicated superficial bursitis may be discharged home. Patients with presumed septic bursitis should be admitted.

SUGGESTED READINGS

2010 ACR/EULAR classification criteria for rheumatoid arthritis. Available at: http://www.rheumatology.org/practice/clinical/classification/ra/ra_2010.asp (last accessed 1/30/2016).

American Geriatrics Society 2012 Beers Criteria Update Expert Panel. American Geriatrics Society updated Beers Criteria for potentially inappropriate medication use in older adults. *J Am Geriatr Soc* 2012;60:616.

Osteoarthritis: National Clinical Guideline for Care and Management in Adults. In: NCCfC, ed. Conditions.. London: Royal College of Physicians, 2008.

Allen KD, Coffman CJ, Golightly YM, et al. Daily pain variations among patients with hand, hip, and knee osteoarthritis. *Osteoarthritis Cartilage* 2009;17:1275.

Choi HK, Niu J, Neogi T, et al. Nocturnal risk of gout attacks. *Arthritis Rheumatol* 2015;67:555.

Goldenberg DL, Reed JI. Bacterial arthritis. *N Engl J Med* 1985;312:764.

Ho G Jr, Su EY. Antibiotic therapy of septic bursitis. Its implication in the treatment of septic arthritis. *Arthritis Rheum* 1981;24:905.

Ho G Jr, Tice AD, Kaplan SR. Septic bursitis in the prepatellar and olecranon bursae: an analysis of 25 cases. *Ann Intern Med* 1978;89:21.

Kortekangas P, Aro HT, Tuominen J, Toivanen A. Synovial fluid leukocytosis in bacterial arthritis vs. reactive arthritis and rheumatoid arthritis in the adult knee. *Scand J Rheumatol* 1992;21:283.

Ko JY, Wang FS. Rotator cuff lesions with shoulder stiffness: updated pathomechanisms and management. *Chang Gung Med J* 2011;34:331.

Lawrence JS, Bremner JM, Bier F. Osteo-arthrosis. Prevalence in the population and relationship between symptoms and x-ray changes. *Ann Rheum Dis* 1966;25:1.

Lee DM, Weinblatt ME. Rheumatoid arthritis. *Lancet* 2001;358:903.

Loeser RF, Goldring SR, Scanzello CR, Goldring MB. Osteoarthritis: a disease of the joint as an organ. *Arthritis Rheum* 2012;64:1697.

Margaretten ME, Kohlwes J, Moore D, Bent S. Does this adult patient have septic arthritis? *JAMA* 2007;297:1478.

Mathews CJ, Coakley G. Septic arthritis: current diagnostic and therapeutic algorithm. *Curr Opin Rheumatol* 2008;20:457.

McQueen FM, Doyle A, Dalbeth N. Imaging in the crystal arthropathies. *Rheum Dis Clin North Am* 2014;40:231.

Rainer TH, Cheng CH, Janssens HJ, et al. Oral prednisolone in the treatment of acute gout: a pragmatic, multicenter, double-blind, randomized trial. *Ann Intern Med* 2016; 164:464.

Roddy E, Choi HK. Epidemiology of gout. *Rheum Dis Clin North Am* 2014;40:155.

Roschmann RA, Bell CL. Septic bursitis in immunocompromised patients. *Am J Med* 1987;83:661.

Rosenthal AK. Crystals, inflammation, and osteoarthritis. *Curr Opin Rheumatol* 2011;23:170.

Sharff KA, Richards EP, Townes JM. Clinical management of septic arthritis. *Curr Rheumatol Rep* 2013;15:332.

Sokka T, Mäkinen H. Drug management of early rheumatoid arthritis–2008. *Best Pract Res Clin Rheumatol* 2009;23:93.

Stell IM, Gransden WR. Simple tests for septic bursitis: comparative study. *BMJ* 1998;316:1877.

Sutaria S, Katbamna R, Underwood M. Effectiveness of interventions for the treatment of acute and prevention of recurrent gout—a systematic review. *Rheumatology (Oxford)* 2006;45:1422.

Terkeltaub RA, Furst DE, Bennett K, et al. High versus low dosing of oral colchicine for early acute gout flare: Twenty-four-hour outcome of the first multicenter, randomized, double-blind, placebo-controlled, parallel-group, dose-comparison colchicine study. *Arthritis Rheum* 2010;62:1060.

Zimmermann B 3rd, Mikolich DJ, Ho G Jr. Septic bursitis. *Semin Arthritis Rheum* 1995;24:391.

54 Musculoskeletal Emergencies: Compression Fractures

Al Lulla

GENERAL PRINCIPLES

Definition

• Compression fractures are deformities of the vertebral bodies that are the most common complication of low bone mineral density and osteoporosis.[1]

Epidemiology/Etiology

• Commonly occur in the midthoracic or thoracolumbar regions of the spine.[2,3]
• Vertebral compression fractures most commonly affect postmenopausal females.
  ○ After the age of 65, men are at increased risk of compression fractures.
  ○ Fractures occur at a lower rate compared to women of the same age.[2,3]
• Other important risk factors are osteoporosis, alcohol abuse, smoking, low calcium intake, vitamin D deficiency, glucocorticoid use, decreased physical activity, Caucasian race, and dementia.[2–4]

Pathophysiology

• Osteoporosis is the major contributor to vertebral compression fractures.[3]
• The vast majority of vertebral compression fractures occur without any history of significant trauma.[3]
• Compression fractures can be associated with other conditions such as malignancy, infection, or hyperparathyroidism.

DIAGNOSIS

- The majority of vertebral compression fractures are found incidentally on imaging, and most patients are asymptomatic at the time of diagnosis.[5]

Clinical Presentation

History
- In the acute setting, patients who are symptomatic may report sudden-onset pain that began after a seemingly benign event. The pain is often severe and localized; however, pain can radiate anteriorly and often times be mistaken for an acute cardiopulmonary process. Pain is usually worse with sitting up and engaging in activity and improved when lying supine.[2,4]

Physical Examination
- In cases of acute fracture, there may be tenderness directly over the corresponding area of the back. A complete neurologic examination, including examination for perineal numbness and rectal tone, should be done to evaluate for any evidence of spinal cord injury.[1,4,5]

Differential Diagnosis

- Osteoarthritis, pathologic fracture, lumbar strain, metastases, Paget's disease of bone, osteomyelitis, pain from tumor compression, epidural abscess, or malignancy.[2]

Diagnostic Criteria and Testing

Laboratories
- There are no laboratory values that are specific for the diagnosis of compression fracture.

Imaging
- The diagnosis of vertebral compression fracture is made using spinal imaging studies. Comparison to prior plain radiographs if available can be beneficial to determine approximate age of the fracture.[1,2,6]
- CT or MRI may also be used in a subset of patients to better assess characteristics of the vertebral body and possible spinal cord injury and to rule out other causes of compression fracture such as malignancy.[2,6]
  - To be classified as a compression fracture, there must be at least a 20% reduction in height of the anterior, middle, or posterior portions of the vertebral body, or a 4 mm reduction in vertebral height as measured compared to baseline.[2,3,6,7]

TREATMENT

Medications

- NSAIDs are often first-line medications.
- Opioid analgesics, muscle relaxants, local anesthetic patches, and intercostal nerve blocks can also be considered in the acute setting.[1,2,4,6]

Other Nonpharmacologic Therapies

- Stable compression fractures are usually treated conservatively.[6] Surgical consultation is required for unstable fractures.
- While immediate bed rest is recommended, prolonged immobility is associated with worse outcomes, especially in the elderly.
- One small randomized trial showed decreased pain and improvement in activities of daily living with the use of a spinal orthotic device.[6]

SPECIAL CONSIDERATIONS

Disposition

- Patients with unstable fractures, neurologic deficits, or uncontrolled pain or those requiring surgical intervention can be admitted.

Complications

- The acute presentation of a compression fracture may be a medical emergency. A fracture may manifest as spinal cord compression, cauda equina, or neurologic complications.[2,7]

REFERENCES

1. Ensrud KE, Schousboe JT. Vertebral fractures. *N Engl J Med* 2011;364:1634–42.
2. Wong CC, McGirt MJ. Vertebral compression fractures: a review of current management and multimodal therapy. *J Multidiscip Healthc* 2013;6:205–14.
3. Alexandru D, So W. Evaluation and management of vertebral compression fractures. *Perm J* 2012;16:46–51.
4. Old JL, Calvert M. Vertebral compression fractures in the elderly. *Am Fam Physician* 2004;69:111–16.
5. Kim DH, Vaccaro AR. Osteoporotic compression fractures of the spine; current options and considerations for treatment. *Spine J* 2006;6:479–87.
6. Pfeifer M, Begerow B, Minne HW. Effects of a new spinal orthosis on posture, trunk strength, and quality of life in women with postmenopausal osteoporosis: a randomized trial. *Am J Phys Med Rehabil* 2004;83:177–86.
7. Francis RM, Baillie SP, Chuck AJ, et al. Acute and long-term management of patients with vertebral fractures. *QJM* 2004;97:63–74.

55 Musculoskeletal Emergencies: Spinal Epidural Abscess

Al Lulla

GENERAL PRINCIPLES

Definition

- A spinal epidural abscess is defined as an infection in the epidural space between the dura mater and vertebral bodies.

Epidemiology/Etiology

- A spinal epidural abscess is a relatively uncommon entity.[1]
- Risk factors include diabetes mellitus, HIV infection, alcoholism, trauma, degenerative joint disease, skin and soft tissue infection, sepsis, osteomyelitis, indwelling catheters, intravenous drug use, or tattooing.[2–6]

- Spinal epidural abscesses occur most commonly in adult patients aged 30–60 years old.[5]

Pathophysiology

- Infection can be introduced to the epidural space via three primary mechanisms: hematogenous dissemination, direct contiguous spread from surrounding structures, or iatrogenic (invasive procedures) means.
- Spinal epidural abscesses extend approximately four vertebral segments on average.[7]
- In roughly two-thirds of cases, the causative organism is *Staphylococcus aureus*, commonly MRSA.[3,6] Other organisms implicated in spinal epidural abscesses include coagulase-negative staphylococci, gram-negative bacilli (*Escherichia coli*, *Pseudomonas aeruginosa*, *Klebsiella* spp.), and streptococci species.[8]

DIAGNOSIS

Clinical Presentation

History

- Patients with a spinal epidural abscess can present to the ED in various different stages of the disease process. These stages are outlined based on their neurologic presentation[2]:
  - Stage 1: Localized back pain at the level of the lesion
  - Stage 2: Radiculopathy with shooting pains in regions that correspond to affected nerve roots
  - Stage 3: Motor deficits, sensory dysfunction, bowel or bladder dysfunction
  - Stage 4: Paralysis
- Back pain is the most common presentation to the ED. The "classic triad" of symptoms for patients with spinal epidural abscess is defined as the following: back pain, fever (temperature ≥100.4°F), and neurologic deficits but only 2-13% of patients will have the "classic triad" at the time of presentation.[7,2,5,9].

Physical Examination

- A full neurologic exam should be performed with special attention paid to the triad of symptoms noted above.[5]
- Potential sources of infection should be investigated, including evidence of skin/soft tissue infection, needle track marks, or evidence of prior surgical interventions.

Differential Diagnosis

- Discitis, meningitis, vertebral osteomyelitis, compression fracture, cauda equina syndrome, and cancer metastasis

Diagnostic Criteria and Testing

Laboratories

- Elevated WBC, erythrocyte sedimentation rate (ESR), and c-reactive protein (CRP) are found in the majority of patients.[9]
- Blood cultures should be obtained.[10]

Imaging

- MRI with gadolinium contrast is the gold standard imaging modality.[2,9]

TREATMENT

- The treatment of choice for a spinal epidural abscess is surgical drainage and systemic intravenous antibiotics.
- Antibiotic therapy should be tailored to cover methicillin-resistant *Staphylococcus aureus* (MRSA) with vancomycin, and gram-negative bacilli with third- or fourth-generation cephalosporins.[8]
- A spine surgeon should be consulted immediately when there is clinical suspicion for spinal epidural abscess or confirmation of diagnosis based on imaging findings.

SPECIAL CONSIDERATIONS

Disposition

- Admit for surgical intervention.

Complications

- Many of the complications are neurologic, including weakness of an extremity, sensory deficit, bowel or bladder dysfunction, and irreversible paralysis.[7]
- Infectious complications include life-threatening sepsis, endocarditis, vertebral osteomyelitis, and psoas abscess.[1,2]

REFERENCES

1. Sendi P, Bregenzer T, Zimmerli W. Spinal epidural abscess in clinical practice. *QJ Med* 2008;101:1–12.
2. Darouiche RO. Spinal Epidural Abscess. *N Engl J Med* 2006;355:2012–20.
3. Sampath P, Rigamonti D. Spinal epidural abscess: a review of epidemiology, diagnosis, and treatment. *J Spinal Disord* 1999;12:89–93.
4. Reihsaus E, Waldbaur H, Seeling W. Spinal epidural abscess: a meta-analysis of 915 patients. *Neurosurg Rev* 2000;23:175–204; discussion 205.
5. Davis DP, Wold RM, Patel RJ, et al. The clinical presentation and impact of diagnostic delays on emergency department patients with spinal epidural abscess. *J Emerg Med* 2004;26:285–91.
6. Patel AR, Alton TB, Bransford RJ, et al. Spinal epidural abscesses: risk factors, medical versus surgical management, a retrospective review of 128 cases. *Spine J* 2014;14: 326–30.
7. Darouiche RO, Hamill RJ, Greenberg SB, et al. Bacterial spinal epidural abscess. Review of 43 cases and literature survey. *Medicine (Baltimore)* 1992;71:369–85.
8. Rigamonti D, Liem L, Sampath P, et al. Spinal epidural abscess: contemporary trends in etiology, evaluation, and management. *Surg Neurol* 1999;52:189–96.
9. Davis DP, Salazar A, Chan TC, Vilke GM. Prospective evaluation of a clinical decision guideline to diagnose spinal epidural abscess in patients who present to the emergency department with spine pain. *J Neurosurg Spine* 2011;14:765–70.
10. Curry WT, Hoh BL, Amin-Hanjani S, Eskandar EN. Spinal epidural abscess: clinical presentation, management, and outcome. *Surg Neurol* 2005;63:364–71.

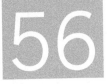

56 Musculoskeletal Emergencies: Hand and Wrist Injuries and Disorders

Louis H. Poppler and Grant Kleiber

GENERAL PRINCIPLES

Epidemiology/Etiology
• Males and working age adults are at increased risk for hand injuries.
• Elderly females are at increased risk for wrist fractures.
• The elderly are at increased risk for burns.

Pathophysiology
• Hand pathology is heterogeneous. A thorough history and examination is essential to identify the source of patients' injury/dysfunction and will guide further studies and treatment in the emergency department.

Clinical Presentation
• Patients typically present with swelling and pain. Often, they will be stiff, sore, or unwilling to move their hand and/or wrist.

History
• Every patient with a hand injury or disorder should be asked about hand dominance, profession, and hand usage.
• The history should also include the timing of the injury, duration of the symptoms, mechanism of the injury, changing or evolving symptoms, and subjective sensory symptoms.
  ○ Ask the patient to identify the most painful point.

Physical Examination
• Assess color, turgor, and capillary refill (with Doppler if needed).
• Check the sensation in the fingers and the back of the hand.
  ○ The "10/10 test" asks patients to rate their level of sensation in the finger relative to the opposite (normal) hand. 10/10 sensation is full sensation. 0/10 sensation would be no sensation.
  ○ Evaluate for tingling, numbness, or pain.
  ○ Assess the median nerve by testing sensation in the thumb, the ulnar by testing sensation in the small finger, and the radial by testing sensation on the back of the hand.
  ○ Ulnar nerve motor function is tested by asking patients to cross their fingers. Inability to do this should raise concerns for ulnar nerve pathology.
• Observe for swelling and palpating along the bones of the finger and hand.

- Check for tendinous injuries by asking the patients to flex each finger, extend each finger, and make a table top (MCP joints flexed, fingers straight). Wrist flexion and extension should also be evaluated.
  - A sensitive test for bony or musculotendinous pathology is to observe a patients finger cascade (the way the fingers move when the wrist is passively extended and flexed). The fingers should extend when the wrist flexes and flex when the wrist extends. The fingers should close in line with one another without crossing or impeding one another. They should also be symmetric to the contralateral hand. If they do not, further evaluation is warranted.
  - Pain with passive movement (especially extension) can be a hallmark of tenosynovitis or compartment syndrome.

Diagnostic Criteria and Testing
Laboratory
- Routine laboratory testing should include a CBC, BMP, and, if indicated, an erythrocyte sedimentation rate (ESR) and c-reactive protein (CRP).
  - A normal white blood count, ESR, or CRP does not rule out hand pathology.

Imaging
- Anytime a patient presents with hand trauma, or bony injury is suspected, a three-view radiograph series of the hand and/or wrist should be obtained.
- CT imaging should be obtained if a deep space infection is suspected.

Diagnostic Procedures
- Suspected septic joints in the hand or wrist should be tapped.

SPLINTING

- Splints can help manage nearly all hand injuries.
  - Sugar-tong splint—used for distal radius and/or ulna fractures or most carpal bone fractures
    - Wraps from the volar hand down the forearm with the wrist neutral, around the elbow, and up the dorsal forearm to the metacarpal–phalangeal joints.
    - The volar splint should not extend past midpalmar crease to allow finger flexion.
  - Intrinsic plus splint—used for all hand fractures (not including carpal bones)
    - It immobilizes the wrist at neutral or 15–30 degree extension, metacarpal phalangeal joints flexed 70 degrees, and interphalangeal joints fully extended. The elbow is free.
    - Can be tailored to include all or just some digits.
    - This places all of the joint support ligaments at their maximum length, minimizing stiffness later.
    - Point of flexion is at the midpalmar crease, not at the level of the web spaces.
    - An ulnar gutter style is not good for intrinsic plus positioning because the point of flexion is different on the volar and dorsal sides.
  - Thumb spica splint—used for thumb or scaphoid fractures
    - Starts midforearm, wrapping up around the thumb holding the wrist neutral and thumb in opposition as if holding a can
- When concerned for a tendon injury, splint the hand so that the injured tendon will be at its shortest possible length (i.e., wrist and MCPs flexed for flexor injury).

Flexor Tenosynovitis

GENERAL PRINCIPLES

Definition
- Infection of the flexor sheath, which surrounds the flexor tendons.
- Tendinitis of the dorsal extensor tendons is common but rarely the result of infection and therefore rarely urgent.[1]

CLINICAL PRESENTATION AND DIAGNOSIS

- Patients typically have a history of trauma to their digit.
  - The site of trauma may be underwhelming compared with the swelling and pain of the digit.
  - Immunocompromised or diabetic patients may have a more indolent course.
- Four "Kanavel" cardinal signs (in order of sensitivity).[2]
  - Fusiform swelling of digit
  - Pain with passive extension of digit (most specific)
  - Finger held in slightly flexed position
  - Pain along flexor sheath up into palm beyond zone of erythema and swelling (often a late finding)
- Patients will not actively move the injured finger.

Laboratories and Imaging
- CBC
- Three-view hand radiographs to rule out foreign body or unrecognized fracture

Differential Diagnosis
- Cellulitis, subcutaneous abscess or felon, or septic or gouty joint

TREATMENT

- Flexor tenosynovitis is a surgical emergency. Hand surgery consult for emergent surgical washout.
- Administer broad spectrum antibiotics as soon as diagnosis is suspected.
- Splint in position of comfort and elevate extremity until taken to OR.

Septic Joint

GENERAL PRINCIPLES

Definition
- Infection of one of the joints in the hand or wrist.

CLINICAL PRESENTATION AND DIAGNOSIS

- Patients typically do not have a history of trauma.
- There is erythema and swelling overlying the joint and extreme pain with movement or loading of the joint.
- Diagnosis requires aspiration of joint fluid for Gram stain and culture, and cell count.

Laboratories and Imaging

- CBC, ESR, and CRP have little value in diagnosing septic wrist or finger joints.
- Three-view hand radiographs to rule out a foreign body, unrecognized fracture, or to sequelae of chronic gout.

Differential Diagnosis

- Gout, pseudogout, arthritis, cellulitis, or abscess of tissues overlying joint

TREATMENT

- A septic joint requires emergent washout and is a surgical emergency.[3]
- Broad spectrum antibiotics should be started as soon as joint culture is obtained.

Paronychia

GENERAL PRINCIPLES

Definition

- Infection of the lateral and proximal fingernail folds usually by *S. aureus*, oral flora, and *S. pyogenes*.
- Risk factors include manicuring/nail biting, DM, chronic water immersion (occupational), and HIV antiretroviral therapy.

CLINICAL PRESENTATION AND DIAGNOSIS

- Pain and erythema of the postural or lateral nail folds with associated superficial abscess

Laboratories and Imaging

- Three-view hand radiographs to rule out foreign body or unrecognized fracture

Differential Diagnosis

- Onychomycosis, herpetic whitlow, psoriasis, or felon

TREATMENT

- If there is no abscess, local compresses/soaks and oral antibiotic therapy may help.
- If an abscess has formed, incision and drainage is indicated by elevation of the cuticle margin or superficial drainage after appropriate anesthesia has been provided.
- Oral antibiotic therapy can be prescribed based on the presumed etiology (oral flora or staph/strep), but incision and drainage is usually sufficient.

Felon

GENERAL PRINCIPLES

Definition

- Infection of the volar pulp of the fingertip

CLINICAL PRESENTATION AND DIAGNOSIS

- Patients typically have a history of trauma to their digit or nail.
- Swelling is focal and limited to the distal finger/volar pulp.
- There should be no pain proximal to the swelling and no pain with passive extension.

Laboratories and Imaging
• Three-view hand radiographs to rule out foreign body or unrecognized fracture

Differential Diagnosis
• Cellulitis, paronychia, or septic or gouty joint

TREATMENT

• Requires drainage under digital block
• Antibiotics to cover skin flora and MRSA[4]
• Follow-up with a hand surgeon within 1 week to ensure the infection is resolving.

Acute Carpal Tunnel Syndrome

GENERAL PRINCIPLES

Definition
• Compression of the median nerve usually caused by displaced distal radius fracture, carpal dislocation (i.e., perilunate injury), or swelling[5]

CLINICAL PRESENTATION AND DIAGNOSIS

• Patients have progressive numbness and pain in the thumb, index, long, and ring fingers.

Laboratories and Imaging
• Three-view wrist radiographs or as indicated by injury pattern

Differential Diagnosis
• Acute nerve injury, chronic carpal tunnel, or other nerve compression

TREATMENT

• Reduce and splint fracture/dislocation as quickly as possible.
• Elevate arm.
• If numbness and pain do not rapidly improve, emergent carpal tunnel release is indicated.

High-Pressure Injection Injuries

GENERAL PRINCIPLES

Definition
• High-pressure injections cause tissue necrosis.
• Injected substances track along tissue planes and the zone of injury can be far more extensive than injection site.

CLINICAL PRESENTATION AND DIAGNOSIS

• Initial presentation is often unimpressive.
• There is rapid and progressive swelling and pain.
• Patients may present with hand compartment syndrome, acute carpal tunnel, flexor tenosynovitis, or a combination of these.

Laboratories and Imaging

- Three-view hand radiographs can demonstrate the extent of subcutaneous emphysema.

Treatment

- Except in rare cases, these injuries require emergent debridement and compartment release.
- While awaiting hand surgeon consultation, splint in a position of comfort, elevate the extremity, and provide pain control.

Compartment Syndrome

GENERAL PRINCIPLES

Definition

- Edema of muscles within their fascial compartment increases compartment pressure beyond mean capillary pressure, arresting perfusion within the compartment and causing ischemia of muscle.

CLINICAL PRESENTATION AND DIAGNOSIS

- Commonly presents following high-energy trauma or following prolonged ischemia and reperfusion.
- The 5P's (pain, paresthesia, pallor, paralysis, pulselessness) are rarely all present.
  - Pain with passive movement and out of proportion to exam is the most sensitive exam finding.[6]
  - Palpably firm compartments are also common.
  - The hand is often held in intrinsic minus position (interphalangeal joints flexed, metacarpal phalangeal joints extended).

Laboratories and Imaging

- Lactate and serum myoglobin
- Radiographs as directed by underlying trauma

SPECIAL CONSIDERATIONS

- Compartment pressures can be measured, and if >30 mm Hg, surgical consultation for fasciotomy is indicated.

TREATMENT

- When present, emergent fasciotomies are indicated.
- While awaiting surgery, splinting in a position of comfort, elevating the extremity, and pain control are indicated.

REFERENCES

1. Adams JE, Habbu R. Tendinopathies of the hand and wrist. *J Am Acad Orthop Surg* 2015;23(12):741–50.
2. Kennedy CD, Huang JI, Hanel DP. In brief: Kanavel's signs and pyogenic flexor tenosynovitis. *Clin Orthop Relat Res* 2016;474(1):280–4.

3. Birman MV, Strauch RJ. Management of the septic wrist. *J Hand Surg Am* 2011;36(2):324–6; quiz 7.
4. Connolly B, Johnstone F, Gerlinger T, Puttler E. Methicillin-resistant Staphylococcus aureus in a finger felon. *J Hand Surg Am* 2000;25(1):173–5.
5. Gillig JD, White SD, Rachel JN. Acute carpal tunnel syndrome: a review of current literature. *Orthop Clin North Am* 2016;47(3):599–607.
6. Oak NR, Abrams RA. Compartment syndrome of the hand. *Orthop Clin North Am* 2016;47(3):609–16.

57 Musculoskeletal Emergencies: Inflammatory Myopathies

Maureen Gross

Myositis: Polymyositis and Dermatomyositis

GENERAL PRINCIPLES

Definition

- Inflammatory myopathies are a group of rare and heterogeneous disorders defined by immune-mediated muscle injury, often referred to as "myositis."[1]

Epidemiology/Etiology

- The inflammatory myopathies are rare.
- The age distribution is bimodal, with a peak between 10 and 15 years and between 40 and 60 years.[2]
- The male to female ratio is ~2:1 for polymyositis and dermatomyositis.[3,4]

Pathophysiology

- The precise pathogenic mechanisms of tissue injury are poorly defined in most cases. The association with other autoimmune disorders (Hashimoto's thyroiditis, myasthenia gravis) as well as response to corticosteroids suggests an autoimmune pathogenesis.[3]
  - In some cases, these inflammatory myopathies are paraneoplastic syndromes associated with malignancy.[1,3,5,6]

DIAGNOSIS

Clinical Presentation

History

- Patients often present with subacute to chronic onset of proximal muscle weakness that can be painful or painless.[5] Patients will often complain of fatigue, difficulty

rising from a chair, lifting objects, or even combing one's hair. Symptoms typically occur relatively slowly, over weeks to months.
- Extramuscular manifestations include rash, dyspnea, dysphagia, cough, or difficulty swallowing.

Physical Examination
- Muscular Manifestations
  - Proximal and frequently symmetric weakness of limb girdle muscles[7] (tested with active resistance).
  - Facial and ocular muscle involvement should bring doubt to this diagnosis.
  - Compartment syndrome and significant muscle body edema can be a rare complication of myositis.[8]
- Extramuscular Manifestations
  - Pulmonary
    - 20–65% of patients exhibit pulmonary manifestations in the form of interstitial lung disease, or dysphagia leading to aspiration pneumonia.[6,9] In rare and advanced cases, respiratory muscles are involved.
  - Cardiac
    - Common cardiac associations with myositis include myocarditis, conduction blockages, arrhythmias, and congestive heart failure.
  - Gastrointestinal
    - Dysphagia or vasculopathy causing gastrointestinal (GI) bleeding
  - Skin
    - The rash of dermatomyositis typically includes an erythematous, photosensitive rash on the neck, back, and shoulders (shawl sign), eyelids (heliotrope rash), and a scaly lichenoid rash over knuckles (Gottron papules).

Differential Diagnosis
- Viral or bacterial myositis (HIV, enterovirus, Epstein-Barr virus [EBV], influenza, hepatitis A and B)
- Drug-induced myopathy (statin, alcohol, colchicine, corticosteroids, cocaine)
- Endocrine/metabolic (hyper/hypothyroidism, hyper/hypoparathyroidism, hypercortisolism, hypokalemia, hypocalcemia)
- Rhabdomyolysis
- Neurologic disorders (Guillain-Barré syndrome, polymyalgia rheumatica, myesthenia gravis, muscular dystrophy)

Diagnostic Criteria and Testing
- The Bohan and Peter Diagnostic criteria include muscle weakness, elevation of muscle enzymes, EMG, biopsy results, and skin rash in the case of DM.[5,7]

Laboratories
- CBC, CMP, magnesium, phosphorus, thyroid panel, creatine phosphokinase (CPK), erythrocyte sedimentation rate (ESR), and c-reactive protein (CRP) should be obtained.

Imaging
- There is no emergent imaging that will diagnose myositis in the ED.

Diagnostic Procedures
- Check a negative inspiratory force (NIF) on dyspneic patients. Values closer to -30 cm H_2O suggest impending respiratory failure.[10]

TREATMENT

Medications
- Prednisone (1 mg/kg/d) is the first-line drug for empiric treatment.[11]
- Methylprednisolone (500–1000 mg IV) may be used for more severe cases.[11]

SPECIAL CONSIDERATIONS

Disposition
- Uncomplicated inflammatory myopathies without cardiopulmonary complaints or aspiration risk can be safely discharged with primary care or neurology follow-up.
- Patients too weak to safely ambulate should be admitted to the floor with fall precautions.
- Patients with cardiopulmonary compromise or hemodynamic instability should be admitted to the ICU.

Complication
- Respiratory failure

REFERENCES

1. Lilleker J, Murphy S, Cooper R. Selected aspects of the current management of myositis. *Ther Adv Musculoskelet Dis* 2016;8(4):136–44. doi: 10.1177/1759720X16655126.
2. Rayavarapu S, Coley W, Kinder TB, Nagaraju K. Idiopathic inflammatory myopathies: pathogenic mechanisms of muscle weakness. *Skelet Muscle* 2013;3:13. doi: 10.1186/2044-5040-3-13.
3. Simms RW. Idiopathic Inflammatory Myopathies. In: Andreoli T, Carpenter C, Griggs R. *Cecil's Essentials of Medicine*. 6th ed. Philadelphia: W.B. Saunders Company, 2004.
4. Schwartz T, Diederichsen LP, Lundberg IE, et al. Cardiac involvement in adult and juvenile idiopathic inflammatory myopathies. *RMD Open* 2016;2(2):e000291. doi: 10.1136/rmdopen-2016-000291.
5. Malik A, Hayat G, Kalia JS, Guzman MA. Idiopathic inflammatory myopathies: clinical approach and management. *Front Neurol* 2016;7:64. doi: 10.3389/fneur.2016.00064.
6. Strauss KW, Gonzalez-Buritica H, Khamashta MA, Hughes GR. Polymyositis-dermatomyositis: a clinical review. *Postgrad Med J* 1989;65(765):437–43.
7. Dalakas MC. Polymyositis, dermatomyositis, and inclusion-body myositis. *N Engl J Med* 1991;325(21):1487–98. doi: 10.1056/NEJM199111213252107.
8. Jo D, Pompa T, Khalil A, et al. *Clin Rheumatol* 2015;34:1813. doi: 10.1007/s10067-014-2657-4.
9. Labirua A, Lundberg IE. Interstitial lung disease and idiopathic inflammatory myopathies: progress and pitfalls. *Curr Opin Rheumatol* 2010;22(6):633–8.
10. Kollef M, Isakow W. *Washington Manual of Critical Care*. 2nd ed. Philadelphia: Wolters Kluwer Lippincott Williams & Wilkins, 2012.
11. Moghadam-Kia S, Aggarwal R, Oddis CV. Treatment of inflammatory myopathy: emerging therapies and therapeutic targets. *Expert Rev Clin Immunol* 2015;11(11):1265–75. doi: 10.1586/1744666X.2015.1082908.

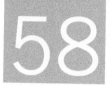

58 Musculoskeletal Emergencies: Osteomyelitis

Daniel C. Kolinsky and Stephen Y. Liang

GENERAL PRINCIPLES

Definition

- Osteomyelitis is an inflammatory reaction of the bone due to an infectious organism, usually bacteria, resulting in bone destruction. Infection can involve the bone marrow, cortex, periosteum, and/or surrounding soft tissues.

Classification

- Acute osteomyelitis develops over days to weeks.
- Chronic osteomyelitis can progress over months or years.

Epidemiology/Etiology

- Local spread occurs from a contiguous focus of infection (e.g., infected ulcer, abscess, overlying cellulitis).
  - In the setting of vascular insufficiency, infection starts almost exclusively in the feet and ascends proximally.
- Direct inoculation of the bone occurs due to an open fracture or infected prosthetic hardware.
- Hematogenous seeding (bacteremia)
  - Hematogenous seeding of vertebral bodies is common (particularly in the thoracic and lumbar spine).[1]
  - Risk factors include diabetes, vascular insufficiency, sickle cell disease, immunocompromised, extremes of age, urinary infection, IV drug use, human or animal bites, abscess/cellulitis/infected ulcer, central venous catheter or other long-term vascular device, or prior orthopedic surgery or indwelling orthopedic hardware.

DIAGNOSIS

Clinical Presentation

History

- Local pain, warmth, swelling, and erythema (may be absent in diabetic patients)[1]

Physical Examination

- Primary signs of infection include redness, warmth, swelling, tenderness, pain, and/or purulent discharge.[2]
  - Other physical findings suggestive for infection may include nonpurulent secretions, friable or discolored granulation tissue, undermining of wound edges, and/or foul odor.[2]

Diagnostic Criteria

- Osteomyelitis is more likely when one of the following is present on physical exam[1]:
  - Bone is visibly exposed in the wound or ulcer bed.
  - Exploration of the wound or ulcer bed with a sterile surgical probe reaches the bone (positive probe-to-bone test).[1]
  - Skin ulcer of the lower extremity with an area larger than 2 cm.[1]
- Hematogenous osteomyelitis (especially of the spine) can be present without any of the aforementioned physical exam findings.

Laboratories

- ESR >70 mm/h is suggestive of osteomyelitis. Both erythrocyte sedimentation rate (ESR) and c-reactive protein (CRP) can be used to trend response to treatment but may be normal.[3]
- WBC and superficial wound culture have little diagnostic utility in osteomyelitis.[3]
- In patients with osteomyelitis who are bacteremic, blood cultures may help identify an offending organism.[3]

Imaging

- Plain radiographs may demonstrate cortical bone deformity and/or destruction, often accompanied by soft tissue swelling.[1] They may also reveal subcutaneous gas or radiopaque foreign bodies serving as a nidus of infection.[2]
  - Although plain films may not show bony erosion until after 2–3 weeks of infection, they should still be obtained for the purposes of comparison at subsequent follow-up visits.
- CT can show periosteal reaction, cortical/medullary bone destruction, and/or adjacent soft tissue infection.

TREATMENT

- Optimal management of osteomyelitis requires both medical and surgical therapies in many instances.
- If the patient is hemodynamically stable, consider delaying empiric antibiotic coverage until after bone biopsy to better guide antibiotic therapy.[3]

Medications

- Empiric coverage will initially require broad-spectrum antibiotics and can be de-escalated once culture and susceptibilities are available.
  - Empiric gram-positive coverage (e.g., MSSA, methicillin-resistant *Staphylococcus aureus* [MRSA], *Streptococcus* sp.) can be achieved with vancomycin (15 mg/kg IV q12h), daptomycin (6 mg/kg IV q24h), or linezolid (600 mg IV q12h).
  - Empiric gram-negative coverage can be achieved using cefepime (2 g IV q12h), meropenem (1 g IV q8h), or piperacillin–tazobactam (3.375 g IV q6h).
  - Appropriate initial broad spectrum should include both gram-positive and gram-negative aerobic and anaerobic coverage. When using cefepime, metronidazole should be added for anaerobic coverage.
- The recommended duration of antibiotic therapy for osteomyelitis is at least 4–6 weeks.
- Consultation with an infectious disease specialist should be considered to help direct appropriate antibiotic therapy.

SPECIAL CONSIDERATIONS

Disposition

- Patients with acute osteomyelitis typically require admission.
- Patients with chronic osteomyelitis whose cultures have resulted, are on appropriate antibiotics, and are without signs of systemic infection or instability may be treated on an outpatient basis.

REFERENCES

1. Butalia S, Palda VA, Sargeant RJ, et al. Does this patient with diabetes have osteomyelitis of the lower extremity? *JAMA* 2008;299:806–13.
2. Lipsky BA, Berendt AR, Cornia PB, et al. Infectious Diseases Society of America clinical practice guideline for the diagnosis and treatment of diabetic foot infections. *Clin Infect Dis* 2012;54:132–73.
3. Berbari EF, Kanj SS, Kowalski TJ, et al. Infectious Diseases Society of America clinical practice guidelines for the diagnosis and treatment of native vertebral osteomyelitis in adults. *Clin Infect Dis* 2015;61:26–46.
4. Lew DP, Waldvogel FA. Osteomyelitis. *Lancet* 2004 Jul 24–30;364(9431):369–79.
5. Kapoor A, Page S, LaValley M, et al. Magnetic resonance imaging for diagnosing foot osteomyelitis: a meta-analysis. *Arch Intern Med* 2007;167:125–32.

59 Musculoskeletal Emergencies: Overuse Syndromes

Mark D. Levine

Tendinopathy

GENERAL PRINCIPLES

Definition

- A syndrome characterized by tendon thickening and chronic pain.
- Tendonitis is indicative of inflammation secondary to overuse.

Epidemiology/Etiology

- Risk factors for overuse include age >35 years, prior tendon injury, type of strain on the tendon, and particular properties of the patient's healing response or innate anatomy and physiology.
- Extrinsic risk factors include training errors, environmental conditions, equipment, ergonomics, and footwear.

Pathophysiology

- An inflammatory response leads to pain, swelling, and decreased flexibility.

DIAGNOSIS

Clinical Presentation

History
- Patients will usually report pain in the area of injury.

Physical Examination
- Evaluate pain with tendon loading and stretch. Range of motion should be tested. Crepitus or fluid may also be palpable.

Differential Diagnosis

- Fracture, strain, sprain, referred pain, or crystallopathies

Diagnostic Criteria and Testing

Laboratories
- There are no laboratory tests that are specific for overuse injuries.

Imaging
- There are no imaging studies that are used specifically in the emergency setting.

TREATMENT

Medications

- NSAIDs or acetaminophen are first-line therapies.

Other Nonpharmacologic Therapies

- Rest, reduction in activity, correction of ergonomic issues, stretching, and physical therapy

SPECIAL CONSIDERATIONS

Disposition

- Patients can be discharged to home with follow-up with their primary physician.

Achilles Tendon Injury

GENERAL PRINCIPLES

Epidemiology/Etiology

- Most patients have preexisting Achilles tendon problems, and tear/rupture occurs during recreational sports.
- Risk factors include male gender, obesity, age > 30 years, cold weather training, and poor body mechanics/footwear.
- Fluoroquinolone antibiotics are rarely associated with tendinopathy or rupture (12 per 100,000 treatment episodes).

Pathophysiology

- Trauma leads to degeneration of the tendon. Decreased vascularity of the tendon prevents adequate healing. Rupture occurs after a sudden stress is applied to a weakened tendon.

DIAGNOSIS

Clinical Presentation

History

- The patient will usually complain of a burning pain in the area of the Achilles. If there is a rupture, the patient will report a sudden pain and "pop" usually secondary to a push-off movement.

Physical Examination

- The examination should evaluate for bruising, swelling, or foot misalignment. The tendon is usually tender and thickened. Point tenderness will be ~2–6 cm proximal to the tendon insertion point.

Differential Diagnosis

- Ankle sprain, calcaneal bursitis, or fracture

Diagnostic Criteria and Testing

Laboratories

- There are no laboratory tests that are specific for Achilles tendon injury.

Imaging

- Ultrasound may provide confirmation of the clinical diagnosis.

Diagnostic Procedures

- The Thompson (calf squeeze) test is an accurate way to diagnose a complete tendon rupture. A lack of plantar flexion when squeezing the gastrocnemius muscle belly is more diagnostic than the inability to actively plantar flex.

TREATMENT

Medications

- Acetaminophen and ibuprofen are mainstays of medication therapy.

Other Nonpharmacologic Therapies

- For tendinopathy: rest, application of ice packs, analgesics, and support with a heel lift or bandaging/taping
- For rupture: rest, analgesics, and immobilization in a splint with mild plantar flexion

SPECIAL CONSIDERATIONS

Disposition

- Patients may be discharged home to follow up with an orthopedic surgeon.
- Athletes and very active patients on fluoroquinolones should decrease their training frequency and intensity and resume activity 2–4 weeks after completion of the antibiotics.

Carpal Tunnel Syndrome

GENERAL PRINCIPLES

Definition

- Symptoms brought on by compression of the median nerve as it passes through the carpal tunnel.

Epidemiology/Etiology
- Risk factors include obesity, female sex, pregnancy, genetic predisposition, diabetes, rheumatoid arthritis (RA), hypothyroidism, connective tissue diseases, and workplace factors (vibrating tools, repetitive hand/wrist use, prolonged wrist extension/flexion).
- There is an increase frequency of carpal tunnel syndrome in industrial settings.

Pathophysiology
- Increased pressure within the intracarpal canal exerts pressure on the median nerve leading to direct nerve injury, nerve ischemia, inflammation, and impairment of nerve transmission.

DIAGNOSIS
Clinical Presentation
History
- Patients may report pain and numbness/tingling primarily in the median nerve distribution of the hand and are reported to be worse at night. Activities that require flexion or extension of the wrist or raising of the arms may provoke symptoms.

Physical Examination
- A full neurologic exam of the extremity should be performed (a loss of sensation over the thenar eminence suggests a median nerve injury proximal to the carpal tunnel).
- The Phalen maneuver, Tinel test, manual carpal compression test, and hand elevation tests may all help to diagnosis carpal tunnel syndrome but are only moderately sensitive and specific.

Differential Diagnosis
- Fracture, strain/sprain, nerve injury proximal to the carpal tunnel, cellulitis, Reynaud disease, motor neuron disease, or compartment syndrome

Diagnostic Criteria and Testing
Laboratories
- There are no laboratory tests that are specific for carpal tunnel syndrome.

Imaging
- There is no imaging study that is diagnostic for carpal tunnel syndrome.

TREATMENT
Medications
- NSAIDs or oral prednisone (20 mg PO daily for 10–14 days) may provide some symptomatic relief.

Other Nonpharmacologic Therapies
- Splinting in the neutral position at night, physical therapy, and occupational therapy may provide some amelioration of symptoms.

SPECIAL CONSIDERATIONS
Disposition
- Patients may be discharged home to follow up with their primary physician for electrodiagnostic studies and possible referral for surgical intervention.

SUGGESTED READINGS

Amirfeyz R, Gozzrd C, Leslie IJ. Hand elevation test for assessment of carpal tunnel syndrome. *J Hand Surg Br* 2005;30:361.

Bland JD. Carpal tunnel syndrome. *BMJ* 2007;335–43.

Corrao G, Zambon A, Bertù L, et al. Evidence of tendinitis provoked by fluoroquinolone treatment: a case-control study. *Drug Saf* 2006;29:889.

Hall MM, Finnoff JT, Smith J. Musculoskeletal complications of fluoroquinolones: guidelines and precautions for usage in the athletic population. *PMR* 2011;3:132.

Holmes GB, Lin J. Etiologic factors associated with symptomatic Achilles tendinopathy. *Foot Ankle Int* 2006;27:952.

Leppilahti J, Puranen J, Orava S. Incidence of Achilles tendon rupture. *Acta Orthop Scand* 1996;67:277.

Leppilahti J, Orava S. Total Achilles tendon rupture. A review. *Sports Med* 1998;25:79.

MacDermid JC, Wessel J. Clinical diagnosis of carpal tunnel syndrome: a systemic review. *J Hand Ther* 2004;17:309.

Maffulli N. The clinical diagnosis of subcutaneous tear of the Achilles tendon. A prospective study in 174 patients. *Am J Sports Med* 1998;26:266.

Maffulli N, Wong J, Almekinders LC. Types and epidemiology of tendinopathy. *Clin Sports Med* 2003;22:675.

Nirschl, RP. Patterns of Failed Hearing in Tendon Injury. In: Leadbetter WB, Buckwalter JA, Gordon SL, eds. *Sports-Induced Inflammation: Clinical and Basic Science Concepts*. Park Ridge, IL: American Academy of Orthopaedic Surgeons, 1990:577.

O'Connor D, Marshall S, Massy-Westropp N. Non-surgical treatment (other than steroid injection) for carpal tunnel syndrome. *Cochrane Database Syst Rev* 2003:CD003219.

Thompson C, Visco C. Lateral epicondylosis: emerging management options. *Curr Sports Med Rep* 2015;14(3):215–20.

60 Musculoskeletal Emergencies: Low Back Pain

Al Lulla

GENERAL PRINCIPLES

Definition

- Acute back pain is defined as 2–4 weeks of pain located between the costal angles and gluteal folds.
- Subacute back pain can be classified as pain lasting up to 12 weeks.
- Chronic low back pain is pain that persists >12 weeks.

Epidemiology/Etiology

- Men and women are both affected by low back pain equally. Symptoms most often present between 30 and 50 years of age.[1]

- Risk factors for development of acute and chronic low back pain include increasing age, strenuous physical work, work dissatisfaction, depression, obesity, smoking, severe scoliosis, and drug abuse.[2]

Pathophysiology

- In ~85% of patients with low back pain, no cause can be identified.[1]
- Mechanical causes of low back pain are usually related to musculoskeletal or ligamentous injury. Some of these mechanical causes are referred to colloquially as "strain" or "sprain."
- Low back pain can be caused by mechanical or nonmechanical causes.

DIAGNOSIS

Clinical Presentation

History
- The initial history of a patient with low back pain in the ED should focus on addressing a possible life-threatening cause for the symptoms. Red flags on history include age <18 or >50, pain lasting longer than 6 weeks, prior history of malignancy, subjective fever or chills, night sweats or unexplained weight loss, pain that does not improve with rest or analgesics, pain that is worse at night, a history of intravenous drug use, a history of immunocompromised status, or a history of trauma.[3]
- General questions in the patient history should assess the onset, location, time course, intensity, character, radiation, and alleviating or exacerbating factors.[3]

Physical Examination
- Red flag findings on physical examination include fever, a patient who is visibly writhing in pain, bowel or bladder incontinence, saddle anesthesia, loss of perianal sensation, a pulsating abdominal mass, or severe neurologic deficit. Examination of rectal sphincter tone is not mandated in patients unless indicated for a red flag symptom.[3,4]
- A comprehensive neurologic exam including flexion and extension of the lumbar spine and straight leg testing should be performed.[2-4]

Differential Diagnosis

- Benign: lumbar strain, isolated sciatica, or spinal stenosis
- Emergent: metastatic disease, infectious causes (spinal epidural abscess, vertebral osteomyelitis, infectious discitis), spinal epidural hematoma, central disk herniation causing cauda equina syndrome, and spinal fracture with cord or root impingement
- Non–spine-related causes: aortic disease (AAA, dissection), genitourinary disease (ureteral colic, nephrolithiasis, pyelonephritis), gastrointestinal disease (pancreatitis, pancreatic cancer, perforated peptic ulcer, cholecystitis, cholangitis), retroperitoneal hemorrhage, endocarditis or psoas abscess.[5]

Diagnostic Criteria and Testing

- Patients with low back pain should be risk stratified into low-, intermediate-, or high-risk categories.[5]
  - Low risk: these patients include those who have no red flag findings on history and a normal neurologic exam. These patients require no further laboratory or radiographic studies.

- ○ Intermediate risk: these patients include those who may have a concerning red flag on history (such as fever) but have no abnormalities on neurologic exam. These patients can be further risk stratified with the aid of laboratory studies and consultation with a neurologist or spine surgeon. Imaging may also be part of their diagnostic workup.
- ○ High risk: these patients have clear red flag findings on history and new or progressive neurologic deficits on examination. These patients should undergo emergent imaging in the ED with appropriate referral to a surgeon if indicated.

Laboratories

- Laboratory testing is only indicated for further risk stratification in patients that are deemed to be intermediate risk. A WBC, erythrocyte sedimentation rate, and c-reactive protein may be considered.

Imaging

- Patients who are intermediate risk may need emergent imaging depending on the clinical context and suspicion.
- All high-risk patients should undergo immediate imaging in the ED without waiting for the results of laboratory testing.
- Plain radiographs should not be routinely ordered in patients with low back pain. Radiographs may be considered as the first step in patients with suspected infection, fracture, or malignancy.
- CT is superior to plain radiographs in the identification of vertebral fractures, and is of particular use in patients with a history of trauma. However, in patients who present with new-onset or progressive neurologic deficits, MRI is the gold standard imaging modality.[3]

TREATMENT

Medications

- NSAIDs and acetaminophen are first-line agents for symptomatic control of acute back pain without any red flag findings.[3,4]
- Muscle relaxants have shown to have similar short-term efficacy comparable to NSAIDs and acetaminophen. Furthermore, studies demonstrate a lack of synergistic effect when combined with NSAIDs.[4,6,7]
- Opioids may be considered as a last-line alternative for patients who have severe acute back pain that has not responded to conservative control measures.
- Systemic steroids have not shown to be effective in the management of low back pain and are currently not recommended.[4,6]

Other Nonpharmacologic Therapies

- For patients determined to be intermediate risk, consultation with a neurologist or spine surgeon may be warranted.[5,7]

SPECIAL CONSIDERATIONS

Disposition

- Patients with benign causes of back pain such as musculoskeletal or ligamentous injury can be discharged home with PMD referral.
- Patients with red flag symptoms should be admitted to the appropriate service for definitive management.

- Patients should be extensively counseled on the importance of physical activity and refraining from bed rest.[6] In addition, patients can be educated on the avoiding heavy lifting and twisting or bending maneuvers, which lead to recurrence or worsening of symptoms.[6]

REFERENCES

1. Deyo RA, Weinstein JN. Low back pain. *N Engl J Med* 2001;344:363–70.
2. Devereaux M. Low back pain. *Med Clin North Am* 2009;93:477–501.
3. Corwell BN. The emergency department evaluation, management, and treatment of back pain. *Emerg Med Clin North Am* 2010;28:811–39.
4. Della-Giustina D. Evaluation and treatment of acute back pain in the emergency department. *Emerg Med Clin North Am* 2015;33:311–26.
5. Edlow JA. Managing nontraumatic acute back pain. *Ann Emerg Med* 2015;66:148–53.
6. Casazza B. Diagnosis and treatment of acute low back pain. *Am Fam Physician* 2012;85: 343–50.
7. Last AR, Hulbert K. Chronic low back pain: evaluation and management. *Am Fam Physician* 2009;79:1067–74.
8. Winters ME, Kluetz P, Zilberstein J. Back pain emergencies. *Med Clin North Am* 2006;90:505–23.

61 Musculoskeletal Emergencies: Sciatica

Al Lulla

GENERAL PRINCIPLES

Definition

- Sciatica refers to radicular pain that originates in the lower back and radiates along lumbar and sacral nerve roots to the posterior or lateral thigh along the distribution of the sciatic nerve.[1,2] Often times, there are motor or sensory deficits.[3]

Epidemiology/Etiology

- The vast majority of cases of sciatica are caused by acute lumbar disk herniation.[1]
- Sciatica is common in the general population.[2]
- The risk factors for development of sciatica include increasing height, age (peak 45–64 years), occupational factors such as frequent bending or lifting, and smoking.[2,4,5]

Pathophysiology

- The sciatic nerve is the largest nerve in the body and is given rise to by the fourth and fifth lumbar nerve roots and the first two sacral nerve roots. Pathology at any location along the course of the sciatic nerve can give rise to the symptoms associated with sciatica.[6]

- The most common cause of sciatica is compression of the lumbosacral nerves by a herniated disk.[3,6]

DIAGNOSIS

Clinical Presentation

History

- A comprehensive history aimed at identifying risk factors for sciatica is essential. The characteristics and distribution of the pain are also an important part of the evaluation.
- The presence of concerning symptoms such as saddle anesthesia, fecal incontinence, and urinary retention should be assessed.[1]
- The pain associated with sciatica may be sudden in onset or develop gradually over time. Often times, the pain has variable aching and sharp characteristics. The pain can radiate from the middle aspect of the buttocks down to dorsolateral surface of the thigh. When lower nerve roots are affected, such as S1, the pain may radiate along the posterior aspect of the thigh.[6]
- Patients may report paresthesias in the dermatomal distribution of the affected nerve root. In addition, a proportion of patients may report lower extremity weakness.[7]

Physical Examination

- Patients should undergo extensive physical examination with a complete neurologic exam. Physical examination often reveals localized neurologic deficit at the level of the affected nerve roots. Rectal examination is not mandatory for all patients with low back pain and should be reserved for patients who have "red flag" symptoms.[3]
- Provocative maneuvers such as the straight leg test are an essential component of the physical examination. A positive result is defined as radiating pain extending from the buttock to below the knee that is reproduced by raising the leg to an angle of 30–70 degrees. The absence of a positive result significantly decreases the likelihood of lumbar disk herniation.[1,6]
- The crossed straight leg test is a variation of the straight leg test and involves performing the same maneuver on the unaffected side. A positive test is defined as the presence of radicular pain on the affected side when the unaffected side is raised.

Differential Diagnosis

- Emergent: cauda equina syndrome, spinal neoplasm, spinal infection (i.e., epidural abscess or vertebral osteomyelitis), or spinal fracture.
- Nonemergent: greater trochanteric bursitis, iliotibial band syndrome, lumbar disk herniation, piriformis syndrome, facet arthropathy, or sacroiliitis.

Diagnostic Criteria and Testing

- Patient history suggestive of radicular leg pain that extends in a dermatomal distribution combined with neurologic maneuvers that indicate nerve root tension or neurologic deficit (such as straight leg raise testing) is sufficient to make a clinical diagnosis of sciatica.[4]

Imaging

- Imaging has limited utility in the evaluation of sciatica unless these symptoms are elicited.[1,4,5,6,7]
- For patients who present with concerning symptoms, MRI is the preferred imaging modality.

TREATMENT

- Conservative treatment is preferred for most patients with sciatica. Initial therapeutic measures should be aimed at pain control via medication and physical therapy.[6]

Medications

- The role of NSAIDs, acetaminophen, and muscle relaxants in the treatment of patients with sciatica remains unclear. While many studies have shown their benefit in patients with generalized low back pain, their efficacy in patients with sciatica does not appear to be significant, and in some cases, no different than placebo.[1,4,6]
- There are many conflicting reports on the efficacy of steroids in the treatment of acute sciatica.[1,2,4,6]

Other Nonpharmacologic Therapies

- Bed rest may provide initial symptomatic relief; however, when compared to physical activity, there appears to be no difference in pain or functional status.[4,6,8]

SPECIAL CONSIDERATIONS

Disposition

- Patients who are diagnosed with uncomplicated sciatica secondary to lumbar disk herniation can be discharged home with outpatient follow-up. Patients who have presence of red flag symptoms should be admitted and immediately referred to a surgical specialist.

REFERENCES

1. Gregory DS, Seto CK, Wortley GC, Shugart CM. Acute lumbar disk pain: navigating evaluation and treatment choices. *Am Fam Physician* 2008;78:835–42.
2. Stafford MA, Peng P, Hill DA. Sciatica: a review of history, epidemiology, pathogenesis, and the role of epidural steroid injection in management. *Br J Anaesth* 2007;99:461–73.
3. Della-Giustina D. Evaluation and treatment of acute back pain in the emergency department. *Emerg Med Clin North Am* 2015;33:311–26.
4. Koes B, van Tulder M, Peul W. Diagnosis and treatment of sciatica. *BMJ* 2007;1:1069–70, 1072–3.
5. Frymoyer JW. Back pain and sciatica. *N Engl J Med* 1988;318:291–300.
6. Ropper AH, Zafonte RD. Sciatica. *N Engl J Med* 2015;372:1240–8.
7. Jarvik J, Deyo R. Diagnostic evaluation of low back pain with emphasis on imaging. *Ann Intern Med* 2002;137:586–97.
8. Vroomen PC, de Krom MC, Wilmink JT, et al. Lack of effectiveness of bed rest for sciatica. *N Engl J Med* 1999;340:418–23.

Musculoskeletal Emergencies: Spinal Stenosis

Al Lulla

GENERAL PRINCIPLES

Definition

- Spinal stenosis refers to narrowing of the spinal canal, lateral recesses, or neural foramina where the spinal nerves exit the spinal cord.[1]
- Cauda equina syndrome is a rare complication of lumbar spinal stenosis; the symptoms of saddle anesthesia, urinary and fecal incontinence, and paraparesis are more often present with standing and walking than while being seated at rest.[1]

Epidemiology

- The most common cause of acquired lumbar spinal stenosis is age-related degenerative arthritis of the spine.[1]
- Patients with lumbar spinal stenosis most commonly become symptomatic after the seventh decade of life, and it is more common in women than in men.[2]

Pathophysiology

- Stenosis of the spinal canal is a result of loss of intervertebral disk height, facet joint arthropathy, and thickening of the ligamentum flavum. Eventual compression of the lumbosacral nerve roots is responsible for the symptoms associated with spinal stenosis.[3,4]
- Spinal stenosis is less frequently iatrogenic.[5]

DIAGNOSIS

Clinical Presentation

History

- The most common symptom associated with lumbar spinal stenosis is neurogenic claudication, present during activity such as standing up and walking and absent during periods of rest.[5,4]

Physical Examination

- Physical examination should be aimed at a very thorough neurologic assessment. Absent or decreased reflexes are a nonspecific finding. Straight leg testing is usually negative. The Romberg maneuver may reveal unsteadiness and wide-based gait in a significant proportion of patients with lumbar spinal stenosis.[5,2,4]
- Examination of the back may demonstrate decreased mobility with lumbar extension being more painful than flexion.[3,5,2]

- Upon briskly walking, the patient may involuntarily assume a stooped posture, which may help to partially alleviate the symptoms (the "stoop test").[2]
- Patients may have bilateral sensory changes such as numbness or tingling and weakness of the lower extremities.[3]

Differential Diagnosis
- Osteoarthritis of the hip, trochanteric bursitis, peripheral neuropathy, vascular claudication, or sciatica secondary to disk herniation.[5,2]

Diagnostic Criteria and Testing
- A presumptive diagnosis of spinal stenosis can often times be made with history and physical examination alone.

Imaging
- MRI is the imaging study of choice to evaluate for the presence of lumbar spinal stenosis and is often done as an outpatient.
- CT images may demonstrate narrowing of the central canal and neural foramina secondary to disk protrusion, hypertrophy of the ligamentum flavum, or hypertrophy of the facet joints with osteophyte formation.[3,5]
- Plain radiographs may have some utility to rule out a traumatic injury, loss of disk height, and presence of osteophytes.[5,2]

TREATMENT

Medications
- Acetaminophen and NSAIDs are recommended as first-line medications.[3,5]

Other Nonpharmacologic Therapies
- Physical therapy, especially in the form of exercises that utilize lumbar flexion such as bicycling, and abdominal strengthening have been shown to be well tolerated.[1,5]

SPECIAL CONSIDERATIONS

Disposition
- Most patients with spinal stenosis can be safely discharged from the emergency department, unless evidence of cauda equina syndrome exists, necessitating admission and emergency consultation with a spinal surgeon.

REFERENCES

1. Binder DK, Schmidt MH, Weinstein PR. Lumbar spinal stenosis. *Semin Neurol* 2002;22:157–66.
2. Lee SY, Kim TH, Oh JK, et al. Lumbar stenosis: a recent update by review of literature. *Asian Spine J* 2015;9:818–28.
3. Corwell BN. The emergency department evaluation, management, and treatment of back pain. *Emerg Med Clin North Am* 2010;28:811–39.
4. Gevenay S, Atlas SJ. Lumbar spinal stenosis. *Best Pr Res Clin Rheumatol* 2010;24:253–65.
5. Katz JN, Harris MB. Lumbar spinal stenosis. *N Engl J Med* 2008;358:818–25.

63 Neurologic Emergencies: Cranial Neuropathies

Matthew C. Loftspring and Robert Bucelli

GENERAL PRINCIPLES

- The normal intracranial pressure (ICP) is between 5 and 25 cm H_2O (equivalent to mm Hg).
- Elevated ICP comes to attention in patients with brain tumors, hemorrhagic or ischemic stroke, meningitis, venous sinus thrombosis, and idiopathic intracranial hypertension (IIH).

Elevated Intracranial Pressure and Cranial Neuropathies

GENERAL PRINCIPLES

Epidemiology/Etiology

- The most common cranial neuropathy present with elevated ICP is a CN VI palsy (unilateral or bilateral), due to its apposition to the dura. CNs III and IV are also commonly affected.

Pathophysiology

- Numerous etiologies of elevated ICP exist as listed in Table 63.1.

DIAGNOSIS

Clinical Presentation

History

- The alert patient may present with double vision, pulsatile tinnitus, or transient visual obscurations. Also inquire about nausea, vomiting, ataxia, and headache. Some patients may be somnolent and/or encephalopathic and unable to provide a history.

Physical Examination

- Essential components of the neurologic exam in an awake patient include the following:
  - Level of alertness, fundoscopic exam, visual fields, and extraocular movements.
  - The presence of papilledema is not 100% specific for elevated ICP.
- In the somnolent or comatose patient, a pertinent cranial nerve exam includes the following:
  - The pupillary light reflex, pupillary asymmetry (>1 mm), oculocephalic reflexes, and the cough test in intubated patient

Differential Diagnosis

- The main differential diagnoses are listed in Table 63.1.

TABLE 63.1   Etiologies of Elevated Intracranial Pressure

Stroke

Hemorrhage
- IPH
- IVH
- SAH
- SDH
- EDH

CVST with/without stroke

Meningoencephalitis
- Infectious
- Noninfectious

Traumatic brain injury

Tumor

Vasculitis

Hydrocephalus
- Communicating
- Noncommunicating

Idiopathic
- IIH

Vitamin A intoxication

Nitroglycerin

Diffuse cerebral edema
- Anoxic/hypoxic injury
- Metabolic (e.g., liver failure)

EDH, epidural hematoma; IPH, intraparenchymal hemorrhage; IVH, intraventricular hemorrhage; SAH, subarachnoid hemorrhage; SDH, subdural hematoma.

Diagnostic Criteria and Testing

Laboratories
- Routine labs, urine drug screen, and ammonia level should be obtained.

Imaging
- A noncontrast head CT or MRI is necessary in any patient who is suspected to have increased ICP, especially if there is an altered mental status.

Diagnostic Procedures

- Lumbar puncture should be done in any patient without a mass lesion or without magnetic resonance venography (MRV) evidence of cerebral venous sinus thrombosis (CVST). An opening pressure should be obtained. The LP may also be of therapeutic benefit with certain etiologies (e.g., IIH).

TREATMENT

Medications

- Mannitol given at 1–1.5 g/kg IV is the initial form of empiric osmotic therapy.
- Hypertonic saline (5%) can be given as a bolus through a peripheral line (3.2 mL/kg), but 23.4% must be given through a central line (0.687 mL/kg).
  - Common diagnoses requiring osmotic therapy include subarachnoid and intra-cerebral hemorrhages.

Other Nonpharmacologic Therapies

- In patients with signs of brain herniation, immediate interventions include hyper-ventilation (temporizing) and elevation of the head of the bed to at least 45 degrees.
- Neurosurgical consultation should be obtained in cases of intracranial hemorrhage or in cases where there is concern for rapidly developing hydrocephalus that may require placement of an external ventriculostomy drain (EVD).

SPECIAL CONSIDERATIONS

Disposition

- Patients with elevated ICP causing an alteration of consciousness require ICU admission. Patients with IIH can be managed as an outpatient unless there is a threat for imminent vision loss.

Optic Neuritis and Optic Neuropathies

GENERAL PRINCIPLES

Epidemiology/Etiology

- Arteritic anterior ischemic optic neuropathy (AAION) is more common in women and uncommon in patients under 60 years of age.

Pathophysiology

- Lesions are most commonly characterized by demyelination or ischemia of the optic nerve.

DIAGNOSIS

Clinical Presentation

History

- Patients with optic neuritis often present with a monocular decrease in visual acuity or abnormal color vision along with painful eye movement.
- Neuromyelitis optica (NMO) can present with bilateral optic neuritis.
- Giant cell arteritis (GCA) presents with headache and acute monocular vision loss in an older patient.

Physical Examination

- Signs of optic neuritis include a monocular decrease in visual acuity, red color desaturation, pain with eye movement, and often decreased central vision with a central scotoma.
- Fundoscopy may reveal blurring of the optic disc margins, but retrobulbar lesions may show no abnormalities acutely.

- Other exam findings include a relative afferent pupillary defect.
- Patients with GCA may have a bulging or painful temporal artery. Retinal exam may be normal or show a pale disc with blurred margins.

Differential Diagnosis

- Acute angle glaucoma, central retinal artery occlusion, branch retinal artery occlusion, other inflammatory optic neuropathies, or tumors/infiltrative lesions

Diagnostic Criteria and Testing

Laboratories
- The erythrocyte sedimentation rate (ESR) is nonspecific but can be helpful in diagnosing GCA, especially if it is >100 mm/h.

Imaging
- An MRI with contrast including fine cuts through the orbits with orbital fat suppression is the imaging test of choice for optic neuritis.

TREATMENT

Medications

- Patients are often treated with high-dose intravenous methylprednisolone (IVMP, 1 g/d for 3–5 days). GCA is also commonly treated with an initial pulse of IVMP for 3–5 days followed by oral prednisone over the course of months.

SPECIAL CONSIDERATIONS

- Initiation of steroids should not be delayed in GCA given the risk of permanent vision loss with delayed treatment.

Disposition

- Almost all patients with a new presentation, and some patients with an established diagnosis, will require admission.

Cavernous Sinus Syndrome

GENERAL PRINCIPLES

Epidemiology/Etiology

- Cavernous sinus lesions are rare but may have high morbidity and mortality, depending on the underlying cause.
- Cavernous sinus thrombosis can affect any age group (mean age of 22 years).

Pathophysiology

- Specific conditions that can affect the cavernous sinus include thrombosis, carotid-cavernous fistula, Tolosa-Hunt syndrome, pituitary apoplexy, and infections including mucormycosis.
- Septic thrombosis can also be caused by *Staphylococcus aureus* and *Streptococcus pneumoniae* spreading from the sphenoid and ethmoid sinuses, teeth/jaw, inner ear, or orbit.
- Nonseptic thrombosis can be caused by prothrombotic states.
- Carotid-cavernous fistulae (CCF) may occur spontaneously, after trauma or after dental procedures (especially upper root canals).

DIAGNOSIS

Clinical Presentation

History

- Patients with septic thrombosis will have fever, double vision, headache, chemosis, and possibly altered mental status.
- CCF present with insidious headache, multiple cranial neuropathies, and often a feeling of "whooshing" or "roaring" in their head.
- Tolosa-Hunt syndrome presents with intermittent orbital pain along with one or more cranial neuropathies.
- Pituitary apoplexy presents with headache and vision loss (typically temporal fields) and can progress to affect cranial nerves in the cavernous sinus.
- Mucormycosis presents with fever, orbital pain, periorbital and facial swelling, and ptosis.

Physical Examination

- Thrombosis: fever, optic disc edema, and venous engorgement along with multiple cranial neuropathies (III, IV and VI, with the latter often the first CN affected).
- CCF: proptosis, chemosis, and conjunctival injection can be observed along with one or more CN palsies.
- Mucormycosis: presents with fever, ophthalmoplegia, eschar of the palate or nasal mucosa, sinusitis, and periorbital and facial swelling.

Differential Diagnosis

- Elevated ICP, tumors, immune-mediated radiculoneuropathies (e.g., Guillain-Barré syndrome [GBS]), and infectious and noninfectious meningoencephalitis

Diagnostic Criteria and Testing

Laboratories

- There are no specific laboratory tests that aid in diagnosis.

Imaging

- All patients need a noncontrast head CT to evaluate for an intracranial bleed or mass. A computed tomographic angiography (CTA) is of additional diagnostic benefit in evaluating for vascular lesions that require urgent treatment. A maxillofacial CT may also be helpful in identification of infectious sources.

TREATMENT

Medications

- The primary form of treatment administered will be empiric thiamine, along with empiric IV antibiotics in cases with a suspected infectious etiology.

SPECIAL CONSIDERATIONS

- Neurology and/or ENT, as well as possible neurosurgical consults are often warranted in these patients.
- CCF and mucormycosis may require surgical intervention.

Disposition

- These patients should be admitted to the hospital.

Trigeminal Neuralgia (Tic Douloureux)

GENERAL PRINCIPLES

Epidemiology/Etiology
- Incidence of ~10 per 100,000

Pathophysiology
- There is often a lesion such as an aberrant vascular loop trapping a portion of CN V. Other causes include tumors, multiple sclerosis (MS) or other central nervous system (CNS) demyelinating disorders, Sjögren syndrome, varicella-zoster virus (VZV) reactivation or postherpetic neuralgia, dental abscess, or other dental pathology affecting divisions of the maxillary or mandibular nerve divisions.

DIAGNOSIS

Clinical Presentation
History
- The pain is episodic and characterized as sharp, stabbing, or an electrical shock in the distribution of cranial nerve V.
- Each attack lasts for seconds though it can occur hundreds of times per day.
- The pain can occur spontaneously, with chewing, speaking, or brushing teeth.

Physical Examination
- Paroxysmal pain is present in one or more divisions of cranial nerve V.
- Sometimes, there is sensory impairment in the affected divisions of CN V or unilateral hearing loss.
- A characteristic herpetic rash may be identified.

Differential Diagnosis
- MS, infectious etiologies including VZV, tumor, or other inflammatory infiltrative lesions including hematologic malignancies

Diagnostic Criteria and Testing
Laboratories
- Dictated by the clinical presentation

Imaging
- No emergent imaging is indicated.

Diagnostic Procedures
- If workup warrants an evaluation for infectious etiologies or MS, a lumbar puncture may be indicated.

TREATMENT

Medication
- The standard of care is carbamazepine, starting at 200 mg bid ER.
  - Use with caution in patients of Asian descent as there is a high incidence of Stevens-Johnson syndrome and toxic epidermal necrolysis with use of carbamazepine.
  - Oxcarbazepine does not carry the same warning and is similarly effective for pain reduction.

SPECIAL CONSIDERATIONS

- VZV infection of the V_1 branch of the trigeminal nerve (i.e., zoster ophthalmicus) carries a high risk of permanent vision loss if there is a delay in diagnosis.

Disposition

- Patients can be discharged with outpatient neurology follow-up.

Intracranial Compressive Lesions Causing Cranial Neuropathies

GENERAL PRINCIPLES

Pathophysiology

- Compressive lesions (pituitary tumors, optic nerve gliomas, posterior communicating artery [PCOM] aneurysm, cavernous sinus meningioma, acoustic neuromas, brainstem gliomas, and inflammatory or infiltrative processes involving the meninges) can cause injury by direct compression of the nerve(s).

DIAGNOSIS

Clinical Presentation

History

- Pituitary tumors classically present with bitemporal vision loss that is often asymmetric early on in its presentation.
- A PCOM aneurysm may present with pain, ptosis, double vision, and a dilated pupil.
- Cavernous sinus meningiomas present with cavernous sinus syndrome as described above.
- Patients with acoustic neuromas may have unilateral tinnitus or hearing loss, while those with meningeal processes may have multiple cranial neuropathies.

Physical Examination

- In patients with a PCOM aneurysm, the exam will show a dilated, poorly reactive pupil on the side ipsilateral to the aneurysm. If the entirety of CN III is involved, the eye will appear "down and out," which is primarily caused by impairment of the medial and superior rectus muscles.
- Brainstem gliomas can cause many signs that develop slowly and may include multiple cranial neuropathies of adjacent cranial nerves, sometimes bilateral.

Diagnostic Criteria and Testing

Laboratories

- Limited utility in most of these conditions

Imaging

- A noncontrast head CT is obtained initially. CTA or MRA may be used to identify aneurysms.
- An MRI with contrast can identify most tumors.

TREATMENT

Medications

- Steroids may be used in conjunction with neurologic or neurosurgical consultation.

SPECIAL CONSIDERATIONS

- Most structural lesions will require neurosurgical consultation but not all will be amenable to surgical interventions.

Disposition
- Highly dependent upon the nature of the lesion.

Complications
- Large aneurysms can result in a fatal subarachnoid hemorrhage.

Horner Syndrome

GENERAL PRINCIPLES

Classification
- First-order Horner syndrome is caused by lesions to the central sympathetic pathways (hypothalamus, brainstem, or spinal cord).
- Second-order Horner involves preganglionic nerves.
- Third order involves postganglionic nerves.

Pathophysiology
- The majority of cases are caused by preganglionic or postganglionic lesions (as opposed to CNS lesions).
- The classic cause of Horner syndrome is an apical lung tumor (second order).
- Occlusion of the vertebral artery by a lesion of the lateral medulla causes an infarct in the posterior inferior cerebellar artery, leading to a Horner syndrome.
- Important causes of third-order Horner syndrome include carotid dissection or aneurysm, cavernous sinus thrombosis, tumor (including meningioma), and trauma to the superior cervical ganglion.

DIAGNOSIS

Clinical Presentation
History
- Lateral medullary syndrome presents with a sudden onset of vertigo, ipsilateral ataxia, dysarthria, and nausea.
- Patients with apical lung tumors may have a history of smoking and ipsilateral arm pain.

Physical Examination
- Isolated Horner syndrome is characterized by ipsilateral ptosis and miosis, with or without anhidrosis.
- Anisocoria is more prominent in the dark.

Diagnostic Criteria and Testing
Laboratories
- Limited utility in most cases.

Imaging
- A chest radiograph can screen for a lung mass.
- A noncontrast head CT can help rule out hemorrhage or large space occupying lesions.
- An MRI is the best study for detecting a lesion resulting in a lateral medullary syndrome.

TREATMENT

Medications
- Aspirin may be started after consultation with neurology and/or vascular surgery.

SPECIAL CONSIDERATIONS

- Dissection of the carotid or vertebral arteries is probably the most common cause of Horner in young patients without other significant cardiovascular risk factors.

Disposition
- Patients with dissections or strokes require admission.

Bell's Palsy

GENERAL PRINCIPLES

Epidemiology/Etiology
- The etiology is thought to be secondary to a viral infection (HSV-1) or a primary immune-mediated process, but a cause is not identified in up to 50% of cases.

Pathophysiology
- Facial nerve dysfunction likely results from a number of different mechanisms including endoneurial edema, perivascular and perineurial inflammation, and direct axonal injury.

DIAGNOSIS

Clinical Presentation
History
- Patients will notice upper and lower facial weakness.
- They may also report ipsilateral change in taste and hyperacusis.

Physical Examination
- Bell's palsy refers to an acute, unilateral, facial mononeuropathy.
- An otoscopic examination and a thorough HEENT examination should be performed to screen for signs/symptoms of a herpes infection or reactivation syndrome.
- Patients with a facial neuropathy or a lesion of the facial nucleus will have notable weakness in upper and lower facial muscles.

Differential Diagnosis
- Stroke, CNS demyelinating disease, acute inflammatory demyelinating polyradiculoneuropathy (AIDP) and other acute immune neuropathy syndromes, brainstem encephalitides (infectious and noninfectious), Lyme disease, other noninfectious inflammatory disorders including sarcoidosis and Sjögren's syndrome, myasthenia gravis, botulism, nerve sheath neoplasms, or compressive lesions along the course of the nerve

Diagnostic Criteria and Testing

Laboratories
- HIV, rapid plasma reagin (RPR), and Lyme serologies (if the patient lives in or has a recent history of travel to endemic areas)

TREATMENT

Medications
- A 10- to 14-day course of corticosteroids (60 mg/d for 5 days followed by a 5-day taper).
- In the absence of an identifiable herpesvirus infection, there is no strong evidence to support the use of acyclovir in addition to corticosteroids.

Other Nonpharmacologic Therapies
- An eye moisture chamber and/or moisturizing ointment may be necessary to prevent desiccation of the affected eye, and resultant corneal damage, if there is incomplete eye closure.

SPECIAL CONSIDERATIONS

Disposition
- Patients can be discharged with close outpatient follow-up.

SUGGESTED READINGS

Amezcua L, Morrow MJ, Jirawuthiworavong GV. Multiple sclerosis: review of eye movement disorders and update of disease-modifying therapies. *Curr Opin Ophthalmol* 2015;26:534–9.

Burgess S, Abu-Laban RB, Slavik RS, et al. A systematic review of randomized controlled trials comparing hypertonic sodium solutions and mannitol for traumatic brain injury: implications for emergency department management. *Ann Pharmacother* 2016;50:291–300.

de Falco FA, de Falco A. Migraine with aura: which patients are most at risk of stroke? *Neurol Sci* 2016;36(Suppl 1):57–60.

Gilhus NE, Skeie GO, Romi F, et al. Myasthenia gravis—autoantibody characteristics and their implications for therapy. *Nat Rev Neurol* 2016;12:259–68.

Headache Classification Committee of the International Headache Society (IHS). The International Classification of Headache Disorders, 3rd ed (beta version). *Cephalalgia* 2013;33:629–808.

Kattaj JC, Talkad AV, Wang DZ, et al. HINTS to diagnose stroke in the acute vestibular syndrome: three-step bedside oculomotor examination more sensitive than early MRI diffusion-weighted imaging. *Stroke* 2009;40(11):3504–10.

Lemos J, Eggenberger E. Neuro-ophthalmological emergencies. *Neurohospitalist* 2015;5:223–33.

Ling JD, Chao D, Al Zubidi N, Lee AG. Big red flags in neuro-ophthalmology. *Can J Ophthalmol* 2013;48:3–7.

MacDonald BK, Cockerell OC, Sander JW, Shorvon SD. The incidence and lifetime prevalence of neurological disorders in a prospective community-based study in the UK. *Brain* 2000;123(Pt 4):665–76.

Patel DK, Levin KH. Bell palsy: clinical examination and management. *Cleve Clin J Med* 2015;82:419–26.

Pereira WL, Reiche EM, Kallaur AP, Kaimen-Maciel DR. Epidemiological, clinical, and immunological characteristics of neuromyelitis optica: a review. *J Neurol Sci* 2015;355:7–17.

Posner JB, Saper CB, Schiff N. *Plum and Posner's Diagnosis of Stupor and Coma.* Cary: Oxford University Press, 2007. ProQuest ebrary. Web. 8/5 2016.

Said G. Diabetic neuropathy—a review. *Nat Clin Pract Neurol* 2007;3:331–40.

Venhovens J, Meulstee J, Verhagen WI. Acute vestibular syndrome: a critical review and diagnostic algorithm concerning the clinical differentiation of peripheral versus central aetiologies in the emergency department. *J Neurol* 2016;263(11):2151–7.

Zakrzewska JM, Linskey ME. Trigeminal neuralgia. *BMJ* 2015;350:h1238.

64 Neurologic Emergencies: Demyelinating Disorders

Elizabeth Silbermann and Robert Bucelli

Multiple Sclerosis (MS)

GENERAL PRINCIPLES

Definition

- Multiple sclerosis is a chronic, inflammatory disease of the central nervous system (CNS) and the most common among this class of disorders.

Classification

- Relapsing-remitting multiple sclerosis (RRMS): most common disease course (85% of patients)
- Primary progressive multiple sclerosis (PPMS): 15% of patients
- Secondary progressive multiple sclerosis (SPMS)

Epidemiology/Etiology

- Average age of symptom onset is between 20 and 40 years of age.
- Women are twice as likely as men to have RRMS or SPMS.[1]
- Smoking is associated with an increased incidence of MS.[1]

Pathophysiology

- The exact mechanism of MS is not understood, but it is believed to be an immune-mediated process.

DIAGNOSIS

- It is important to recognize signs and symptoms that may represent MS in an undiagnosed patient and to be able to distinguish manifestations of active disease (i.e., "an attack") from unrelated or comorbid systemic disorders (e.g., "pseudoexacerbation") in patients with an established diagnosis.

Clinical Presentation

History

The patient may present with:

- Optic neuritis: vision changes.
- Transverse myelitis: weakness, numbness, bladder/bowel dysfunction.
- Lhermitte sign: an electrical sensation, which runs down the back with neck flexion.
- Uhthoff phenomenon: worsening of neurologic symptoms in a warm environment.

- Pseudoexacerbation: patients with known MS with a worsening of their prior symptoms in the setting of an infection or significant metabolic disturbance.

Physical Examination
- A careful, comprehensive neurologic exam is always indicated in this patient population including detailed cranial nerve, motor, and sensory exam.

Differential Diagnosis

- Infections: HIV, human T-cell leukemia virus type 1 (HTLV-1), syphilis, Lyme disease, cytomegalovirus/varicella-zoster virus (CMV/VZV) vasculitis, progressive multifocal leukoencephalopathy (PML)
- Inflammatory conditions: lupus, Sjögren syndrome, Behçet disease, sarcoidosis, antiphospholipid antibody syndrome
- Vascular conditions: vasculitis, multifocal strokes
- Other demyelinating conditions: neuromyelitis optica (NMO), acute demyelinating encephalomyelitis (ADEM), idiopathic transverse myelitis
- Malignancy: primary or metastatic brain tumor, CNS lymphoma
- Others: leukodystrophies, nutritional deficiencies (B_{12}, thiamine, copper), mitochondrial encephalopathies, Leber hereditary optic neuropathy

Diagnostic Criteria and Testing

Laboratories
- Complete blood count (CBC), basic electrolytes, HIV, rapid plasma reagin (RPR), and urinalysis should be obtained to evaluate for infection or metabolic disturbance.
- Oligoclonal bands should be ordered in both cerebrospinal fluid (CSF) and serum.

Imaging
- MRI with and without contrast including FLAIR and fine cuts through the orbits.
- Any patient with evidence of transverse myelitis warrants emergent MRI imaging to rule out a structural/compressive lesion that may require an urgent surgical intervention.

Diagnostic Procedures

- Lumbar puncture is indicated for suspected MS.

TREATMENT

Medications

- There are currently 13 FDA-approved disease-modifying treatments for MS.[2] Initiation should be done in consultation with a neurologist.

Other Nonpharmacologic Therapies

- Any patient with new dysarthria or significant drooling should be kept NPO and monitored closely for aspiration.
- Intubation may be needed for any patient with clinical evidence of impending respiratory failure (e.g., negative inspiratory force [NIF] <-20 cm H_2O or forced vital capacity [FVC] < 1 L).

SPECIAL CONSIDERATIONS

Disposition

- Patients with new neurologic symptoms or deficits resulting in significant morbidity should be admitted to the hospital. ICU admission is required for any patient at risk for respiratory compromise.
- Patients with an established diagnosis without new neurologic symptoms who have an infection or metabolic disturbance are typically safe for discharge after consultation with a neurologist.

Progressive Multifocal Leukoencephalopathy (PML)

GENERAL PRINCIPLES

- PML is a very rare, life-threatening disease caused by reactivation of the JC virus in patients who are immune compromised. Certain MS medications cause an increased risk of PML.
- Presentation is varied but can include subacute weakness, aphasia, personality change, seizures, neglect, or ataxia.
- Any patient with suspected PML should immediately be evaluated by a neurologist to determine the most appropriate treatment and disposition.

Neuromyelitis Optica (NMO)

GENERAL PRINCIPLES

Definition

- NMO is a rare, severe, and often debilitating autoimmune demyelinating disorder with a monophasic or relapsing-remitting course that affects the optic nerves, brainstem, and spinal cord.
- Classically, this disorder is defined as episodes of optic neuritis (typically bilateral) and longitudinally extensive transverse myelitis.

Epidemiology/Etiology[3-5]

- It is much more common in women (80%) than in men.
- Typical onset is in the fifth decade of life but also manifests in pediatric and elderly populations.

Pathophysiology

- 70% of patients with NMO have serum antibodies that cross the blood–brain barrier, resulting in cell damage, inflammation, and demyelinating lesions.

DIAGNOSIS

Clinical Presentation

History

- Optic neuritis: patients will complain of new eye pain that is worse with eye movement, vision loss, and loss of color vision.

- Transverse myelitis: patients will report a new symmetric paraplegia and new sensory loss (with presence of a sensory level), with evolving symptoms.

Physical Examination
- A full ophthalmologic and neuro exam should be performed on any patient with suspected ON or transverse myelitis.

Differential Diagnosis
- As listed for MS, optic neuritis, and transverse myelitis

Diagnostic Criteria and Testing
- Diagnosis of NMO requires a combination of specific clinical symptoms, laboratory abnormalities, and/or radiographic findings including presence of one of the following: optic neuritis, transverse myelitis, acute area postrema syndrome, or acute brainstem dysfunction.

Laboratories
- Basic chemistry and urinalysis, HIV, RPR, ESR, and CRP
- Cerebrospinal fluid[6]
  - Elevated protein and pleocytosis >50 cells/μL are frequently seen.
  - Viral studies to rule out infectious etiologies.

Imaging
- MRI
  - To evaluate for ON, brain MRI must be ordered with fine cuts through the orbit, with and without contrast.
  - NMO classically results in minimal brain lesions initially.
  - Spine MRI classically reveals longitudinally extensive lesions.

TREATMENT

Medications
- Corticosteroids and plasma exchange are indicated for an acute attack of NMO.
- Immunomodulatory medication should be recommended by a neurologist.

SPECIAL CONSIDERATIONS

Disposition
- Any patient with suspected NMO should be admitted.

Complications
- Patients may have residual visual loss.

Isolated Optic Neuritis

GENERAL PRINCIPLES

Definition
- Optic neuritis refers to inflammation of the optic nerve with resultant loss of vision.
- This is commonly the initial presentation of MS or NMO or other autoimmune condition. It can also exist as a clinically isolated syndrome.

Epidemiology/Etiology
- Average age of onset is 20–40 years old.
- Over 60% of those affected are women.[7]

Pathophysiology
- In patients with ON and MS, there is T-cell infiltration of the nerve followed by myelin sheath destruction and retinal ganglion cell death.
- While the exact cause of ON is unknown, associated conditions include demyelinating diseases, systemic autoimmune inflammatory diseases, infections, and neoplasms.

DIAGNOSIS

Clinical Presentation
History
- Periorbital pain: eye pain, which worsens with eye movement
- Vision loss: loss of central vision and color vision[7]
- Uhthoff phenomenon (worsening symptoms when overheating)

Physical Examination
- Relative afferent pupillary defect (Marcus Gunn pupil).
- Field cut deficits including a central scotoma.
- One-third of patients may have papillitis (swollen disc).

Diagnostic Criteria and Testing
Laboratories
- There are no specific lab tests that will diagnose optic neuritis.

Imaging
- Patients presenting with new clinical features suggestive of optic neuritis should have MRI of the brain with and without contrast.

TREATMENT

- Patients with isolated optic neuritis are most commonly treated with high-dose corticosteroids (IV methylprednisolone 250 mg q6h)[7].

SPECIAL CONSIDERATIONS

Disposition
- Any patient with optic neuritis should be admitted to the hospital for administration of high-dose steroids.

Transverse Myelitis (TM)

GENERAL PRINCIPLES

Definition
- Describes a number of diseases, which result in inflammation of the spinal cord with resultant disruption of sensory, motor, and autonomic pathways

Epidemiology/Etiology
- Bimodal peak in incidence at 10–19 years of age and 30–39 years.
- Causes of transverse myelitis are demyelinating diseases, autoimmune/inflammatory disorders, or parainfectious diseases.[8]

Pathophysiology
- TM results in inflammation within the affected spinal cord that leads to demyelination and axonal destruction.
- Adults tend to have upper motor neuron involvement.[7]

DIAGNOSIS

Clinical Presentation
History
- Patients present with evidence of a new myelopathy: weakness, sensory, and/or autonomic dysfunction that localizes to an anatomic level.
- Classically, symptoms are bilateral but can be unilateral or asymmetric.
- Symptoms evolve over hours to days.
- Neuropathic pain is common and may have a dermatomal distribution.[27]
- In cases of isolated transverse myelitis, there is often a history of preceding illness or vaccination.

Physical Examination
- A complete neurologic exam should be done.
- Patients may present with hyperreflexia/positive Babinski, areflexia, or flaccid paralysis.[9]

Differential Diagnosis
- Structural lesions (compressive myelopathy), vascular issues (spinal cord stroke, AVM), or metabolic myelopathy

Diagnostic Testing
Laboratories
- Basic labs including B12, HIV, RPR, and TSH should be sent.
- CSF should be evaluated for cell count, glucose, protein, oligoclonal bands, VDRL, fungal cultures, and cryptococcal antigen.
- VZV, HSV, and CMV if immunocompromised.
- West Nile virus IgM and/or enterovirus PCR if presenting in summer/fall.

Imaging
- All patients with suspected TM warrant urgent MRI of the spine (cervical, thoracic, and lumbar) with and without contrast.

Diagnostic Procedures
- An LP should be performed.

Longitudinally Extensive Transverse Myelitis (LETM)[3]

GENERAL PRINCIPLES

- Refers to inflammation spanning 3 or more consecutive spinal levels.
- Treatment is with intravenous steroids (methylprednisolone 250 mg q6h).
- Plasma exchange may be necessary.[7,9–11]

SPECIAL CONSIDERATIONS

Disposition
- All patients should be admitted.

Complications
- Deep vein thromboses, pulmonary embolus, urinary retention, constipation, and autonomic instability are all complications of TM.

REFERENCES

1. Tullman MJ. Overview of the epidemiology, diagnosis, and disease progression associated with multiple sclerosis. *Am J Manage Care* 2013;19(2 Suppl):S15–20. Available at: http://www.ajmc.com/publications/supplement/2013/ace008_13feb_ms/ACE008_13feb_MS_TullmanS15toS20\n and http://www.ncbi.nlm.nih.gov/pubmed/23544716.
2. Sellner J, Boggild M, Clanet M, et al. EFNS guidelines on diagnosis and management of neuromyelitis optica. *Eur J Neurol* 2010;17(8):1019–32. doi: 10.1111/j.1468-1331.2010.03066.x.
3. Saiz A, Zuliani L, Blanco Y, et al. Revised diagnostic criteria for neuromyelitis optica (NMO). *J Neurol* 2007;254(9):1233–7. doi: 10.1007/s00415-007-0509-8.
4. Sahraian MA, Radue EW, Minagar A. Neuromyelitis optica. Clinical manifestations and neuroimaging features. *Neurol Clin* 2013;31(1):139–52. doi: 10.1016/j.ncl.2012.09.010.
5. Balcer LJ, Miller DH, Reingold SC, Cohen JA. Vision and vision-related outcome measures in multiple sclerosis. *Brain* 2014;138(Pt 1):11–27. doi: 10.1093/brain/awu335.
6. Beck RW, Cleary PA, Anderson MM, et al. A randomized, controlled trial of corticosteroids in the treatment of acute optic neuritis. The Optic Neuritis Study Group. *N Engl J Med* 1992;326(9):581–8. doi: 10.1056/NEJM199202273260901.
7. Bhat A, Naguwa S, Cheema G, Gershwin ME. The epidemiology of transverse myelitis. *Autoimmun Rev* 2010;9(5):A395–9. doi: 10.1016/j.autrev.2009.12.007.
8. Kimbrough DJ, Fujihara K, Jacob A, et al. Treatment of neuromyelitis optica: review and recommendations. *Mult Scler Relat Disord* 2012;1(4):180–7. doi: 10.1016/j.msard.2012.06.002.
9. Frohman EM, Wingerchuk DM. Clinical Practice. Transverse myelitis. *N Engl J Med*. 2010 Aug 5;363(6):564–72.
10. Beh SC, Greenberg BM, Frohman T, Frohman EM. Transverse myelitis. *Neurol Clin* 2013;31(1):79–138. doi: 10.1016/j.ncl.2012.09.008.

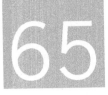

65 Neurologic Emergencies: Dizziness and Vertigo

Matthew C. Loftspring and Robert Bucelli

GENERAL PRINCIPLES

Definition

- Patients may have individual descriptions of dizziness.
- Light-headedness implies the sensation of presyncope.
- Vertigo denotes the sensation of spinning or of motion.
- Disequilibrium may be used as descriptors of general imbalance and can result from sensory, motor, visual, vestibular, or coordination deficits.

Pathophysiology

- Light-headedness is often caused by hypotension, infection, or other toxic and metabolic etiologies.
- True vertigo and disequilibrium are more likely to have a primary neurologic or neurootologic etiology.
- True syncope and presyncope may be due to cardiac/cardiovascular, neurogenic, or systemic etiologies.
- Vestibular neuritis and labyrinthitis are thought to be consequences of viral infection or postviral inflammation.
- Benign paroxysmal positional vertigo (BPPV) is caused by calcium buildup in the semicircular canals (most commonly the posterior semicircular canal).
- Ménière's disease is caused by increased endolymphatic pressure.
- Posterior circulation strokes are due to occlusion or hemorrhage of the vertebral or basilar arteries or their deep penetrating branches.

DIAGNOSIS

Clinical Presentation

History

- Patients with syncope or presyncope often have preceding symptoms of tunneling of vision, muffling of sounds, sweating, palpitations, and a sense of an impending "fainting spell."
- Vestibular neuritis and labyrinthitis will present with severe vertigo, nausea, and vomiting.
  - Labyrinthitis involves hearing loss, whereas vestibular neuritis does not.
  - BPPV commonly involves several minutes of vertigo often precipitated by a change in position, though central causes of vertigo (i.e., stroke) can also worsen with change in position.
- The double vision of peripheral vertigo is often horizontal (images are side by side) or vertical with central causes (images stacked on top of each other).

- Patients with Ménière's disease will endorse unilateral hearing loss. Attacks are often preceded by a feeling of ear fullness followed by vertigo.
- Vertigo and nausea of peripheral disorders are more marked than with central causes.
- While patients with vestibular migraine can present with isolated vertigo in the absence of headache, there should be great hesitation in making a new diagnosis of vestibular migraine in the ED before a thorough evaluation for alternative etiologies has been performed.

Physical Examination

- In vestibular neuritis and labyrinthitis, there is often horizontal and/or torsional nystagmus that can be suppressed by fixation on an object and does not change with shifting the direction of gaze. If there is nystagmus in primary gaze away from the involved side, the examiner should screen for nystagmus in all cardinal directions of gaze to determine whether any direction-changing or vertical nystagmus is present.
- The head impulse test involves turning the head quickly toward the side of the lesion that causes a corrective saccade, and if present unilaterally, this can be used as part of the HINTS criteria in evaluating patients in the ED.
- HINTS stands for "Head Impulse, Nystagmus, Test of Skew" and is a three step process that looks for the following findings in distinguishing peripheral from central vertigo: (1) the corrective saccade mentioned above with a rapid head impulse test suggestive of unilateral impairment of the vestibuloocular reflex; (2) unidirectional, often horizontal or rotational, nystagmus with the features mentioned above and localizing to the same side as the deficit suggested by the head impulse test; and (3) the absence of ocular misalignment on cover–uncover testing. Failure to meet all of these criteria warrants an evaluation for a central lesion.
- Patients with peripheral causes of vertigo should not have other craniobulbar deficits or ataxia. They may have an unsteady gait but are able to ambulate.

Differential Diagnosis

- Posterior circulation stroke, syncope/presyncope, infection, vestibular neuritis, labyrinthitis, BPPV, migraine, or Ménière's disease

Diagnostic Criteria and Testing

Imaging

- CT head is indicated in most cases to rule out hemorrhage or a space-occupying lesion.

Diagnostic Procedures

- BPPV of the posterior semicircular canal can be diagnosed with the Dix-Hallpike maneuver.

TREATMENT

Medications

- Vestibular neuritis and labyrinthitis are typically treated with steroids. One approach is prednisone 60 mg for 7 days followed by a rapid taper over 3 days. Acyclovir is of minimal additional benefit in most cases.
- Meclizine (25–100 mg daily in divided doses) can be used for symptomatic relief of vertigo.
- Vestibular migraine is treated similarly to classic migraine.

Other Nonpharmacologic Therapies
• The Epley maneuver can be administered in the ED or self-administered at home.

SPECIAL CONSIDERATIONS

• An important and often challenging differential diagnosis is a posterior circulation stroke. True vertigo without any other neurologic signs is unlikely to represent a stroke. However, neurologic consultation and a brain MRI should be obtained if there remains any question of a central etiology.

Disposition
• In the absence of a stroke or alternative central etiology warranting inpatient evaluation or treatment, patients with peripheral vertigo can often be discharged if they are able to maintain adequate oral hydration and nutrition.

66 Neurologic Emergencies: Headache in the ER

Peter Kang and Robert Bucelli

GENERAL PRINCIPLES

Classification
Primary Headache Syndromes
• Primary headaches are divided into migraine with and without aura, tension-type headache (TTH), cluster headache and other trigeminal autonomic cephalalgias (TACs), and other primary headaches (e.g., hemicrania continua).
  ○ Migraine with and without aura
    ▪ Migraine without aura: at least five recurrent headaches manifesting as episodes lasting between 4 and 72 hours. Typical features are unilateral location, pulsating quality, moderate to severe intensity, and worsening with physical exertion. There must be associated nausea or photophobia and/or phonophobia.
    ▪ Migraine with aura: at least two attacks that meet criteria for migraine without aura as above but also includes episodes of reversible focal neurologic symptoms (e.g., scintillating scotoma) that develop slowly over 5–20 minutes but last <1 hour. Auras typically precede or begin simultaneously with the onset of headache. Migraines may rarely present with an aura alone without headache (acephalgic migraine).
    ▪ Chronic migraine is defined as 15 or more days of headache a month for at least 3 months.

- Status migrainosus is a debilitating migraine headache lasting >72 hours with or without treatment.
  - Tension-type headache (TTH)
    - TTH is the most common form of primary headache. Headache episodes last between 30 minutes and 7 days. It is typically bilateral and described as pressure or tightening around the head. It is of mild to moderate intensity and not exacerbated by routine physical activity. By definition, nausea or vomiting should be absent. There may be photo- or phonophobia but not both.
  - Trigeminal autonomic cephalalgias
    - Cluster headaches consist of episodes of severe, unilateral facial pain with associated autonomic symptoms lasting between 15 and 180 minutes and can occur in the range of every other day to 8 times per day. Patients may be restless and agitated during episodes. Clusters can last weeks to months, typically with months to years of remission in between clusters. There is a male predominance.
    - Paroxysmal hemicrania and hemicrania continua present similarly to cluster headache but is shorter lasting (2–30 minutes) and more frequent. By definition, these headaches respond to indomethacin.
    - Activity/Valsalva-induced headache disorders are also indomethacin sensitive and include primary cough headache, primary exercise headache, and primary headache associated with sexual activity (i.e., coital headache). These headache syndromes often present with a severe headache that is maximal at onset (i.e., "thunderclap"). At first presentation, these syndromes warrant a thorough screen for subarachnoid hemorrhage.

Secondary Headache Syndromes

- Subarachnoid hemorrhage (SAH): most patients with SAH will endorse a sudden-onset, severe headache that is maximal at onset or soon after onset (i.e., "thunderclap"). SAH should be excluded in anyone presenting with thunderclap headache. Most hemorrhages are related to ruptured saccular aneurysms of the cerebral vasculature and will require either clipping or coiling of the lesion.
- Giant cell arteritis (GCA): GCA should be considered in adults over the age of 50 who present with new headache. Associated symptoms are fatigue, jaw claudication, and visual disturbances. Inflammatory biomarkers (erythrocyte sedimentation rate [ESR] and C-reactive protein [CRP]) are elevated.
- Reversible cerebral vasoconstrictive syndrome (RCVS): patients with RCVS also classically present with a severe "thunderclap headache," although some may present with milder headaches. They may develop ischemic strokes, convexity SAH, and lobar hemorrhages. Patients may also present with seizure. Angiography shows segmental narrowing of cerebral vasculature in the absence of a ruptured aneurysm or other vascular lesion. Risk factors include vasoactive or sympathomimetic drug use, antidepressant use, and pregnancy.
- Posterior reversible encephalopathy syndrome (PRES): PRES, also known as reversible posterior leukoencephalopathy is a clinicoradiologic diagnosis and may present with headache, encephalopathy, seizures, and cortical visual deficits. Risk factors are hypertension, chemotherapeutic and immunosuppressive agents, and sepsis. MRI is necessary for the diagnosis and may be abnormal. In addition to supportive care, treatment of the underlying abnormality is key.
- Meningitis/encephalitis: this should be considered in patients presenting with new-onset headache and associated symptoms of focal neurologic deficits, neck stiffness, seizure, fever, and constitutional symptoms.

- Idiopathic intracranial hypertension (IIH): this is also referred to as pseudotumor cerebri. IIH presents with headache, diplopia, vision loss, transient visual obscurations, and photopsias. Lumbar puncture demonstrates elevated cerebrospinal fluid (CSF) pressure (>25 cm H_2O in adults), but can be falsely elevated or low if not in the correct positioning. Venography should be done to rule out cerebral venous sinus thrombosis (CVST).
- Hypertensive emergency: this is defined as elevated blood pressure with evidence of end-organ damage. Neurologic involvement of hypertensive emergency may include headache and encephalopathy, even without imaging evidence of PRES.
- Medication overuse headache (MOH): MOH is a complication of many headache disorders and is defined as a headache that occurs >15 days per month in association with overutilization of abortive headache treatments.

DIAGNOSIS

Clinical Presentation

History

- History should focus on:
  - Frequency, intensity, and duration of attacks
  - Location and quality of pain
  - Triggers, associations, and associated symptoms
  - Number of total headaches per month and number of disabling headaches
  - Family history of headaches
  - Lifestyle factors (sleep, diet, caffeine intake, stress)
  - Frequency of analgesic use, including over-the-counter medications
- "Red flags"
  - "Thunderclap" headache or severe headache
  - Age >50 without a known preexisting primary headache disorder
  - Immunocompromised state
  - History of recreational drug use or anticoagulants
  - New headache type
  - Worsening with activity or worse in the morning
  - Worse with Valsalva maneuver
  - Visual changes other than typical aura
  - Fever or other constitutional symptoms
  - Focal neurologic signs/deficits
  - Encephalopathy
  - Seizure
  - Meningismus
  - Papilledema on fundoscopic exam

Physical Examination

- Check for neck stiffness and meningismus.
- Perform a careful fundoscopic examination looking for papilledema, suggesting increased intracranial pressure of any cause.
- Perform a full neurologic and ocular examination.
- Autonomic symptoms may be seen in trigeminal autonomic cephalgias.

Differential Diagnosis

- Central nervous system (CNS)-related causes: subdural hematoma, intracerebral hemorrhage, arteriovenous malformation, brain abscess, vasculitis, obstructive

hydrocephalus (especially with known history of shunt for chronic CSF diversion), cerebral infarction, or CVST
- Other causes: sinusitis, glaucoma, dental disease (including temporomandibular joint syndrome), and disorders of the spine ("cervicogenic" headache)
- Systemic causes: fever, viremia, hypoxia, carbon monoxide poisoning, hypercapnia, anemia, caffeine withdrawal, or vasoactive or toxic chemicals (e.g., nitrites)

Diagnostic Criteria and Testing
Laboratories
- Complete blood count (CBC) and inflammatory markers should be sent if suspecting infection or GCA.

Imaging
- Neuroimaging is generally not indicated for known primary headache syndromes.
- CT: a noncontrast CT scan can detect blood better than MRI for hyperacute presentations of intracerebral hemorrhage (ICH).
- MRI may show small/early infarcts on diffusion-weighted imaging.
- CT and MR angiography may help rule out a vascular lesion, hematoma expansion, or dissection in ICH.
- Venography: CT or MR venography (MRV) is useful for evaluating for CVST.

Diagnostic Procedures
- Lumbar puncture is indicated for diagnosis of suspected meningitis, subarachnoid hemorrhage (if CT negative and >6 hours from onset), or IIH. An opening pressure should be obtained.

TREATMENT

Medications
- If meningitis is suspected, ceftriaxone (2 g every 12 hours) or cefotaxime (3 g every 6 hours) and vancomycin (15–20 mg/kg every 8 hours) ± dexamethasone 10 mg IV prior to lumbar puncture (LP) or imaging, followed by dexamethasone 10 mg q6h.
- If GCA is suspected, intravenous methylprednisolone at a dose of 250 mg q6h should be started as soon as clinical suspicion of GCA is established.
- For medication overuse headache (MOA), treatment is withdrawal of the offending analgesic. Transitional therapy with IV medications may be needed (e.g., prochlorperazine, metoclopramide, valproate, methylprednisolone).

Abortive Migraine Treatment
- Acute treatment of migraine is directed at aborting the headache prior to it being well established. Emergent treatments include serotonin agonists and other parenteral medications.
  - Scheduled intravenous NSAID (e.g., ketorolac at 15–30 mg IV q6h) in combination with antiemetics (typically prochlorperazine 5–10 mg IV q6h or metoclopramide 20 mg IV ± diphenhydramine 25 mg IV), magnesium (2 g of IV magnesium sulfate), and IV fluids is an effective first-line regimen in many cases.
  - Antidopaminergic therapies including haloperidol (single dose 5 mg IV) and droperidol (1–2.5 mg IV q6h × 2–3 doses) are also effective first-line therapies. A baseline ECG should be obtained to evaluate for a prolonged QT_c.

○ Triptans are effective abortive medications and may be effective even in a protracted attack. Triptans should not be used in patients with coronary artery disease, cerebrovascular disease, uncontrolled hypertension, hemiplegic migraine, or vertebrobasilar migraine given the concern for vasospasm. If the patient does not have any contraindications, a one-time dose of 100 mg of oral sumatriptan followed by a repeat at dose at 2 hours, if needed, can be considered.

○ Dihydroergotamine (DHE) is a potent venoconstrictor with minimal peripheral arterial constriction. The patient should be on a cardiac monitor, have a baseline ECG, and have a negative pregnancy test prior to initiating DHE. This medication is contraindicated when there is a history of angina, MI or peripheral vascular disease, or if there is any concern for RCVS. A test dose of 0.5 mg IV over 3–5 minutes should be administered followed by repeat ECG and another dose of 0.5 mg IV if no evidence of cardiac ischemia. The medication can then be continued at a dose of 1 mg IV q8h.

○ Ergotamine (1 spray = 0.5 mg in each nostril with max of four sprays per headache) is a vasoconstrictive agent effective for aborting migraine headaches, particularly if administered during the prodromal phase. This medication is also contraindicated in patients with a history of angina, MI, or peripheral vascular disease (PVD).

○ Narcotic analgesia should be avoided in headaches.

Trigeminal Autonomic Cephalalgias

• Paroxysmal hemicranias, hemicrania continua, and the activity/Valsalva-related headache syndromes mentioned above are robustly responsive to indomethacin (50 mg PO tid to start), while cluster headaches are not.
• Cluster headache treatment includes high flow oxygen.

SPECIAL CONSIDERATIONS

Disposition

• Severe debilitating headaches refractory to abortive medication may require inpatient admission for more advanced therapy and monitoring.

Follow-Up

• Patients should follow up with a primary care physician, general neurologist, or headache specialist.
• Patients should be advised on common triggers of headaches such as stress, poor sleep, general health status, and certain foods such as chocolate, caffeine, artificial sweeteners, processed meat products, aged cheeses, red wine, and monosodium glutamate (MSG).
• Patients should be advised on "red flags" for their headaches that should prompt emergency evaluation.

Prognosis

• Reasonable expectation for headache relief should be considered (the goal of a 50% improvement usually represents success).

SUGGESTED READINGS

Becker WJ. Acute migraine treatment in adults. *Headache* 2015;55(6);778–93.

Chiang CC, Schwedt TJ, Wang SJ, Dodick DW. Treatment of medication-overuse headache: a systematic overview. *Cephalalgia* 2016;36(4):371–86.

De Coo IF, Wilbrink LA, Haan J. Symptomatic trigeminal autonomic cephalalgias. *Curr Pain Headache Rep* 2014;19(8):39. doi: 10.1007/s11916-015-0514-z.

Dodick DW. Indomethacin-responsive headache syndromes. *Curr Pain Headache Rep* 2004;8(1):19–26.

Marmura MJ, Goldberg SW. Inpatient management of migraine. *Curr Neurol Neurosci Rep* 2015;15(4):13. doi: 10.1007/s11910-015-0539-z/.

Marmura MJ, Silberstein SD, Schwedt TJ. The acute treatment of migraine in adults: the American Headache Society evidence assessment of migraine pharmacotherapies. *Headache* 2015;55(1):3–20.

Nagy AJ, Ghandhi S, Bhola R, Goadsby PJ. Intravenous dihydroergotamine for inpatient management of refractory primary headaches. *Neurology* 2011;77(20):1827–32.

Rozen TD. Trigeminal autonomic cephalalgias. *Neurol Clin* 2009;27(2):537–56.

Schwedt TJ. Chronic migraine. *BJM* 2014;348:g1416. doi: 10.1136/bmj.g1416.

Taggart E, Doran S, Kokotillo A, et al. Ketorolac in the treatment of acute migraine: a systematic review. *Headache* 2013;53(2):227–87.

VanderPluym J. Indomethacin-responsive headaches. *Curr Neurol Neurosci Rep* 2015;15(2):516.

Weatherall MW. Drug therapy in headache. *Clin Med (Lond)* 2015 Jun;15(3):273–9. http://ihs-classification.org/en/

67 Neurologic Emergencies: Hydrocephalus and Shunt Malfunction

Mark D. Levine

GENERAL PRINCIPLES

Definition

- Hydrocephalus is defined as a pathologic enlargement of the ventricles within the brain.
  - There are four types: communicating, noncommunicating, ex vacuo, and normal.
- Ventricular shunts will divert CSF into either the peritoneum or the heart via one-way valves.

Epidemiology/Etiology

- Hydrocephalus can occur in all age groups and is equally common in both sexes. Idiopathic normal pressure hydrocephalus (NPH) is more common in adults over the age of 60.
- Causes may be due to congenital issues, infection, tumor, TBI, and hemorrhage, whereas idiopathic NPH is usually secondary to abnormal absorption of cerebrospinal fluid (CSF).
- Shunt malfunctions may be due to infection, drainage issues (too slow or too rapid), or bleeding.

Pathophysiology
- When CSF production exceeds drainage/absorption, intracranial pressure (ICP) is increased.

DIAGNOSIS

Clinical Presentation

History
- The usual complaints of a patient with altered ventricular pressure may range from morning headache and malaise to nausea and vomiting, blurry or double vision, light sensitivity, auditory hyperesthesia, vertigo, seizures, and the classic triad of gait disturbance, altered mental status, and incontinence in NPH.
- In the patient that has an indwelling ventricular shunt, the complaint may also be compared with a history of the patient's symptoms prior to shunt placement or symptoms that the patient has had in the past with prior shunt malfunctions.

Physical Examination
- A full physical exam should be performed on the patient with special attention paid to a full neurologic exam and cognitive tests such as the Mini-Mental State Examination.
- Papilledema and nerve palsies may be present.
- Increased reflexes and Babinski response in one or both feet may be seen in NPH.

Differential Diagnosis
- Dementia, delirium, ophthalmologic issues, neurologic or obstructive symptoms of the GU tract, Parkinson disease, infection, tumor, or shunt malfunction

Diagnostic Criteria and Testing

Laboratories
- No laboratory tests are confirmatory for hydrocephalus or shunt failure.

Imaging
- CT and MRI can evaluate ventricular size with the hallmark finding of ventriculomegaly out of proportion to enlargement of the sulci.
  ○ CT changes may not be obvious if the ventricles are draining too quickly.
- A "shunt series" should be performed in any patient with a history of a ventricular shunt. This usually includes radiographs of the path of the shunt to evaluate for discontinuity of the tubing as well as a CT scan of the head to evaluate for increased intraventricular size.

Diagnostic Procedures
- In the patient that has a ventricular shunt malfunction, neurosurgery should be consulted.

TREATMENT

Medications
- Medications are used mainly to alleviate symptoms until the etiology of the disease process can be discovered. Analgesics and antiemetics are frequently administered.

Other Nonpharmacologic Therapies

• Reduction of CSF and possible replacement of the shunt will be performed by neurosurgery.

SPECIAL CONSIDERATIONS

Disposition

• These patients should be admitted to the hospital in consultation with the neurosurgical service.
• If symptoms can be alleviated in the emergency department, discharge home is appropriate with close follow-up.

SUGGESTED READINGS

Hebb AO, Cusimano MD. Idiopathic normal pressure hydrocephalus: a systemic review of diagnosis and outcome. *Neurosurgery* 2001;49:1166.
Hydrocephalus Fact Sheet. NINDS. 2016. Retrieved on December 14, 2016.
Pople IK. Hydrocephalus and shunts: what the neurologist should know. *J Neurol Neurosurg Psychiatry* 2002;73(Suppl I):i17–22.

Neurologic Emergencies: Infections of the Central Nervous System

Maia Dorsett and Stephen Y. Liang

Meningitis

GENERAL PRINCIPLES

Definition

• Meningitis refers to inflammation of the meninges due to infection.

Epidemiology/Etiology

• The average age of the patient with meningitis is 35 years of age has changed because of to the introduction of the *Haemophilus influenzae* type b (Hib) vaccine in 1998.[1–3]
• The causative organism in bacterial meningitis varies with patient age, immune status, history of hospitalization, or neurosurgical procedure (Table 68.1).

TABLE 68.1	Etiologic and Recommended Antimicrobial Therapy by Age and Clinical Context	
Subgroup	Most common bacterial pathogen	Initial intravenous therapy
Adults	S. pneumoniae, Neisseria meningitidis	Ceftriaxone (2 g every 12 h) or cefotaxime (3 g every 6 h) and vancomycin (15–20 mg/kg every 8 h)
Elderly	S. pneumoniae, N. meningitidis, Listeria monocytogenes	Ceftriaxone (2 g every 12 h) or cefotaxime (3 g every 6 h) and vancomycin (15–20 mg/kg every 8 h) and ampicillin (2 g every 4 h)
Immunocompromised	S. pneumoniae, N. meningitidis, H. influenzae, L. monocytogenes, aerobic gram-negative bacilli	Vancomycin (15–20 mg/kg every 8 h) and ceftazidime (2 g every 8 h) or cefepime (2 g every 8 h) or meropenem (2 g every 8 h) and ampicillin (2 g every 4 h)
Nosocomial	S. aureus, S. epidermidis, aerobic gram-negative bacilli	Vancomycin (15–20 mg/kg every 8 h) and ceftazidime (2 g every 8 h) or cefepime (2 g every 8 h) or meropenem (2 g every 8 h)

- Enteroviruses (Coxsackie A and B, echovirus) are the most common cause of viral meningitis. Herpes simplex virus (HSV), cytomegalovirus (CMV), Epstein-Barr virus (EBV), varicella-zoster virus (VZV), and HIV may cause viral meningitis.[4]
- Causes of fungal meningitis include *Cryptococcus neoformans*, *Coccidioides immitis*, or *Histoplasma capsulatum*.[5,24]
- In patients with impaired cell-mediated immunity (CD4+ count < 200 cells/μL), there is a predisposition to infection.[27]

Pathophysiology

- Organisms access the subarachnoid space through contiguous spread from dental or sinus infections, bacteremia, neurosurgical procedures, or traumatic or congenital communications with the exterior.
- Meningitis leads to brain and meningeal edema and eventually increases intracranial pressure.
- Fungal meningitis is usually seen in patients with an underlying immunocompromised condition and originates from infection somewhere else in the body.[5]

DIAGNOSIS

Clinical Presentation

History
- The classic symptoms include fever, headache, nuchal rigidity, altered mental status, and nausea/vomiting. While the combination is present in only the minority patients, 99–100% of patients with bacterial meningitis will have at least one of these symptoms.[6,7]

Physical Examination

- Kernig and Brudzinski maneuvers have low sensitivity so should not be used to the rule out the diagnosis of meningitis[8–10] but are highly specific for predicting cerebrospinal fluid (CSF) pleocytosis.
- Patients with an underlying immunocompromised condition or advanced age are more likely to present with non-specific symptoms (altered mental status, stupor, or coma).

Differential Diagnosis

- Fever and altered mental status have a broad differential diagnosis, including:
  - Sepsis, sympathomimetic toxicity, neuroleptic malignant syndrome, salicylate toxicity, or serotonin syndrome
- Headache with/without altered mental status:
  - Subarachnoid hemorrhage (especially with neck stiffness), intracranial mass, migraine headache, hypertensive encephalopathy, or pseudotumor cerebri

Diagnostic Criteria and Testing

Imaging

- Patients who are immunocompromised and have pre-existing central nervous system disease, new-onset seizure, altered level of consciousness, papilledema, or focal neurologic deficit at risk for intracranial mass or midline shift should have a head CT performed prior to the LP.[11]

Diagnostic Procedures

- In the absence of contraindications, a lumbar puncture should be performed.

Laboratories

- Blood tests should be obtained including coagulation studies and platelet count.
- CSF should be sent for cell count, glucose, protein, and culture. Fungal or mycobacterial testing in the right clinical setting (Table 68.2).

TABLE 68.2	Typical CSF Fluid Profiles for Bacterial, Viral, and Fungal Meningitis			
Parameter	Normal	Bacterial	Viral[a]	Fungal[a]
CSF opening pressure	<170 mm	Elevated	Normal	Normal or elevated
Cell count	<5 cells/mm^3	>1000/mm^3	<1000 mm^3	<500/mm^3
Cell predominance	—	Neutrophils	Lymphocytes	Lymphocytes
CSF glucose	>0.66 × serum	Low	Normal	Low
CSF protein	<45 mg/dL	Elevated	Normal	Elevated

[a]Findings may not be adequate to rule out bacterial disease in an individual patient.

Data from Fitch MT, Abrahamian FM, Moran GJ, Talan DA. Emergency department management of meningitis and encephalitis. *Infect Dis Clin North Am* 2008;22(1):33–52.

TREATMENT

Medications

- Empiric antibiotics should not be delayed until after the head CT or lumbar puncture are performed.[12,19]
- Antibiotic recommendation by patient age and clinical history is provided in Table 68.1.
- In cases of suspected bacterial meningitis, corticosteroids should be considered as adjunctive therapy as they have the potential to reduce hearing loss and other subsequent neurologic sequelae.[13] Ideally, they should be administered before or with antibiotics.
- Treatment is supportive for viral meningitis.

SPECIAL CONSIDERATIONS

Disposition

- Patients with bacterial meningitis often require care in an intensive care unit. Patients in whom the CSF profile is benign and who are otherwise clinically well appearing or improved can generally be discharged home with follow-up.

Encephalitis

GENERAL PRINCIPLES

Definition

- Encephalitis is inflammation of the brain parenchyma.
- Postinfectious encephalomyelitis (disseminated encephalomyelitis) is an autoimmune phenomenon that may follow a disseminated viral illness or vaccination, usually in children or young adults.[14]

Epidemiology/Etiology

- The most common cause of viral encephalitis is HSV and has a bimodal age distribution affecting the very young and the elderly.[15,16]

Pathophysiology

- Viral encephalitis stems from direct infection of the brain parenchyma as a result of viremia or reactivation of latent virus within neuronal tissues.[14]

DIAGNOSIS

Clinical Presentation

History

- The patient may report a fever and may present with altered mental status.
- Patients may present with personality changes, psychosis, and olfactory and gustatory hallucinations and may be initially misdiagnosed as a psychiatric disorder.[14,17,18]
- A social history, including tick exposures and travel history, is important to assess.

Physical Examination

- The neurologic findings vary with the underlying infectious agent (Table 68.3).
- A full physical exam with special focus on rash or arthropod bites can be helpful in making the diagnosis.

TABLE 68.3 Demographics, Clinical Presentation, and Treatment of Select Etiologies of Viral Encephalitis

Pathogen	Demographics	Neurologic symptoms (headache, fever, altered mental status and...)	Non-neurologic symptoms	Diagnostic test	Treatment
Herpes simplex virus (HSV)	Usually young and elderly; no seasonal predilection	Seizures, olfactory/gustatory hallucinations, aphasia, personality changes, hemiparesis (face/arm/leg), upper visual field cut	Rash	HSV-1, HSV-2 PCR (CSF)	Acyclovir 10 mg/kg every 8 h (adjust for renal function)
Varicella-zoster virus (VZV)	Most common in immunocompromised	Cranial nerve palsies, cerebellitis	Shingles	VZV PCR (CSF)	Acyclovir 10 mg/kg every 8 h (adjust for renal function)
Cytomegalovirus (CMV)	Immunocompromised	Behavior changes, coma	Pneumonitis, retinitis, myelitis	CMV PCR (CSF)	Ganciclovir 5 mg/kg every 12 h
Enterovirus	Usually young	Rhombencephalitis (myoclonus, tremors, ataxia, cranial nerve palsies), polio-like acute flaccid paralysis, neurogenic shock	Hand–foot–mouth disease, rash, myocarditis, pericarditis, conjunctivitis, pulmonary edema	Enterovirus PCR (CSF)	Supportive care
Arboviruses	Summer months			IgG and IgM (CSF and serum)	Supportive care

Flaviviridae					
West Nile virus (80% infections asymptomatic)	US, Africa, Europe, Middle East, Asia	Tremors, parkinsonism, asymmetric flaccid paralysis	Insect bite, myalgias, hepatitis, pancreatitis, myocarditis, rhabdomyolysis, orchitis, rash		
St. Louis encephalitis virus	Widespread in US; adults (> 50 y old)	Vomiting, confusion, disorientation, stupor, coma	Insect bite, malaise, myalgias, syndrome of inappropriate antidiuretic hormone secretion (SIADH)		
Togaviridae			Myalgias, malaise		
Eastern equine encephalitis virus	Eastern and gulf coasts of USA, Caribbean, and South America; children and adults	Seizures			
Western equine encephalitis virus	West, Midwest USA, and Canada; infants and adults	Seizures	Myalgias, malaise		
Rabies virus	Exposure to infected animal	Agitation, bizarre behavior, coma, stupor	Hydrophobia, fever, malaise, anxiety, pain or itching at site of the bite wound	Rabies virus RNA by rtPCR (saliva)	Post exposure vaccination, once infected supportive care but universally fatal

IgG, immunoglobulin G; IgM, immunoglobulin M; PCR, polymerase chain reaction.

Differential Diagnosis

- Infectious/postinfectious, metabolic, toxic, autoimmune, or paraneoplastic causes
- Intracranial hemorrhage, nonhemorrhagic stroke, Todd's paralysis, or intracranial mass/abscess

Diagnostic Criteria and Testing

Imaging

- Patients who are immunocompromised and have pre-existing central nervous system disease, new-onset seizure, altered level of consciousness, papilledema, or focal neurologic deficit at risk for intracranial mass or midline shift should have a head CT performed.[11]

Diagnostic Procedures

- Unless contraindicated, a lumbar puncture (LP) should be performed.

Laboratories

- HIV should be drawn.
- CSF should be sent for cell count, protein, glucose, and culture. CSF findings in HSV encephalitis can vary greatly.[15,16]
- CSF should be sent for polymerase chain reaction (PCR) for HSV and VZV.

TREATMENT

Medications

- Management of encephalitis is directed toward the underlying etiology (Table 68.3).
- Patients should receive immediate empiric treatment with intravenous acyclovir pending confirmatory testing, as a delay in acyclovir initiation is associated with poor outcome (Table 68.4).[20–22]

SPECIAL CONSIDERATIONS

Disposition

- Patients with severe presentations typically require ICU admission. For patients with less severe presentations, admission to the floor with seizure precautions may be appropriate.

Brain Abscess

GENERAL PRINCIPLES

Definition

- A brain abscess is a collection of purulent material resulting from infection within the brain parenchyma.

Epidemiology/Etiology

- More commonly, patients are male, immunocompromised, and in their third or fourth decade of life.[18,22]
- The majority of brain abscesses are caused by *Streptococcus* and *Staphylococcus* species, although gram-negative bacteria have been found in a subset of cases. Up to a quarter of all cases are polymicrobial.[22]
- Less common etiologies of brain abscess, such as *Nocardia*, fungal, and parasitic, may be seen in the setting of severe immunocompromise.

TABLE 68.4 Clinical Presentation, Diagnosis, and Treatment of Opportunistic Infections in HIV Disease

Infection	Typical CD4+ cell count at presentation (cells per µL)	Clinical presentation	Temporal evolution	Special CSF tests [sensitivity/ specificity]	Typical radiographic appearance	Treatment: antiretroviral therapy AND
Cytomegalovirus (CMV) encephalitis	<50	Altered mental status, seizures	Days	CMV PCR [>90%/>90%]	Usually normal; may have evidence of ventriculitis with ventriculomegaly and periventricular enhancement on MRI	Ganciclovir
Cryptococcal meningitis	<50 (rarely up to 200)	Fever, headache, altered mental status, vomiting	Days	Elevated opening pressure; cryptococcal antigen	May be normal; "punched-out" cystic lesions on MRI if cryptoccocomas develop	Amphotericin B and flucytosine
Progressive multifocal leukoencephalopathy (PML)	<100	Altered mental status, focal neurologic deficits	Weeks to months	JC virus PCR [50–90%/90–100%]	Hyperintense areas in white matter on T2-FLA1R imaging	–
Central nervous system (CNS) lymphoma	<100	Altered mental status, focal neurologic deficits, headache	Weeks to months	EBV PCR [100%/50% specific]	Usually solitary, heterogeneously enhancing lesions with mass effect	–

(continued)

TABLE 68.4 Clinical Presentation, Diagnosis, and Treatment of Opportunistic Infections in HIV Disease (CONTINUED)

Infection	Typical CD4+ cell count at presentation (cells per μL)	Clinical presentation	Temporal evolution	Special CSF tests [sensitivity/specificity]	Typical radiographic appearance	Treatment: antiretroviral therapy AND
Toxoplasma encephalitis	<200	Fever, headache, altered mental status	Days	*Toxoplasma gondii* PCR [50–80%/100%]	Multiple ring-enhancing lesions with mass effect	Pyrimethamine, folinic acid, and sulfadiazine OR trimethoprim-sulfamethoxazole
Tuberculous meningitis	<200	Altered mental status, cranial neuropathies	Days to weeks	Culture and acid-fast bacilli stain [>80%]	Rarely basilar enhancement; possibly abscesses or tuberculomas	Rifampin, isoniazid, pyrazinamide, ethambutol
Acute syphilitic meningitis	<350	Headache, photophobia, emesis; ocular manifestations (CN palsies, uveitis, optic neuritis) commonly associated	Within 12 months (chronic neurosyphilis 5-20 years)	CSF VDRL [CSF FTA-ABS more sensitive but less specific]	No pathognomonic findings	Penicillin G 3-4 million units q 4 h × 10-14 days

FTA-ABS, fluorescent treponemal antibody absorption test; VDRL, Venereal Disease Research Laboratory.

Pathophysiology

- Most bacterial brain abscesses are due to a spread of a congruous focus, hematogenous seeding, or traumatic inoculation.[22]
- Initial infection leads to focal inflammation and edema (early cerebritis). Over days, this expands to a wider inflammatory response in the white matter surrounding an increasingly necrotic core (late cerebritis). Over a period of weeks, a collagenous capsule can surround the wall of the core, but surrounding edema and inflammation may still persist.

DIAGNOSIS

Clinical Presentation

History
- Headache may be the only initial symptom of a brain abscess, particularly in the earliest stages.

Physical Examination
- Fever is present only in half of all cases, and the classic triad of headache, fever, and focal neurologic deficit is present in only 20%.[22]
- Onset of neurologic symptoms, such as hemiparesis, cranial nerve palsy, gait disorders, and altered mental status, may develop over days to weeks.

Differential Diagnosis

- See Encephalitis.

Diagnostic Criteria and Testing

Laboratories
- Blood cultures are commonly obtained in patients that are thought to have a brain abscess.
- If operative intervention is expected, coagulation studies and a type and screen/cross would be appropriate.

Imaging
- A head CT with contrast can reveal ring-enhancing lesions in the late stages of cerebritis as the lesion encapsulates.
- A maxillofacial CT can be ordered if mastoiditis or sinusitis is believed to be the source of infection.
- MRI with contrast is the most sensitive modality for diagnosis. It helps distinguish abscess from metastatic disease.

TREATMENT

- Brain abscesses are treated using a multidisciplinary approach involving neurosurgical and medical therapy.

Medications

- Vancomycin, a third- or fourth-generation cephalosporin, and metronidazole will target the most common etiologies.

SPECIAL CONSIDERATIONS

Disposition

- Patients with brain abscess are almost uniformly critically ill and usually go to the operating room or ICU directly from the emergency department.

REFERENCES

1. Centers for Disease Control and Prevention (CDC). Progress toward elimination of *Haemophilus influenzae* type b invasive disease among infants and children—United States, 1998–2000. *MMWR Morb Mortal Wkly Rep* 2002;51(11):234–7.
2. Castelblanco RL, Lee M, Hasbun R. Epidemiology of bacterial meningitis in the USA from 1997 to 2010: a population-based observational study. *Lancet Infect Dis* 2014;14(9):813–9.
3. Brouwer MC, Tunkel AR, van de Beek D. Epidemiology, diagnosis, and antimicrobial treatment of acute bacterial meningitis. *Clin Microbiol Rev* 2010;23(3):467–92.
4. Gottfredsson M, Perfect JR. Fungal meningitis. *Semin Neurol* 2001;20(03):307–22.
5. Smith RM, Schaefer MK, Kainer MA, et al. Fungal infections associated with contaminated methylprednisolone injections. *N Engl J Med* 2013;369(17):1598–609.
6. Durand ML, Calderwood SB, Weber DJ, et al. Acute bacterial meningitis in adults. A review of 493 episodes. *N Engl J Med* 1993;328(1):21–8.
7. Sigurdardóttir B, Björnsson OM, Jónsdóttir KE, et al. Acute bacterial meningitis in adults. A 20-year overview. *Arch Intern Med* 1997;157(4):425–30.
8. Nakao JH, Jafri FN, Kaushal S, et al. Jolt accentuation of headache and other clinical signs: poor predictors of meningitis in adults. *Am J Emerg Med* 2014;32(1):24–8.
9. Thomas KE, Hasbun R, Jekel J, Quagliarello VJ. The diagnostic accuracy of Kernig's sign, Brudzinski's sign, and nuchal rigidity in adults with suspected meningitis. *Clin Infect Dis* 2002;35(1):46–52.
10. Waghdhare S, Kalantri A, Joshi R, Kalantri S. Accuracy of physical signs for detecting meningitis: a hospital-based diagnostic accuracy study. *Clin Neurol Neurosurg* 2010;112(9):752–7.
11. Wang AY, Machicado JD, Khoury NT, et al. Community-acquired meningitis in older adults: clinical features, etiology, and prognostic factors. *J Am Geriatr Soc* 2014;62(11):2064–70.
12. Viallon A, Desseigne N, Marjollet O, et al. Meningitis in adult patients with a negative direct cerebrospinal fluid examination: value of cytochemical markers for differential diagnosis. *Crit Care* 2011;15(3):R136.
13. Aronin SI, Peduzzi P, Quagliarello VJ. Community-acquired bacterial meningitis: risk stratification for adverse clinical outcome and effect of antibiotic timing. *Ann Intern Med* 1998;129(11):862–9.
14. Greenlee JE. Encephalitis and postinfectious encephalitis. *Continuum (Minneap Minn)* 2012;18:1271–89.
15. Proulx N, Fréchette D, Toye B, et al. Delays in the administration of antibiotics are associated with mortality from adult acute bacterial meningitis. *QJM* 2005;98(4):291–8.
16. Brouwer MC, McIntyre P, Prasad K, van de Beek D. Corticosteroids for acute bacterial meningitis. *Cochrane Database Syst Rev* 2013;(6):CD004405.
17. Whitley RJ, Lakeman F. Herpes simplex virus infections of the central nervous system: therapeutic and diagnostic considerations. *Clin Infect Dis* 1995;20(2):414–20.
18. Hjalmarsson A, Blomqvist P, Sköldenberg B. Herpes simplex encephalitis in Sweden, 1990–2001: incidence, morbidity, and mortality. *Clin Infect Dis* 2007;45(7):875–80.
19. Auburtin M, Wolff M, Charpentier J, et al. Detrimental role of delayed antibiotic administration and penicillin-nonsusceptible strains in adult intensive care unit patients with pneumococcal meningitis: the PNEUMOREA prospective multicenter study. *Crit Care Med* 2006;34(11):2758–65.
20. Granerod J, Ambrose HE, Davies NW, et al. Causes of encephalitis and differences in their clinical presentations in England: a multicentre, population-based prospective study. *Lancet Infect Dis* 2010;10(12):835–44.
21. Johnson RT. Acute encephalitis. *Clin Infect Dis* 1996;23(2):219–24; quiz 225–6.
22. Whitley RJ. Herpes simplex encephalitis: clinical assessment. *JAMA* 1982;247(3):317.
23. Logan SA, MacMahon E. Viral meningitis. *BMJ* 2008;336(7634):36–40.
24. Tan, I. L., Smith, B. R., von Geldern, G., Mateen, F. J. & McArthur, J. C. HIV-associated opportunistic infections of the CNS. *Lancet Neurol.* 11, 605–617 (2012).

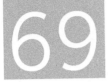

69 Neurologic Emergencies: Neuromuscular Disorders

Matthew Burford and Robert Bucelli

GENERAL PRINCIPLES

Definition
- Myasthenia gravis (MG) is an autoimmune neuromuscular junction disorder.
- Myasthenic crisis is a complication of MG characterized by worsening bulbar weakness and respiratory compromise.
  - Cholinergic crisis may mimic myasthenic crisis and is characterized by increased weakness secondary to cholinergic excess.

Epidemiology/Etiology
- MG has a bimodal age distribution, affecting young women and older men.
- 15–20% of MG patients will develop a myasthenic crisis at some point over the course of their disease, and the crisis may be the initial presentation of MG.[1]
- Myasthenic crisis is often associated with a precipitating event.

Pathophysiology
- Antibodies directed toward the postsynaptic nicotinic acetylcholine receptor (AChR) complex in skeletal muscle lead to destruction and decreased function of AChR.
- Acetylcholine (ACh) released by motor neurons is then less effective at depolarizing the muscle membrane. This failure of neuromuscular transmission leads to fatigable weakness.
- Thymoma and autoimmune thyroid disease are associated with MG.[2-4]

DIAGNOSIS

Clinical Presentation
History
- In addition to worsening diplopia, ptosis, and dysarthria, patients may also present with complaints of morning headaches, daytime somnolence, orthopnea, dyspnea on exertion, and hyperhidrosis that may indicate worsening respiratory function.

Physical Examination
- MG
  - 90% of patients will present with oculobulbar weakness. Fatigability can often be demonstrated, such as fatigable ptosis with prolonged upgaze.
  - Facial, jaw, tongue, and proximal limb weakness may be present.

TABLE 69.1	Neuromuscular Respiratory Failure	
Signs/symptoms		Objective measures
Staccato speech	Morning headaches	Breath count < 20 (~ <2 L FVC)
Weak cough	Excessive daytime somnolence	FVC < 20 mL/kg[a]
Tachypnea	Frequent nocturnal arousals	MIP (NIF) > −30 cm H$_2$O[a]
Tachycardia	Lack of restful sleep	MEP < 40 cm H$_2$O[a]
Accessory muscle use	Orthopnea	Hypoxemia (late sign)
Paradoxical breathing	Dyspnea on exertion	Hypercapnia (late sign)
Difficulty handling secretions	Hyperhidrosis	
Weak neck flexion/ extension	Restlessness	

[a]These three parameters make up the "20/30/40" rule.

FVC, forced vital capacity; MEP, maximum expiratory pressure; MIP, maximum inspiratory pressure; NIF, negative inspiratory force.

- Myasthenic crisis
  ○ In addition to several typical features of MG, signs of neuromuscular respiratory failure are also present (Table 69.1).
- Cholinergic crisis
  ○ SLUDGE symptoms may be present.

Differential Diagnosis
- Guillain-Barré syndrome (GBS), botulism, inflammatory myopathies, braintem ischemic stroke, medication-induced exacerbation, or thyroid disorders

Diagnostic Criteria and Testing
- Testing should focus on identification of neuromuscular respiratory failure, precipitating causes of crisis, and confirmatory evidence of MG.

Laboratories
- There are no rapid serum tests that will specifically identify MG.

Imaging
- CXR may be helpful, as the most commonly reported precipitating event is respiratory infection.

Diagnostic Procedures
- Negative inspiratory force (NIF) and forced vital capacity (FVC) can be performed at the bedside and should be done serially (but not to excess so as to avoid exhausting the patient) (Table 69.1).

TREATMENT

- In patients with known MG, pyridostigmine is typically stopped.
- AChE inhibitors are halted to avoid the risk of increased secretions that may complicate respiratory status and to remove the possibility of a component of cholinergic crisis.
- Immunosuppressant medications may be temporarily held until infection is ruled out or treated although this is not always necessary.
- Initial treatment must focus on stabilization of respiratory status.
  - Implement BiPAP early in patients with mild respiratory dysfunction and relatively preserved bulbar strength.
    - Neuromuscular blocking agents should be avoided if possible.[5]
- Precipitating illness.
  - Treatment of metabolic, endocrinologic, or infectious insults is the key to stabilizing the patient's MG.

Medications

- Immunomodulatory Therapy
  - Intravenous immunoglobulin (IVIg) (2 g/kg divided over 2–5 days)
  - Therapeutic plasma exchange (PLEX)

SPECIAL CONSIDERATIONS

Disposition

- These patients will almost always need admission to the hospital and possibly the ICU depending on their respiratory status.

Guillain-Barré Syndrome

GENERAL PRINCIPLES

Definition

- GBS is a heterogeneous group of immune-mediated, acute polyradiculoneuropathies. GBS represents a neuromuscular emergency as it may produce respiratory failure and/or life-threatening autonomic instability.

Epidemiology/Etiology

- Acute inflammatory demyelinating polyradiculoneuropathy (AIDP) is the most common form of GBS in the United States and Europe.
- GBS is the most common cause of acute flaccid paralysis (AFP) in developed countries.[7]
  - Two-thirds of GBS cases have an identifiable preceding upper respiratory or diarrheal illness.[8]
  - The risk of developing GBS increases with age.

Pathophysiology

- GBS is caused by a primarily antibody-mediated autoimmune reaction to components of peripheral nerve myelin.
- Autoantibodies are thought to be generated following exposure to an infectious organism (*Cytomegalovirus* [CMV], Epstein-Barr virus [EBV], *Mycoplasma*).

DIAGNOSIS

- The presenting signs and symptoms in GBS may be mild or atypical.
- If not diagnosed early, there is an increased risk of intubation.[9]

Clinical Presentation

History

- The classic presentation of GBS consists of a progressive, symmetric, ascending, flaccid paralysis, as well as pain (especially in the low back or lower extremities), distal paresthesias, and intermittent autonomic instability.

Physical Examination

- Weakness is typically symmetric.
  - While mild asymmetry in weakness may be seen, prominent asymmetry should prompt an investigation for alternative diagnoses.
- Facial or oropharyngeal weakness occurs in up to 70% of AIDP.[10]
- Reflexes are often hypoactive or absent, but may be preserved or even exaggerated early in the disease course.
- While positive sensory symptoms (paresthesias) are common, sensory loss on exam is uncommon.
- Perform thorough screening for signs of impending respiratory failure (Table 69.1).
- Altered mental status should prompt consideration of complications associated with GBS including respiratory failure or posterior reversible leukoencephalopathy syndrome (PRES).[11]

Differential Diagnosis

- See Table 69.2.

TABLE 69.2 Differential Diagnosis of GBS[31]
Fulminant/confluent mononeuritis multiplex (e.g., vasculitic neuropathy)
Infectious polyradiculoneuropathy—HIV, Lyme disease
Infectious poliomyelitis/acute flaccid paralysis—West Nile virus, polioviruses, enteroviruses
Acute presentation of chronic inflammatory demyelinating polyneuropathy (CIDP) or multifocal motor neuropathy (MMN)
Acute myelopathy/myeloradiculopathy
Diabetic/nondiabetic lumbosacral radiculoplexopathy
Inflammatory polyradiculoneuropathy—sarcoidosis
Biologic toxin—botulism, diphtheria, tick paralysis
Chemical toxin—thiamine (deficiency, particularly in patients with suspected Miller Fisher Syndrome or Bickerstaff's brainstem encephalitis), lead, arsenic, gold, hexacarbons, organophosphate
Medication induced—lithium, ifosfamide, nitrofurantoin, captopril
Infectious neuropathy—rabies
See http://neuromuscular.wustl.edu/time/nmacute.htm for further details.

Diagnostic Testing

Laboratories
- There are no specific laboratory values that diagnose GBS.

Imaging
- MRI of the spine with and without contrast may be helpful to rule out a structural cause of weakness.

Diagnostic Procedures
- NIF and FVC should be performed serially (Table 69.1).

TREATMENT

- Autonomic instability should be treated conservatively.
- Respiratory failure
  - Signs of impending respiratory failure (Table 69.1) should prompt early, elective intubation.
  - BiPAP is not effective at preventing the need for intubation.[12]
    - Avoid paralytic agents.

Medications
- Immunomodulatory treatment with PLEX or IVIg is warranted in patients who cannot walk independently.
- Corticosteroids are ineffective for AIDP.

SPECIAL CONSIDERATIONS

Disposition
- Patients with mild weakness and normal and/or stable respiratory parameters may be monitored outside the ICU, though a close monitoring unit is preferable given the likelihood of continued progression.
- Any patient with pending respiratory failure or intubation needs to be in the intensive care unit.

Prognosis
- Weakness typically progresses for 2–4 weeks before reaching a plateau phase that may last for weeks, with the majority of patients recovering within a year.

Infectious Motor Neuronopathy/Acute Flaccid Paralysis (AFP)

GENERAL PRINCIPLES

Definition
- AFP is a limited form of myelitis that preferentially involves the lower motor neurons or ventral roots of the brainstem and/or spinal cord.

Epidemiology
- GBS remains the most common cause of AFP worldwide.
- West Nile virus (WNV) is the most common cause of infectious AFP and occurs almost exclusively between July and September in the United States.

Pathophysiology
• The syndrome is caused by direct viral infection of the lower motor neurons.

DIAGNOSIS

Clinical Presentation

History
• AFP is often preceded by a systemic prodrome (fever, malaise, nausea/vomiting, lymphadenopathy, and headache) with weakness emerging days (2–8) later.
  ○ Neuroinvasive WNV is typically preceded by fever and a generalized, nonpruritic, maculopapular rash.

Physical Examination
• Weakness is typically proximal and asymmetric.
• Reflexes are hypoactive or absent.
• Respiratory muscles may be affected.
• Encephalitis may preclude detection of subtle motor deficits on exam.

Differential Diagnosis
• See Table 69.2.

Diagnostic Criteria and Testing

Laboratories
• There are no serum laboratory values that definitively diagnose AFP in the emergency department. CSF testing may reveal pleocytosis (mean 200 cells/L), elevated protein early in the disease course, and identification of poliovirus (via PCR) or WNV IgM in the CSF (which is diagnostic).[13,14]

Diagnostic Procedures
• Lumbar puncture is helpful in differentiating from GBS and in obtaining a specific viral diagnosis.

Imaging
• Spine MRI is abnormal in a minority of WNV-associated AFP cases.

TREATMENT

• Treatment is primarily supportive. If intubation is necessary, no paralytics should be used.

SPECIAL CONSIDERATIONS

Disposition
• Patients should be admitted to the hospital and may need the intensive care unit if having respiratory compromise.

Botulism

Definition
• Botulism is a rare presynaptic neuromuscular junction disorder caused by a neurotoxin produced by *Clostridium botulinum*.

Epidemiology

- Higher risk of developing botulism include:
  - Infants
  - Intravenous drug users
  - Consumers of inadequately prepared canned foods
  - Adults with immunosuppression or long-term antibiotic use
  - Patients receiving therapeutic administration of botulinum toxin

Pathophysiology

- The common mode of action of botulinum toxin is prevention of the release of ACh from peripheral nerve terminals by irreversible binding and cleavage of the molecular machinery.
  - The pathophysiology occurs in both motor nerve terminals and autonomic nerve terminals.

DIAGNOSIS

Clinical Presentation

History
- Time from ingestion to symptom onset varies from 2 hours to 8 days, but most cases present between 12 and 72 hours after exposure.[16]
- The incubation for botulism from a wound averages 5 days.[17]

Physical Examination
- Clinical features are similar despite mode of acquisition.
  - Weakness may be preceded by prominent GI symptoms.
  - Autonomic dysfunction is common.
  - Weakness typically begins with cranial nerves and descends symmetrically to involve the limbs and respiratory muscles.
    - The pentad of nausea/vomiting, dysphagia, diplopia, dry mouth, and fixed, dilated pupils has been suggested as a "classic" combination of signs and symptoms but only 2% of cases will present with all five features.[18]
  - Patients should be afebrile, have normal mental status, and have no sensory deficits.

Differential Diagnosis

- See Table 69.2.

Diagnostic Testing

Laboratories
- The diagnostic consideration of botulism is primarily clinical.
- Toxin should be obtained from stool, wound, serum, or nares depending on the route of exposure.

TREATMENT

- Initial treatment focuses on prompt recognition of respiratory failure (Table 69.1).
- Toxin elimination.
  - For recent ingestion of contaminated food, cathartics may be used to aid in removal of unabsorbed toxin after ileus has been ruled out.

- Antitoxin administration.
  - Antitoxin should be initiated promptly upon suspicion of the diagnosis.
    - Due to risk of anaphylaxis, skin testing should be performed prior to antitoxin administration.
- Treatment of infection.
  - Wound botulism
    - Penicillin G (10–20 million units IV per day [divided])
      □ Metronidazole, tetracycline, and chloramphenicol may be effective alternatives.[15,17]
    - Aminoglycosides may potentiate neuromuscular blockade and should be avoided if possible.[19]
    - Wound debridement is necessary in conjunction with antibiotics.

SPECIAL CONSIDERATIONS

Disposition

- Patients should be admitted to the hospital and may need the intensive care unit if having respiratory compromise.

Tick Paralysis

Definition

- Tick paralysis (TP) is a rare disorder affecting motor axon signaling and neuromuscular transmission due to envenomation by neurotoxins of gravid female hard ticks (Ixodidae).

Epidemiology

- The majority of reported TP cases have occurred in the United States and Australia.
  - Cases typically occur during Spring and Summer months during tick breeding seasons and typically affect females under 8 and >60 years of age.[20]
- The most commonly implicated tick species are the Rocky Mountain wood tick (*Dermacentor andersoni*) and American dog tick (*Dermacentor variabilis*).

Pathophysiology

- The neurotoxin in TP causes disruption of axon sodium channels and prevention of release of ACh at the neuromuscular junction.

DIAGNOSIS

Clinical Presentation

History

- The disease course occurs with a nonspecific prodromal phase within 24–48 hours of tick attachment and is followed by ataxia and symmetric ascending flaccid paralysis with craniobulbar involvement.

Physical Examination

- A tick is most frequently found around the head or scalp, often behind the ear.
- Facial weakness, dysphonia, or dysphagia may be present.
- Symmetric extremity weakness with reduced reflexes is the most common finding.

Differential Diagnosis
• See Table 69.2.

Diagnostic Criteria and Testing
• There are no specific diagnostic tests for tick paralysis in the ED.

TREATMENT
• Proper tick removal is the only specific treatment for TP and leads to prompt recovery.

SPECIAL CONSIDERATIONS

Disposition
• Patients should be admitted to the hospital and may need the intensive care unit if having respiratory compromise.

Tetanus

GENERAL PRINCIPLES

Definition
• The neurotoxin produced by *Clostridium tetani* causes a failure of inhibitory neurotransmitter release.

Epidemiology/Etiology
• In the United States, tetanus has become increasingly uncommon since implementation of vaccination programs and regular tetanus toxoid prophylaxis.
  ○ Sporadic cases still occur in those unvaccinated or undervaccinated or those with age-related waning immunity.
• Approximately 250,000 deaths occur from tetanus each year worldwide.

Pathophysiology
• Tetanospasmin is released by *C. tetani* and is taken up by motor nerve terminals. The toxin is then transported (retrograde) to the spinal cord anterior horn where it is released and binds to inhibitory interneuron terminals, preventing the release of inhibitory neurotransmitter, leading muscle rigidity and spasm.

DIAGNOSIS

• The diagnosis of tetanus remains clinical and focuses on recognition of the typical clinical presentation.

Clinical Presentation
History
• Symptom onset is, on average, 7–10 days after an injury but may range from 1 to 60 days.[21]

Physical Examination
• Though not present in all cases, the "classic" triad of rigidity, muscle spasm, and autonomic dysfunction should prompt consideration of tetanus.

- ○ Classic signs include rigidity of masseter (lockjaw or trismus), facial (risus sardonicus), and axial (opisthotonus) muscles.[22]
  - In the first week, spasm (including laryngospasm) may be provoked by movement or other stimuli such as touch, sound, or emotion.
- ○ Autonomic dysfunction begins days after spasms and is characterized by a hyperadrenergic state.

Differential Diagnosis

- Myelopathy, neuroleptic malignant syndrome, serotonin syndrome, tetanus, rabies, strychnine intoxication
- Other neurologic conditions: neuromyotonia, atypical parkinsonism, primary lateral sclerosis, generalized dystonia, and spastic paraplegia

Diagnostic Criteria and Testing

- Diagnosis of tetanus is clinical and there are no specific ED tests that will diagnose tetanus.[23]

TREATMENT

- Toxin neutralization
  - ○ Human tetanus immune globulin (500 units intramuscularly) should be given as soon after injury as possible.[22]
  - ○ Passive immunization is via immune globulin or antitoxin. Active immunization is also required and may be initiated concurrently with immune globulin but should be administered at a different inoculation site to avoid interaction (Table 69.3).
  - ○ Early administration of tetanus toxoid may provide additional benefit by saturating the binding sites for tetanus toxin.[22]
- Organism elimination
  - ○ Penicillin and metronidazole are considered effective against *C. tetani*.[24]
  - ○ Wound debridement should also occur along with antibiotic administration.
- Symptomatic control
  - ○ Rigidity and spasm
    - Benzodiazepines remain the most widely used form of sedation and muscle relaxant for tetanus.

TABLE 69.3	Tetanus Prophylaxis[32]			
Vaccination history	Clean, minor wounds		All other wounds	
	Tdap or Td[a]	TIG	Tdap or Td[a]	TIG
Unknown or < three doses	Yes	No	Yes	Yes
Three or more doses	No[b]	No	No[c]	No

[a]Tdap is preferred in adults who have never received Tdap in the past. Otherwise, Td is used.
[b]Yes if more than 10 years since last dose of tetanus toxoid–containing vaccine.
[c]Yes if more than 5 years since last dose of tetanus toxoid–containing vaccine.
Tdap, tetanus–diphtheria–acellular pertussis; TIG, tetanus immune globulin.

- Baclofen, magnesium sulfate, dantrolene, and nondepolarizing neuromuscular blockade also may be used.

SPECIAL CONSIDERATIONS

Disposition
- Patients should be admitted to the hospital and may need the intensive care unit if having respiratory compromise.

Complications
- Rhabdomyolysis, fracture, respiratory compromise, or autonomic dysfunction

Amyotrophic Lateral Sclerosis

GENERAL PRINCIPLES

Definition
- Amyotrophic lateral sclerosis (ALS) is a progressive, neurodegenerative disease of unknown etiology that leads to loss of motor neurons within the brain and spinal cord.
  - Complications
    - The most concerning complication related to ALS is hypercapnic respiratory failure related to weakening of respiratory muscles.
    - Dysphagia and weak cough may increase the risk of pneumonia.

Epidemiology
- The lifetime risk of developing ALS is estimated at 1/350 men and 1/500 women.[24]

Pathophysiology
- While the etiology of ALS is unknown, studies have suggested abnormal protein aggregation, excitotoxicity, mitochondrial dysfunction, accumulation of reactive oxygen species, and dysfunction of axonal transport.

DIAGNOSIS

- The diagnosis of ALS is typically made based on accepted sets of diagnostic criteria:
  - The revised El Escorial criteria are primarily clinical criteria.[25]
  - The Awaji criteria are primarily electrophysiologic criteria.[26]
- ALS presentations to the ER are likely to be related to respiratory complications.

Clinical Presentation
History
- Respiratory failure will typically begin to manifest with nocturnal hypoventilation, so history should focus on symptoms (morning headache, confusion, restless sleep, orthopnea).
- Other systemic symptoms that may indicate worsening respiratory function in ALS patients include decreased appetite and rapid weight loss.

Physical Examination
- In general, ALS is characterized by asymmetric weakness with variable combinations of lower motor neuron signs (flaccidity, atrophy, fasciculations) and upper motor neuron signs (spasticity, hyperreflexia, etc.) affecting any body region (bulbar, cervical, thoracic, and lumbosacral).

Differential Diagnosis

- The differential should focus on alternative or precipitating causes of hypercapnic respiratory failure.
- Since neuromuscular respiratory failure should be primarily hypercapnic, hypoxemia should prompt investigation for an underlying cause (aspiration, pneumonia, pulmonary embolism, etc.).
- For undiagnosed cases that present with respiratory failure, consideration may be given to other disorders such as cervical myelopathy, phrenic neuropathy (including neuralgic amyotrophy), MG, GBS, Pompe disease, amyloidosis, or other hereditary/acquired myopathies associated with early respiratory failure.

Diagnostic Criteria and Testing

Laboratories
- Arterial blood gas is likely to show hypercapnia with a respiratory acidosis.

Imaging
- An elevated diaphragm on chest plain radiograph is not a sensitive indicator of diaphragmatic weakness in ALS[27]
- A chest plain radiograph may show pneumonia as a source of respiratory failure.

TREATMENT

- Intubation has a high rate of morbidity and mortality rate in ALS patients.[28]
  ○ A careful discussion with the patient and family should explore the patient's advanced directives and goals of care to ensure that the patient's wishes are carried out.
- Short of intubation or in patients that are DNI, noninvasive positive pressure ventilation may be considered as an initial, alternative, or palliative treatment option. In combination with cough assist, noninvasive ventilation may be effective at avoiding the need for intubation.[29]

SPECIAL CONSIDERATIONS

Disposition

- ALS patients with respiratory compromise or failure should be admitted to a monitored or ICU bed.

Complications

- The most concerning complication related to ALS is hypercapnic respiratory failure related to weakening of respiratory muscles. Dysphagia and weak cough may increase the risk of pneumonia.

REFERENCES

1. Wendell LC, Levine JM. Myasthenic crisis. *Neurohospitalist* 2011;1(1):16–22.
2. Okumura M, Fujii Y, Shiono H, et al. Immunological function of thymoma and pathogenesis of paraneoplastic myasthenia gravis. *Gen Thorac Cardiovasc Surg* 2008;56(4):143–50.

3. Romi F. Thymoma in myasthenia gravis: from diagnosis to treatment. *Autoimmune Dis* 2011;2011:5.
4. Chen YL, Yeh JH, Chiu HC. Clinical features of myasthenia gravis patients with autoimmune thyroid disease in Taiwan. *Acta Neurol Scand* 2013;127(3):170–4.
5. Baraka A. Anaesthesia and myasthenia gravis. *Can J Anaesth* 1992;39(5):476–86.
6. Frenzen PD. Hospital admission for Guillain-Barré syndrome in the United States, 1993–2004. *Neuroepidemiology* 2007;29(1–2):83–8.
7. Yuki N, Hartung HP. Guillain-Barré syndrome. *N Engl J Med* 2012;366:2294–304.
8. Kuwabara S, Yuki N. Axonal Guillain-Barré syndrome: concepts and controversies. *Lancet Neurol* 2013;12(12):1180–8.
9. Chen A, Kim J, Henderson G, Berkowitz A. Posterior reversible encephalopathy syndrome in Guillain-Barré syndrome. *J Clin Neurosci* 2014;22(5):914–6.
10. Zochodne DW. Autonomic involvement in Guillain-Barré syndrome: a review. *Muscle Nerve* 1994;17(10):1145–55.
11. Cho T, Vaitkevicius H. Infectious myelopathies. *Continuum* 2012;18(6):1351–73.
12. Maiti J, Bucelli R. Atypical CSF findings in West Nile neuroinvasive disease: a diagnostic and therapeutic conundrum. *Neurol Neuroimmunol Neuroinflamm* 2014;1:e8.
13. Lindsey NP, Erin Staples J, Lehman JA, Fischer M. Surveillance for human West Nile virus disease—United States, 1999–2008. *MMWR Surveill Summ* 2010;59(SS-2):1–6. Available at: http://www.cdc.gov/mmwr/pdf/ss/ss5902.pdf.
14. Dembek ZF, Smith LA, Rusnak JM. Botulism: cause, effects, diagnosis, clinical and laboratory identification, and treatment modalities. *Disaster Med Public Health Prep* 2007;1(2):122–34.
15. Werner SB, Passaro D, McGee J, et al. Wound botulism in California, 1951–98: recent epidemic in heroin injectors. *Clin Infect Dis* 2000;31(4):1018–24.
16. Varma JK, Katsitadze G, Moiscrafishvili M, et al. Signs and symptoms predictive of death in patients with foodborne botulism—Republic of Georgia, 1980–2002. *Clin Infect Dis* 2004;39:357–62.
17. Santos JI, Swensen P, Glasgow LA. Potentiation of *Clostridium botulinum* toxin aminoglycoside antibiotics: clinical and laboratory observations. *Pediatrics* 1981;68(1):50–4.
18. Diaz JH. A comparative meta-analysis of tick paralysis in the United States and Australia. *Clin Toxicol* 2015;53(9):874–83.
19. Cook TM, Protheroe RT, Handel JM. Tetanus: a review of the literature. *Br J Anaesth* 2001;87(3):477–87.
20. Farrar JJ, Yen LM, Cook T, et al. Tetanus. *J Neurol Neurosurg Psychiatry* 2000;69:292–301.
21. Bunch TJ, Thalji MK, Pellikka PA, Aksamit TR. Respiratory failure in tetanus: case report and review of a 25-year experience. *Chest* 2002;122(4):1488–92.
22. Govindaraj GM, Riyaz A. Current practice in the management of tetanus. *Crit Care* 2014;18(3):145–6.
23. Chiò A, Logroscino G, Traynor BJ, et al. Global epidemiology of amyotrophic lateral sclerosis: a systemic review of the published literature. *Neuroepidemiology* 2013;41(2):118–30.
24. Brooks BR, Miller RG, Swash M, et al. El Escorial revisited: revised criteria for the diagnosis of amyotrophic lateral sclerosis. *Amyotroph Lateral Scler Other Motor Neuron Disord* 2000;1(5):293–99.
25. De Carvalho M, Dengler R, Eisen A, et al. Electrodiagnostic criteria for diagnosis of ALS. *Clin Neurophysiol* 2008;119:497–503.
26. Chen R, Grand'Maison F, Strong MJ, et al. Motor neuron disease presenting as acute respiratory failure: a clinical and pathological study. *J Neurol Neurosurg Psychiatry* 1996;60:455–8.
27. Bradley MD, Orrell RW, Clarke J, et al. Outcome of ventilatory support for acute respiratory failure in motor neurone disease. *J Neurol Neurosurg Psychiatry* 2002;72:752–6.
28. Rabenstein AA. Noninvasive ventilation for neuromuscular respiratory failure: when to use and when to avoid. *Curr Opin Crit Care* 2016;22(2):94–9.

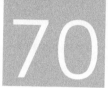

Neurologic Emergencies: Seizure

Sahar Morkos El Hayek, Laura Heitsch and
Peter Panagos

GENERAL PRINCIPLES

Definition

- Seizures occur due to abnormal electrical activity in the brain.
- Primary seizures occur without a clear cause. Two or more unprovoked seizures, >24 hours apart, is the diagnosis of epilepsy.
- Provoked or secondary seizures usually have an identifiable cause.
- Focal seizures involve a single hemisphere or brain region and manifest with unilateral symptoms.
- Generalized seizures are characterized by abnormal neuronal firing in both brain hemispheres, leading to bilateral symptoms. They are often associated with alteration of mental status, amnesia to the event and ongoing postictal confusion. They can be convulsive or nonconvulsive depending on the degree of motor involvement.
- Status epilepticus (SE): Seizures with more than 30 minutes of continuous seizure activity or two or more sequential seizures without full recovery of consciousness between seizures. This is a medical emergency with significant morbidity and mortality. As many as 40% of SE cases occur in patients with a preexisting seizure disorder.[1]
- Pseudoseizures, also called psychogenic seizures, manifest with seizure-like symptoms with no evidence of abnormal electrical activity on EEG.

Epidemiology/Etiology

- Males are more commonly affected. The incidence of seizure is higher in African Americans and the middle aged.[2]
- Seizures are largely classified as being caused by structural, metabolic, or genetic abnormalities, with the majority being of unknown cause. Primary seizures are due to inherent abnormalities in signal propagation from one neuronal circuit to the other.
- Less than one-half of seizure cases have an identifiable cause. The elderly are more likely to have a vascular, degenerative, or neoplastic cause. Seizures in younger adults are more often due to congenital brain malformations.

Potential sources of provoked/secondary seizures:

- Metabolic abnormalities including hypoglycemia, hyperglycemia, hyponatremia, hypomagnesemia, hypocalcemia, uremia, hepatic encephalopathy, and hypoxia
- Intracranial infection, trauma, mass, or hemorrhage
- Stroke (seizure can occur both at onset of a large stroke or in the poststroke period)
- Intoxication and withdrawal syndromes
- Inborn errors of metabolism
- Eclampsia

Pathophysiology
- Any pathophysiologic process that alters neuronal membrane stability will provoke an electrical abnormality that propagates the seizure.

DIAGNOSIS
Clinical Presentation
History
- Patients with true generalized seizures usually have no recollection of the event. Patients with epilepsy typically experience the same aura prior to every seizure. Most collateral information is provided by bystanders who witnessed the event. Details about the onset, progression, and duration of the seizure help identify its type.
- The patient's past medical history, including prior seizures, intake of antiepileptic drugs, illicit drug use, alcohol use, head trauma, and immunologic status, should all be elicited.
- Illness, stress, sleep deprivation, and alcohol can all lower the seizure threshold in an epileptic patient who is normally well controlled on a medication regimen.

Physical Examination
- Any patient presenting with seizures should receive a complete physical exam to document any neurologic deficit.
- Some physical exam findings should alert the physician to more dangerous underlying causes of seizure. Document the presence or absence of focal neurologic deficit, neck stiffness, rash, or fever and abnormal vital signs.
- Look for urinary or bowel incontinence, signs of head trauma, tongue or lip lacerations, or posterior shoulder dislocations.
- If the patient is still seizing on presentation, the seizure pattern and the involved limbs should all be documented.

Differential Diagnosis
- Elderly: transient ischemic attack (TIA), transient global amnesia (TGA), and syncope
- Young adults: syncope, psychological disorders, sleep disorders, migraine, miscellaneous neurologic events, eclampsia, and drug/alcohol intoxication

Diagnostic Criteria and Testing
Laboratories
- Fingerstick blood sugar rules out hypoglycemia as an easily reversible cause of seizures.
- Complete blood count (CBC) and basic metabolic panel (BMP) looking for metabolic derangements, especially hyponatremia as it is the most common electrolyte imbalance causing seizures.
- Antiepileptic drug (AED) levels in any patient being treated for epilepsy.
- Pregnancy test urine human chorionic gonadotropin (HCG) (female of child-bearing age).
- Both white blood count and lactate may be elevated in the acute setting, especially following a tonic–clonic seizure. These labs may need to be repeated after IV fluids to determine if persistent abnormalities indicate a potential underlying cause of the seizure.

- Elevated serum prolactin levels and lactate have been shown to have limited diagnostic utility.
- Creatine phosphokinase (CPK) levels are often elevated after a generalized tonic–clonic seizure but no defined threshold for abnormality exists.

Imaging

- A noncontrast head CT is used to rule out large bleeds, strokes, or other space-occupying lesions.[3]
- CT with contrast or MRI may be recommended in immunocompromised patients.

Diagnostic Procedures

- A lumbar puncture is performed in adults with febrile seizure to rule out central nervous system (CNS) infections, immunocompromised patients with a first-time seizure, or to rule out subarachnoid hemorrhage that is not detected on initial CT scan. Patients with signs of hydrocephalus and history of brain malignancy or surgery should have neuroimaging done prior to lumbar puncture (LP).
- Emergent EEGs are recommended in patients with prolonged SE, persistent altered mental status concerning for nonconvulsive seizures, and patients who require intubation and paralysis. Less than one-third of patients have significant electroencephalogram (EEG) abnormalities. If performed early, EEG helps to clarify type of seizure.

TREATMENT

- Upon presentation, the initial management should focus around airway, breathing, and circulation.
- Most seizures are self-limited. Fall/trauma precautions should be instituted. Placing the patient in the left lateral decubitus position minimizes the risk of aspiration.

Medications

- Benzodiazepines (lorazepam 1–2 mg/min IV, IM, IO up to 10 mg or diazepam 1–2 mg/min IN, IV, IO, IM, or rectally up to 20 mg) are the first-line treatment.
- If benzodiazepines do not break the seizure, phenytoin 18–20 mg/kg IV or fosphenytoin 15–20 PE/kg IV or IM may be administered if benzodiazepines do not break the seizure.
- Barbiturates are administered as the third line of treatment. The dose of IV phenobarbital is 20 mg/kg.
- SE may require paralysis and endotracheal intubation.
- In the event of alcohol withdrawal seizures, continuous benzodiazepine loading is the mainstay of management.
- In patients with known history of tuberculosis, intractable seizures may be due to isoniazid (INH) toxicity and should be treated with pyridoxine.

SPECIAL CONSIDERATIONS

Disposition

- Most patients with first-time seizures can be discharged home without antiepileptic medications once they reach their normal neurologic baseline. They should be provided with appropriate follow-up with neurology. Patients with provoked seizures may be admitted on case-by-case basis.

Patient Education

- Patients should be warned about the possibility of seizure recurrence and should be provided with clear return precautions. The importance of compliance to the antiepileptic drug regimen should be highlighted. They should also be warned against driving or operating heavy machinery until cleared by neurology.

Complications

- Todd's paralysis is a neurologic deficit that persists in the postictal period and may last from half an hour to 36 hours, with the average of 15 hours. Paralysis may be partial or complete, usually occurs on just one side of the body, and may also affect vision or speech. It is expected to resolve completely. The etiology is unknown. It is important to distinguish Todd's paralysis from a stroke because stroke requires a completely different treatment.

STATUS EPILEPTICUS

- A life-threatening condition characterized by a seizure lasting 5–30 minutes or 2 or more seizures in succession without return to baseline.
- Overall mortality rate is 22%.
- Causes of status in adults are subtherapeutic antiepileptic levels, stroke, electrolyte abnormalities, alcohol withdrawal, hypoxia, CNS infection, tumors, trauma, or idiopathic causes.[4,6]
- The excessive neuronal firing eventually leads to cell death. Patients will suffer from lactic acidosis, rhabdomyolysis, aspiration pneumonia, and possible respiratory failure.
- Airway protection should take priority.
- A subset of SE is the nonconvulsive status, where patients do not have any muscle contractions, but experience prolonged altered mental status (should be a consideration for any AMS presentation or postarrest patient). This is an indication for an emergent EEG.
- Attempts at breaking SE should proceed, starting with benzodiazepines and phenytoin, with paralytics being the last resort.

REFERENCES

1. Wu YW, Shek DW, Garcia PA, et al. Incidence and mortality of generalized convulsive status epilepticus in California. *Neurology* 2002;58:1070–6.
2. Pallin DJ, et al. Seizure visits in US emergency departments: epidemiology and potential disparities in care. *Int J Emerg Med* 2008;1(2):97–105.
3. Krumholz A, Shinnar S, Gronseth G, et al. Evidence-based guideline: management of an unprovoked first seizure in adults: report of the Guideline Development Subcommittee of the American Academy of Neurology and the American Epilepsy Society. *Neurology* 2015;85(17):1526–7. doi:10.1212/01.wnl.0000473351.32413.7c.
4. Martindale J. Emergency department seizure epidemiology. *Emerg Med Clin N Am* 2011;29: 15–27.
5. Grover EH, Nazzal Y. Treatment of Convulsive Status Epilepticus. *Curr Treat Options Neurol* 2016;18(3):11. doi:10.1007/s11940-016-0394-5.

71 Neurologic Emergencies: Stroke

Laura Heitsch, Peter Panagos and
Sahar Morkos El Hayek

GENERAL PRINCIPLES

Definition

- An ischemic stroke occurs when a cerebral vessel is occluded, preventing blood flow to a region of the brain. A thrombus can form in the artery or embolize from a proximal source, usually the heart. Branches and bifurcations of the internal carotid artery are most commonly implicated.
- Lacunar strokes occur when small terminal arteries are occluded, usually in the basal ganglia, internal capsule, and thalamus. They are more common in the setting of diabetes and hypertension.
- Hemorrhagic strokes occur when blood leaks into brain parenchyma from a ruptured blood vessel, resulting in intracerebral hemorrhage (ICH). Subarachnoid hemorrhage (SAH) normally results from rupture of an existing aneurysm.
- Transient ischemic attacks (TIA) represent any transient neurologic deficit without infarction on imaging. TIA can be a harbinger of a future stroke. The highest risk of stroke following a TIA is in the first 30 days with the majority occurring within the first 24–48 hours.[1–5]
- Strokes are classified as anterior or posterior, depending on the vessels involved.

Epidemiology/Etiology

- Stroke can be ischemic (87%) or hemorrhagic (13%) in nature.[6]
- Strokes are more common in the elderly population and African Americans.[7,8] Risk factors predisposing to stroke are hypertension, diabetes, smoking, dyslipidemia, and cardiac arrhythmias. Stroke may still occur in younger patients, especially in the setting of coagulopathies, pregnancy, sickle cell disease, or oral contraceptive use.

Pathophysiology

- Occlusion of cerebral arteries results in rapid brain tissue ischemia. Atherosclerotic plaques in large arteries accumulate platelets and debris, eventually causing arterial stenosis and occlusion (large artery atherosclerotic stroke). Thrombi may also embolize and occlude smaller, more distal arteries (cardioembolic stroke).
- Embolic strokes originate mainly from the heart, most commonly in patients with atrial fibrillation or recent myocardial infarction.
- Hemorrhagic strokes occur either due to hypertensive vasculopathy, amyloid angiopathy (primarily in the elderly), or ruptured arteriovenous malformations. Hemorrhagic transformation (HT) of ischemic strokes with or without thrombolytic therapy can also occur, with the former being more common.
- Carotid and vertebral artery dissections may also lead to brain ischemia and present with stroke symptoms. They are usually seen in younger patients, following trauma, or due to preexisting vascular abnormalities.

DIAGNOSIS

Clinical Presentation

History

- The patient may report motor and/or sensory deficit in one or more limbs, speech difficulty, or inability to perform daily tasks. Family members provide important collateral information if the patient is unable to express complaints. A key piece in the history is to identify the timing of the last known normal state of the patients because it guides eligibility for treatment.
- Patients with ICH may also present with sudden onset severe headache, nausea, vomiting, and severe hypertension.

Physical Examination

- A complete neurologic examination should be performed as soon as the patient presents. The NIH stroke scale (NIHSS) is the recommended screening tool. Scoring is from 0 to 42, with a score of 0 indicating no deficits and a score >20 indicating a severe stroke.[9]
- Vascular evaluation: carotid bruits, peripheral pulses for symmetry, and heart exam for rhythm and murmurs.
- Symptoms depend on the location of the brain ischemia. Middle cerebral artery (MCA) strokes (80%) are characterized by contralateral sensory–motor deficits, more severe in the upper extremities, with facial involvement, and aphasia if the dominant hemisphere is affected. Posterior strokes (20%) are frequently associated with ataxia and visual changes, among other symptoms, and may be more challenging to diagnose.[10,11]

Differential Diagnosis

- Trauma, epidural/subdural hematoma, seizure, postictal state, Todd's paralysis, or Bell's palsy
- Aortic dissection with carotid involvement, syncope, hypertensive encephalopathy, complicated migraines, metabolic abnormalities (especially hypoglycemia), and acute intoxication

Diagnostic Criteria and Testing

- Timely diagnosis of stroke in the emergency department (ED) greatly impacts prognosis and recovery.

Laboratories

- Glucose (preferably fingerstick).
- Complete blood count (CBC), basic metabolic panel (BMP), cardiac enzymes, and prothrombin time/partial thromboplastin time (PT/PTT) (unless an abnormality is suspected by history or medications, it is not recommended to wait for results of these tests prior to making a treatment decision about thrombolysis if the patient is otherwise eligible).

Electrocardiography

- ECG is done to evaluate for underlying atrial fibrillation.

Imaging

- Noncontrast head CT is done immediately at presentation to rule out hemorrhage. Most commonly in an ischemic stroke, the CT is grossly normal in an early presentation.

- CT angiography (CTA) and CT perfusion (CTP) imaging provide additional information and are usually performed in order to determine eligibility for endovascular intervention or treatment outside of the standard time window.
- MRI/magnetic resonance angiography (MRA) are more sensitive than CT in detecting acute strokes.

TREATMENT

- A streamlined protocol-driven approach is key to the evaluation of potential strokes so as to reduce time to treatment in eligible patients.
- It is recommended by the American Heart Association (AHA) that at least 80% of eligible stroke patients are treated with IV tPA within 60 minutes of arrival.[1]
- Stroke management should initially aim at stabilizing the patient. Patients who rapidly deteriorate, are comatose, or cannot protect their airway should be intubated.
- Oxygen supplementation is recommended only in hypoxic patients (O_2 Sat <94%).
  - Treat hypoglycemia, hyperglycemia, and hyperthermia
- In ischemic strokes, systolic blood pressure (SBP) should be lowered below 185 mm Hg (and diastolic blood pressure [DBP] < 110 mm Hg) before tPA administration.[12] Labetalol and nicardipine are considered first-line treatment. In hemorrhagic strokes patients presenting with SBP between 150 and 220 mm Hg and without contraindication to acute BP treatment, acute lowering of SBP to 140 mm Hg and is safe and may be effective for improving functional outcome.[13,14]
- For ischemic stroke, the type of intervention depends on the timing from symptom onset. Acute treatments include intravenous thrombolysis and mechanical thrombectomy.

Medications

Acute Ischemic Stroke

- Intravenous tissue plasminogen activator (tPA) can be administered to eligible ischemic stroke patients presenting within the 0- to 3-hour window with FDA approval and up to 4.5 hours in other patients, though with slightly more stringent inclusion/exclusion criteria.[15,16] Dose of IV tPA is 0.9 mg/kg (max dose of 90 mg), with 10% given as a bolus over 1 minute and the rest as a continuous infusion over an hour.
- It is recommended that a brief discussion of benefit versus risk of treatment be conducted with the patient and family members prior to administration of any therapy.
- Anticoagulation should not be administered within the first 24 hours to patients receiving thrombolytic therapy.[12] Oral aspirin administration is recommended at 24–48 hours after stroke onset regardless of thrombolytic therapy.

Hemorrhagic Stroke

- For a hemorrhagic stroke in association with anticoagulation therapy, it is recommended that an elevated international normalized ratio (INR) be corrected with intravenous vitamin K and vitamin K–dependent factors. For patients who are taking a factor Xa antagonist or direct thrombin inhibitor, treatment is considered on an individual basis and dependent on availability of reversal agents as well as hospital protocols.

Transient Ischemic Attack

- Antiplatelet therapy is the mainstay of secondary stroke prevention in noncardio-embolic TIA with several potential regimens (monotherapy with aspirin, dual therapy with either aspirin + extended-release dipyridamole or aspirin + clopidogrel) being appropriate for initiation within 24 hours.[17]

Other Nonpharmacologic Therapies

- Patients within 6 hours of symptom onset may be eligible for endovascular interventions, such as clot retrieval. CTA should not delay time to tPA administration. To be eligible for endovascular therapy with a stent retriever, patients should meet all the following criteria: have limited to no disability at baseline (measured as a prestroke modified Rankin scale [mRS] score of 0–1), receive tPA within 4.5 hours of symptom onset (if eligible), have an occlusion of the proximal MCA or internal carotid artery, be 18 years or older, have an NIHSS score of ≥6, have an ASPECTS score of ≥6, and be able to undergo the procedure within 6 hours of symptom onset.[18] A patient who meets eligibility criteria but is not at a facility that can provide endovascular intervention should be transferred to a center that is capable of performing endovascular treatment.

SPECIAL CONSIDERATIONS

Disposition

- Patients with an ischemic stroke who received tPA and hemorrhagic strokes and patients who have been intubated should be admitted to a monitored setting/ICU for observation. Otherwise, they may be admitted to a regular floor for serial exams and risk factor modification. It is strongly recommended that patients with a (confirmed or suspected) TIA be admitted.

Complications

- Stroke patients are at high risk of aspiration pneumonia due to swallowing difficulties. Patients should receive a screening study in the ED and be made NPO if they fail. Ischemic stroke patients who receive tPA should be monitored for any signs suggesting hemorrhagic transformation: change in mental status, headache, worsening neurologic symptoms, poorly controlled blood pressure, and tachycardia. If hemorrhagic transformation is suspected, the tPA infusion should be immediately stopped and a repeat NCCT obtained.

REFERENCES

1. Johnston SC, Gress DR, Browner WS, Sidney S. Short-term prognosis after emergency department diagnosis of TIA. *JAMA* 2000;284:2901–6.
2. Chandratheva A, Mehta Z, Geraghty OC, et al. Population-based study of risk and predictors of stroke in the first few hours after a TIA. *Neurology* 2009;72:1941–7.

3. Lovett JK, Dennis MS, Sandercock PA, et al. Very early risk of stroke after a first transient ischemic attack. *Stroke* 2003;34:e138–40.

4. Lisabeth LD, Ireland JK, Risser JM, et al. Stroke risk after transient ischemic attack in a population-based setting. *Stroke* 2004;35:1842–6.

5. Giles MF, Rothwell PM. Risk of stroke early after transient ischaemic attack: a systematic review and meta-analysis. *Lancet Neurol* 2007;6:1063–72.

6. Go AS, Mozaffarian D, Roger VL, et al. Heart disease and stroke statistics—2014 update: a report from the American Heart Association. *Circulation* 2014;129:e28–292.

7. Kleindorfer DO, Khoury J, Moomaw CJ, et al. Stroke incidence is decreasing in whites but not in blacks: a population-based estimate of temporal trends in stroke incidence from the Greater Cincinnati/Northern Kentucky Stroke Study. *Stroke* 2010;41: 1326–31.

8. Howard G, Moy CS, Howard VJ, et al. Where to focus efforts to reduce the black-white disparity in stroke mortality: incidence versus case fatality? *Stroke* 2016;47:1893–8.

9. Lyden P, Brott T, Tilley B, et al. Improved reliability of the NIH Stroke Scale using video training. NINDS TPA Stroke Study Group. *Stroke* 1994;25:2220–6.

10. Schulz UG, Fischer U. Posterior circulation cerebrovascular syndromes: diagnosis and management. *J Neurol Neurosurg Psychiatry* 2017;88(1):45–53.

11. Nouh A, Remke J, Ruland S. Ischemic posterior circulation stroke: a review of anatomy, clinical presentations, diagnosis, and current management. *Front Neurol* 2014;5:30.

12. Jauch EC, Saver JL, Adams HP Jr, et al. Guidelines for the early management of patients with acute ischemic stroke: a guideline for healthcare professionals from the American Heart Association/American Stroke Association. *Stroke* 2013;44:870–947.

13. Anderson CS, Heeley E, Huang Y, et al. Rapid blood-pressure lowering in patients with acute intracerebral hemorrhage. *N Engl J Med* 2013;368:2355–65.

14. Hemphill JC 3rd, Greenberg SM, Anderson CS, et al. Guidelines for the management of spontaneous intracerebral hemorrhage: a guideline for healthcare professionals from the American Heart Association/American Stroke Association. *Stroke* 2015;46: 2032–60.

15. Del Zoppo GJ, Saver JL, Jauch EC, Adams HP Jr; American Heart Association Stroke C. Expansion of the time window for treatment of acute ischemic stroke with intravenous tissue plasminogen activator: a science advisory from the American Heart Association/American Stroke Association. *Stroke* 2009;40:2945–8.

16. Demaerschalk BM, Kleindorfer DO, Adeoye OM, et al. Scientific rationale for the inclusion and exclusion criteria for intravenous alteplase in acute ischemic stroke: a statement for healthcare professionals from the American Heart Association/American Stroke Association. *Stroke* 2016;47:581–641.

17. Kernan WN, Ovbiagele B, Black HR, et al. Guidelines for the prevention of stroke in patients with stroke and transient ischemic attack: a guideline for healthcare professionals from the American Heart Association/American Stroke Association. *Stroke* 2014;45:2160–236.

18. Powers WJ, Derdeyn CP, Biller J, et al. 2015 American Heart Association/American stroke association focused update of the 2013 guidelines for the early management of patients with acute ischemic stroke regarding endovascular treatment: a guideline for healthcare professionals from the American Heart Association/American Stroke Association. *Stroke* 2015;46:3020–35.

Neurologic Emergencies: Space-Occupying Lesions and Pseudotumor Cerebri

Mark D. Levine

GENERAL PRINCIPLES

Definition

- Space-occupying lesions (solid mass, hemorrhage) expand in size and may displace normal brain structure leading to increased intracranial pressure.
- Pseudotumor cerebri is a form of idiopathic intracranial hypertension.

Epidemiology/Etiology

- Meningiomas represent 36% of primary brain tumors and gliomas represent 27%.
- Pseudotumor cerebri is classically seen with young obese females on birth control but has an unknown etiology.

Pathophysiology

- Mass effect causes obstruction of normal cerebrospinal fluid (CSF) flow and may also increase intracranial pressure, leading to decreased perfusion of the brain. The brain tissue may also be compressed, leading to focal neurologic deficits, seizure, or respiratory and circulatory compromise.
- Pseudotumor is characterized by increased intracranial pressure in the absence of a tumor.

DIAGNOSIS

Clinical Presentation

History

- Patients will usually report headaches, vomiting, or focal neurologic deficits. Seizures or personality changes may be reported by significant others or bystanders.
- Headaches may be increased in the early morning.
- Pseudotumor cerebri patients may also report vision change or loss.

Physical Examination

- In addition to a full physical examination, special attention should be paid to focal neurologic deficits, cranial nerve changes, and papilledema.
- Vital signs may be consistent with Cushing triad (hypertension, bradycardia, irregular respirations).
- Altered mentation, blown unilateral pupil, or decerebrate posturing is consistent with uncal herniation.

- Miosis, decorticate posturing, and Cheyne-Stokes breathing are consistent with central herniation.
- Bradycardia and respiratory arrest are consistent with tonsillar herniation.

Differential Diagnosis
- Primary or metastatic cancer, trauma, infectious process, cephalalgia, hemorrhage, multiple sclerosis

Diagnostic Criteria and Testing
Laboratories
- There are no specific laboratory tests that will diagnose an intracranial mass in the emergency department.

Imaging
- A noncontrast CT scan of the head is the usual first radiographic study to obtain.
- MRI may be more diagnostic for the type of lesion but is not indicated as emergent.

Diagnostic Procedures
- A lumbar puncture (LP) with opening pressure >20 mm Hg may assist in the diagnosis of pseudotumor cerebri.

TREATMENT

Medications
- Antiepileptics are frequently begun in the emergency department on new finding of brain mass with or without vasogenic edema or intracranial hemorrhage.
- Dexamethasone is usually ordered in conjunction with neurosurgical consultation to decrease mass-related swelling.
- Acetazolamide, corticosteroids, and primary headache prophylaxis are indicated in pseudotumor cerebri.

Other Nonpharmacologic Therapies
- The head of the bed should be raised to 30 degrees to improve cerebral perfusion.
- Emergent neurosurgical consultation is indicated for decompressive procedures or definitive operative management.
- In patients with pseudotumor cerebri, an LP is usually performed and CSF is drained until a closing pressure of 15–20 cm H_2O is obtained.

SPECIAL CONSIDERATIONS

Disposition
- Patients with a space-occupying lesion should be admitted to the hospital.
- Patients with pseudotumor cerebri can frequently be discharged with appropriate neurologic follow-up after resolution of their symptoms.

Complications
- Seizure, vital sign instability, or respiratory arrest

SUGGESTED READINGS

Burgett RA, Purvin VA, Kawasaki A. Lumboperitoneal shunting for pseudotumor cerebri. *Neurology* 1997;49(3):734–9.

Gurol ME, St Louis EK. Treatment of cerebellar masses. *Curr Treat Options Neurol* 2008;10:138.

Rosner MJ, Coley IB. Cerebral perfusion pressure, intracranial pressure, and head elevation. *J Neurosurg* 1986;65:636–41.

Wall M. Idiopathic intracranial hypertension. *Neurol Clin* 2010;28(3):593–617.

Wall M, McDermott MP, Kieburtz KD, et al. Effect of acetazolamide on visual function in patients with idiopathic intracranial hypertension and mild visual loss: the idiopathic intracranial hypertension treatment trial. *JAMA* 2014;311(16):1641–51.

73 Obstetric and Gynecologic Emergencies: Complications of Pregnancy

P. Gabriel Miranda Gomez and Mark D. Levine

Preeclampsia

GENERAL PRINCIPLES

Definition

- Preeclampsia is defined as a syndrome of new onset of elevated blood pressure and proteinuria or thrombocytopenia, impaired liver function, new renal insufficiency, pulmonary edema, or cerebral/visual disturbances anytime from 20 weeks of gestational age to 6 weeks postpartum.

Epidemiology/Etiology

- Risk factors include diabetes mellitus, primary hypertension, obesity, age >35 years or <20 years, personal or family history of preeclampsia (including that of the baby's father), hydatidiform pregnancy, fetal chromosomal abnormality, or multiple gestation (e.g., twins).

Pathophysiology

- It is thought that there is hypoperfusion of the placenta leading to maternal endothelial dysfunction and diffuse vasospasm and multiorgan damage.

DIAGNOSIS

Clinical Presentation

History
- Classic symptoms include severe headache, visual disturbance, abdominal pain, and swelling.

Physical Examination
- Generalized edema may or may not be seen.
- A neurologic screening examination should be performed to rule out lateralizing neuro deficits of an intracranial mass lesion or bleed, which could present similarly with hypertension and headache.

Differential Diagnosis

- Primary hypertension, gestational hypertension, elevated intracranial pressure, "white coat" hypertension, or nephrotic syndrome

Diagnostic Criteria and Testing

Laboratories
- Urine dipstick to screen for proteinuria
- Complete blood count (CBC) and comprehensive metabolic panel (CMP) including liver enzymes to screen for HELLP syndrome
- Serum lactate dehydrogenase (LDH) and uric acid levels

Imaging
- Women with lateralizing neurologic signs should have a noncontrast CT of the head to rule out intracranial hemorrhage or a mass lesion.
- An US to document fetal viability by sonographic measurement of fetal heart tones should be part of the workup, although this is not a test for preeclampsia.

TREATMENT

- Blood pressure should be gradually lowered to <160 mm Hg systolic and <105 mm Hg diastolic. Magnesium sulfate therapy should be initiated in the emergency department for seizure prophylaxis.

Medications

- Hydralazine starting dose 5–10 mg IV push; repeat as needed
- Labetalol starting dose 5–10 mg IV push; repeat as needed
- Magnesium sulfate 4 mg IV over 10 minutes once prior to transfer or admission

SPECIAL CONSIDERATIONS

Disposition

- Stable patients with severe preeclampsia should be transferred/admitted to an obstetrics ward for continuous maternal and fetal vital signs monitoring.
- Outpatient management for women with nonsevere range blood pressure and proteinuria is acceptable, as long as short-term follow-up with an obstetrician can be reliably obtained.

Complications
- Complications include seizure (eclampsia), HELLP syndrome, (hemolysis, elevated liver enzymes, low platelet count), liver failure, kidney failure, pulmonary edema, abruptio placenta, cerebrovascular accident, or death.

Hyperemesis Gravidarum

GENERAL PRINCIPLES

Definition
- Nausea and vomiting of pregnancy, causing weight loss exceeding 5% of prepregnancy body weight and ketonuria, usually within the first trimester

Epidemiology/Etiology
- Risk factors include young, primigravid women, women with a history of motion sickness or migraines, and multiple gestations.

Pathophysiology
- Increased estrogen and progesterone levels and gastric mobility abnormalities are thought to play a role in hyperemesis.

DIAGNOSIS

Clinical Presentation
History
- The patient usually reports episodes of nausea and vomiting occurring at any time during the day, beginning during the 5th or 6th week of gestation.

Physical Examination
- Patients may exhibit abdominal discomfort, hypotension, or signs of dehydration.

Differential Diagnosis
- UTI, pyelonephritis, viral syndrome, or food borne illness

Diagnostic Criteria and Testing
Laboratories
- A basic metabolic panel and urinalysis should be obtained.

TREATMENT

Medications
All of the medications below may be administered for nausea and vomiting but have varying side effects. Studies have shown relative safety in pregnancy (see references), but choices should be tailored to individual practice and comfort.

- Pyridoxine (vitamin B_6) 10–25 mg PO q6–8h
- Doxylamine succinate and pyridoxine (10 mg/10 mg) at bedtime
- Diphenhydramine 25–50 mg IV/PO q4–6h
- Metoclopramide 10 mg IV/PO
- Promethazine 12.5–25 mg IV/PO q4h
- Prochlorperazine 5–10 mg IV/PO q6h
- Ondansetron 4 mg IV/PO q8h

SPECIAL CONSIDERATIONS

Disposition

- Patients may be discharged home with follow-up if their symptoms and laboratory abnormalities have resolved.

Placenta Previa

GENERAL PRINCIPLES

Definition

- Placental tissue that extends over the cervical os

Epidemiology/Etiology

- A decrease in vascularity of the upper endometrium promotes implantation in the lower uterus.
- Risk factors include prior placenta previa, prior cesarean section, multiple gestation, multiparity, smoking, cocaine use, nonwhite race, and advanced maternal age.

Pathophysiology

- Bleeding occurs as shearing occurs at the placental attachment site.

DIAGNOSIS

Clinical Presentation

History

- Patients may report painless vaginal bleeding after 20 weeks of gestation.

Physical Examination

- Digital examination should be performed only after an ultrasound has been obtained to confirm placenta location.

Differential Diagnosis

- Trauma, placenta accreta, urinary tract infection, or preterm labor

Diagnostic Criteria and Testing

Laboratories

- There are no specific laboratory values that are diagnostic for placenta previa.

Imaging

- Ultrasound should be performed in consultation with an obstetrician to determine location, size, and severity of the placenta previa.

TREATMENT

- Resuscitation of the mother should be performed if there is any question of hemodynamic instability.

Medications

- Tocolytics and magnesium may be indicated but should be used in conjunction with obstetrical consultation.

Other Nonpharmacologic Therapies
- Emergent delivery may be indicated.

SPECIAL CONSIDERATIONS

Disposition
- Depending on the size and the location of the placenta, the patient may be discharged home with close follow-up or may need admission to the obstetrical service. Active bleeding is an obstetrical emergency.

Complications
- Hemorrhagic shock, intrauterine growth restriction, fetal demise, or death of mother

Placental Abruption (Abruptio Placentae)

GENERAL PRINCIPLES

Definition
- Total placental detachment at the decidual–placental interface prior to fetal delivery

Epidemiology/Etiology
- A complication of <1% of pregnancies, the majority occuring prior to 37 weeks.
- Trauma or uterine decompression leads to shearing of the placenta from the uterine wall.
- Risk factors include trauma, cocaine use, smoking, hypertension, preeclampsia/eclampsia, premature rupture of membranes, and uterine abnormalities.

Pathophysiology
- Bleeding occurs secondary to abnormalities in the early development of the spiral arteries, leading to decidual necrosis, inflammation, and infarction.
- Any process that leads to further vasoconstriction or disruption of vascular integrity leads to bleeding that separates the placenta from the uterine wall.

DIAGNOSIS

Clinical Presentation
History
- Patients usually complain of abdominal or back pain and uterine contractions. Vaginal bleeding is not always present.

Physical Examination
- The uterus is firm, rigid, or tender, and contractions are typical of a labor pattern.

Differential Diagnosis
- Placenta previa, labor, uterine rupture, subchorionic hemorrhage

Diagnostic Criteria and Testing
Laboratories
- Fibrinogen levels of ≤200 mg/dL have 100% positive predictive value.
- Coagulation studies and a complete metabolic panel are indicated due to potential for renal dysfunction and HELLP.

Imaging
- Ultrasound is the modality of choice to evaluate abruption.

TREATMENT

Medications
- Magnesium, tocolytic medication, or antenatal steroids should be administered in conjunction with obstetrical consultation.

Other Nonpharmacologic Therapies
- Tocometric monitoring of the fetus
- Emergent delivery
- Treatment of hemorrhage and disseminated intravascular coagulation (DIC)

SPECIAL CONSIDERATIONS

Disposition
- These patients need to be admitted to the hospital.

Complications
- Hemorrhage, DIC, uterine rupture, fetal demise, or maternal death

Eclampsia

GENERAL PRINCIPLES

Definition
- New onset, generalized, tonic–clonic seizure in a pregnant patient with preeclampsia that can occur before, during, or after labor

Epidemiology/Etiology
- Occurs in <3% of pregnant women (usually in weeks 20–30) but may also occur usually within the first 48 hours following delivery but eclampsia may be seen up to 23 days postpartum.
- Risk factors include chronic hypertension, renal disease, diabetes, obesity, nulliparity, nonwhite race, lower socioeconomic status, prior preeclampsia, and women in adolescence/early 20s and over the age of 35.

Pathophysiology
- Two models have been proposed with the common end point being cerebral edema.

DIAGNOSIS

Clinical Presentation
History
- Patients may report headache, visual disturbances, or upper abdominal pain prior to seizure.
- Patients may not have a history of hypertension during the pregnancy.

Physical Examination
- Classically, the patient will present with a seizure.
- Hypertension and ankle clonus may be present.
- Neurologic findings may include memory deficits, altered mentation, cranial nerve deficits, and increased deep tendon reflexes.

Differential Diagnosis
- Molar pregnancy (seizure prior to 20 weeks gestation), stroke, space-occupying lesion, metabolic abnormality, infection, ingestion, thrombotic thrombocytopenic purpura (TTP), hemolytic uremic syndrome (HUS), or trauma

Diagnostic Criteria and Testing
Laboratories
- As eclampsia is a clinical diagnosis, there are no specific laboratory tests.
- Magnesium levels should be monitored.

Imaging
- Imaging is not acutely required and is used to rule out differentials.

TREATMENT

Medications
- Supplemental oxygen should be administered.
- Antihypertensive therapy should be tailored in consultation with the obstetrics service.
- Magnesium sulfate 4–6 g IV over 15–20 minutes should be administered with a maintenance dose of 2 g/h (in consultation with renal service if renal insufficiency exists).
  ○ Calcium gluconate 1 g IV may be administered to counteract magnesium toxicity.
- Benzodiazepines may also be administered if seizures do not cease with magnesium or if signs of magnesium toxicity occur (loss of patellar reflex, respirations <12/min).

Other Nonpharmacologic Therapies
- Place the patient in a lateral position to relieve the vena cava from pressure from the fetus.
- Delivery.

SPECIAL CONSIDERATIONS

Disposition
- This is an obstetrical emergency. These patients must be admitted.

Complications
- Magnesium sulfate toxicity, respiratory failure, fetal demise, maternal death

HELLP

GENERAL PRINCIPLES

Definition
- A syndrome characterized by *h*emolysis, *e*levated *l*iver enzymes, and *l*ow *p*latelet counts

Epidemiology/Etiology
- Risk factors include a prior history of HELLP, preeclampsia, or first-degree family members with the same.
- Patients may not have hypertension or proteinuria.

Pathophysiology
- HELLP is thought to stem from abnormal placental development and function, leading to hepatic inflammation.

DIAGNOSIS

Clinical Presentation
History
- Most patients will present with epigastric/right upper quadrant tenderness with associated nausea, vomiting, and malaise. Patients may also complain of headache or visual changes. Typically, these complaints will occur between 28 and 36 weeks of gestation.

Physical Examination
- Jaundice or ascites may be present, and epigastric or right upper quadrant abdominal tenderness will be elicited.

Differential Diagnosis
- Hepatitis, gastroenteritis, appendicitis, cholecystitis, lupus, idiopathic thrombocytopenic purpura ITP, TTP, HUS

Diagnostic Criteria and Testing
Laboratories
- Obtain a CBC and comprehensive metabolic panel.
  - Microangiopathic hemolytic anemia with schistocytes on smear.
  - Platelets count will be ≤100,000 cells/μL.
  - Total bilirubin ≥1.2 mg/dL (indirect bilirubin is also elevated).
  - Serum AST >2 times upper limit of normal.

TREATMENT

Medications
- Antihypertensive medications (labetalol, hydralazine, nifedipine, or nitroprusside) may be administered to control blood pressure.
- Magnesium sulfate is administered to prevent seizures.

Other Nonpharmacologic Therapies
- Delivery is the mainstay of treatment.

SPECIAL CONSIDERATIONS

Disposition
- Patients must be admitted.

Complications
- Hepatic hematoma, hepatic infarction, hepatic rupture, DIC, abruptio placentae, pulmonary edema, acute renal failure, maternal or fetal demise

SUGGESTED READINGS

Abildgaard U, Heimdal K. Pathogenesis of the syndrome of hemolysis, elevated liver enzymes, and low platelet count (HELLP): a review. *Eur J Obstet Gynecol Reprod Biol* 2013;166:117.

American College of Obstetricians and Gynecologists, Task Force on Hypertension in Pregnancy. Hypertension in pregnancy. Report of the American College of Obstetricians and Gynecologists' Task Force on Hypertension in Pregnancy. *Obstet Gynecol* 2013;122(5):1122–31.

Ananth VV, Getahun D, Peltier MR, et al. Placental abruption in term and preterm gestations: evidence for heterogeneity in clinical pathways. *Obstet Gynecol* 2006;107:785.

Berhan Y, Berhan A. Should magnesium sulfate be administered to women with mild preeclampsia? A systematic review of published reports on eclampsia. *J Obstet Gynaecol Res* 2015;41:831.

Braude D, Crandall C. Ondansetron versus promethazine to treat acute undifferentiated nausea in the emergency department: a randomized, double-blind, noninferiority trial. *Acad Emerg Med* 2008;15:209.

Brewer J, Owens MY, Wallace K, et al. Posterior reversible encephalopathy syndrome in 46 of 47 patients with eclampsia. *Am J Obstet Gynecol* 2013;208:468.e1.

Carstairs SD. Ondansetron use in pregnancy and birth defects: a systematic review. *Obstet Gynecol* 2016;127:878.

Charbit B, Mandelbrot L, Samain E, et al. The decrease of fibrinogen is an early predictor of the severity of postpartum hemorrhage. *J Throb Haemost* 2007;5:266.

Clark SL. Placentae Previa and Abruptio Placentae. In: Creasy RK, Resnik R, eds. *Maternal Fetal Medicine*. 4ᵗʰ ed. Philadelphia: WB Saunders Company, 1999:623.

Coetzee EJ, Dommisse J, Anthony J. A randomized controlled trial of intravenous magnesium sulphate versus placebo in the management of women with severe preeclampsia. *Br J Obstet Gynaecol* 1998;105:300–3.

Duley L, Adadevoh S, Atallah A, et al. Which anticonvulsant for women with eclampsia? Evidence from the collaborative eclampsia trial. *Lancet* 1995;345:1455–63.

Faiz AS, Ananth CV. Etiology and risk factors for placenta previa: an overview and meta-analysis of observational studies. *J Matern Fetal Neonatal Med* 2003;13:175.

Fitzgerald JP. The effect of promethazine in nausea and vomiting of pregnancy. *N Z Med J* 1955;54:215.

Kallen B. Hyperemesis Gravidarum during Pregnancy and Delivery: A Registry Study. In: Koren G, Bishai R, eds. *Nausea and Vomiting of Pregnancy: State of the Art 2000*. Toronto: Motherisk, 2000:36.

Lacasse A, Rey E, Ferrereira E, et al. Epidemiology of nausea and vomiting during pregnancy: prevalence, severity, determinants, and the importance of race/ethnicity. *BMC Pregnancy Childbirth* 2009;9:26.

Lagiou P, Taminim R, Mucci LA, et al. Nausea and vomiting in pregnancy in relation to prolactin, estrogens, and progesterone: a prospective study. *Obstet Gynecol* 2003;101:639.

Lee NM, Saha S. Nausea and vomiting of pregnancy. *Gastroenterol Clin North Am* 2011;40:309.

Mackay AP, Berg CJ, Atrash HK. Pregnancy-related mortality from preeclampsia and eclampsia. *Obstet Gynecol* 2001;97(4):533–8.

Matok I, Gorodischer R, Koren G, et al. The safety of metoclopramide use in the first trimester of pregnancy. *N Engl J Med* 2009;360:2528.

Matthews A, Haas DM, O'Mathúna DP, Dowswell T. Interventions for nausea and vomiting in early pregnancy. *Cochrane Database Syst Rev* 2015:CD007575.

Melamed N, Aviram A, Silver M, et al. Pregnancy course and outcome following blunt trauma. *J Matern Fetal Neonatal Med* 2012;25:1612.

Mouer JR. Placenta previa: antepartum conservative management, inpatient versus outpatient. *Am J Obstet Gynecol* 1994;170:1683.

Pasternak B, Svanström H, Mølgaard-Nielsen D, et al. Metoclopramide in pregnancy and risk of major congenital malformations and fetal death. *JAMA* 2013;310:1601.

Rosenberg T, Pariente G, Sergienko R, et al. Critical analysis of risk factors and outcome of placenta previa. *Arch Gynecol Obstet* 2011;284:47.

Sharma A, Suri V, Gupta I. Tocolytic therapy in conservative management of symptomatic placenta previa. *Int J Gynaecol Obstet* 2004;84:109.

Sibai BM. Diagnosis, controversies, and management of the syndrome of hemolysis, elevated liver enzymes, and low platelet count. *Obstet Gynecol* 2004;103:981.

Sibai BM. Magnesium sulfate prophylaxis in preeclampsia: lessons learned from recent trials. *Am J Obstet Gynecol* 2004;190:1520.

Sibai BM, Ramadan MK, Usta I, et al. Maternal morbidity and mortality in 442 pregnancies with hemolysis, elevated liver enzymes, and low platelets (HELLP syndrome). *Am J Obstet Gynecol* 1993;169:1000.

Stone JH. HELLP syndrome: hemolysis, elevated liver enzymes, and low platelets. *JAMA* 1998;280:559.

Tikkanen M. Placental abruption: epidemiology, risk factors, and consequences. *Acta Obstet Gynecol Scand* 2011;90:140.

Towers CV, Pircon RA, Heppard M. Is tocolysis safe in the management of third-trimester bleeding? *Am J Obstet Gynecol* 1999;180:1572.

74 Obstetric and Gynecologic Emergencies: Ectopic Pregnancy

Stephanie Charshafian, Rebecca Bavolek and
SueLin M. Hilbert

GENERAL PRINCIPLES

Definition

- Ectopic pregnancy: implantation of the fertilized egg outside the body of the uterus.
- Heterotopic pregnancy: a state in which both extrauterine and intrauterine pregnancies occur simultaneously.

Epidemiology/Etiology

- Ectopic pregnancy occurs in ~2% of all pregnancies.
- Ectopic pregnancy remains the leading cause of maternal death in the first trimester.
- 40–50% of patients with ectopic pregnancy receive an initial misdiagnosis.
- Risk factors include African American women, women over the age of 35, patients with a history of tubal surgery, prior ectopic, in utero exposure to diethylstilbestrol (DES), current IUD use, known tubal pathology, prior STIs, or multiple sex partners at a young age.
- The risk of heterotopic pregnancy is as high as 11.7% when assisted reproductive techniques are used.

DIAGNOSIS

Clinical Presentation

History
- The patient may report a history of missed or irregular menses, abdominal or low back pain, abnormal vaginal bleeding, nausea, light-headedness, or syncope.

Physical Examination
- Exam findings of lower abdominal pain, rebound tenderness, cervical motion tenderness, vaginal bleeding, tachycardia, or hypotension may be present.
  - An open os and/or passage of blood or clots on pelvic exam does not exclude ectopic pregnancy.

Differential Diagnosis

- The differential diagnosis of ectopic pregnancy is based on the clinical presentation and includes an intrauterine pregnancy, urinary tract infection (UTI), STI/pelvic inflammatory disease (PID), ovarian torsion, tuboovarian abscess (TOA), ovarian cyst, miscarriage, or uterine cancer.

Diagnostic Criteria and Testing

Laboratories
- Urine hCG testing should be performed and, if positive, should be followed by a quantitative measurement.
  - See table 74.1 for hCG ranges and expected characteristics visible on ultrasound.
    - In an abnormal or ectopic pregnancy, beta hCG levels do not correlate well with fetal age; therefore, a low beta hCG (or any hCG level) does not rule out ectopic pregnancy.
    - <1500: normal intrauterine pregnancy (IUP) is not expected to be visible on TV ultrasound, but does not rule out ectopic pregnancy.
    - >1500: gestational sac (at a minimum) expected to be seen on TV ultrasound.
- Rh status, complete blood count (CBC), coagulation profile, and urinalysis should be obtained on all pregnant patients in whom an ectopic is suspected.

Imaging
- Ultrasound, either transabdominal or transvaginal, is the test of choice for differentiating intrauterine pregnancy from ectopic pregnancy.

TABLE 74.1	Ultrasound Findings by Gestational Age and hCG Level		
	Transabdominal	Transvaginal	hCG level
Gestational sac	5.5–6 wk	4.5–5 wk	1700–6000
Yolk sac	6–6.5 wk	5–5.5 wk	8000–15,000
Fetal pole	7 wk	5.5–6 wk	13,000–15,000
Fetal heart tone	7 wk	6 wk	16,000–25,000
Fetal parts	>8 wk	8 wk	29,000–39,000

- To confirm an intrauterine pregnancy, a yolk sac, fetal pole, fetal heartbeat, or identifiable fetal parts must be seen within the uterus.
- Because the intrauterine pseudosac of an ectopic pregnancy is easily confused with a gestational sac, ultrasound diagnosis of IUP can only be confirmed when, at a minimum, the yolk sac is seen.
- While a double decidual sign decreases the likelihood that the intrauterine sac is a pseudosac, it does not rule out ectopic.
- At least 8 mm of myometrium should surround the fetus to confirm a viable pregnancy. If the myometrial rim is too narrow, this can be a sign of cornual or irregularly placed ectopic.

TREATMENT

- All patients with confirmed or suspected ectopic pregnancy require consultation with an obstetrician for confirmation of diagnosis and further management.

Medications

- Methotrexate may be administered in consultation with OB.

SPECIAL CONSIDERATIONS

Disposition

- Stable patients that have no adnexal tenderness, no pelvic free fluid, are hemodynamically stable, and have an hCG <1500 may be safe for discharge without OB consultation. These patients need follow-up in 48 hours for repeat ultrasound and hCG levels. This is up to the comfort level of the treating clinicians and depends of the patient's ability to reliably follow up in 48 hours.

Complications

- Rupture, hypotension, or death

SUGGESTED READINGS

Adhikari S, Blaivas M, Lyon M. Diagnosis and management of ectopic pregnancy using bedside transvaginal ultrasonography in the ED: a 2-year experience. *Am J Emerg Med* 2007;25(6):591–96.

Durham B, Lane B, Burbridge L, Balasubramaniam S. Pelvic ultrasound performed by emergency physicians for the detection of ectopic pregnancy in complicated first-trimester pregnancies. *Ann Emerg Med* 1997;29(3):338–47.

Kriebs J, Fahey J. Ectopic pregnancy. *J Midwifery Women Health* 2006;51:431–9.

Lozeau A, Potter S. Diagnosis and management of ectopic pregnancy. *Am Fam Physicians* 2005;72(9):1707–14.

Murray H, Baakdah H, Bardell T, Tulandi T. Diagnosis and treatment of ectopic pregnancy. *CMAJ* 2005;173(8):905–12.

Saul T, Lewiss R. ACEP. Focus On. ACEP News, July 2008. Web. 13 July 2014.

Stead L, Behara S. Ectopic pregnancy. *J Emerg Med* 2007;32(2):205–6.

Stein JC, Wang R, Adler N, et al. Emergency physician ultrasonography for evaluating patients at risk for ectopic pregnancy: a meta-analysis. *Ann Emerg Med* 2010;56(6):674–83.

75

Obstetric and Gynecologic Emergencies: Female Genital Tract

SueLin M. Hilbert and Rebecca Bavolek

GENERAL PRINCIPLES

- Always obtain a pregnancy test on any woman of child bearing age, regardless of LMP, who presents with any abdominal, pelvic, or urogenital complaint.
- A complete pelvic exam (speculum and bimanual) is essential for evaluation and diagnosis.
  - Samples may be obtained for wet prep slides and other microbiologic testing.
- Disposition is usually home with PMD or OB/GYN follow-up as needed.

VULVA

Vulvovaginal Candidiasis

GENERAL PRINCIPLES

Epidemiology/Etiology
- Risk factors include recent antibiotic use, immune-compromised state, or pregnancy.

DIAGNOSIS

Clinical Presentation
History
- The patient may report vaginal itching, abnormal vaginal discharge, dyspareunia, or dysuria.

Physical Examination
- The external exam will show vulvar erythema or edema, excoriation, or satellite lesions.
- The pelvic exam will show a white, curd-like discharge.

Diagnostic Criteria and Testing
Laboratories
- Slides prepared with saline and 10% KOH wet prep will show budding yeast, hyphae, or pseudohyphae ("spaghetti and meatballs" appearance).

TREATMENT

Medication

- Topical agents
  - Clotrimazole or miconazole according to label directions
- Oral agents
  - Fluconazole 150 mg orally in a single dose

SPECIAL CONSIDERATIONS

- Topical treatments may weaken latex condoms or diaphragms.
- Pregnant patients should only receive topical treatment.
- Immunocompromised patients or patients with recurrent cases should receive longer therapies.

Vulvar Abscesses

GENERAL PRINCIPLES

Epidemiology/Etiology

- Methicillin-resistant staphylococcus aureus (MRSA) is the most common pathogen.
  - Other pathogens: *Proteus mirabilis*, *Escherichia coli*, group B streptococcus (GBS), and *Enterococcus* sp.
- Risk factors include diabetes, obesity, pregnancy, immunosuppression, recent waxing or shaving, or recent trauma/surgery/delivery.

DIAGNOSIS

Clinical Presentation

History
- The patient may report vulvovaginal pain or swelling, dyspareunia, urinary urgency, urinary frequency, or dysuria.

Physical Examination
- There may be unilateral erythema, edema, induration, tenderness, and/or fluctuance.
- The presence of skin discoloration/necrosis or crepitus suggests necrotizing fasciitis.

Differential Diagnoses

- Bartholin cyst/abscess, vulvar cellulitis, or necrotizing fasciitis

Diagnostic Criteria and Testing

Laboratories
- Standard culture and Gram stain of fluid after I&D can help guide antibiotic management but is not required.

TREATMENT

- Small, ill-defined abscesses: sitz baths, oral antibiotics, and follow-up if not improving.
- Larger, well-defined abscesses: I&D on the mucosal side of the labia and oral antibiotics.
- Extensive or complicated abscesses or high suspicion for necrotizing fasciitis will require Gyn consultation, IV antibiotics, and possible operative drainage.

Medications
- Oral antibiotics: trimethoprim–sulfamethoxazole (TMP-SMX) DS bid or doxycycline 100 mg bid for 7–10 days
- IV antibiotics: vancomycin, clindamycin

SPECIAL CONSIDERATIONS

Disposition
- Admit patients if there is evidence of failed outpatient management or evidence of systemic infection.

Bartholin Cyst/Abscess

Epidemiology/Etiology
- Most commonly seen among women in their 20s
  - Starting around age 30, the glands begin to involute, making obstruction and infection less likely.
  - Any vaginal mass in a woman age 40 or older is concerning for malignancy.
- Typically polymicrobial—aerobic and anaerobic pathogens

DIAGNOSIS

Clinical Presentation
History
- The patient may report posterior vulvovaginal pain or swelling, vaginal discharge or drainage from the lesion, dyspareunia, or urinary urgency, frequency, or dysuria.

Physical Examination
- Unilateral tenderness, tense swelling, and fluctuance of posterior labia majora—usually at 5 or 7 o'clock position will be present without induration or erythema.

Differential Diagnoses
- Vulvar abscess/cellulitis
- Necrotizing fasciitis

Diagnostic Criteria and Testing
Laboratories
- No routine labs are necessary.

TREATMENT

- Small, asymptomatic cysts do not require intervention.
- Painful cysts and abscesses should undergo I&D.
- Regular sitz baths may aid with pain and discomfort.

Procedure
- I&D is performed using standard technique but includes insertion of a Word catheter to create an epithelialized tract for continued drainage.
  - After anesthetizing the area with local anesthetic, such as lidocaine, make a small (<5 mm) incision on the mucosal surface of the abscess.

- ○ Use universal precautions as lesions are often tense and fluid may extrude with a fair amount of pressure.
- ○ Once the fluid has completely drained, irrigate the abscess cavity and place a Word catheter, which is a small, rubber catheter with a Foley balloon at the tip.
- ○ Inflate the catheter balloon with 2–3 mL of saline through the catheter hub and gently tug the catheter to ensure it remains in the cavity.
- ○ After the catheter is securely placed, the protruding portion may be tucked up into the vagina for the patient's comfort.
- The Word catheter should remain in place for 4–6 weeks.

Medications

- Oral antibiotics may be prescribed if significant overlying cellulitis is present; otherwise, I&D and Word catheter placement is sufficient.

UTERUS AND VAGINA

Vaginal Foreign Body

DIAGNOSIS

Clinical Presentation

- Generally, a clinical diagnosis based on history and physical exam

History
- Adult patients will present with a chief complaint of a vaginal foreign body.
- Rarely, the patient will not be forthcoming with the history, but there will be a vaginal-related complaint such as abnormal bleeding or discharge.

Physical Examination
- Pelvic examination with speculum is diagnostic.
  - ○ After removal of foreign body, inspect the vaginal canal for any resultant trauma.
- Extraction of larger foreign bodies may be needed to be performed under sedation or anesthesia.

Diagnostic Criteria and Testing
Laboratories
- There are no specific laboratory values to diagnose a foreign body.

TREATMENT

- Removal is often therapeutic; if significant injury is present, consult gynecology for further management.
- If the patient is systemically ill from retained foreign body (i.e., tampon and toxic shock), resuscitate and treat accordingly.

Vaginal Bleeding

Definitions

- Abnormal uterine bleeding (AUB) covers a spectrum of conditions and has replaced the prior nomenclature of "menorrhagia, menometrorrhagia," etc.

- Normal limits of menstruation and the menstrual cycle:
  - Frequency of menses: 24–38 days
  - Regularity of menses (cycle to cycle): 2–20 days
  - Duration of flow: 4.5–8.0 days
  - Volume of blood loss monthly: 5–80 mL

Epidemiology/Etiology

- Heavy menstrual bleeding affects more than 20% of premenopausal women over the age of 35.
- Risk factors vary by underlying etiology of AUB.
- The classification of AUB is stratified into nine categories based around the acronym "PALM-COEIN."
  - PALM (structural abnormalities)—polyp, adenomyosis, leiomyoma, malignancy/hyperplasia
  - COEIN (structurally normal uteri)—coagulopathy, ovulatory disorders, endometrium, iatrogenic, and not classified

DIAGNOSIS

Clinical Presentation

History

- Patients may complain of acute or indolent onset of lower abdominal pain.
- Patients with significant bleeding may report symptoms consistent with symptomatic anemia.
- It is important to characterize the timing, duration, and amount of bleeding.
- Establish if the patient is on contraception, if concurrent sexually transmitted diseases (STDs) are present, or if the patient is on any medication that may interfere with coagulation.

Physical Examination

- A pelvic examination should be performed to assess for amount of bleeding and a search for possible etiologies such as masses or lacerations.

Differential Diagnosis

- Menstrual cycle, ectopic pregnancy, miscarriage, vaginal bleeding of pregnancy

Diagnostic Criteria and Testing

Laboratories

- Complete blood count (CBC) to assess for anemia.
- Type and screen/crossmatch if significant bleeding is suspected and the patient may require a blood transfusion.
- Consider coagulation studies and platelet function studies if the patient has risk factors based on history.

Imaging

- Routine imaging is not necessary in the emergency department.

TREATMENT

- Hemodynamically stable
  - If the patient is asymptomatic, follow up with gynecology as an outpatient.
  - Symptomatic treatment for pain; usually NSAIDs are sufficient.

- Hemodynamically unstable
  - Blood transfusion and emergent gynecologic consultation

Medications

- Medical therapy for acute bleeding is usually done in conjunction with a gynecologist.
  - Estrogen and combination oral contraceptives
    - Conjugated estrogen—2.5 mg by mouth every 6 hours or 25 mg IV every 6 hours
    - Combination pills—monophasic combined oral contraceptive that contains 25 μg of ethinyl estradiol three times per day for 7 days
  - Tranexamic acid
    - Tranexamic acid 1.3 g by mouth or 10 mg/kg IV (maximum 600 mg/dose) three times per day for 5 days
    - Use with caution in patients with a history of thrombosis
  - Progesterone
    - Medroxyprogesterone acetate 20 mg by mouth three times per day for 7 days

Surgical Management

- If bleeding cannot be controlled, the patient may require surgical intervention.

SPECIAL CONSIDERATIONS

- Postmenopausal vaginal bleeding is always pathologic in nature and must always be referred for gynecologic follow-up for further testing.

Disposition

- Admit hemodynamically unstable patients with continued significant bleeding.

Complications

- Significant anemia

Bacterial Vaginosis

GENERAL PRINCIPLES

Epidemiology/Etiology

- Most common cause of vaginal discharge.
- Caused by an alteration in the normal vaginal flora (*Lactobacillus* sp.) that results in an overgrowth of anaerobic bacteria.
- Risk factors include multiple or new sexual partners or douching.

DIAGNOSIS

Clinical Presentation

History

- Patients may present with and report a vaginal discharge with a "fishy" odor that is more apparent after sexual intercourse.
- 50% of patients are asymptomatic and diagnosis is made incidentally.

Physical Examination
- There is a homogenous, thin, white discharge that coats the vaginal walls.
- Vaginal fluid pH >4.5.

Differential Diagnoses
- Trichomoniasis or other STD

Diagnostic Criteria and Testing
Laboratories
- Amsel Diagnostic Criteria (3 characteristics = positive for BV)
  - Characteristic discharge
  - pH >4.5
  - Wet prep microscopy:
    - Amine/"fishy" odor before or after the application of KOH (positive whiff test)
    - Epithelial cells covered in coccobacilli ("clue cells")

TREATMENT

- Treat if symptomatic.
- Treatment of sexual partners is not indicated.

Medications
- Metronidazole 500 mg PO bid × 7 days
  - In order to avoid a disulfiram-like reaction, patients should be counseled to abstain from alcohol during and for 24 hours after completion of treatment.
- Metronidazole gel 0.75%, one full applicator (5 g) intravaginally daily × 5 days
- Clindamycin cream 2%, one full applicator (5 g) intravaginally at bedtime × 7 days

OVARIAN PATHOLOGY

GENERAL PRINCIPLES

Classification
- Ovarian cysts—sudden onset of materializing pelvic pain, right greater than left secondary to normal rupture in the course of ovulation.
  - Cysts may be hemorrhagic if a blood vessel in the wall also ruptures.
  - Dermoid cysts—multicystic masses continuing various tissue types. Most are benign, but malignancy must be considered in patients over 45, diameter over 8 cm, or rapid growth.
- Mittelschmerz—mild pain that occurs mid cycle at the time of ovulation, usually lasting a few hours to days.
- Ovarian neoplasm—patients usually present with nonspecific symptoms such as anorexia, early satiety, bloating, and ascites. Ovarian masses in postmenopausal women should be considered a malignancy until proven otherwise.
- Ovarian hyperstimulation syndrome—complication of ovulation induction. Patients may have enlarged ovaries with multiple cysts and can present with a wide range of complications including ascites and complications of systemic thrombosis.

- Ovarian torsion—classically described as acute onset of severe abdominal pain that may be constant or intermittent. The right adnexa is preferentially affected. It may be accompanied by nausea (70%) and vomiting (45%).
  - Risk factors—ovulation induction, ovarian hyperstimulation syndrome, polycystic ovarian syndrome, and pregnancy.
  - Usually, enlarged ovaries or ovaries with cysts are at risk for torsion; however, up to 46% of cases of torsion involve a normal ovary.
  - Up to 50% of cases are initially misdiagnosed due to the variable presentation and intermittent nature of the torsion process.

Epidemiology

- Ovarian torsion and cysts are more common in women of child bearing age.
- Ovarian torsion, a surgical emergency, has an annual prevalence of 2–6%.
- Women undergoing fertility treatments have higher risk of ovarian pathology due to ovarian stimulation techniques and ovarian hyperstimulation syndrome.

DIAGNOSIS

Clinical Presentation

History

- Patients may report an acute onset of unilateral pelvic pain, with associated symptoms of vaginal bleeding, discharge, and signs/symptoms of shock.

Physical Examination

- Evaluate for laterality of pain or masses, cervical motion tenderness, vaginal bleeding, or discharge.

Differential Diagnoses

- Appendicitis, urinary tract infection, diverticulosis or diverticulosis, intra-abdominal abscess, or ectopic pregnancy

Diagnostic Testing

Laboratories

- Laboratory testing is often not necessary unless there is evidence of significant bleeding.

Imaging

- Pelvic ultrasound is the test of choice for patients with acute onset of pelvic pain with a suspected gynecologic etiology.
  - Doppler flow studies for ovarian torsion are highly specific.
- Contrast CT can detect findings of ovarian torsion.

TREATMENT

Medications

- The majority of ovarian issues require only supportive care.

Surgical Management

- Ovarian torsion is a surgical emergency. If torsion is highly suspected, immediate gynecologic consultation is necessary for emergent surgical detorsion of the affected ovary.

- Complicated cyst rupture with concomitant significant bleeding may require surgery if the patient is unstable.

SPECIAL CONSIDERATIONS

- If Doppler studies are negative, but suspicion remains high for torsion, proceed with gynecologic consultation.

Complications

- Delay in diagnosis and treatment of ovarian torsion can lead to loss of an ovary and diminished fertility.
- Ruptured cysts can cause intra-abdominal bleeding and hemorrhagic shock, although rarely.

SUGGESTED READINGS

Amirbekian S, Hooley RJ. Ultrasound evaluation of pelvic pan. *Radiol Clin N Am* 2014;52: 1215–35.

Bhavsar AK, Gelder EJ, Shorma R. Common questions about the evaluation of acute pelvic pain. *Am Fam Physician* 2016;93(1):41–9.

Birnbaumer DM. *"Sexually Transmitted Diseases"* In: Marx JA, Hockerberger RS, Walls RM, eds. Rosen's Emergency Medicine. 8th ed Philadephia PA: Saunders-Elsevier 2014, Chapter 98, 1312–25.e1

Cirilli AR, Capot SJ. Emergency evaluation and management of vaginal bleeding in the non-pregnant patient. *Emerg Med Clin N Am* 2012;30:991–1006.

Heniff M, Fleming HRB. Chapter 97 Abdominal and Pelvic Pain in the Nonpregnant Female. In: Tintinalli JE, Stapczynski J, Ma O, Yealy DM, Meckler GD, Cline DM. eds. *Tintinalli's Emergency Medicine: A Comprehensive Study Guide.* 8th ed. McGraw Hill, 2015.

Kruszka PS, Kruska SJ. Evaluation of acute pelvic pain in women. *Am Fam Physician* 2010;82(2):141–7.

ACOG committee opinion no. 557: management of acute abnormal uterine bleeding in non-pregnant reproductive-aged women. *Obstet Gynecol* 2013 Apr;121(4):891–6.

Munro MG. Classification of menstrual bleeding disorders. *Rev Endor Metab Disord* 2012;13: 225–34.

Omole F, Simmons BJ, Hacker Y. Management of Bartholin's duct cyst and gland abscess. *Am Fam Physician* 2003;68(1):135–40.

Sasaki KJ, Miller CE. Adnexal torsion: review of the literature. *J Minim Invasive Gynecol* 2014;21(2):196–202.

Swenson DW, Lourenco AP, Beaudoin FL, et al. Ovarian torsion: case-control study comparing the sensitivity and specificity of ultrasonography and computed tomography for the diagnosis in the emergency department. *Eur J Radiol* 2014;83:733–8.

Wood SC. Clinical Manifestations and Therapeutic Management of Vulvar Cellulitis and Abscess: Methicillin-resistant Staphylococcus aureus, Necrotizing Fasciitis, Bartholin Abscess, Crohn Disease of the Vulva, Hidradenitis Suppurativa. *Clin Obstet Gynecol* 2015;58(3): 503–11.

76

Obstetric and Gynecologic Emergencies: Stages of Labor, Delivery, and Delivery Complications

Chandra Aubin

STAGES OF LABOR

GENERAL PRINCIPLES

First Stage
- The time from onset of labor to complete cervical dilation
  - Latent phase: gradual cervical change to ~4–6 cm, at a rate of ~1 cm/h
  - Active phase: rapid cervical change
- Median times: nulliparas 5.3 hours, multiparas 3.8 hours, and longer with induced labor

Second Stage
- Time from complete cervical dilation to delivery of infant, including the changes in fetal station and descent
  - Passive phase: complete cervical dilation to onset of active maternal pushing
  - Active phase: active maternal pushing to delivery of infant
- Median times without epidural anesthesia: nulliparas 0.6 hours and multiparas 0.2 hours

Third Stage
- Time from delivery of infant to delivery of placenta
- Median time 4 minutes with the risk of postpartum hemorrhage increased after 20 minutes

NORMAL DELIVERY MANEUVERS

Maternal Position
- One of maternal comfort, with semi upright position having shown some benefit.
- Routine episiotomy should not be performed.
- "Hands off": Passive perineal support with support of the crowning head.
- "Hands on": One hand maintains the head in a flexed position controlling the speed of crowning and one hand easing the perineum over the head.
- Once the head is delivered, external rotation occurs spontaneously. No benefit has been shown to performing routine oropharyngeal suctioning in healthy term newborns, even in the presence of meconium.
- Check for the nuchal cord and reduce it over the head if possible.

- If not possible to reduce cord, double clamp and cut.
- After the head has delivered, place a hand on either side of the head and deliver the anterior shoulder during the next contraction by using gentle downward traction; the posterior shoulder is then delivered by gentle upward traction.
- Cord clamping: Benefit has been shown in delaying for at least 30–60 seconds in vigorous term infants.
- Dry the infant and place on the mother's skin.
- Placenta delivery: Active management including oxytocin, a hand on the uterine fundus, and gentle cord traction will reduce the risk of severe postpartum hemorrhage. Inspect for completeness of the placenta once delivered.
- Postpartum bleeding may be limited by oxytocin administration and uterine fundus massage.
- Examine the cervix, rectum, and vagina for evidence of birth injury and repair any lacerations.

DIFFICULT DELIVERY MANEUVERS

Shoulder Dystocia

- A subjective clinical diagnosis in 0.2–3% of births, suspected when fetal head retracts into the perineum—"turtle sign." Complications include brachial nerve injuries from traction.
- Announce dystocia when it is suspected, call for help, and instruct the mother not to push. Place the mother's buttocks at edge of bed to facilitate delivery maneuvers, avoid fundal pressure, and release the nuchal cord if present. Do not place any traction on the fetus and insert a Foley catheter to drain bladder.
- The objective is to release the impacted anterior shoulder from underneath the pubic symphysis.

McRoberts Maneuver

- Assistants hyperflex the maternal thighs up and back against the abdomen. This optimizes the pelvic outlet position and relieves dystocia up to 42% of the time.
- The assistant presses down firmly with fist just above symphysis.
- Deliver the posterior fetal arm after analgesia by inserting hand into vagina, locating posterior arm following it to the elbow, applying pressure to antecubital fossa to flex arm while grabbing the hand or wrist and pulling across fetal chest and out of vagina. If anterior shoulder still will not deliver, rotate anterior shoulder down and deliver now posterior shoulder in similar fashion.
- Menticoglou maneuver/delivery of posterior shoulder: if unable to grasp the arm, locate the posterior shoulder and insert physician's middle fingers in front and back of the fetal axilla, sliding the shoulder down the sacrum to bring the posterior arm into reach. Then proceed with posterior arm delivery.

Rubin Maneuver

- Insertion of the physician's hand into the vagina along the posterior aspect of the posterior or anterior fetal shoulder rotating the shoulder anteriorly toward the fetal chest

Woods Screw Maneuver

- Apply anterior pressure on the posterior shoulder to rotate the fetus and release the anterior shoulder. It can be combined with applying posterior pressure to the anterior shoulder of the fetus.

Gaskin All-Fours Maneuver

- Place mother on her hands and knees, apply gentle downward traction on posterior shoulder against the sacrum, and then gentle upward traction on anterior shoulder underneath the symphysis.

Zavanelli Maneuver

- Replacement of fetal head into the pelvis and prepare for cesarean section. Rotate head into occiput anterior position, flex the head, and push as far cephalad as possible.

Symphysiotomy

- Only if all other maneuvers have failed and a c-section is not possible—Incision of the cartilaginous portion of the symphysis after local anesthesia will allow the pubic bones to separate. There can be multiple post procedure complications.

Breech Delivery

- Avoid assisting the delivery until the baby is spontaneously delivered to the umbilicus or more. The fetal body should be supported at or below the level of the vagina.

Pinard Maneuver

- If the legs are extended after delivery of the trunk, apply pressure to the back of the knee away from the trunk to extract the foot and leg. Repeat for the other leg.
- Check cord pulsation and pull a small loop down to prevent traction on the cord.
- Ask the mother to push again to deliver the shoulders and arms, usually flexed across the chest, in the anterior posterior plane.
- If the arms do not deliver spontaneously, the fetus is held by its hips and rotated 180 degrees to deliver the shoulders.
- If rotation does not deliver the shoulders, slide a finger along the anterior surface of the shoulder into the antecubital fossa, flex the arm, and then sweep the elbow down and across the chest to deliver the arm. Repeat for the other side.

Bracht Maneuver/Delivery of the Head

- If the hairline is not visible after shoulders are delivered, rotate the fetus' body to face the floor, apply maternal suprapubic pressure to flex the fetus' head down, and encourage pushing by the mother and avoiding fetal traction.
- Once the hairline is visible, swing the fetal legs upward and support the perineum with the other hand control head delivery.
- Alternatively, use the Mauriceau-Smellie-Veit maneuver.

Mauriceau-Smellie-Veit Maneuver

- Support the baby's trunk on the forearm with its legs straddling on the physician arm, place the physician's fingers in the vagina and on the maxilla of the fetus to flex the head down and promote delivery; apply gentle pressure on the occiput of the fetus with the other hand.

SUGGESTED READINGS

Berghella V, Baxter JK, Chauhan SP. Evidence based labor and delivery management. *Am J Obstet Gynecol* 2008;199:445.

Zhang J, Troendle J, Mikolajczyk R, et al. The natural history of the normal first stage of labor. *Obstet Gynecol* 2010;116:1281.

Zhang J, Landy HJ, Branch DW, et al. Contemporary patterns of spontaneous labor with normal neonatal outcomes. *Obstet Gynecol* 2010;116:1281.

77

Obstetric and Gynecologic Emergencies: Normal Pregnancy

P. Gabriel Miranda Gomez

GENERAL PRINCIPLES

Definition

- Gravidity: all normal and abnormal pregnancies, including current, in a mother's lifetime
- Parity: all expectant and surgical births, beyond 20 weeks' gestational age, regardless of outcome, in a mother's lifetime
- Gestational age: time since the mother's last menstrual period

DIAGNOSIS

Clinical Presentation

History

- Common symptoms of early pregnancy include breast swelling and tenderness, nausea, anorexia, fatigue, and cessation of menses.
- Vaginal bleeding, discharge, and abdominal cramping that are intermittent and not associated with any pathologic lesion are commonplace within the first trimester.
- Perception of fetal movements ("quickening") is thought to occur no earlier than 16 weeks' gestation.
- In the second and third trimesters, patients may begin to report abdominal distention, heartburn, leg swelling, and stretching and darkening of the skin.
- Abdominal contractions may occur normally at any time during the pregnancy.
  - Braxton Hicks contractions, or "false labor," are synchronous uterine contractions occurring beyond 30 weeks' gestation that do not progress in frequency or duration, nor do they produce any associated cervical dilatation or effacement.
  - True labor consists of cyclical uterine contractions that progress in frequency, duration, and severity.

Physical Examination

- Expected vital signs changes include an increase in pulse rate by 10–15 beats per minute and a decrease in mean arterial blood pressure of 6–10 mm Hg below baseline, both returning to prepregnancy levels by 36 weeks' gestation.
- Respiratory rate declines slightly during mid gestation.
- A systolic ejection murmur and S3 gallop is common.
- Skin changes include melasma gravidarum (increased skin pigment) and abdominal striae.
- Breast changes include overall engorgement, prominence of superficial venules, areolar darkening, and presence of colostrum at the nipple.

- Uterine fundal height reaches the pubic symphysis at ~12 weeks, the umbilicus at 16–20 weeks, and the xiphoid beyond 36 weeks. The fetal outline may be palpated in the third trimester but is often unreliable.
- Transabdominally, fetal heart tones may be auscultated as early as 17 weeks while the uterine fundus can be palpated to approximate the gestational age.
- Vaginal speculum examination may reveal hyperemia from pelvic congestion, causing bluish color of the vaginal walls.

Differential Diagnosis
- Ectopic or heterotopic pregnancy
- Uterine molar pregnancy
- hCG-secreting neoplasms (germ cell tumor, teratoma, choriocarcinoma)

Diagnostic Criteria and Testing
Laboratories
- Urine hCG, qualitative, is an adequate screening test in early pregnancy.
- Serum hCG, quantitative, will allow determination of approximate gestational age and progression of pregnancy.
- There is a dilutional anemia in pregnancy; Hgb during pregnancy drops to ~11.5 g/dL. WBC count increases and platelet count decreases during gestation.

Imaging
- Ultrasound is used to evaluate presence and progression of pregnancy.
- Classically, the hCG cutoffs for visualizing a gestational sac was 1000–2000 mIU/mL on a transvaginal ultrasound and 3000–6000 mIU/mL transabdominally. These may change with afvances in technology.
- Transabdominal Doppler ultrasonography can detect fetal heart tones at 8–10 weeks.
- Transvaginal ultrasonography can detect fetal heart tones as early as 6 weeks.

TREATMENT

Medications
WHO-Recommended Supplementation
- Folic acid 400 µg daily
- Elemental iron 30–60 mg daily

Antiemetics
- Metoclopramide 5–10 mg tid PRN
- Prochlorperazine 5–10 mg every 6–8 hours PRN
- Ondansetron 4–8 mg IV or PO every 4–6 hours PRN
- Pyridoxine (B6) 25 mg PO tid PRN
- Doxylamine 25 mg PO daily PRN

SPECIAL CONSIDERATIONS

- Pregnancy should not be excluded on the basis of historical factors alone.
- Pregnant patients may be asymptomatic or have poor recall of their sexual and menstrual histories.
- Pregnancy is a strong risk factor for intimate partner violence.

Disposition

- Following confirmation of live, intrauterine pregnancy, most patients can be discharged to home after safely addressing the patient's chief complaint. Patients in active labor should be transferred, time permitting, to the immediate care of an obstetrician. Precipitous delivery requires emergency department expectant management.

Complications

- Braxton Hicks contractions, vaginal bleeding, placental abruption, placenta previa, or hyperemesis gravidarum

SUGGESTED READINGS

Connolly A, Ryan DH, Stuebe AM, Wolfe HM. Reevaluation of discriminatory and threshold levels for serum β-hCG in early pregnancy. *Obstet Gynecol* 2013;121(1):65–70.

Daily iron and folic acid supplementation during pregnancy. Guidance summary. WHO recommendations. e-Library of Evidence for Nutrition Actions (eLENA) (last accessed: 09/06/2016).

Morrison L, Toma A, Gray S. General Approach to the Pregnant Patient. In: Marx JA, Hockerberger RS, Walls RM, eds. *Rosen's Emergency Medicine: Concepts and Clinical Practice*. 8th ed Philadephia PA: Saunders-Elsevier 2014 p 2271–2281

78 Obstetric and Gynecologic Emergencies: Postpartum Hemorrhage

P. Gabriel Miranda Gomez

GENERAL PRINCIPLES

Definition

- Primary postpartum hemorrhage (PPH) is a potential life-threatening complication of all deliveries that is defined as blood loss exceeding 500 mL within 24 hours of vaginal delivery.
- Secondary postpartum hemorrhage is abnormal or excessive bleed from the birth canal for up to 12 weeks postpartum.

Epidemiology/Etiology

- Risk factors for PPH include a prolonged third stage of labor, multiple gestations, fetal macrosomia, episiotomy, and a history of multiple cesarean incisions.
- The vast majority of PPH is caused by uterine atony. Retained placenta, vaginal or perineal laceration, and uterine rupture and inversion are other causes.

Pathophysiology

- Postpartum hemorrhage can occur if the vessels supplying the placental bed are not compressed by myometrial contraction, if the placenta does not separate fully, or if there are bleeding diatheses that interfere with the clotting pathway.

DIAGNOSIS

Clinical Presentation

History
- Severe hemorrhage after delivery in the ED or as a complication of home delivery.

Physical Examination
- Blood loss cannot be approximated by direct visualization.
- Signs of shock may be present.
- Transabdominal fundal massage may reveal a soft, "boggy" uterus due to uterine atony.
- A pelvic exam should be performed looking for uterine inversion.

Differential Diagnosis

- Uterine atony
- Retained uterine products
- Vaginal or perineal laceration
- Uterine rupture
- Uterine inversion

Diagnostic Criteria and Testing

Laboratories
- Complete blood count (CBC), prothrombin time (PT)/partial thromboplastin time (PTT), and type and screen should be drawn to evaluate for bleeding diathesis and need for blood product administration.

Imaging
- Ultrasound may be used in conjunction with obstetrical consultation to evaluate uterine sources of bleeding.

TREATMENT

- Active management of the third stage of labor decreases the risk of PPH without increasing the risk of retained placenta.
  - Administer a uterotonic agent soon after delivery of the anterior shoulder.
  - Place gentle traction on the umbilical cord.
  - Perform transabdominal uterine fundus massage.
  - In the case of uterine atony, perform bimanual uterine massage to induce uterine contraction and tamponade bleeding. Administer uterotonic agents. Examine the placenta and, if it is incomplete or torn, manually sweep the uterus for retained

placenta and blood that may be physically preventing the uterus from contracting down.

- ○ Uterine inversion may present with shock. Perform immediate manual reduction and administer uterotonic agents.
- ○ Obtain early emergent consultation from obstetrics in all cases to guide medical management. Life-threatening bleeding refractory to medication and manual tamponade will require operative hemostasis by uterine packing, vessel ligation, embolization, or hysterectomy.

Medications

- Oxytocin (10 international units IM; or 10–30 international units in 500 mL crystalloid infused over 10 minutes) is the uterotonic drug of choice.
- Second-line agents include the following:
  - ○ Misoprostol (1000 µg per rectum)
  - ○ Carboprost (250 µg IM)
  - ○ Methylergonovine (200 µg IM)

SPECIAL CONSIDERATIONS

Disposition

- All patients who meet the diagnostic definition of PPH should receive emergent consultation from an obstetric physician. Patients with ongoing life-threatening hemorrhage may require direct transportation to the OR for surgical hemostasis. Patients in disseminated intravascular coagulation (DIC) should be admitted to an ICU.

Complications

- Disseminated intravascular coagulation, postpartum pituitary gland necrosis (the Sheehan syndrome), and delayed complications including rebleeding at 24–48 hours

SUGGESTED READINGS

Elbourne DR, Prendiville WJ, Carroli G, et al. Prophylactic use of oxytocin in the third stage of labour. *Cochrane Database Syst Rev* 2001;(4):CD001808.

Prendiville WJ, Elbourne D, McDonald S. Active versus expectant management in the third stage of labour. *Cochrane Database Syst Rev* 2000;(3):CD000007.

Psychiatric Emergencies: Addiction

Evan Schwarz

GENERAL PRINCIPLES

Definitions

- Substance use disorder refers to recurrent use of alcohol or other drugs, which causes clinically and functionally significant impairment. This can be classified as mild, moderate, or severe. Substance use disorder encompasses both substance abuse and dependence.
- Addiction is a term that denotes a level of substance use disorder in which there is a substantial loss of self-control despite the desire to stop taking the drug or substance of abuse. In the *Diagnostic and Statistical Manual of Mental Disorders (DSM-5)*, addiction is synonymous with substance use disorder.
- According to the Centers for Disease Control, binge drinking is defined as 4 or more drinks on a single occasion for a woman and 5 or more for a man. Heavy drinking is defined as 8 or more drinks per week for women and 15 or more for men.
- Tolerance is the need for markedly increasing amounts of the substance to achieve intoxication or the desired effects.
- Tolerance and withdrawal are not considered as part of the criteria for substance abuse disorder if the patient is using opioids under medical supervision.
- Dependence is a state in which someone only functions normally in the presence of the substance or drug. This usually manifests by a withdrawal syndrome or physical or psychological disturbance when the drug is removed.

Pathophysiology

- Addiction involves increased and compulsive drug use even after significant medical and social consequences.
- Drug addiction and alcohol addiction are conceptualized as a reward deficit disorder. Positive and negative reinforcement transitions drug use from an impulsive intake to a compulsive intake in people with substance use disorders. Once transitioned to compulsive use, negative reinforcement plays a substantial role in continued drug use and escalation. In negative reinforcement, the negative emotional state precipitated by drug withdrawal or abstinence is improved by continued substance use.
- While many neurotransmitters are implicated in drug abuse, dopamine is consistently associated with reinforcing the effects of most drugs.
- Drugs of abuse increase dopamine concentrations in the limbic system, which reinforce their potential for abuse. Drugs and alcohol increase the duration and magnitude of dopamine released in the limbic system.
- Surges of dopamine cause drug craving and result in drug-seeking behavior.[1] These responses become deeply ingrained and trigger strong cravings even while patients are facing negative consequences of their continued drug use.
- Over time, the release of dopamine is attenuated resulting in people not feeling the same degree of euphoria as they did when their drug use first began. This results in people using drugs not to "get high" but to avoid dysphoria.

- Compulsive drug use also damages the prefrontal cortex, causing poor inhibitory control and poor executive function. Studies estimate that 40–60% of the vulnerability to addiction is attributable to genetic factors or mental illness.[2]

Epidemiology/Etiology

- Nearly 20 million people over 12 years of age in the United States are addicted to alcohol or other drugs.[3]
- Over 10 million people used prescription opioids for nonmedical reasons in 2014.[3]
- Heroin use increased from 2007 to 2014 by 145%, while mortality following a heroin overdose quintupled.[4]

SCREENING FOR SUBSTANCE USE DISORDERS

- Brief intervention (BI) is a time-limited counseling session designed to reduce substance use. When added to screening and treatment referral, it is referred to as screening, brief intervention, and referral to treatment (SBIRT).
- Studies suggest that factors such as needing multiple BI sessions, as opposed to a single session to be effective, or a patient's readiness to change when the BI occurs influence the effectiveness of BIs, limiting their utility in the emergency department.[5]
- Screening and brief intervention (SBI) can consist of using the 5A's.
  - *Ask* refers to screening and assessment of the risk level followed by an intervention consisting of the remaining A's. There are a variety of validated tools that are used to screen patients for alcohol and substance use disorders.
  - *Advise* refers to direct personal advice about substance use.
  - *Assess* refers to evaluating the patient's willingness or readiness to change their substance use.
  - *Assist* involves assisting the patient in developing a treatment plan.
  - *Arrange* refers to coordinating a follow-up visit and specialty referral.

Opioid Withdrawal

- Opioid withdrawal occurs following the abrupt discontinuation of opioids.
- Signs and symptoms of withdrawal may begin as early as 4–6 hours after the last dose of a short-acting opioid and up to 24–48 hours after cessation of a long-acting opioid such as methadone. Opioid withdrawal is extremely unpleasant, but generally not life threatening in otherwise healthy adults.[6]
- Typical signs and symptoms of opioid withdrawal include:
  - Flulike symptoms and myalgias
  - Rhinorrhea and lacrimation
  - Nausea, vomiting, and diarrhea
  - Diaphoresis and hot and cold flashes
  - Insomnia, anxiety, and irritability
  - Intense drug craving
  - Pruritus
  - Mydriasis
  - Piloerection
  - Yawning
  - Hyperactive bowel sounds
  - Tachycardia and hypertension
  - Alternatively, hypotension may be present if volume depletion has resulted from vomiting and diarrhea.
  - Patients may be agitated but should have a clear sensorium.

- The Clinical Opioid Withdrawal Scale (COWS) (Table 79.1) or a similar withdrawal scale is used to monitor patients for signs of opioid withdrawal.
- Medication-Assisted Treatment (MAT) is used to treat or prevent opioid withdrawal. Methadone and buprenorphine are both effective treatments. Any provider can administer either medication in the emergency department. However, only those with proper licensing can prescribe them at discharge. Consultation with a specialist in addiction medicine is advised prior to starting either medication in the emergency department.
  - Methadone prolongs the QTc interval. It is not mandatory to acquire an ECG before administering methadone in patients without other risk factors for QTc prolongation.
  - Methadone has a very long half-life. As such, dosing adjustments should only be made in 3–5 day intervals.
- Consultation with pain management or an addiction specialist and obstetrics should be obtained in pregnant patients with signs of opioid withdrawal, as withdrawal can be detrimental to the fetus and fetal viability needs to be documented. In addition, neonates born to mothers on opioids require special care and treatment.
  - Methadone is used in pregnancy to treat opioid withdrawal as its benefits outweigh its potential for fetal risk, despite being pregnancy category C.
  - The initial dose of methadone is 20–30 mg daily with an additional 5–10 mg given after 2–4 hours if the patient is symptomatic. The dose is titrated to a goal of preventing symptoms for 24 hours.[4] Further stacking of doses is not recommended due to the long half-life of methadone.
  - Obstetrics or pain management can guide methadone dosing and titration in pregnancy.
  - Buprenorphine is also indicated for the treatment of opioid withdrawal. In general, it is recommended to prescribe a combination buprenorphine/naloxone product to prevent misuse.
  - In pregnancy, only buprenorphine products without naloxone should be administered. Buprenorphine is as effective as methadone in pregnancy.[7]
- Clonidine can treat symptoms of opioid withdrawal.
  - Given at an initial dose of 0.1–0.2 mg orally, clonidine is increased to a maximum of 1 mg/d as needed until resolutions of symptoms.
- Benzodiazepines should only be used sparingly if at all to treat opioid withdrawal and should not be used in pregnancy.
- Additional symptom-specific therapies include:
  - Ondansetron 4–8 mg PO or IV q6h or prochlorperazine 5–10 mg PO or IV q6h, both PRN for nausea
  - Loperamide 4 mg PO then 2 mg PO PRN diarrhea up to 16 mg/d as needed for diarrhea

Ethanol Withdrawal

- Ethanol withdrawal is a form of sedative/hypnotic withdrawal.
- It occurs following the abrupt discontinuation of alcohol.
- Signs and symptoms of alcohol withdrawal begin within a few days of stopping drinking.
- Future episodes are more severe and become more resistant to treatment.
- Typical signs and symptoms include:
  - Anxiety
  - Tachycardia

TABLE 79.1 Clinical Opiate Withdrawal Scale (COWS)

For each item, circle the number that best describes the patient's signs or symptom. Rate on just the apparent relationship to opiate withdrawal. For example, if heart rate is increased because the patient was jogging just prior to assessment, the increased pulse rate would not add to the score.

Patient's Name:_____ Date and Time ____/____/____:_____

Reason for this assessment:_____

Resting Pulse Rate _____beats/minute *Measured after patient is sitting or lying for 1 minute* 0 pulse rate 80 or below 1 pulse rate 81–100 2 pulse rate 101–120 4 pulse rate greater than 120	**GI Upset** *over last 1/2 hour* 0 no GI symptoms 1 stomach cramps 2 nausea or loose stool 3 vomiting or diarrhea 5 multiple episodes of diarrhea or vomiting
Sweating *over past 1/2 hour not accounted for by room temperature or patient activity.* 0 no report of chills or flushing 1 subjective report of chills or flushing 2 flushed or observable moistness on face 3 beads of sweat on brow or face 4 sweat streaming off face	**Tremor** *observation of outstretched hands* 0 no tremor 1 tremor can be felt, but not observed 2 slight tremor observable 4 gross tremor or muscle twitching
Restlessness *Observation during assessment* 0 able to sit still 1 reports difficulty sitting still, but is able to do so 3 frequent shifting or extraneous movements of legs/arms 5 unable to sit still for more than a few seconds	**Yawning** *Observation during assessment* 0 no yawning 1 yawning once or twice during assessment 2 yawning three or more times during assessment 4 yawning several times/minute
Pupil Size 0 pupils pinned or normal size for room light 1 pupils possibly larger than normal for room light 2 pupils moderately dilated 5 pupils so dilated that only the rim of the iris is visible	**Anxiety or Irritability** 0 none 1 patient reports increasing irritability or anxiousness 2 patient obviously irritable or anxious 4 patient so irritable or anxious that participation in the assessment is difficult
Bone or Joint Aches *If patient was having pain previously, only the additional component attributed to opiates withdrawal is scored* 0 not present 1 mild diffuse discomfort 2 patient reports severe diffuse aching of joints/muscles 4 patient is rubbing joints or muscles and is unable to sit still because of discomfort	**Gooseflesh Skin** 0 skin is smooth 3 piloerrection of skin can be felt or hairs standing up on arms 5 prominent piloerrection
Runny Nose or Tearing *Not accounted for by cold symptoms or allergies* 0 not present 1 nasal stuffiness or unusually moist eyes 2 nose running or tearing 4 nose constantly running or tears streaming down cheeks	Total Score _____ The total score is the sum of all 11 items Initials of person completing assessment: _____

Score: 5–12 = mild; 13–24 = moderate; 25–36 = moderately severe; more than 36 = severe withdrawal
Adapted from: Wesson R, Ling W. The Clinical Opiate Withdrawal Scale (COWS). *J Psychoactive Drugs* 2003; 35(2):253–9.

- ○ Diaphoresis
- ○ Nausea and vomiting
- ○ Hypertension
- ○ Tremors
- ○ Seizures
- ○ Hallucinations
- ○ Delirium
- There are multiple stages of alcohol withdrawal, which include the following:
  - ○ Autonomic hyperactivity: Patients typically develop autonomic instability and tremors but have a clear sensorium.
  - ○ Alcoholic hallucinosis: Patients actively hallucinate but are aware that the hallucinations are not real.
  - ○ Seizures: The seizures can be isolated or patients may develop status epilepticus. Only ~1/3 of patients with alcohol withdrawal seizures will develop delirium tremens.
  - ○ Delirium tremens: Patients are generally delirious and sympathomimetic.
  - ○ Although alcohol withdrawal is a spectrum disorder, patients do not necessarily progress through all stages. For instance, seizures may be some patients only sign of withdrawal.
- Using validated withdrawal scales to determine when additional medication is needed is preferred to placing patients on a scheduled regimen or administering medications on an as needed basis without using a scale. Potential scales include the Clinical Institute Withdrawal Assessment of Alcohol Scale, Revised (CIWA-Ar) (Table 79.2) and Richmond Agitation-Sedation Scale (RASS) for intubated patients (Table 79.3).
  - ○ CIWA-Ar:
    - Can be administered in <2 minutes by providers.
    - Categories include nausea/vomiting, tremors, anxiety, agitation, paroxysmal diaphoresis, orientation and sensorium disturbances, tactile disturbances, auditory disturbances, visual disturbances, and headache.
- Treatment is with sedatives such as benzodiazepines, barbiturates, and propofol. More recent literature suggests ketamine or dexmedetomidine as treatment adjuncts, although neither agent is recommended as monotherapy.[8,9]
- Benzodiazepines are the recommended therapy for treating ethanol withdrawal. Lorazepam and diazepam are both effective intravenous options. Dosing should be aggressively increased until symptoms are controlled.[10] Administration of large doses effectively treats patients, minimizes complications, and lowers intubation rates.
- Barbiturates and propofol are effective in treating patients with benzodiazepine-resistant withdrawal.
- Antipsychotics and nodal blockers should be avoided.
- Patients in withdrawal may need thiamine, magnesium, folate, and vitamin supplementation.
  - ○ Wernicke encephalopathy is a rare occurrence but occasionally can be seen in this patient population.

URINE DRUG SCREENS

- Positive urine drug screens (UDS) serve as markers of exposure but do not prove intoxication. Some screens are still positive days to weeks after the exposure.

TABLE 79.2   CIWA

Clinical Institute Withdrawal Assessment - Alcohol (CIWA-A)

Patient:_____   Date: (yy/mm/dd) _____   Time: (24 hr)_____

Pulse or heart rate: _____   Blood Pressure: _____

Nausea and Vomiting
Ask: *"Do you feel sick to your stomach? Have you vomited?"*
Observation:
- O 0—None
- O 1—Mild nausea with no vomiting
- O 2
- O 3
- O 4—Intermittent nausea with dry heaves
- O 5
- O 6
- O 7—Constant nausea, frequent dry heaves and vomiting

Paroxysmal Sweats
Observation:
- O 0—No sweat visible
- O 1—Barely perceptible sweating, palms moist
- O 2
- O 3
- O 4—Beads of sweat obvious on forehead
- O 5
- O 6
- O 7—Drenching sweats

Anxiety
Ask: *"Do you feel nervous"*
Observation:
- O 0—No anxiety, at ease
- O 1—Mildly anxious
- O 2
- O 3
- O 4—Moderately anxious, or guarded, so anxiety is inferred
- O 5
- O 6
- O 7—Equivalent to acute panic states as seen in severe delirium or acute schizophrenic reactions

Orientation and Clouding of Sensorium
Ask: *"What day is this? Where are you? Who am I?"*
Observation:
- O 0—Oriented and can form serial additions
- O 1—Cannot do serial additions or is uncertain about date
- O 2—Disoriented for date by no more than 2 calendar days
- O 3—Disoriented for date by more than 2 calendar days
- O 4—Disoriented for place and/or person

Agitation
Observation:
- O 0—Normal activity
- O 1—Somewhat more than normal activity
- O 2
- O 3
- O 4—Moderately fidgety and restless
- O 5
- O 6
- O 7—Paces back and forth during most of the interview, or constantly thrashes about

Tremor
Arms extended and fingers spread apart
Observation:
- O 0—None
- O 1—Not visible, but can be felt fingertip to fingertip
- O 2
- O 3
- O 4—Moderate, with patient's arms extended
- O 5
- O 6
- O 7—Severe, even with arms not extended

Headache/Fullness in Head
Ask: *"Does your head feel different? Does it feel like there is a band around your head?"* Do not rate dizziness or lightheadedness. Otherwise rate severity.
Observation:
- O 0—Not present
- O 1—Very mild
- O 2—Mild
- O 3—Moderate
- O 4—Moderately severe
- O 5—Severe
- O 6—Very severe
- O 7—Extremely severe

Auditory Disturbances
Ask: *"Are you more aware of sounds around you? Are they harsh? Do they frighten you? Are you hearing anything that is disturbing to you? Are you hearing things that you know aren't there?"*
Observation:
- O 0—None
- O 1—Very mild harshness or ability to frighten
- O 2—Mild harshness or ability to frighten
- O 3—Moderate harshness or ability to frighten
- O 4—Moderately severe hallucinations
- O 5—Severe hallucinations
- O 6—Extremely severe hallucinations
- O 7—Continuous hallucinations

Tactile Disturbances
Ask: *"Do you have any itching, pins and needles sensations, any burning, numbness, or do you feel bugs crawling on or under your skin?"*
Observation:
- O 0—None
- O 1—Very mild itching, pins and needles, burning or numbness
- O 2—Mild itching, pins and needles, burning or numbness
- O 3—Moderate itching, pins and needles, burning or numbness
- O 4—Moderately severe hallucinations
- O 5—Severe hallucinations
- O 6—Extremely severe hallucinations
- O 7—Continuous hallucinations

Visual Disturbances
Ask: *"Does the light appear too bright? Is its color different? Does it hurt your eyes? Are you seeing things that you know aren't there?"*
Observation:
- O 0—None
- O 1—Very mild
- O 2—Mild
- O 3—Moderate
- O 4—Moderately severe
- O 5—Severe
- O 6—Very severe
- O 7—Extremely severe

Rater's Initials: _____

Total CIWA-A Score:_____
Maximum Possible Score: 67

- Positive screens are then confirmed with further testing such as gas chromatography/mass spectrometry or tandem mass spectrometry.
- The standard ELISA UDS tests for the following drugs:
  - Opioids
    - Tests for morphine.
    - Morphine, codeine, and heroin cause a positive screen. 6-monoacetylmorphine (6-MAM) is a metabolite of heroin and what is normally reported for heroin confirmation due to the extremely short half-life of heroin.
    - Oxycodone and hydrocodone inconsistently cause positive screens and frequently result in negative screens.
    - Methadone, fentanyl, and other synthetic opioids do not cause positive screens.

TABLE 79.3	Richmond Agitation-Sedation Scale (RASS)
+4	Combative, violent, of immediate danger to himself and staff
+3	Very agitated, aggressive, pulls or removes tubes or catheters
+2	Agitated frequent nonpurposeful movement, dyssynchronous with the ventilator
+1	Restless, anxious but not aggressive
0	Alert and calm
−1	Drowsy, not fully alert, but has sustained eye-opening/eye contact to voice **(>10s)**
−2	Light sedation—briefly awakens with eye contact to voice **(<10 s)**
−3	Moderate sedation—moves or opens eyes to voice **(but no eye contact)**
−4	Deep sedation—No response to voice. Movement or eye opening to physical stimulation
−5	Unarousable—No response to voice or physical stimulation

- Benzodiazepines
  - Tests for oxazepam.
  - Diazepam and chlordiazepoxide cause a positive screen.
  - Lorazepam, alprazolam, and clonazepam do not cause a positive screen.
- Amphetamines
  - Tests for amphetamine.
  - Amphetamine, methamphetamine, selegiline, and pseudoephedrine cause a positive screen.
  - Ecstasy (methylenedioxymethamphetamine [MDMA]) and designer amphetamines such as cathinones (bath salts) do not produce a positive test.
- Cannabinoids
  - Tests for an inactive metabolite of tetrahydrocannabinol (THC).
  - Synthetic cannabinoids do not turn the test positive.
  - In chronic users, the test can remain positive for a month.
- Cocaine
  - Tests for benzoylecgonine, an inactive metabolite.
  - False positives are very unlikely.
- Phencyclidine (PCP)
  - Ketamine, diphenhydramine, and dextromethorphan cause false-positive testing.

REFERENCES

1. Volkow ND, Wang GJ, Telang F, et al. Cocaine cues and dopamine in dorsal striatum: mechanism of craving in cocaine addiction. *J Neurosci* 2006;26:6583–8.
2. Uhl GR, Grow RW. The burden of complex genetics in brain disorders. *Arch Gen Psychiatry* 2004;61:223–9.
3. Center for Behavioral Health Statistics and Quality. *2014 National Survey on Drug Use and Health: Detailed Tables*. Rockville, MD: Substance Abuse and Mental Health Services Administration, 2015.

4. Nicholls L, Bragaw L, Ruetsch C. Opioid dependence treatment and guidelines. *J Manag Care Pharm* 2010;16:S14–21.
5. Field CA, Baird J, Saitz R, et al. The mixed evidence for brief intervention in ED, trauma care centers and inpt hospital settings. *Alcohol Clin Exp Res* 2010;34(12):2004–10.
6. Farrell M. Opiate withdrawal. *Addiction* 1994;89:1471–5.
7. Jones HE, Kaltenbach K, Heil SH, et al. Neonatal abstinence syndrome after methadone or buprenorphine exposure. *N Engl J Med* 2010;363(24):2320–31. PMID: 21142534.
8. Wong A, Benedict NJ, Armahizer MJ, Kane-Gill SL. Evaluation of adjunctive ketamine to benzodiazepines for management of alcohol withdrawal syndrome. *Ann Pharmacother* 2015;49(1):14–9.
9. Rayner SG, Weinert CR, Peng H, et al. Dexmedetomidine as adjunct treatment for severe alcohol withdrawal in the ICU. *Ann Intensive Care* 2012;2(1):12.
10. Gold JA, Rimal B, Nolan A, Nelson LS. A strategy of escalating doses of benzodiazepines and phenobarbital administration reduces the need for mechanical ventilation in delirium tremens. *Crit Care Med* 2007;35(3):724–30.

Psychiatric Emergencies: Delirium and Dementia

Christopher P. Miller

GENERAL PRINCIPLES

Definition[1]

- Delirium—a disturbance in attention and awareness that develops over hours to a days that fluctuates and is a change from the patient's baseline. There should be evidence that the clinical manifestations are a physiologic response to another medical condition, such as medication, toxin, or patient environment.
- Dementia—modest cognitive decline from a prior state that typically occurs over months to years that progressively worsens. The condition must exist outside of a state of delirium and cannot be better explained by another mental disorder. Conditions that cause dementia are now referred to by the *Diagnostic and Statistical Manual of Mental Disorders (DSM-5)* as neurocognitive disorders.

Epidemiology

- Delirium
  - Incidence may range from 6 to 87% in patients that are in the hospital, ED, or ICU.[2]
  - Older age, underlying neurocognitive disorder, and having a low functional level of activity place patients at higher risk for delirium.[1]

- Dementia
  - Incidence is ~1–2% by age 65 and as high as 30% by 85 years of age.[1]
  - Risk factors are varied and tend to increase with age. Normal pressure hydrocephalus is also associated with an increased rate of dementia.

Pathophysiology

- Delirium—alteration in cerebral metabolic activity and neurotransmitter regulation[3]
- Dementia—varies based on disease process being considered

DIAGNOSIS

- In order to diagnose dementia, delirium must first be excluded; however, patients with dementia may also suffer from intermittent episodes of delirium.

Clinical Presentation

- Usually, the patient presents with an acute or chronic confusional state.

History

- Gather information from caregivers or family members to determine if the change in the patient's mental state has been progressive worsening over months, developed in the past few days, or possibly an acute on chronic exacerbation.

Physical Examination

- Complete a thorough exam including neurologic testing. Assess the patient for orientation and cognition. The Mini-Mental State Exam can be used to assess cognition. A higher score indicates a higher likelihood of dementia.[4] Note that many delirious patients may not be able to complete any of this exam.

Differential Diagnosis

- Alzheimer's disease, Huntington's chorea, cerebrovascular disease, head trauma intracranial mass, infectious (neurosyphilis, HIV), normal pressure hydrocephalus (NPH), or electrolyte/nutritional (thiamine) abnormalities
- Medication use, injury, pain, stress, or environmental changes

Diagnostic Criteria and Testing

Laboratories

- There is no specific laboratory test to diagnose delerium or dementia.

Imaging

- There is no specific imaging study performed in the ED that will diagnose delerium or dementia.

Diagnostic Procedures

- Mini-Mental State Examination (MMSE) (Table 80.1)

TREATMENT

- Delirium—any identified reversible cause should be addressed.

Medications

- Pharmacologic restraint—often needed for either condition to prevent self-harm and staff safety
  - Benzodiazepines—lorazepam 1–2 mg IM or IV.

TABLE 80.1 Mini-Mental State Exam

Maximum score	Score	
		Orientation
5	____	What is the (year) (season) (date) (day) (month)?
5	____	Where are we: (state) (country) (town or city) (hospital) (floor)?
		Registration
3	____	Name three common objects (e.g., "apple," "table," "penny"): Take one second to say each. Then ask the patient to repeat all three after you have said them. Give one point for each correct answer. Then repeat them until he or she learns all three. Count trials and record.
		Trials: ____
		Attention and calculation
5	____	Spell "wold" backwards. The score is the number of letters in correct order. (D___L___R___O___W___)
		Recall
3	____	Ask for the three objects repeated above. Give one point for each correct answer. (Note: recall cannot be tested if all three objects were not remembered during registration.)
		Language
2	____	Name a "pencil" and "watch."
		Repeat the following: "No ifs, ands or buts."
1	____	Follow a three-stage command:
3	____	"Take a paper in your right hand, fold it in half and put it on the floor."
		Read and obey the following:
1	____	Close your eyes.
1	____	Write a sentence.
1	____	Copy the following design.

Total score: ____	

- Antipsychotics[5]—haloperidol 5–10 mg IM or IV is the most commonly used in the ED.
- Dementia
  - Long-term pharmacologic treatment will vary based on underlying cause, and it is not recommended to be started in the emergency department.

Other Nonpharmacologic Therapies

- Environment—try to normalize when possible. Reorient patient, expose to natural sunlight, and try to keep noises (other patients, alarms) to a minimum.
- Restraints—avoid physical restraints when at all possible, as this has been associated with patient injury and death.[6]
- Activity—try to keep sleep/wake cycles consistent with patient's natural circadian rhythm. This includes limiting naps during the day. This will help keep the patient from getting disoriented.

SPECIAL CONSIDERATIONS

Disposition

Patients may be discharged home if the offending cause is found and corrected. It is not acceptable to discharge a delirious patient home. A patient who is suffering from dementia without acute delirium may be appropriate for discharge home. However, this patient must have a caregiver (whether family or nursing facility) who is able to ensure the care and safety of the patient. The patient should be evaluated by their primary care physician who can see to appropriate modifications to avoid delirium recurrence or to arrange neuropsychiatric testing to evaluate for dementia.

REFERENCES

1. American Psychiatric Association. *Diagnostic and Statistical Manual of Mental Disorders: DSM-5*. Washington, DC: American Psychiatric Association, 2013.
2. Hustey FM, Meldon SW. The prevalence and documentation of impaired mental status in elderly emergency department patients. *Ann Emerg Med* 2002;39(3):248–53.
3. Marx JA, Rosen P. *Rosen's Emergency Medicine: Concepts and Clinical Practice*. Philadelphia: Elsevier/Saunders, 2014.
4. Lonergan E, Britton AM, Luxenberg J, Wyller T. Antipsychotics for delirium. *Cochrane Database Syst Rev* 2007:CD00594.
5. Stratton SJ, Rogers C, Brickett K, Gruzinski G. Factors associated with sudden death of individuals requiring restraint for excited delirium. *Am J Emerg Med* 2001;19(3):187–91.

81 Psychiatric Emergencies: Factitious (Somatoform, Factitious, and Malingering) Disorders

Christopher P. Miller and Gregory M. Polites

GENERAL PRINCIPLES

Definition

- Somatoform disorder[1]—a condition where psychological distress is manifested as one or more physical symptoms that are not feigned by the patient.
  - Conversion—otherwise unexplained neurologic symptom associated with psychological stressors

- Psychogenic nonepileptic seizures (PNES)—formally "pseudoseizures." No abnormal electrical discharges in the brain are noted on electroencephalography (EEG) evaluation.
  ○ Hypochondriasis—fear and preoccupation with having a serious medical condition
- Factitious disorders[2]—symptoms intentionally feigned or produced by the patient in the absence of external incentives. The patient has pathologic need for the "sick role" and is willing to undergo unnecessary medical procedures or treatments.
  ○ Munchausen syndrome—symptoms are feigned or induced by the patient.
  ○ Munchausen syndrome by proxy—symptoms of a child are feigned or induced by the parent in order for the parent to assume the sick role through their child's treatment.[3]
- Malingering—intentional feigning or exaggerating of symptoms for purpose of external incentives including financial, work avoidance, housing, and prescription medications.[4]

Epidemiology

- Somatoform Disorders[1]
  ○ Thought to be 5–7% in the adult population with a female predominance.
- Factitious Disorders
  ○ Approximately 1200 new cases of Munchausen syndrome by proxy are thought to occur in the United States annually with a female predominance.[5]
- Malingering
  ○ Estimates of 1% of mental health patients, 10–20% of patients who threaten litigation at presentation, and associated with antisocial personality disorder.[4]

DIAGNOSIS

Clinical Presentation

- Patients present with symptoms or complaints of other medical conditions, although the motive is what separates these diagnoses.
  ○ Somatoform disorders—the patient is not consciously deceiving clinician.
  ○ Factitious disorders—the patient is consciously deceiving clinician for purpose or receiving medical attention.
  ○ Malingering—the patient is consciously deceiving clinician for purpose of secondary gain (place to sleep, avoiding work, litigation).

History

- Somatoform Disorders
  ○ Be sure to address the patients psyche in regard to stress, anxiety, and depression.
  ○ Prior records should be obtained to see what previous workup has been done for the same complaints (consults, imaging, and other diagnostic testing on prior visits).
- Factitious Disorders
  ○ Patients are often willing to submit themselves to diagnostic testing or treatment even if significant morbidity is associated (painful procedures, surgery, etc.).[6]
- Malingering
  ○ Vague history.
  ○ Feigned symptoms are often related to mental health because they are subjective in nature. Diagnostic testing can be skewed in the patient's favor.

Physical Examination
- Somatoform Disorders
  - While all complaints and symptoms should be examined as appropriate, the sheer number may be overwhelming to the clinician. It may be helpful to focus on the symptom(s) most concerning to the patient.
- Factitious Disorder
  - Perform a thorough examination focusing on the patient's symptoms and complaints.
  - Patients will be cooperative.
- Malingering
  - Perform a thorough examination focusing on the patient's symptoms and complaints.
  - Patients are often not cooperative.

Differential Diagnosis

- Anxiety or depression in patients with somatoform disorder.[7]
- Other differential diagnoses are those associated with the reported complaint.

TREATMENT

- Initial treatment should be based on clinical findings. If no explanation for the patient's symptoms and complaints is found, consideration can be given to trying to relay the clinician's concerns of underlying psychiatric disease.
  - Somatoform disorders—carefully explain to the patient that their symptoms may be a physical manifestation of underlying emotion and stress (even if the patient denies feeling this). Be sure to relay to the patient that you are not invalidating their symptoms, but merely giving another possible explanation.
  - Factitious disorders—there is no consensus as to the appropriate approach to discussing this diagnosis with the patient.
  - Malingering—provide clinical reassurance and try to avoid reinforcing the behavior (prolonged ED stay, food, prescriptions, etc.).

Medications

- There are no medications that are recommended to treat this spectrum of disorders.

SPECIAL CONSIDERATIONS

Disposition

- To home in the absence of new objective findings of organic disease.

REFERENCES

1. American Psychiatric Association. *Diagnostic and Statistical Manual of Mental Disorders: DSM-5.* Washington, DC: American Psychiatric Association, 2013.
2. Sutherland AJ, Rodin GM. Factitious disorders in a general hospital setting. *Psychosomatics* 1990;31(4):392–99.
3. Rosenberg DA. Web of deceit: a literature review of Munchausen syndrome by proxy. *Child Abuse Negl* 1987;11(4):547–63.
4. Sadock BJ, Sadock VA. *Kaplan & Sadock's Comprehensive Textbook of Psychiatry.* Philadelphia: Lippincott Williams & Wilkins, 2000.
5. Feldman MD. Munchausen by proxy and malingering by proxy. *Psychosomatics* 2004;45(4):365–66.
6. Stonnington C. Conversion disorder. *Am J Psychiatry* 2006;163(9):1510–7.
7. Rogers MP, Weinshenker NJ, Warshaw MG, et al. Prevalence of somatoform disorders in a large sample of patients with anxiety disorders. *Psychosomatics* 1996;37(1):17–22.

Psychiatric Emergencies: Suicidal Ideation and Homicidal Ideation

A. Benjamin Srivastava

Suicidal Ideation

GENERAL PRINCIPLES

Definitions[1]

- Suicide: the act of an individual intentionally ending his or her life
- Suicidal behavior: thoughts and actions related to an individual intentionally taking his or her own life
- Suicidal ideation: thoughts of an individual regarding intentionally taking his or her own life
- Suicide plan: formulation of a specific plot by an individual to end his or her own life
- Suicide attempt: engagement in potentially self-injurious behavior with at least some intention of dying as the result of that behavior

Epidemiology/Etiology[2]

- Risk factors include previous suicide attempt,[3] concomitant psychiatric diagnosis,[4–10] women ages 45–64 (by poison), men ages >75 (by poisoning)[11] (younger people have highest rates of ideation and attempts),[12] Native American/Native Alaskan, Caucasian,[2] family history of suicide, history of violence, childhood trauma, social factors of unemployment, low education level, single, and personality factors (impulsivity, perfectionism, high neuroticism, low extroversion, low optimism, and resilience).[1]

Pathophysiology[13]

- Complex gene–environment interactions
- Impairments in serotonin neurotransmitter system and hypothalamic–pituitary–adrenocortical (HPA) axis stress response

DIAGNOSIS

Clinical Presentation

History[4]
- Thorough history regarding past psychiatric history, diagnoses, and hospitalization, suicide attempts (severity, disposition, means, methods), and current psychiatric symptomatology:
  - Ask about current suicidal ideation, homicidal ideation, and planning for the future.
  - Ask specifically about current intent, current plans, and means.
- Family history of suicide attempts and psychiatric pathology
- Psychosocial history includes a thorough substance history, access to firearms, and level of psychosocial support.
- Collateral informants are indispensable.

Physical Examination
- Mental status exam is crucial
  - Objective signs of depression, mania, psychosis, substance intoxication, or withdrawal.
  - Dissimulation may present if the patient has clear, secondary gain.

Diagnostic Criteria

- Thorough risk assessment discussing risk and protective factors.[14]
- Assessment of risk and disposition is ultimately a clinical judgment (i.e., not a utilitarian measure of risk vs. benefits).[14]
- Beck Hopelessness and Beck Suicidal Intent Scales may be helpful.[4]
- The SADPERSONS score, though widely used, fails to consistently identify individuals requiring either inpatient psychiatric hospitalization or psychiatric aftercare, nor does it predict future hopelessness.[15]

TREATMENT

- Patient should always be in view of treatment staff and should not have access to potentially dangerous items.[16]
- Risk factor mitigation.[4,14,16]
  - Should involve family members and social support.
- Disposition planning: involuntary inpatient hospitalization versus voluntary inpatient hospitalization versus outpatient care.
  - Chronically suicidal patients, though at elevated risk, often benefit when denied admission, as admission would promote regression.
  - Substance use disorder treatment
  - Removal of firearms and limiting access to potentially dangerous items
- Risk assessment should be clearly documented.
- Consultation with psychiatry as necessary.

SPECIAL CONSIDERATIONS

Disposition

- Contingent upon clinical evaluation and risk assessment (involuntary inpatient hospitalization vs. voluntary inpatient hospitalization vs. outpatient treatment)

Homicidal Ideation and Risk of Violence Toward Others

GENERAL PRINCIPLES

Risk Factors for Violence

- Past history of violence, peaks in teenage years, dropping in the 30s and 40s, nonwhite individuals, male sex, lower socioeconomic status/employment stability, substance abuse, impulsivity/antisocial personality disorder, or a history of childhood trauma[14]

DIAGNOSIS

Clinical Evaluation

History
- A patient may have past psychiatric history, diagnoses, and hospitalizations.
- The patient should be questioned about a history of violence and suicide attempts—severity, disposition, means, methods.

- Current psychiatric symptomatology.
  - Ask specifically about current intent, current plans, and means.
- Psychosocial history including thorough substance history, access to firearms, and level of psychosocial support.
- Collateral informants are indispensible.

Physical Examination
- Mental status exam is crucial.
  - Objective signs of depression, mania, psychosis, substance intoxication, or withdrawal
  - Dissimulation may present if the patient has clear, secondary gain.

MANAGEMENT

- Perform an assessment discussing risk and protective factors.
- Assessment of risk and disposition is ultimately a clinical judgment (i.e., not a utilitarian measure of risk vs. benefits).
- If the patient's violent intentions are the result of treatable psychiatric illness, inpatient hospitalization (either voluntarily or involuntarily) is warranted.[14]
  - In certain circumstances (stable psychosocial support, access to care, dangerous means of attack removed, identifiable victim notified), outpatient treatment may be warranted.
- If the violent intent or actions are not derived from treatable psychopathology, contacting law enforcement is the appropriate intervention.[14]
- If the patient names a readily identifiable victim, may invoke Tarasoff Warning[14]
  - Physicians have a duty to protect a readily-identifiable victim.
  - Varies between states whether this is duty to warn or duty to protect, required or optional.
  - Physicians should have knowledge of state law and best practice.
- Clear documentation and risk assessment.
- Psychiatric consultation may be warranted.

SPECIAL CONSIDERATIONS

Disposition

- Contingent upon clinical evaluation and risk assessment (involuntary inpatient hospitalization vs. voluntary inpatient hospitalization vs. outpatient treatment)

REFERENCES

1. O'Connor RC, Nock MK. The psychology of suicidal behaviour. *Lancet Psychiatry* 2014;1: 73–85.
2. Web-Based Injury Statistics Query and Reporting System (WISQARS). National Center for Injury Prevention and Control, CDC (producer). 2013, Available at: http://www.cdc.gov/injury/wisqars/index.html
3. Bostwick JM, Pabbati C, Geske JR, et al. Suicide attempt as a risk factor for completed suicide: even more lethal than we knew. *Am J Psychiatry* 2016;173:1094–100.
4. American Psychiatric Association. Practice guideline for the assessment and treatment of patients with suicidal behaviors. *Am J Psychiatry* 2003;160:1–60.
5. Bostwick JM, Pankratz VS. Affective disorders and suicide risk: a reexamination. *Am J Psychiatry* 2000;157:1925–32.
6. Inskip HM, Harris EC, Barraclough B. Lifetime risk of suicide for affective disorder, alcoholism and schizophrenia. *Br J Psychiatry* 1998;172:35–7.
7. Pompili M, Amador XF, Girardi P, et al. Suicide risk in schizophrenia: learning from the past to change the future. *Ann Gen Psychiatry* 2007;6:10.

8. Schneider B. Substance use disorders and risk for completed suicide. *Arch Suicide Res* 2009;13:303–16.

9. Nepon J, Belik S-L, Bolton J, et al. The relationship between anxiety disorders and suicide attempts: findings from the National Epidemiologic Survey on Alcohol and Related Conditions. *Depress Anxiety* 2010;27:791–8.

10. Oldham JM. Borderline personality disorder and suicidality. *Am J Psychiatry* 2006;163:20–6.

11. National Center for Health Statistics. *About Underlying Cause of Death 1999–2014. CDC WONDER Online Database*; 2016.

12. Substance Abuse and Mental Health Services Administration. *Results from the 2013 National Survey on Drug Use and Health: Mental Health Findings*. Rockville, MD: Substance Abuse and Mental Health Services Administration, 2014.

13. van Heeringen K, Mann JJ. The neurobiology of suicide. *Lancet Psychiatry* 2014;1:63–72.

14. Appelbaum PS, Gutheil TG. *Clinical Handbook of Psychiatry & the Law*. 4th ed.: Lippincott Williams & Wilkins, 2007.

15. Saunders K, Brand F, Lascelles K, et al. The sad truth about the SADPERSONS scale: an evaluation of its clinical utility in self-harm patients. *Emerg Med J* 2014;31:796–8.

16. Riba MB, Rvindranath D, Winder GS. *Clinical Manual of Emergency Psychiatry*. 2nd ed. Arlington: American Psychiatric Association, 2016.

Psychiatric Emergencies: Acute Psychosis: Schizophrenia and Bipolar Disorder

A. Benjamin Srivastava

GENERAL PRINCIPLES

Definitions

Schizophrenia

- A chronic, debilitating brain illness affecting emotion, volition, and cognition, characterized by hallucinations, delusions, and disorganization of speech and/or behavior. Anhedonia, avolition, alogia, inattention, poor executive functioning, or deficits in working memory may also be present and not attributable to the physiologic affects of a substance or another medical condition.[1,2]

Bipolar Affective Disorder, Type 1

- A disorder characterized by the presence of at least one manic episode for a period lasting 1 week with three additional symptoms (grandiosity, increased goal-directed behavior, impulsive/reckless/dangerous behavior, hypertalkativity, flight of ideas, distractibility) or irritable mood with four of the additional symptoms[1]

    ○ Must cause marked impairment in functioning, result in hospitalization, and/or contain psychotic symptoms.
- Can also have major depressive episodes lasting at least 2 weeks (depressed mood or anhedonia) with at least four of the following symptoms (appetite changes, insomnia, hypersomnia, psychomotor agitation or retardation, loss of energy, worthlessness, guilt, impaired concentration, indecisiveness, suicidality, or thoughts of death)

Catatonia
- A volitional disorder that is characterized by three of the following:[1,3]
  - Stupor (absence of psychomotor activity or responsiveness)
  - Catalepsy (passive, even resistance against gravity)
  - Waxy flexibility (even resistance to passive, positional changes)
  - Mutism (minimal expressive speech)
  - Negativism (oppositional or absent response to instructions)
  - Posturing (spontaneous initiation/maintenance of antigravity posture)
  - Mannerism (odd, circumstantial conduction of normal movements)
  - Stereotypy (repetitive, frequent, nongoal directed movements)
  - Agitation (internally derived)
  - Grimacing
  - Echolalia (repetition of another's speech)
  - Echopraxia (repetition of another's behavior)
- More common in bipolar disorder (during both manic and depressed phases) but can be seen in neurodevelopmental (autism), infections, metabolic, or autoimmune disorders.

Epidemiology/Etiology
Schizophrenia
- Males are more likely than females to be affected; males typically present in their mid to early 20s and females are more likely to present in their late 20s.[1,4]

Bipolar Disorder
- Males and females are equally affected.[1]

Pathophysiology
Schizophrenia
- Complex gene and environmental stressor interaction: neonatal insults, urban rearing, childhood trauma, intellectual disability, and marijuana.[4,5]
- Dopamine hypothesis: Striatal hyperdopaminergia is thought to be linked to positive symptoms; cortical hypopaminergia to negative and cognitive symptoms.
- NMDA hypofunction

Bipolar Disorder
- Pathophysiology poorly characterized as there is inconsistency in data and findings[6]

DIAGNOSIS

Clinical Presentation
History
- A longitudinal history is essential for discernment between bipolar disorder and schizophrenia (the Kraepelinian Dichotomy).[7]

- Schizophrenia
  - Prodromal phase (social withdrawal, loss of interest, inattention)
  - Can have periods of mania and major depression
  - Terminal state of some degree of loss of volition
- Bipolar disorder
  - Episodic periods of mania and/or depression
  - Often have stable inter-episodic functioning
  - Psychotic symptoms can appear during either mania or depression

Physical Examination
- Acutely, bipolar disorder and schizophrenia can appear identical and may share symptoms of each disorder.
- Diagnosis should not be made solely based on mental status examination; it requires knowledge of longitudinal history, delineation from other illness, family history, and biomarkers.[8]

Differential Diagnosis
- Schizoaffective disorder[10]
- Major depressive disorder
  - Delusional disorders, anxiety disorders, attention deficit, or hyperactivity disorder
  - Decompensated borderline or antisocial personality disorders
  - Paranoid, schizoid, or schizotypal personality disorders
  - Thyroid disease, Cushing disease, multiple sclerosis, and autoimmune encephalitis
  - Dementia, delirium acute intermittent porphyria, Wilson disease, Huntington disease, B_{12} deficiency, HSV, HIV, syphilis, or intoxication[1,9]

Diagnostic Criteria and Testing
- Formal diagnosis should be confirmed by a psychiatrist.

Laboratories
- On the initial presentation, a full lab workup should be performed including RPR and urine drug screen.

TREATMENT

Medications
- Typical antipsychotics:[11]
  - High potency: Haloperidol 5 mg q6h PRN PO or IM
    - Maximum daily dose 20 mg.
    - Recommend telemetry if given IV because of risk of QTc prolongation and torsades de pointes.
    - Give with lorazepam 1–2 mg PO q6h PO or IM.
    - Monitor for extrapyramidal symptoms (acute dystonia, parkinsonism, akathisia): Treat with benztropine 1–2 mg IM or PO or Benadryl 25–50 mg PO (if pregnant).
  - Low potency: chlorpromazine 25–50 mg q4h PRN PO or IM
    - Maximum daily dose 200 mg
    - Monitor for QTc prolongation and hypotension.
    - Can cause excess sedation and rebound agitation/hypertension
- Atypical neuroleptics:
  - Olanzapine 5–10 mg PO or IM q4–8h
    - Monitor for excess sedation.

- Avoid giving IM olanzapine with IM benzodiazepines (increased risk for respiratory depression).
  - Monitor blood pressure (can cause orthostatic hypotension).
  - Ziprazidone and aripiprazole are available in parenteral formulations
- Lithium (for acute mania): 600 mg starting dose, can increase to TID 900 mg (in two doses)
  - Check TSH and BMP.
  - Avoid NSAIDs and diuretics.
- Catatonia[3,12]
  - Antipsychotics and electroconvulsive therapy are the treatments of choice.
  - Benzodiazepines work ~30% of the time.

Nonpharmacologic Interventions

- Risk assessment for suicide and violence toward others
- Structured, safe environment.
- Avoid physical restraints if possible.

SPECIAL CONSIDERATIONS

Disposition

- Often will require psychiatric consult to determine if the patient meets criteria for inpatient admission if cleared medically.

REFERENCES

1. American Psychiatric Association. *Diagnostic and Statistical Manual of Mental Disorders: DSM-5.* Arlington: American Psychiatric Association, 2013.
2. Zorumski CFR. *E.H. Psychiatry and Clinical Neuroscience.* New York: Oxford University Press, 2011.
3. Peralta V, Campos MS, de Jalon EG, et al. DSM-IV catatonia signs and criteria in first-episode, drug-naive, psychotic patients: psychometric validity and response to antipsychotic medication. *Schizophrenia Res* 2010;118:168–75.
4. Insel TR. Rethinking schizophrenia. *Nature* 2010;468:187–93.
5. Millan MJ, Andrieux A, Bartzokis G, et al. Altering the course of schizophrenia: progress and perspectives. *Nat Rev Drug Discov* 2016;15:485–515.
6. Ozerdem A, Ceylan D, Can G. Neurobiology of risk for bipolar disorder. *Curr Treat Options Psychiatry* 2016;3:315–29.
7. Kendler KS. Kraepelin and the differential diagnosis of dementia praecox and manic-depressive insanity. *Compr Psychiatry* 1986;27:549–58.
8. Feighner JP, Robins E, Guze SB, et al. Diagnostic criteria for use in psychiatric research. *Arch Gen Psychiatry* 1972;26:57–63.
9. Riba MB, Rvindranath D, Winder GS. *Clinical Manual of Emergency Psychiatry.* 2nd ed. Arlington: American Psychiatric Association, 2016.
10. Kotov R, Leong SH, Mojtabai R, et al. Boundaries of schizoaffective disorder: revisiting kraepelin. *JAMA Psychiatry* 2013;70:1276–86.
11. Stahl SM. *Essential Psychopharmacology Prescriber's Guide.* 5th ed. New York: Cambridge University Press, 2014.
12. England ML, Öngür D, Konopaske GT, et al. Catatonia in psychotic patients: clinical features and treatment response. *J Neuropsychiatry Clin Neurosci* 2011;23:223–6.

84 Psychiatric Emergencies: Anxiety and Panic

Christopher P. Miller

GENERAL PRINCIPLES

Definition

- Anxiety is defined as an emotional response to anticipation of future threat, which can be contrasted to fear which is an emotional response to real or perceived imminent threat.[1]
- Panic attacks are defined by abrupt onset of extreme fear which are often unexpected and may not have any clear triggering event.[1]
- Anxiety disorders cover a large spectrum of disease ranging from generalized anxiety disorder (GAD), panic disorder, phobias (agoraphobia, social phobia, among others), obsessive–compulsive disorder (OCD), posttraumatic stress disorder (PTSD), separation anxiety disorder, and substance-induced anxiety.

Epidemiology

- The conditions tend to present before the third or fourth decade of life.
- Anxiety disorders are more prevalent in women, and those who have a strong family history, and those who have suffered traumatic life events. In addition, patients who suffer from comorbid chronic conditions such as migraines and irritable bowel syndrome are more likely to have an anxiety disorder.[3]

Pathophysiology

- Believed to be related to low serotonin system activity, elevated noradrenergic system activity, and γ-aminobutyric acid (GABA) receptors.

DIAGNOSIS

Clinical Presentation

History
- Patients will describe a gradual or sudden onset of a fear and panic-producing state.

Physical Examination
- Should be tailored to the presenting symptoms

Differential Diagnosis

- Primary anxiety disorders[4]
  - GAD, panic attack, PTSD, or OCD
  - Bipolar disorder, schizophrenia, and somatoform disorders
- Medical illness that have symptoms that may present as anxiety:
  - Cardiac—myocardial infarction, arrhythmias
  - Endocrine—hyperthyroidism, pheochromocytoma, hyper/hypoglycemia

- ○ Pulmonary—asthma, chronic obstructive pulmonary disease (COPD)
- ○ Neurologic—seizure, transient ischemic attack, cerebrovascular accident
- ○ Substance use—amphetamines, cocaine, caffeine, and other sympathomimetics.

Diagnostic Criteria and Testing
- Formal diagnosis should be deferred to an outpatient psychologist or psychiatrist.

TREATMENT
- Medication can be administered to help with anxiolysis, which may be necessary before initial evaluation is even performed.
- If an underlying medical condition is diagnosed, it should be treated as indicated.

Medications
- Benzodiazepines
  - ○ Lorazepam: 1–2 mg IV or PO
  - ○ A short PRN course can be prescribed for durations of no >1 week to help patients until they can arrange follow-up with their primary care provider or psychiatrist.[4]
- Selective Serotonin Reuptake Inhibitors (SSRIs), serotonin-norepinephrine receptor inhibitors (SNRIs), monoamine oxidase inhibitors (MAOIs), tricyclic antidepressants (TCAs)
  - ○ Typically deferred to the outpatient setting

SPECIAL CONSIDERATIONS

Disposition
- These patients can usually be discharged; however, in severe situations, it may be necessary to consult psychiatry for evaluation in the emergency department for medication management and to help arrange follow-up.

Complications
- Anxiety and panic states can often overlap with organic disease and differentiation between the two is imperative.

REFERENCES

1. American Psychiatric Association. *Diagnostic and Statistical Manual of Mental Disorders: DSM-5*. Washington, DC: American Psychiatric Association, 2013.
2. McPheeters R, Tobias JL. Anxiety Disorders In: Marx JA, Hockberger RS, Walls RM, eds. *Rosen's Emergency Medicine*. 8th ed Philadephia PA: Saunders-Elsevier 2014. pp 1474–1480
3. Rowney J, Hermida T, Malone D. *Anxiety Disorders*. Cleveland Clinic, 2016.

85 Personality Disorders

Christopher P. Miller

GENERAL PRINCIPLES

Definitions

- Personality disorder—a consistent pattern of thought and behavior that is outside the normal expectations of a person's culture, persistent and unchanging, develops before early adulthood, and leads to distress and impairment.[1]
  - Cluster A—odd and eccentric
    - Paranoid—suspicion and distrust of others and the assumption that others' actions are deliberate acts to exploit, deceive, or harm the patient
    - Schizoid—detachment and avoidance form social relationships
    - Schizotypal—avoidance of social relationships as well as cognitive distortions, often described as having "magical thinking"
  - Cluster B—hyperemotional and dramatic in emotions and behavior
    - Antisocial—disregards and violates the rights of others, deceitful and manipulative, often described as "psychopathic." These patients are often seen in the ED.
    - Borderline—unstable personal relationships, labile moods, impulsive, and practice self-harm for attention. These patients are often seen in the ED.
    - Histrionic—attention seeking, flirtatious, dramatic, "life of the party"
    - Narcissistic—grandiose, lacks empathy, desire to be admired
  - Cluster C—anxious and fearful
    - Avoidant—social inhibition, feeling inadequate, desires to be social unlike schizotypal
    - Dependent—desire/need to be taken care of resulting in submissive behavior and fear of being separated. Passive, allowing others to make their decisions
    - Obsessive–compulsive—preoccupation with order and control that negatively affects the patient's personal life

Epidemiology

- Antisocial
  - Risk factors for antisocial personality disorder (ASPD) are low socioeconomic status[1] and first-degree family members with the disease.
- Borderline
  - Risk factors for a borderline personality disorder include a first-degree family member with the disease and a history of childhood trauma.[2]
  - Among patients in the clinical setting, women are three times more common than men to have this disorder, even though it is likely equivalent in the general population.[3]

DIAGNOSIS

- Should not be made upon one visit or interaction with a patient but if necessary should be made by a psychiatrist or psychologist.

Clinical Presentation

History
- Patients with ASPD may describe wanting to commit violent acts, whereas borderline patients may describe a desire for self-harm or complain of acute pain.

Physical Examination
- Attention should be paid to evidence of self-harm with borderline personality disorder.

Differential Diagnosis
- Psychotic disorder—schizophrenia, mania
- Anxiety, depression, PTSD, substance abuse
- Other nonpsychiatric medical condition—dementia, brain lesion

TREATMENT

- No acute treatment is indicated for patients with a personality disorder. However, if the patient consents, psychiatric follow-up should be provided.

SPECIAL CONSIDERATIONS

Disposition
- Patients may be discharged to home with psychiatric follow-up, unless felt to be at risk to themselves or others.

REFERENCES

1. American Psychiatric Association. *Diagnostic and Statistical Manual of Mental Disorders: DSM-5.* Washington, DC: American Psychiatric Association, 2013.
2. Zanarini MC, Williams AA, Lewis RE, et al. Reported pathological childhood experiences associated with the development of borderline personality disorder. *Am J Psychiatry* 1997;154(8): 1101–6.
3. Grant BF, Chou SP, Goldstein RB, et al. Prevalence, correlates, disability, and comorbidity of DSM-IV borderline personality disorder. *J Clin Psychiatry* 2008;69(4):533–45.

86 Psychiatric Emergencies: Tardive Dyskinesia

Christopher P. Miller

GENERAL PRINCIPLES

Definition
- Abnormal involuntary movements of the tongue, face, and cheek after chronic exposure to dopamine receptor blocking agents that persists after medication withdrawal[1]

Epidemiology

- Twenty percent of patients treated with neuroleptic drugs will develop tardive dyskinesia (TD) at some point during treatment.[2]
  - There is a higher incidence and lower remission[3] of tardive dyskinesia in elderly patients.
  - First-generation antipsychotics such as haloperidol carry a higher incidence[1] of dyskinesia.
  - A longer exposure to the offending agent carries a greater risk of development.[1]

Pathophysiology

- Chronic blocking of the dopamine receptor leads to more receptors being produced and an up-regulation in their sensitivity.[4]
  - Medications most frequently associated with TD include levodopa, cocaine, amphetamines, tricyclic antidepressants (TCAs), antihistamines, and lithium.

DIAGNOSIS

Clinical Presentation

- This is primarily a clinical diagnosis based on history, review of patient medication exposure, and physical examination.

History

- The patient will present with a history of the slow development of repetitive facial movements after a long-term use of a dopamine blocking agent, such as haloperidol or metoclopramide.

Physical Examination

- Abnormal, involuntary facial twitching of face, lips, and tongue
  - Can be suppressed by having patient talk or eat
  - The facial movements are repetitive and extinguishable.

Differential Diagnosis

- Huntington disease, central nervous system (CNS) tumor, stroke, hyperthyroidism, electrolyte disturbance[1]

TREATMENT

- Removal of the offending agent.
  - No emergent indication for treatment; it is best handled by patient's primary care physician or psychiatrist.

Medications

- Clozapine—although an atypical antipsychotic, it is a weak blocker of D2 dopamine receptors and has been shown to decrease tardive symptoms by as much as 30%.[1] This medication should be started by the patient's neurologist or psychiatrist who can follow therapy long term.
- Benzodiazepines[5] and vitamin E[6] have been inconsistently shown to be helpful in reducing a patient's symptoms.

SPECIAL CONSIDERATIONS

Disposition

- Patients with TD can usually be discharged home. The practitioner should attempt to contact the patient's primary care physician or primary psychiatrist to make medication changes prior to discharge.

Complications

- Removal of offending agent may exacerbate underlying disease medication is treating. Consultation with prescriber is highly recommended.

REFERENCES

1. Fernandez HH, Friedman JH. Classification and treatment of tardive syndromes. *Neurologist* 2003;9(1):16–27.
2. Kane JM, Woerner M, Lieberman J. Tardive dyskinesia. *J Clin Psychopharmacol* 1988;8(4 Suppl):52S–56S.
3. Muscettola G, Pampallona S, Barbato G, et al. Persistent tardive dyskinesia: demographic and pharmacological risk factors. *Acta Psychiatr Scand* 1993;87(1):29–36.
4. Klawans HL, Tanner CM, Goetz CG. Epidemiology and pathophysiology of tardive dyskinesias. *Adv Neurology* 1988;49:185–97.
5. Walker P, Soares KVS. Benzodiazepines for neuroleptic-induced tardive dyskinesia. *Cochrane Database Syst Rev* 2003;(2):CD000205.
6. McGrath JJ, Soares KV. Vitamin E for neuroleptic-induced tardive dyskinesia. *Cochrane Database Syst Rev* 2001;(4):CD000209.

87 Renal and GU Emergencies: Acid–Base Disturbances

Lucy Yang Hormberg and S. Eliza Dunn

GENERAL PRINCIPLES

- Suspect an acid–base abnormality in any patient who has abnormal vital signs (especially abnormal respiratory rate or breathing pattern), altered mental status, or signs of impaired perfusion.[1]
- Several studies have shown a close correlation between pH and pCO_2 values from an arterial blood gas (ABG) or venous blood gas (VBG).[2] However, studies have not yet evaluated the correlation between ABG and VBG values in patients with hemodynamic shock.

- A patient may have multiple, coexisting problems that can simultaneously cause acid–base disturbances.
  - Changes in pCO_2 through respiratory ventilation, directly changes the $[H^+]$ of plasma and plasma pH.[3]
  - A patient may have several coexisting metabolic disturbances because there are multiple etiologies or mechanisms that can produce and/or maintain the metabolic acid and base disturbances.
  - Unlike pCO_2, which directly changes $[H^+]$ and thus plasma pH, the $[HCO_3^-]$ does not necessarily directly change the plasma pH because of the presence of other buffers in the blood. While plasma pH is primarily determined by H_2CO_3/HCO_3^- buffer system, bicarbonate is an important alkali buffer in human blood, but it is not the only buffer. Understanding the limitations of using this bicarbonate buffer system as a proxy for all the acidic and basic components of human blood is crucial to understanding the limitations of the Henderson–Hasselbalch approach in patients, especially those who are critically ill.

Definition

- The normal human extracellular (plasma) pH is ~7.40 ± 0.03.
- Acidosis is a pathologic process that causes the normal plasma pH of 7.40 to decrease. Conversely, an alkalosis is the process that drives plasma pH above 7.40.

Epidemiology/Etiologies

- Acid–base disturbances are not uncommon in the ED and common in ICUs.[4] Metabolic alkalosis is the most common acid–base disturbance seen in critically ill patients.
- Etiologies—See Figure 87.1.

Pathophysiology

- A typical "Western" diet can generate 1 mEq of acid/kg/d from sulfur containing amino acids. Normal blood pH is maintained through intracellular and extracellular chemical buffering, respiratory ventilation of pCO_2, and renal physiology.

DIAGNOSIS

Respiratory Acidosis

History

- Patients with acute CO_2 retention, or "CO_2 narcosis," may present with generalized weakness, tremors, headaches, and/or blurry vision.

Physical Examination

- Patients may have altered mental status including drowsiness, be bradypneic or have shallow respirations, and manifest other neurologic symptoms such as tremors and papilledema.

Diagnostic Criteria

Laboratories

- Patients with chronic respiratory acidosis may have a normal pH. At about 6–12 hours of sustained respiratory acidosis, the kidneys contribute to acid–base homeostasis by excreting ammonium and chloride into the urine to generate bicarbonate

Steps	Etiologies		Problem List and DDx
	Finding	Acid–Base Disturbance	
STEP 1: Obtain labs • Blood gas (VBG or ABG) • Electrolytes • As indicated: CBC, albumin, lactate, ketones (point of care, urine, or serum), serum osmolality, ethanol		**Evaluate each disturbance as a separate problem**	Narrow the differential diagnosis based on the clinical context
STEP 2: Look at the pCO_2 Normal $pCO_2 \approx 40$ mm Hg	High pCO_2	**Respiratory acidosis**	Any etiology of hypoventilation
	Low pCO_2	**Respiratory alkalosis**	Any etiology of hyperventilation
STEP 3: Look at the HCO_3^-: Normal $HCO_3^- \approx 22–28$ mmol/L	High HCO_3^-	**Metabolic alkalosis**	▪ Volume loss ▪ Gastric loss ▪ Diuretics ▪ Mineralocorticoid effects on the kidneys
	Low HCO_3^-	*Metabolic acidosis*	
STEP 3A: Calculate an anion gap (AG)[1,2] $AG = Na^+ - Cl^- - HCO_3^-$ Normal AG ≈ 12 • Albumin	Normal AG[3]	**Nonanion gap, hyperchloremic** metabolic acidosis	▪ Diarrhea ▪ Renal loss (RTA) ▪ Administration of chloride containing fluids or compounds
STEP 3B: Calculate osmolar gap (OG) $OG = $ Serum osmolality $-$ $2Na^+ + BUN/2.8 +$ glucose/18 + EtOH/4.6	AG > 12 • Ketones • Lactate • Serum osmolality • Ethanol	**Anion gap** metabolic acidosis	"KULT"[4] ▪ Ketoacidosis ▪ Uremia ▪ Lactic acidosis ▪ Toxic alcohols
STEP 3C: Calculate AG – 12+ HCO_3^-	AG – 12+ $HCO_3^- < 24$	Presence of additional **nonanion gap** metabolic acidosis	
	AG – 12+ $HCO_3^- > 26$	Presence of coexisting **metabolic alkalosis**	

[1]May correct for hypoalbuminemia, although controversial (see Suggested Readings). Adjusted AG = observed AG + 0.25 × (normal albumin – patient's albumin), where albumin concentrations are in g/L. If albumin is given in g/dL, the factor is 2.5.

Figge J, Jabor A, Kazda A, et al. Anion gap and hypoalbuminemia. *Crit Care Med* 1998; 26:1807–10.

Dinh CH, Ng R, Grandinetti A, et al. Correcting the anion gap for hypoalbuminaemia does not improve detection of hyperlactataemia. *Emerg Med* 2006;23(8):627–9. doi: 10.1136/emj.2005.031898.

[2]For anion gap calculations, do not correct sodium concentration for hyperglycemia. The measured serum sodium is a true value. NB To help physicians assess the degree of dehydration present in severely hyperglycemic patients. Katz et al. originally suggested a "correction" of the measured serum sodium to the sodium concentration that would be present after the resolution of the hyperglycemia.

Varon J, Jacobs MB, Mahoney CA. Reflections on the anion gap in hyperglycemia. *West J Med* 1992;157(6):670–2.

[3]What about a low anion gap? See Suggested Readings.

[4]Simplification, and more importantly, the actual types of acidosis underlying the mnemonics "MUDPILES" and "GOLDMARK."

Figure 87.1. Calculation and Etiologies of Acid-Base Disturbances.

for reabsorption. This regenerated bicarbonate is then an additional buffering capacity in the blood, helping to normalize plasma pH.

• Chronic hypochloremia is common in patients with chronic respiratory acidosis because excretion of Cl^- anion balances the negative charges of the additional reabsorbed plasma HCO_3^- anions.

Differential Diagnosis

- Causes of acute or acutely worsening respiratory acidosis include any disorder that decreases lung ventilation or central nervous system (CNS) control of ventilation—acute airway obstruction, lung parenchymal disease, neuromuscular disorders, and CNS depression.

TREATMENT

- Any etiology that leads to respiratory fatigue and consequent respiratory acidosis should prompt the emergency provider to consider intubation for mechanical ventilation.
- Additional treatment consists of identifying and correcting the acute or acutely exacerbated underlying etiologies.

Respiratory Alkalosis

History

- Patients with acute respiratory alkalosis may present with spasm (secondary to increased protein binding of calcium (tetany)), report numbness and tingling in the lips and extremities, and complain of light-headedness.

Physical Examination

- These patients may be tachypneic and may have carpopedal spasms.

Diagnostic Criteria and Testing

Laboratories

- An ABG may show hypoxia, an important etiology of respiratory alkalosis.
- Consider infectious, metabolic, toxicologic, and other laboratory workup as indicated.

Differential Diagnoses

- Hypoxia may be the cause of tachypnea and consequential respiratory alkalosis.
- Other etiologies that affect CNS respiratory control centers: fever/infection, head trauma/stroke/mass, and toxins such as aspirin.
- Other etiologies from CNS stimulation include pain, anxiety, voluntary or iatrogenic mechanical hyperventilation, and increased progesterone or thyroid hormone states.

TREATMENT

- Identify and treat the underlying etiology.
- Acute respiratory alkalosis from voluntary hyperventilation can be treated with rebreathing from a paper bag.
- Regardless of etiology, when a patient begins to fatigue, a "normalizing" respiratory alkalosis or developing respiratory acidosis in this clinically ill patient suggests impending respiratory failure and should prompt mechanical ventilation.

Metabolic Acidosis

History

- A history should include questions about diabetes, infectious symptomatology, chronic kidney disease, toxic ingestions, diarrhea, and other potential etiologies.

Physical Examination

- Patients with metabolic causes of acidemia, in general, will exhibit compensatory hyperventilation. The deep, regular, sighing respirations are called Kussmaul respirations. Kussmaul respirations can be of any rate—slow, normal, or fast. Tachypnea in some of these patients may also be characterized as "quiet" or tachypnea without signs of respiratory distress.

Differential Diagnosis

- Anion gap metabolic acidoses:
  - Increased anion gap represents the concentration of anions that were historically unable to be measured or not routinely measured with serum electrolytes (lactates, phosphates, sulfates, other organic acids, albumin, and other proteins, etc.).
  - Etiology of elevated anion gap metabolic acidoses can be divided into four subtypes:
    - Ketoacidosis (diabetic, starvation, alcoholic, some inborn errors of metabolism)
    - Lactic acidosis from anaerobic metabolism from global or cellular hypoxia or from tissue hypoperfusion
    - Renal failure with plasma accumulation of phosphates, sulfates, and other products of protein metabolism and with other significant electrolyte abnormalities and fluid retention
    - Toxins (salicylates, acetaminophen, ethanol, toxic alcohols—methanol and ethylene glycol)
      - Salicylate poisoning initially exerts a toxic effect on the respiratory center producing a respiratory alkalosis. In addition, salicylates cause the uncoupling of oxidative phosphorylation, leading eventually to accumulation of other acidotic metabolites.
      - Ethanol is metabolized to acetate, which is then used up in the tricyclic antidepressant (TCA) cycle, so ethanol intoxication alone would not be expected to cause an anion gap metabolic acidosis. Chronic ethanol abuse may produce two forms of increased anion gap acidoses: (1) alcoholic ketoacidosis can result from binge drinking with prolonged period of decreased food intake or with vomiting and (2) alcoholic lactic acidosis can result from increased lactate production during ethanol ingestion and decreased liver clearance by diseased liver.
      - Methanol is converted to formatic acid; ethylene glycol to glycolic acid (and oxalic acid). These toxic metabolites cause an increased anion gap. Oxalate causes acute renal failure through the precipitation of calcium oxalate crystals. Glycolic acid may be misinterpreted by some point of care blood gas analyzers as lactic acid.
      - Ethanol, methanol, and ethylene glycol also increase the measured plasma osmolality. The osmolar gap is the difference between the measured and the calculated expected plasma osmolality created by these alcohols.
- Hyperchloremic, nonanion gap metabolic acidoses:
  - Caused by GI or renal bicarbonate loss or administration of Cl^- containing solutions/medications
    - Normal saline resuscitation, $CaCl_2$, $MgCl_2$, NH_4Cl, and cholestyramine.
    - Diarrheal, biliary, pancreatic, and small bowel fluids contain high concentrations of bicarbonate, potassium, and relatively low concentrations of chloride. Thus, loss from these sites results in imbalance of bicarbonate and chloride ions, leading to metabolic acidosis without an anion gap since both of these anions are routinely measured electrolytes. An ileal conduit or other condition in which urine has prolonged contact with the bowel mucosa may result in an active secretary loss of bicarbonate and passive urinary absorption of chloride, leading to an acidosis.
    - In renal tubular acidosis (RTA), acetazolamide therapy, and hypoaldosteronism, an acidosis is created by renal loss of bicarbonate (or, in case of distal RTA, the inability to excrete acid loads).

TREATMENT

- Identify and treat underlying cause.
- Administering bicarbonate for severe acidemia for purpose of correcting the acidemia alone is controversial. In general, sodium bicarbonate should be used when either the sodium or the bicarbonate addresses an underlying problem (such as tricyclic overdose, other medication overdoses causing sodium channel blockade, aspirin overdose, or hyperkalemia) or as a temporizing measure until hemodialysis (such as in methanol or ethylene glycol ingestions). Otherwise, therapy should first be directed at optimizing respiratory status (fixing pCO_2) and treating the underlying etiology in these acidemic patients.

Metabolic Alkalosis

History

- Symptoms may relate to any coexisting hypokalemia, hypocalcemia, or inhibition of the respiratory center in the medulla. Patient may report dyspnea, muscular and cardiac symptoms such as weakness, global paralysis, muscle cramps, and syncope (hypokalemia) or spasms, perioral numbness/tingling, and fatigue (hypocalcemia). History should inquire into vomiting and diuretic use.

Physical Examination

- Patients may present with weakness, arrhythmias, tetany, and hypoventilation.

Differential Diagnosis

- Any process that causes a relatively lower concentration of $[H^+]$ and $[Cl^-]$ compared to $[HCO_3^-]$ and $[Na^+]$ in the plasma can cause a metabolic alkalosis. Renal mechanisms contribute to the creation or maintenance of the disturbance.
  - Vomiting or suctioning of gastric content, due to loss of gastric fluid that has a relatively high $[H^+]$ and $[Cl^-]$
  - Diuretics
  - Mineralocorticoid activity (aldosterone, natural licorice, etc.)
  - Plasma volume contraction
  - Hypoproteinemia

Diagnostic Criteria and Testing

Laboratories

- Hypokalemia, hypocalcemia, and hypochloremia may be seen.

TREATMENT

- Replace volume and identify and treat underlying cause.

SUGGESTED READING

Rutledge TF. Acid-base disturbances in the emergency department: Part 2: making the diagnosis. *Can Fam Physician* 1991;37:2469–75.

REFERENCES

1. Rutledge TF. Acid-base disturbances in the emergency department: Part 2: making the diagnosis. *Can Fam Physician* 1991;37:2469–75.

2. Kelly AM. Review article: can venous blood gas analysis replace arterial in emergency medical care. *Emerg Med Australas* 2010;22:493–498. doi: 10.1111/j.1742-6723.2010.01344.x.
3. Kishen R, Honoré PM, Jacobs R, et al. Facing acid–base disorders in the third millennium–the Stewart approach revisited. *Int J Nephrol Renovasc Dis* 2014;7:209–17. doi: 10.2147/IJNRD.S62126.
4. Gunnerson KJ. Clinical review: the meaning of acid–base abnormalities in the intensive care unit part I–epidemiology. *Crit Care* 2005;9(5):508–16. doi: 10.1186/cc3796.

88 Renal and GU Emergencies: Acute Kidney Injury and Chronic Kidney Disease

S. Eliza Dunn and Carol Faulk

GENERAL PRINCIPLES

Definition and Classification

Acute Kidney Injury
- AKI is defined as:
  - An increase in serum creatinine that is equal to or more than 0.3 mg/dL within 48 hours; or
  - Increase in serum creatinine to 1.5 × baseline, which is known or presumed to have occurred within the prior 7 days; or
  - Urine volume < 0.5 mL/kg/h for 6 hours[1]
- Classifying AKI based on urine output
  - Oliguric AKI: <500 mL/d
  - Anuric AKI: <50 mL/d[2]

Chronic Kidney Disease
- CKD can be defined as an abnormality of kidney structure or function lasting for more than 3 months.[3]
- CKD includes renal abnormalities such as a glomerular filtration rate (GFR) < 60 mL/min/1.73 m², microalbuminuria, casts in the urine, a history of kidney transplant, abnormalities detected by a previous kidney biopsy, or structural abnormalities (e.g., horseshoe kidney).[3]

- End-stage renal disease is defined as the complete loss of kidney function for longer than 3 months.[4]

Epidemiology/Etiology
AKI
- Acute critical illness, older age, and a history of previous AKI are all risk factors.[4,5]

CKD
- The major risk factors for development of CKD include AKI, older age, diabetes, hypertension, cardiovascular disease, and higher body mass index.[5]

Pathophysiology
- Prerenal AKI: This type of AKI is due to reduced blood flow to the kidneys secondary to hypovolemia or vasodilation or intra-abdominal compartment syndrome.[4]
  - Renal artery stenosis, cardiorenal syndrome, and hepatorenal syndrome can also cause AKI.[6,7]
  - Medications that cause intrarenal vasoconstriction include NSAIDs, ACE Inhibitors/angiotensin receptor blockers (ARBs), cyclosporine, and tacrolimus.
- Intrinsic renal failure
  - Acute interstitial nephritis is defined by histologic findings of interstitial inflammation, edema, and tubulitis and is most commonly caused by medications.[8,9,13]
  - Drug-induced acute interstitial nephritis most commonly occurs 7–10 days after exposure.
- Postrenal causes of AKI are a result of increased pressure on the renal tubules from inability of patients to void.[10]
  - Benign prostatic hyperplasia (BPH), obstructing mass from cancer, postsurgical changes (usually after a hysterectomy), renal stones, or blood clots in the bladder or urethra are common causes.

DIAGNOSIS

Clinical Presentation
- Renal failure often presents asymptomatically and is incidentally noted on the patient's lab values.[10]

History
- Ask patients about nephrotoxins including contrast administration and over-the-counter NSAID use.
- Patients should be questioned about diuretic overuse and symptoms of anemia, infection, pancreatitis, DKA, or gastroenteritis.
- Obstructive AKI patients may give a history of BPH or pelvic or genitourinary cancers.
- A history of pharyngeal infection, HIV, lupus, and diabetes or a history of other nephropathies should be obtained.

Physical Examination
- Hypovolemic renal failure: orthostatic hypotension, dry mucous membranes, poor skin turgor, and low jugular venous pressure
- Hypervolemic renal failure: jugular venous distention, an S_3 gallop, lower extremity edema, and pulmonary rales
  - Patients with glomerulonephritis can have moderate edema and hypertension.

- Obstructive renal failure: a feeling of fullness and palpable bladder on exam
- Nephritic renal failure: mild edema, hypertension, hematuria, and oliguria that can occur with certain types of acute glomerulonephritis
- Nephrotic renal failure: severe edema from proteinuria

Diagnostic Testing

Laboratories
- Diagnostic testing for anyone with known or suspected AKI or CKD includes serum electrolyte levels (including potassium, magnesium, and phosphorous) and urinalysis.
- BUN to creatinine ratio (>20 suggests prerenal AKI; <10–15 suggests intrinsic AKI) and urine specific gravity may help determine whether a patient has a prerenal AKI or an intrinsic renal AKI.[11]
- Findings from a urinalysis can suggest different diagnoses.
  - Interstitial nephritis can often present with hematuria and pyuria on urinalysis.
  - Postrenal AKI from nephrolithiasis can present with hematuria.
  - Red blood cell casts are a very specific finding of glomerulonephritis and nephritic syndrome. White blood cell casts and cellular casts may be present in glomerulonephritis.
  - Pigmented "muddy-brown" or granular casts are characteristic of ATN. You can also see tubular epithelial casts in patients with ATN.
  - Urine eosinophils are classically elevated in allergic interstitial nephritis.

Electrocardiography
- An ECG needs to be obtained in all patients with suspected hyperkalemia. Do not wait for lab results.

Imaging
- Renal and bladder ultrasounds may show hydronephrosis and bladder distention.[11]
- Small, shrunken kidneys (<10 cm) is often seen with CKD.
- Enlarged kidneys may be seen with diabetic nephropathy, HIV-associated nephropathy, and infiltrative diseases such as multiple myeloma.
- A CT scan without contrast can be obtained to evaluate for nephrolithiasis.

TREATMENT

- Treatment of CKD is done as an outpatient.
- Prerenal AKI: Treated with either hydration or diuresis.[11]
  - Hydration: Patients with prerenal AKI who are hypovolemic need prompt volume resuscitation.
  - Patients with decreased effective circulating volume from severe heart failure will benefit from diuresis as opposed to volume resuscitation. A typical starting dose would be 40 mg of IV furosemide.
- Intrinsic renal AKI
  - Acute interstitial nephritis is generally treated with discontinuation of the offending drug.
  - ATN has no specific treatment and these patients should be admitted to the hospital and managed supportively.
  - Rhabdomyolysis is treated with infusion of 0.9% normal saline at a rate of 1.5 L/h to maintain a urine output of 200–300 mL/h.

- ○ Patients with tumor lysis syndrome (i.e., with a uric acid level > 8 mg/dL and serum creatinine > 1.6 mg/dL) can be treated with rasburicase 0.2 mg/kg IV. In addition, they should be given hydration with IV fluids.[11]
- Postrenal AKI is treated with relief of obstruction. If this cannot be achieved with Foley catheter placement, a urology consult is recommended.
- Treating AKI involves helping to ameliorate the effects of kidney failure including hyperkalemia, hypervolemia, and acidosis.
- Dialysis should be considered if patients have hypervolemia, electrolyte abnormalities, or acid–base abnormalities that are not responsive to medical management. It is also indicated if a patient has ingested a dialyzable toxin or in patients who are having symptoms from uremia such as impaired cognition, serositis, or pruritus.[3]

SPECIAL CONSIDERATIONS

Renal Transplant Complications

- Renal transplant can be complicated by immunologic rejection, which can be detected by a rise in serum creatinine, hypertension, fever, reduced urine output, or graft tenderness.[11]

Disposition

- Patients who have AKI from dehydration and treated in the emergency department should be informed that NSAIDs are nephroxic and should be avoided for a brief period of time.
- Patients with a new elevation in creatinine should be admitted to the hospital.
- Patients with CKD and indications for dialysis should be admitted.
- Patients with CKD and uncontrolled diabetes or hypertension may be discharged home but should follow up with their PMD or nephrologist.[11]

Complications

- Postobstructive and post-ATN diuresis
  - ○ Significant diuresis may follow resolution of urinary obstruction or acute tubular necrosis. Hypotension and electrolyte disturbances should be treated.[4]
- Contrast nephropathy risk factors:
  - ○ GFR < 60, diabetes, dehydration, congestive heart failure (CHF), age > 70, other nephrotoxic exposures (e.g., NSAIDs), and large doses of contrast.
  - ○ To avoid contrast nephropathy, hydration with either 0.45% or 0.9% saline before a contrast load is recommended. Use of N-acetylcysteine has not been proven to consistently prevent AKI.[3]

REFERENCES

1. Khwaja A. KDIGO clinical practice guidelines for acute kidney injury. *Nephron Clin Pract* 2012;120:179–84.
2. Dixon BS, Anderson RJ. Nonoliguric acute renal failure. *Am J Kidney Dis* 1985;6(2): 71–80.
3. Eknoyan G, Lameire N, Eckardt KU, et al. KDIGO 2012 clinical practice guidelines for the evaluation and management of chronic kidney disease. *Official J Int Soci Nephrol* 2013;3(1):1–150.
4. Lameire N, Van Biesen W, Vanholder R. Acute renal failure. *Lancet* 2005;365:417–30.

5. U.S. Renal Data System, USRDS 2013 annual data report: atlas of chronic kidney disease and end-stage renal disease in the United States, National Institutes of Health, National Institute of Diabetes and Digestive and Kidney Diseases. Bethesda, 2013.
6. Hadjiphilippou S, Kon SP. Cardiorenal syndrome: review of our current understanding. *J R Soc Med* 2016;109(1):12–17.
7. Baraldi O, Valentini C, Donati G, et al. Hepatorenal syndrome: update on diagnosis and treatment. *World J Nephrol* 2015;4(5):511–20.
8. Perazella MA, Markowitz GS. Drug-induced acute interstitial nephritis. *Nat Rev Nephrol* 2010;6(8):461–70.
9. Praga M, Sevillano A, Aunon P, Gonzalez E. Changes in the aetiology, clinical presentation, and management of acute interstitial nephritis, an increasingly common cause of acute kidney injury. *Nephrol Dial Transplant* 2015;30:1472–79.
10. Rahman M, Shad F, Smith MC. Acute kidney injury: a guide to diagnosis and management. *Am Fam Physician* 2012;86:631–639.
11. Moroni G, Ponticelli C. Rapidly progressive crescentic glomerulonephritis: early treatment is a must. *Autoimmun Rev* 2014;13:723–29.
12. Liano F, Pascual J. Epidemiology of acute renal failure: a prospective, multicenter, community-based study. *Kidney Int* 1996;50:811–18.

89 Renal and GU Emergencies: Dialysis Complications

Carla Robinson-Rainey

Catheter-Related Infections

GENERAL PRINCIPLES

Epidemiology/Etiology
- Risk factors for catheter-related infection include advanced age, diabetes, and femoral vein access.
- Access of the fistula or graft is the source of 50–80% of infections.
- ~50% of catheter infections are gram-positive cocci and 25% gram-negative bacilli, and 20% are polymicrobial infections.

Pathophysiology
- The peritoneal dialysis catheter acts as a foreign body and provides portal of entry for pathogen from the external environment. Hemodialysis catheter-related bloodstream infections result when the same organism is grown from a peripheral blood culture and the catheter tip.

DIAGNOSIS

Clinical Presentation

History
- Important aspects of the history include length of catheter utilization, previous history of catheter-related issues or infections in the past, and complaints of fever, warmth, pain, malaise, and skin changes near the catheter site.

Physical Examination
- Specific attention should be focused on the dialysis port site or the fistula site.
- Infection is indicated by inflammation within 2 cm of site or inflammation and swelling along the catheter tract.
- Fever, purulent drainage, or skin changes at the catheter site or erythema over the tunnel should be noted.

Diagnostic Criteria and Testing

Laboratories
- A complete blood count (CBC) and blood cultures taken from two separate sites, one of which should be drawn from the hemodialysis catheter should be obtained.

TREATMENT

- Removal of the catheter is case dependent.
- 90% of skin site infections respond to oral antibiotics.
- Broad-spectrum antibiotics should be started in the case of suspected peritonitis.

SPECIAL CONSIDERATIONS

Disposition
- Patients should be admitted to the hospital.

Bacterial Peritonitis

GENERAL PRINCIPLES

Definition
- Bacterial peritonitis is defined as >100 wbc/mm^3 of peritoneal fluid or >50% polymorphonuclear neutrophils after a "dwell time" of 2 hours.

Epidemiology/Etiology
- The leading cause of bacterial peritonitis is failure to follow sterile technique.
- Staphylococcus epidermis account for 95% of cases of contamination.
- Gram-positive bacteria account for 50–80% of episodes of infection.
- Gram-negative bacteria account for 20–30% of episodes of infection.
- <5% of infections are caused by fungal species.

Pathophysiology
- The catheter acts as a foreign body and provides a portal of entry for pathogens from the external environment.

Clinical Presentation

History
- Special attention should be paid to how long the catheter has been in place, how long/often it has been utilized for dialysis, a history of prior episodes of peritonitis, compliance with sterile technique, and any recent gastrointestinal (GI) or GU procedures.
- Any history of fever, purulent drainage, skin changes, abdominal pain, nausea, vomiting, or diarrhea should be obtained.

Physical Examination
- Assess skin around the peritoneal dialysis (PD) catheter for redness, warmth, purulent drainage, or swelling.
- Tunnel infections may have erythema, edema, or tenderness over the subcutaneous tract.
- The patient may present with abdominal pain, guarding, or rebound tenderness and it is usually generalized. Bowel sounds may be diminished.

Differential Diagnosis

- Abdominal wall abscess, cellulitis, appendicitis, diverticulitis, acute intestinal perforation, peptic ulcer disease, constipation, renal or biliary colic, gynecologic issue, or pancreatitis.

Diagnostic Criteria and Testing

Laboratories
- Common laboratory studies include CBC and basic metabolic panel (BMP).
- A cell count with differential, Gram stain, and culture of the effluent should be obtained.
- Blood cultures are not necessary unless bowel perforation or sepsis is suspected.

Imaging
- Ultrasonography can be used to assess for an abscess along the tract of the tunnel.
- A CT scan may help rule out other differential diagnoses.
- Plain radiographs can identify free air if bowel perforation is a consideration.

TREATMENT

Medications

- Empiric therapy should always cover for Staphylococcus aureus; a first-generation cephalosporin can be used as initial treatment and vancomycin should only be used for suspected methicillin-resistant staphylococcus aureus (MRSA) infection.
- If there is a history of pseudomonas infection, empirically treat with an oral fluoroquinolone (levofloxacin).
  - Intraperitoneal antibiotic treatment may be initiated after consultation with a nephrologist.

SPECIAL CONSIDERATIONS

Disposition

- Patients with suspected peritonitis should be admitted to the hospital.

Aneurysm of Arteriovenous Fistula/Graft

GENERAL PRINCIPLES

Definition

• An aneurysm is defined as an abnormal dilation of the vessel (threefold increase dilation of the native-vessel diameter with minimal size >2 cm).

Epidemiology/Etiology

• Aneurysms are a common complication seen with arteriovenous fistulas.

Pathophysiology

• Causes of an aneurysm include dilation of the vessel due to trauma from frequent needle punctures or infiltration/hematoma secondary to improper technique.
• A pseudoaneurysm results when blood leaks around the lumen from the anastomosis site.

Clinical Presentation

History

• The patient may present with swelling and discomfort at the affected site.

Physical Examination

• Assess skin around the fistula, evaluating for thinning, atrophy, ulcer formation, shiny skin, or other signs of infection.
• The vascular access site should be examined for thrill and bruit to detect stenosis, infection, arterial steal syndrome, or aneurysm.

Differential Diagnosis

• Stenosis, thrombosis, and infection.

Diagnostic Criteria and Testing

Laboratories

• No specific laboratory tests are diagnostic for A-V graft aneurysms.

Imaging

• Ultrasonography or venography can be performed to evaluate an aneurysm.

Diagnostic Procedure

• Patients can be referred for thrombectomy or emergency surgical ligation if imminent rupture is present.

TREATMENT

• Based upon consultation with a vascular surgeon

SPECIAL CONSIDERATIONS

Disposition

- These patients will usually be admitted for graft revision, but consultation with a vascular surgeon is indicated.

SUGGESTED READINGS

Cacho Carolyn P. Complications of Peritoneal Dialysis. In: Donald H, Tyler MR, Sedor JR. *Nephrology Secrets. 2nd ed. Questions and Answers Reveal the Secrets to Effective Treatment of Patients with Renal Disorders.* Philadelphia: Hanley & Belfus, 2003:197–201.

Lai A, Neng K. Acute and Chronic Catheter in Hemodialysis, Technical Problems in Patients on Hemodialysis. 2011. InTech. Available at: Http://www.intechopen.com/books/technical-problems-in-patinets-on-hemodialysis/acute-and-crhonic-catheter-in-hemodialsis (last accessed: 4/15/2016).

Li P, Szeto C, Piraino B, et al. Peritoneal dialysis-related infections recommendations: 2010 update. *Periot Dial Int* 2010;30:393–423. doi:10.3747/pdi.2010.00049

Mudoni A, Cornacchiari M, Gallieni M, et al. Aneurysms and pseudoaneurysms in dialysis access. *Clin Kidney J* 2015;4:363–67. http://www.ncbi.nlm.gov/pm/articles/PMC4515897 (last accessed: 4/15/2016).

Navuluri R, Regalado S. The KDOQI 2006 vascular Access Update and Fistula First Program Synopsis. *Semin Intervent Radiol J* 2009;2:122–24. Available at: http://www.ncbi.nlm.nih.gov/pmc/articles/PMC3036429 (last accessed: 4/15/2016).

Negrea Lavinia A. Complications of Hemodialysis. In: Donald H, Tyler MR, Sedor JR. Tyler, Sedor, John R. *Nephrology Secrets. 2nd ed. Questions and Answers Reveal the Secrets to Effective Treatment of Patients with Renal Disorders.* Philadelphia: Hanley & Belfus, 2003:P183–5.

Shroff G, Frederick P, Herzog C. Renal failure and acute myocardial infarction: clinical characteristics in patients with advanced chronic kidney disease, on dialysis and without chronic kidney disease. A collaborative project of the United States Renal Data System/National Institutes of Health and the National Registry of myocardial Infarction. *Am Heart J* 2012;163(3):399–406. doi: 10.1016/j.ahj.2011.12.002.

Tzanakaki E, Boudouri V, Stavropoulou A, et al. Causes of complications of chronic kidney disease in patients on dialysis. *Heal Sci J* 2014;8:343–7.

Wang K, Wang P, Liang X, et al. Epidemiology of haemodialysis catheter complications: a survey of 865 dialysis patients from 14 haemodialysis centers in Henan province in China. *BMJ Open* 2015;5:e007136. doi: 10.1136/bmjopen-2014-007136.

Weber E, Liberek T, Wolyniec W, et al. Survival of tunneled hemodialysis catheters after percutaneous placement. *Acta Biochem Pol* 2016;63:139–43.

Renal and GU Emergencies: Hematuria

Mark D. Levine

GENERAL PRINCIPLES

Definition
- Hematuria is the presence of red blood cells in the urine.
- As little as 1 mL of blood per liter of urine may be noticeable to the naked eye.

Epidemiology/Etiology
- The most common cause of hematuria is inflammation or infection of the urinary tract. Other causes of hematuria include malignancy, benign prostatic hyperplasia (BPH), trauma, and kidney stones.
- Risk factors include a history of smoking, urinary tract infection (UTI), pelvic radiation, overuse of analgesics, or exposure to certain chemicals or dyes and age > 40 years.

Pathophysiology
- Any disruption of the epithelium of the urinary tract may cause blood loss into the urine.
- If the kidney is the source of bleeding, hematuria is due to disruption of the filtration barrier in the glomerulus. Casts may be seen.

DIAGNOSIS

Clinical Presentation
History
- Hematuria may be of varying intensity, from a light pink to dark brown. There may be associated complaints of abdominal, back, flank pain, or pain with voiding or intercourse. If the stream remains bloody or increases/decreases with course of urination, this should be noted.
- A family history of renal failure, renal stones, bleeding disorders, or polycystic kidney disease should be elicited.
- A medication history, dietary history, and history of extreme exertion should also be obtained.

Physical Examination
- A full physical examination, paying attention to signs of trauma, potential sources of bleeding, abnormal bruising, and presence of blood at the meatus, should be performed. A pelvic exam may be indicated in females, and a rectal exam is indicated in males.

Differential Diagnosis
- Rhabdomyolysis, hyperbilirubinemia, porphyria, lupus, Henoch-Schonlein Purpura prostatitis, or menstruation

Diagnostic Testing

Laboratories
- A urinalysis should be obtained. Casts and proteinuria can localize a renal source of bleeding.
- Significant bleeding may need a complete blood count, basic metabolic panel (BMP), coagulation studies, and a type/cross but will not be helpful in evaluating hematuria specifically.

Imaging
- Ultrasound of the bladder may show a clot, mass, or trauma.
- Ultrasound of the kidney may show hydronephrosis (secondary to renal stone) or other abnormality of the kidney.
- CT scan of the abdomen/pelvis, focusing on location of a kidney stone, malignancy, or ureteral, urethral, or renal abnormality may be helpful but may not be needed on an emergent basis.

TREATMENT

- Continuous bladder irrigation (CBI) and urologic consultation may be needed.

Medications
- There are no specific medications for the ED treatment of hematuria.

SPECIAL CONSIDERATIONS

Disposition
- Patients may be discharged home with PMD and/or urology follow-up. If a Foley catheter was placed, urology recommendations regarding removal should be followed.
- Patients who are unstable, have continued significant bleeding, or have grossly abnormal laboratory values may require admission.

Complications
- Clot formation may cause outflow obstruction of the urine.

SUGGESTED READINGS

Grossfeld GD, Wolf JS Jr, Litwan MS, et al. Asymptomatic microscopic hematuria in adults: summary of the AUA best practice policy recommendations. *Am Fam Physician* 2001;63:1145–54.

Grossfeld GD, Wolf JS, Litwin MS, et al. Evaluation of asymptomatic microscopic hematuria in adults: the American Urological Association best practice policy recommendations. *Urology* 2001;57:599–610.

Rose BD, Fletcher RH. Evaluation of hematuria. Available at: UpToDate Online, http://www.uptodate.com

Sokolosky MC. Hematuria. *Emerg Med Clin North Am* 2001;19(3):621–32.

Renal and GU Emergencies: Urinary Tract Infection

Steven Hung and Stephen Y. Liang

GENERAL PRINCIPLES

Definitions
- Cystitis
  - Infection of the bladder or lower urinary tract in a healthy nonpregnant woman
- Complicated cystitis
  - Any infection in a man, pregnant woman, or any patient with an anatomic abnormality or history of immunosuppression, renal failure, renal transplant, indwelling device, or recent instrumentation of the urinary tract
- Pyelonephritis
  - Ascending infection from the lower urinary tract involving the kidneys
- Catheter-associated urinary tract infection (CAUTI)
  - Infection of the bladder or lower urinary tract associated with an indwelling urinary catheter
- Asymptomatic bacteriuria
  - Evidence of pyuria on urinalysis or recovery of a microorganism from urine culture in the absence of clinical signs or symptoms of infection

Acute Cystitis

GENERAL PRINCIPLES

Epidemiology/Etiology
- Uncomplicated cystitis in women is common due to a shorter urethra, allowing periurethral bacteria to ascend and access the bladder more readily than in men.
- *Escherichia coli* is the most common cause of uncomplicated cystitis. Other microorganisms may include *Proteus mirabilis*, *Klebsiella pneumoniae*, and *Staphylococcus saprophyticus*.
- Complicated cystitis may also be caused by *Pseudomonas aeruginosa*, *Serratia*, *Providencia*, and fungi.
- Patients with a history of recurrent urinary tract infection (UTI) may be at risk for infection due to antibiotic-resistant organisms (*e.g.*, *Proteus*, *Klebsiella*, *Enterobacter*, *Pseudomonas*).
- Most frequently seen in females, those with a history of recurrent UTIs, and those with decreased urine flow (*e.g.*, obstruction, neurogenic bladder, inadequate fluid intake), increased urinary tract colonization (*e.g.*, sexual activity, diaphragm or spermicide use, atrophic vaginitis), or presence of an indwelling device

DIAGNOSIS

Clinical Presentation

History
- Symptoms may include dysuria, urgency, frequency, suprapubic pain, and/or hematuria.
- Some patients may also experience nausea or vomiting.
- In older patients, cystitis may present as generalized weakness or altered mental status rather than irritative voiding symptoms.

Physical Examination
- Suprapubic tenderness may be elicited on abdominal examination.

Differential Diagnosis
- Sexually transmitted disease, appendicitis (sterile pyuria may be present), colitis, or ovarian/uterine issue

Diagnostic Testing

Laboratories
- A properly collected, clean-catch or catheter urine specimen is necessary to accurately diagnose acute cystitis.
- Urinalysis (UA)
  - Macroscopic analysis:
    - Positive leukocyte esterase: pyuria
    - Positive nitrite: bacteriuria
  - If the macroscopic analysis is abnormal, a microscopic analysis should be performed:
    - Leukocytes: >10 leukocytes per high-powered field denotes pyuria.
    - Presence of bacteria denotes bacteriuria.
- Urine culture
  - While not routinely indicated in most cases of uncomplicated cystitis, urine culture is recommended for patients who are over the age of 65 years, have had symptoms >7 days, or have a history of diabetes mellitus, recurrent UTIs, or indwelling devices.
- Blood cultures should be obtained in those with severe disease requiring hospitalization.

TREATMENT

- Uncomplicated cystitis can be treated empirically without testing in women with prior UTIs who report a history of similar symptoms and diagnosis.
- Empiric antibiotic therapy may consist of the following, depending on local antibiotic resistance patterns (Table 91.1):
  - Uncomplicated cystitis:
    - Nitrofurantoin for 5–7 days
    - Trimethoprim–sulfamethoxazole (TMP-SMX) for 3 days
    - Fluoroquinolone (ciprofloxacin, levofloxacin) for 3 days
    - Cephalexin for 3 days
  - Complicated cystitis:
    - Fluoroquinolone or TMP-SMX for 7–14 days

SPECIAL CONSIDERATIONS

Disposition
- Uncomplicated infections may be discharged home with follow-up with a PMD.

Complications

- Recurrent infections, renal insufficiency, strictures, sepsis, perinephric abscess, and renal abscess
  - Untreated bacteriuria in pregnancy may result in complications with pregnancy.
  - Fluoroquinolones may predispose patients to tendon rupture or renal insufficiency.
  - TMP-SMX may cause hyperkalemia or Stevens-Johnson syndrome.

Pyelonephritis

GENERAL PRINCIPLES

Epidemiology/Etiology

- Acute pyelonephritis is less common than cystitis but shares the same risk factors.
- *E. coli* and *Enterococcus* are common causes of pyelonephritis.
- Patients with a history of recurrent UTI may also be at risk for infection with antibiotic-resistant organisms (*e.g.*, *Proteus*, *Klebsiella*, *Enterobacter*, and *Pseudomonas*).

DIAGNOSIS

Clinical Presentation

History

- Patients may report flank pain, fevers, chills, nausea, vomiting, and/or malaise in addition to irritative voiding symptoms.

Physical Examination

- The patient may present with fever, tachycardia, and/or tachypnea.
- Costovertebral angle tenderness may be present on examination.

Diagnostic Testing

Laboratories

- Both urinalysis and urine culture should be obtained not only to establish the diagnosis of pyelonephritis but to determine the adequacy of empiric antibiotic therapy.

Imaging

- Renal ultrasonography or computed tomography may be helpful in evaluating the urinary tract and excluding sequelae of pyelonephritis (*e.g.*, renal abscess), particularly when symptoms have not improved after 48–72 hours of appropriate antibiotic therapy.

TREATMENT (TABLE 91.1)

- Duration of therapy should be 7–14 days, with recent literature supporting shorter durations to treat pyelonephritis. Empiric antibiotic therapy may consist of the following:
  - Mild-to-moderate disease:
    - Fluoroquinolone (ciprofloxacin, levofloxacin)
    - TMP-SMX
  - Severe disease:
    - Fluoroquinolone or a 3rd- or 4th-generation cephalosporin with or without aminoglycoside
    - β-lactam/β-lactamase inhibitor, carbapenem, or aminoglycoside, if an antibiotic-resistant organism is suspected

TABLE 91.1	Common Antibiotics Used to Treat Urinary Tract Infections	
Class	Oral	Parenteral
Folate inhibitors	TMP-SMX DS 160/800 mg PO q12h	N/A
Fluoroquinolone	Ciprofloxacin 250–500 mg PO q12h	Ciprofloxacin 400 mg IV q12h
	Levofloxacin 250–750 mg PO daily	Levofloxacin 250–750 mg IV qd
Cephalosporins	Cephalexin 500 mg PO bid	Cefazolin 1 g IV q8h
		Ceftriaxone 1 g IV qd
		Cefepime 1 g IV q8h
Nitrofurantoin	100 mg PO bid	N/A
Fosfomycin	3 g PO	N/A
β-lactam/β-lactamase inhibitor	Amoxicillin–clavulanate 500/125 mg PO bid-tid	Ampicillin/sulbactam 1.5–3 g IV q6h
		Piperacillin–tazobactam 3.375–4.5 g IV q6h
Carbapenems	N/A	Ertapenem 1 g IV q8h
		Imipenem 500 mg IV q6h
		Meropenem 1 g IV q8h
Aminoglycoside	N/A	Gentamicin 5 mg/kg qd

- Patients with severe disease, those unable to tolerate oral medications, and pregnant women with pyelonephritis should receive intravenous antibiotics and be hospitalized.

SPECIAL CONSIDERATIONS

Disposition
- Patients with pyelonephritis, sepsis, or those who are pregnant should be admitted to the hospital.

Complications
- See cystitis complications

Catheter-Associated Urinary Tract Infection

GENERAL PRINCIPLES

Epidemiology/Etiology
- Most patients with urinary catheters will develop asymptomatic bacteriuria, within 30 days of catheter insertion, and this can progress to symptomatic CAUTI.

- *E. coli* is the most common cause of CAUTI.
- *Enterococcus* species, *Pseudomonas*, *Klebsiella*, and *Candida* may likewise be implicated.
- Duration of urinary catheterization, older age, and female sex are the primary risk factors.

DIAGNOSIS

Clinical Presentation

History
- Patients may report suprapubic discomfort, flank pain, and other symptoms similar to cystitis or pyelonephritis.

Physical Examination
- Suprapubic or costovertebral angle tenderness may be present.

Diagnostic Testing

Laboratories
- Specimens for urinalysis and urine culture should be obtained from the drainage catheter (*e.g.*, via a needleless port) and not the drainage bag.
- A single catheter urine specimen or a clean-catch urine specimen obtained from a patient whose catheter was removed in the past 48 hours with $\geq 10^3$ colony-forming units (CFU)/mL of ≥ 1 bacterial species coupled with signs and symptoms of cystitis or pyelonephritis establishes the diagnosis of CAUTI.

TREATMENT

- The infected urinary catheter should be removed or exchanged whenever possible in a symptomatic patient.
- Antibiotic therapy should be guided by past urine cultures whenever available for a duration of 7–14 days. Otherwise, empiric antibiotic therapy should consist of the following:
  - Mild-to-moderate disease: Fluoroquinolone or 3rd-generation cephalosporin
  - Severe disease: IV fluoroquinolone or 4th-generation cephalosporin. If an antibiotic-resistant organism is suspected, a carbapenem may also be considered in place of the cephalosporin.
- Antifungal therapy to treat candiduria (usually *Candida albicans*) is only indicated in immunocompromised patients and those at high risk for developing candidemia. In all other cases, catheter removal alone is sufficient.

Asymptomatic Bacteriuria

GENERAL PRINCIPLES

Epidemiology/Etiology
- Asymptomatic bacteriuria is more common in women, and prevalence increases with age.
- *E. coli* is the most common cause of asymptomatic bacteriuria.
- In men, other gram-negative microorganisms, *Enterococcus*, and coagulase-negative *Staphylococcus* may also be encountered.

- In addition to age and female sex, diabetes mellitus, spinal cord injury with voiding dysfunction, immunosuppression, and presence of an indwelling device are also risk factors for asymptomatic bacteriuria.

DIAGNOSIS

Diagnostic Testing

Laboratories

- A clean-catch midstream urine specimen is preferred to establish the diagnosis of asymptomatic bacteriuria.
  - Pyuria (>10 leukocytes per high-powered field) on urinalysis should prompt a urine culture.
  - Asymptomatic bacteriuria is defined as $\geq 10^5$ CFU/mL of a single microorganism in two consecutive clean-catch urine samples from a woman or one sample from a man. If a straight catheter urine specimen is obtained, the threshold drops to $\geq 10^2$ CFU/mL in a single urine sample.

TREATMENT

- Asymptomatic bacteriuria in a pregnant woman warrants antibiotic therapy in the emergency department (ED).
- Antibiotic therapy is also warranted in patients undergoing urologic surgery where mucosal bleeding is expected.
- Do not treat asymptomatic bacteriuria in nonpregnant premenopausal women, the elderly, nursing home residents, diabetics, patients with spinal cord injury, or those with a urinary catheter.

SUGGESTED READINGS

Aubin C. Does this woman have an acute uncomplicated urinary tract infection? *Ann Emerg Med* 2007;49(1):106–8.

Eliakim-Raz N, Yahav D, Paul M, Leibovici L. Duration of antibiotic treatment for acute pyelonephritis and septic urinary tract infection—7 days or less versus longer treatment: systematic review and meta-analysis of randomized controlled trials. *J Antimicrob Chemother* 2013;68:2183–91.

Grigoryan L, Trautner BW, Gupta K. Diagnosis and management of urinary tract infections in the outpatient setting: a review. *JAMA* 2014;312(16):1677–84.

Gupta K, Hooton TM, Naber KG, et al. International clinical practice guidelines for the treatment of acute uncomplicated cystitis and pyelonephritis in women: a 2010 update by the Infectious Diseases Society of America and the European Society for Microbiology and Infectious Diseases. *Clin Infect Dis* 2011;52(5):e103–20.

Hooton TM, Bradley SF, Cardenas DD, et al. Diagnosis, prevention, and treatment of catheter-associated urinary tract infection in adults: 2009 international clinical practice guidelines from the Infectious Diseases Society of America. *Clin Infect Dis* 2010;50:625–63.

Lo E, Nicolle LE, Coffin SE, et al. Strategies to prevent catheter-associated urinary tract infections in acute care hospitals: 2014 update. *Infect Control Hosp Epidemiol* 2014;35(5):464–79.

Mody L, Juthani-Mehta M. Urinary tract infections in older women: a clinical review. *JAMA* 2014;311(8):844–54.

Nicolle LE, Bradley S, Colgan R, et al. Infectious Diseases Society of America guidelines for the diagnosis and treatment of asymptomatic bacteriuria in adults. *Clin Infect Dis* 2005;40(5):643–54.

Stamm WE. Measurement of pyuria and its relation to bacteriuria. *Am J Med* 1983;75(1B):53.

Vazquez JC, Abalos E. Treatments for symptomatic urinary tract infections during pregnancy. *Cochrane Database Syst Rev* 2011;(1):CD002256.

92 Renal and GU Emergencies: Male Genitourinary

Steven Hung and Reuben D. Johnson

Acute Urinary Retention

GENERAL PRINCIPLES

Definition
• Acute urinary retention (AUR) is the inability to voluntarily urinate.

Epidemiology/Etiology
• More common in elderly men and rare in women
• Obstructive/mechanical: Benign prostatic hypertrophy (most common cause), stones, neoplasm, trauma, urethral stricture, urethral inflammation postprocedure, cystitis, prostatitis, and hematoma
• Medication: Anticholinergics, alpha adrenergic agonists, antihistamines, antidepressants, antipsychotics, antiparkinsonian medication, antidysrhythmics, anticonvulsants, antiemetics, antihypertensive, muscle relaxants, and pain medications
• Neurologic impairment: Spinal cord injury and disease

Pathophysiology
• Mechanical obstruction of outflow by either narrowing or blockage of the urethra
• Incomplete relaxation of urinary sphincter as seen in neurologic diseases
• Incomplete contraction of detrusor muscle
• Disruption by trauma

DIAGNOSIS

• The diagnosis of AUR is mainly clinical with confirmation of postvoid residual.

Clinical Presentation
History
• The patient will typically complain of associated lower abdominal/suprapubic distention/discomfort as well as the inability to void or void completely.
• There may a be history of prior urinary retention or urinary tract symptoms.
• Recent pelvic trauma, pelvic surgery, or Foley placement should be elicited.
• Recent changes in medication should also be noted.
• Low back pain and neurologic symptoms may also be reported by the patient.

Physical Examination
- Perform a physical and neurologic exam looking for decreased sphincter tone; a normal prostate examination does not rule out obstruction caused by benign prostatic hypertrophy.

Diagnostic Testing
Laboratories
- Urinalysis and/or culture should be sent to look for infection or blood.
- A basic metabolic panel (BMP) should be obtained to evaluate kidney damage.

Imaging
- Bedside ultrasound can be used to assist in diagnosis
  - Volumes >300–400 mL on postvoid bedside ultrasound suggests urinary retention.

TREATMENT

Medications
- Tamsulosin (0.4 mg) qD until seen by urology or PMD

Other Nonpharmacologic Therapies
- Urethral catheterization
  - Intermittent catheterization—fewer complications than indwelling catheter
    - Appropriate for AUR expected to resolve over time (e.g., medication induced)
    - Appropriate for patients comfortable with self-catheterization
  - Indwelling catheter
    - For patients expected to have prolonged retention
    - If suspected benign prostatic hyperplasia (BPH), may need specially shaped catheter (e.g., Coude) or larger catheter (allows more firm pressure) to pass the prostate
    - If postsurgery, may need smaller catheter due to strictures
- Suprapubic catheter
  - Needed if patient has contraindications to catheter placement (recent urologic surgery, trauma with suspected disruption of urethra, artificial urinary sphincter) or failed urethral catheterization. Urology should be consulted.

SPECIAL CONSIDERATIONS

Disposition
- Consult urology in the emergency department if unable to drain the bladder.
- If patient undergoes successful catheterization, he can follow up with urology as an outpatient with the Foley left in place until removed by a urologist.
- If a new acute neurologic cause is suspected, admission is indicated.
- If retention is caused by medication, patients should be instructed to discontinue the medication.
- Instruct on proper catheterization technique or care of an indwelling catheter.

Complications
- Hematuria—resolves over time; minimized by proper Foley placement techniques
- Transient hypotension
- Postobstructive diuresis—more of a problem in those with chronic obstruction

Testicular Torsion

GENERAL PRINCIPLES

Definition
- Testicular torsion occurs when the testis twists on the spermatic cord producing ischemia.

Epidemiology
- There is a bimodal distribution, occurring predominantly and spontaneously in neonates and postpubertal boys; however, it can occur at any age and can be as a direct result of trauma.

Pathophysiology
- Results from the abnormal fixation of the testis to the tunica vaginalis allowing the testis to twist upon itself, reducing arterial and venous flow.

DIAGNOSIS

Clinical Presentation
History
- The patient will complain of acute and severe pain in the testicle, usually after physical activity or trauma and may be associated with nausea and vomiting.

Physical Examination
- The affected testis is usually firm and tender.
- It is typically higher than the contralateral testis with a horizontal lie.
- Shortening of the spermatic cord may cause the "bell clapper deformity."
- There may be a reactive hydrocele and absence of a cremasteric reflex.

Differential Diagnosis
- Torsion of the appendix testis
  - Typically occurs in childhood
  - Onset of pain is typically more gradual.
  - Inspection of the scrotal wall may reveal the classic "blue dot" sign.
  - Ultrasound will show a torsed appendage with normal flow in the testis.
- Epididymitis
  - Onset of pain is more gradual.
  - Bacterial infection is most common cause.
  - Causes a large, tender scrotal mass associated with abdominal/scrotal/testicular pain
  - Relief of pain with scrotal elevation
  - Treatment is with oral antibiotics, scrotal support, and no heavy lifting
- Orchitis
  - Inflammation of testicle alone is rare.
  - Can occur with mumps or other viral illness.
  - Presents initially unilaterally and then contralaterally a few days later
- Scrotal trauma
- Testicular cancer
  - Usually presents as a firm, nontender mass

- Inguinal hernia
- Soft tissue infection

Diagnostic Testing

Laboratories
- Urinalysis may help with the differential diagnosis if torsion is ruled out.

Imaging
- Color Doppler ultrasonography can help differentiate testicular torsion from other causes.
  - Intermittent torsion may cause a false-negative result.

TREATMENT

- The definitive management for testicular torsion is urgent urologic consult for surgery.

Other Nonpharmacologic Therapies

- Detorsion:
  - Typically rotate medial to lateral (as if opening a book).
  - Should try to rotate one and a half turns (540 degrees).
  - Relief of pain demonstrates success.
    - Patient still needs admission for surgery.
  - If pain becomes worse, attempt to detorse the other direction.

SPECIAL CONSIDERATION

Disposition
- All patients with testicular torsion should be admitted to the hospital.

Complications
- Testicular ischemia resulting in death of testis and risk of fertility issues.
- The testis suffers irreversible damage after 12 hours.

Fournier Gangrene

GENERAL PRINCIPLES

Definition
- Fournier gangrene is a necrotizing fasciitis of the perineal, genital, and/or perianal area.

Epidemiology
- More common in elderly males and diabetics/immunocompromised patients

Pathophysiology
- Fournier gangrene usually begins with local trauma or with urinary/perianal infection.

- Usually, it is a polymicrobial infection with aerobic and/or anaerobic organisms. Most common bacteria include *Escherichia coli*, *Proteus*, *Enterococcus*, and *Bacteroides fragilis*.
- The infection spreads along fascial planes and causes vascular thrombosis resulting in tissue necrosis and gangrene of the skin.

DIAGNOSIS

Clinical Presentation
History
- The patient will complain of severe pain and foul smell in the groin.
- The patient may report rapid progression and spread of pain and redness.

Physical Examination
- There will be tense edema of the skin with blisters/bullae or crepitus over the perineal, genital, and/or perianal area with odor and drainage.
- Fever, tachycardia, and hypotension will be present.

Differential Diagnosis
- Scrotal abscess, scrotal edema, or cellulitis

Diagnostic Testing
Laboratories
- There are no specific laboratory values that will diagnose Fournier gangrene; however, preoperative labs will normally be required.
- If sepsis is suspected, trending of lactate may be appropriate.

Imaging
- CT of the abdomen and pelvis with contrast may assist in diagnosis and delineating the extent of the infection; however, it should not delay emergent surgical evaluation and treatment.

TREATMENT

Medications
- Broad-spectrum antibiotics covering aerobic and anaerobic bacteria should be initiated.
- Aggressive fluid resuscitation should be administered.

Surgical Management
- Patient will require emergent surgical debridement by surgery and/or urology.

SPECIAL CONSIDERATIONS

Disposition
- Patients should be admitted to the hospital and possibly the intensive care unit.

Complications
- Sepsis and/or septic shock
- Cystostomy, colostomy, and/or orchiectomy

Foreskin Emergencies

GENERAL PRINCIPLES

Definitions
- Paraphimosis is a urologic emergency that occurs when foreskin is retracted and cannot be returned to its normal position causing restricted blood flow and resultant damage.
- Phimosis is when the opening of the foreskin is so small that when retracted for any reason, the patient's glans is at high risk for entrapment.

Epidemiology
- Can occur in all ages in patients with an uncircumcised penis.
- Risk factors for paraphimosis include having an uncircumcised penis and/or phimosis, sexual activity, failure to retract after urination or cleaning, or iatrogenic after a urologic procedure.

Pathophysiology
Paraphimosis
- Foreskin entrapment behind the coronal sulcus leads to impaired venous and lymphatic flow. Eventually, engorgement causes the arterial flow to be compromised resulting in necrosis.

DIAGNOSIS

Clinical Presentation
History
- The patient may have a history of pain or swelling occurring after urination, cleaning, or sexual activity.

Physical Examination
- Paraphimosis
  - Patients will usually be in significant pain.
  - Examine for any constricting foreign bodies (e.g., hair, rubber bands, piercings).
  - The retracted foreskin will appear as a circular band of painful swelling.
  - The glans penis will be swollen and tender.
  - In late presentations, there might be ischemic changes.

Differential Diagnosis
- Inflammation/infection
  - Balanitis (inflammation of glans penis)
  - Posthitis (inflammation of the foreskin)
  - Balanoposthitis (inflammation of both glans penis and foreskin)
- General edematous state
- Trauma

TREATMENT

- Patient will need adequate local or systemic analgesia prior the manipulation.

- Reduction of paraphimosis
  - Manual reduction—Use index and middle fingers to pull the foreskin while pushing on the glans penis with the thumbs.
  - Puncture method—After adequate analgesia and antiseptic cleaning, multiple punctures are made to the edematous foreskin using a 25-gauge needle, and the foreskin is then reduced manually as above.
  - Dorsal slit—Usually performed by a urologist

SPECIAL CONSIDERATIONS

Disposition

- Avoid retracting foreskin for ~1 week.
- Prevent iatrogenic paraphimosis by returning foreskin position after procedure.
- Patient may be discharged to follow up with a urologist at the completion of the procedure unless taken to the OR for circumcision.

Complications

- Injury to foreskin or glans penis

Priapism

GENERAL PRINCIPLES

Definition

- Priapism is a urologic emergency generally lasting longer than 4 hours without any associated sexual stimulation or desire.

Epidemiology

- Bimodal distribution, between 5–10 years and 20–50 years
  - Side effect of medication such as phosphodiesterase type 5 inhibitors, intracavernous injections, antihypertensives, alpha blockers, cocaine, or trazodone
- Side effect of sickle cell, other hematologic diseases, spinal shock, or trauma

Pathophysiology

- Decreased venous outflow from the corpora cavernosa causes priapism.
- Generally divided into two subclasses:
  - Low flow (ischemic)
    - Impaired relaxation and paralysis of cavernosal smooth muscle.
    - Prolonged erection leads to edema and tissue damage, resulting in fibrosis and erectile dysfunction.
  - High flow (nonischemic)
    - Less common, usually related to penile trauma
    - Fistula between cavernosal artery and corpus cavernosum

DIAGNOSIS

Clinical Presentation

History
- Patients with ischemic priapism will complain of pain with the erection.
- Obtain history on duration of erection, prior episodes, any medication use, or trauma.
- Obtain history about sickle cell or other hematologic diseases.

Physical Examination
- In low-flow (ischemic) priapism, the penis is normally firm, erect, and tender, with the glans penis and corpus spongiosum usually soft.
- In high-flow (nonischemic) priapism, the penis will be erect but rarely rigid.

Differential Diagnosis
- Fracture of the penis
- Peyronie disease (abnormal curvature of erect penis due to thickened plaque)

Diagnostic Testing
Laboratories
- Complete blood count may reveal hematologic abnormalities.
- Blood gas analysis of aspirated blood will indicate ischemic or nonischemic priapism.
  - Ischemic will have a blood gas similar to venous blood and will appear dark.
  - Nonischemic will have a blood gas similar to arterial blood.

TREATMENT

Medications
- Provide adequate analgesia via local block or conscious sedation.
- Injection of phenylephrine (100–500 µg/mL)
  - Inject 1 mL of phenylephrine into the corpus cavernosum.
  - Inject every 3–5 minutes until resolution or up to an hour.

Other Nonpharmacologic Therapies
- Aspiration with/without irrigation
  - After analgesia, needle is inserted into corpus cavernosum and blood is drained.
  - Normal saline can be used for irrigation.
  - Can inject phenylephrine as above after aspiration/irrigation.

SPECIAL CONSIDERATIONS

Disposition
- Discharge home unless failure of local drainage.
- Treatment for high-flow (nonischemic) priapism is nonemergent and should be referred to urology as an outpatient.
- Emergent treatment of low-flow (ischemic) priapism is required since as more time passes, there is increased risk of damage to the penis.

Complications
- Bleeding, sexual dysfunction
- Phenylephrine injection may cause hypertension, bradycardia, headache, or cardiac arrhythmia.

SUGGESTED READINGS

al Mufti RA, Ogedegbe AK, Lafferty K. The use of doppler ultrasound in the clinical management of acute testicular pain. *Br J Urol* 1995;76(5):625.
Dubin J, Davis JE. Penile emergencies. *Emerg Med Clin North Am* 2011;29(3):485–99.

Dunne PJ, O'Loughlin BS. Testicular torsion: time is the enemy. *Aust N Z J Surg* 2000; 70(6):441.

Marshall JR, Haber J, Josephson EB. An evidence-based approach to emergency department management of acute urinary retention. *Emerg Med Pract* 2014;16(1):1.

Montague DK, Jarow J, Broderick GA, et al. American Urological Association guideline on the management of priapism. *J Urol* 2003;170(4 Pt 1):1318–24.

Shyam DC, Rapsang AG. Fournier's gangrene. *Surgeon* 2013;11(4):222–32.

Vilke GM, Ufberg JW, Harrigan RA, Chan TC. Evaluation and treatment of acute urinary retention. *J Emerg Med* 2008;35(2):193–8.

Zhao LC, Lautz TB, Meeks JJ, Maizels ML. Pediatric testicular torsion epidemiology using a national database: incidence, risk of orchiectomy, and possible measures toward improving the quality of care. *J Urol* 2011;186:2009.

93 Renal and GU Emergencies: Rhabdomyolysis

Matthew Burford and Robert Bucelli

GENERAL PRINCIPLES

Definition

- Rhabdomyolysis is defined as striated muscle breakdown with release of intracellular components leading to acute renal failure.
  - The presence of myoglobinuria is characteristic of rhabdomyolysis.

Epidemiology/Etiology

- Approximately 26,000 cases of rhabdomyolysis are reported each year in the United States.[1]
- Rhabdomyolysis may be caused by traumatic injury (crush, immobilization, electrical), exertion, illicit drug use, toxins, infection, endocrine, or temperature extremes.

Pathophysiology

- Rhabdomyolysis is caused by increased intracellular calcium and muscle fiber necrosis leading to a release of intracellular components into the blood.
- Renal failure results from the myoglobin released from muscle fibers causing renal vasoconstriction, renal tubular obstruction, free radical release, and hypovolemia.[3]

DIAGNOSIS

Clinical Presentation

History
- The history should attempt to elicit a precipitating cause such as trauma, prolonged immobilization, drug/toxin exposure, infection, or history of a predisposing medical condition.
- Other nonspecific symptoms, including nausea/vomiting, fever, and malaise, are common.

Physical Examination
- Classic presenting features are acute to subacute myalgia, transient weakness, and pigmenturia (tea- or cola-colored urine).
  - This full triad is only seen in up to 10% of patients.[1]

Differential Diagnosis
- See acute renal failure chapter.

Diagnostic Testing

Laboratories
- Electrolytes, serum creatine kinase (CK), urinalysis (with microscopy), calcium, and lactate should be obtained.

TREATMENT

- Acute management should focus on maintenance of renal function and restoring metabolic derangements.

Medications
- Intravenous hydration improves renal perfusion and dilutes myoglobin concentration.
  - Hydration should occur to maintain urine output of 200–300 mL/h and until serum CK has declined.[1]
  - In addition to volume repletion, diuretics and urine alkalinization with sodium bicarbonate (2 amps of bicarb in 1 L D5W at 100 mL/h) may help correct acidosis and hyperkalemia and may improve clearance of myoglobin[2]
- Treatment of hypocalcemia should be avoided unless severe symptoms are present.[3]

SPECIAL CONSIDERATIONS

Disposition
- Patients should be admitted to the hospital and may need the intensive care unit if having respiratory compromise.

Complications
- Long-term dialysis for renal failure[3]
- Fasciotomy may be required if compartment syndrome develops.

REFERENCES

1. Zutt R, van der Kooi AJ, Linthorst GE, et al. Rhabdomyolysis: review of the literature. *Neuromuscul Disord* 2014;24:651–9.
2. Ward MM. Factors predictive of acute renal failure in rhabdomyolysis. *Arch Intern Med* 1988;148(7):1553–7.
3. Bosch X, Poch E, Grau JM. Rhabdomyolysis and acute kidney injury. *N Engl J Med* 2009;361(1):62–72.

94

Renal and GU Emergencies: Acute Urinary Retention

Emily Harkins and S. Eliza Dunn

GENERAL PRINCIPLES

Definition

- The inability to pass urine voluntarily leads to distension of the bladder and subsequent extreme discomfort.

Epidemiology/Etiology

- Urinary retention is most often seen in older men with benign prostatic hyperplasia (BPH).[1,2]
- When it occurs in women, it is usually due to medication side effects or pelvic organ prolapse/dysfunction.[2]
- Medications most frequently implicated are antihistamines, anticholinergics sympathomimetics, antipsychotics, muscle relaxants, antidepressants, antiarrhythmics, antiparkinsonian agents, and muscle relaxants.[1,2]

Pathophysiology

- The most common cause is obstruction.[1–3] Less common causes are medications, neurologic impairment, infection, trauma, and postanesthesia.

DIAGNOSIS

Clinical Presentation

History

- Patients may complain of abdominal pain and distension, back pain, flank pain, genital pain, or dribbling.[1]
- Obtain a full list of patient medications, including over-the-counter medication, and supplements.

Physical Examination
- The patient with urinary retention will present with a distended abdomen that is dull to percussion.[4]
- Perform a digital rectal exam (DRE) and neurologic exam in all patients.
  - Previous practice recommended caution with DRE if suspicious of prostatitis due to concern for inducing bacteremia, but there has been no evidence to support this.[1]
  - DRE findings may inform you as to the cause of the urinary retention.
  - Saddle anesthesia and voluntary pelvic floor contraction should be assessed.[2]
- Perform a pelvic exam in women to assess for obstructive causes, in particular rectal and vaginal prolapse.[1,2]

Diagnostic Testing

Laboratories
- Send urinalysis and urine cultures.[4,5]
- Creatinine may be checked to evaluated renal function.
- Prostate specific antigen testing is not recommended.[4]

Imaging
- Bladder ultrasound can evaluate postvoid residual, bladder stones, or urethral stones causing obstruction.[4]
  - Bladder ultrasound with ≥300 mL in a patient with trouble voiding is consistent with the diagnosis of acute urinary retention (AUR).[1]
  - Postvoid residual urine volume >50 mL is indicative of retention.[6]
- Renal ultrasound to evaluate for hydronephrosis.[2]
- A CT of the abdomen and pelvis with contrast should be performed if there is concern for an abdominal, pelvic, or retroperitoneal mass.[2]

Diagnostic Procedures

- Urinary bladder catheterization is both diagnostic and therapeutic.
  - >400 mL output in 15 minutes is consistent with AUR.[1]
  - Leave the catheter in place.

TREATMENT

Medications

- Begin an alpha-1 adrenoreceptor antagonist in the ED, such as alfuzosin 10 mg, tamsulosin 0.4 mg, or doxazosin 1 mg.[1–3,5]
- 5-alpha reductase inhibitors such as finasteride 5 mg[7] and dutasteride 0.5 mg[8] significantly reduce recurrences of AUR in men with BPH.
- Reserve antibiotics for treatment of infection discovered via urinalysis, sepsis, and pregnancy or if going to the operating room.[1]

Other Nonpharmacologic Therapies

- Decompress the bladder by catheterization.
  - Attempt with 16- to 20-French catheter initially.[1]
  - If this is unsuccessful and obstruction is likely secondary to enlarged prostate, attempt with 20- to 22-French Coude tip catheter.[1]
  - Coude catheters are not indicated for women.
  - Urethral catheterization is contraindicated in patients with recent urologic surgery or urethral trauma.[1]

- If urethral catheterization fails or is contraindicated, a suprapubic catheter may need to be placed with urologic consultation.[1]
- Rapid decompression of the bladder has not shown to increase complication rate.[9]

SPECIAL CONSIDERATIONS

Disposition

- Most patients can be managed as outpatients, as long as there is follow-up established within 1–3 days.[3]
- Admit if there is a concern for sepsis from a urinary source, gross hematuria, acute renal impairment, obstruction related to malignancy, or acute myelopathy, if catheterization yields >1 L, or if postcatheterization diuresis is so severe that it requires prolonged IV fluid support.[5]
- Upon discharge, teach the patient catheter and bag care, and explain the common side effects of alpha 1-blockers, such as dizziness, hypotension, and sexual dysfunction.[1]

Complications

- Bladder decompression can lead to hematuria, hypotension, and massive diuresis.
- Urethral catheterization carries a risk of infection and urethral damage, stricture, or bladder perforation.
- Suprapubic catheterization has a higher risk of bowel perforation and must be performed by an experienced provider.[5]

REFERENCES

1. Marshall JR, Haber J, Josephson EB. An evidence-based approach to emergency department management of acute urinary retention. *Emerg Med Pract* 2014;16(1):1–20.
2. Selius BA, Subedi R. Urinary retention in adults: diagnosis and initial management. *Am Fam Physician* 2008;77(5):643–50.
3. Fitzpatrick JM, Kirby RS. Management of acute urinary retention. *BJU Int* 2006;97(s2):16–20.
4. Kuppusamy S, Gillatt D. Managing patients with acute urinary retention. *Practitioner* 2011;255(1739):21–3, 2–3.
5. Yoon P, Chalasani V, Woo H. Systematic review and meta-analysis on management of acute urinary retention. *Prostate Cancer Prostatic Dis* 2015;18(4):297–302.
6. Asimakopoulos AD, De Nunzio C, Kocjancic E, et al. Measurement of post-void residual urine. *Neurourol Urodyn* 2016;35(1):55–7. doi: 10.1002/nau.22671.
7. Roehrborn CG, Bruskewitz R, Nickel JC, et al. Sustained decrease in incidence of acute urinary retention and surgery with finasteride for 6 years in men with benign prostatic hyperplasia. *J Urol* 2004;171(3):1194–8.
8. Debruyne F, Barkin J, van Erps P, et al. Efficacy and safety of long-term treatment with the dual 5 alpha-reductase inhibitor dutasteride in men with symptomatic benign prostatic hyperplasia. *Eur Urol* 2004;46(4):488–94.
9. Nyman MA, Schwenk NM, Silverstein MD. Management of urinary retention: rapid versus gradual decompression and risk of complications. *Mayo Clin Proc* 1997;72(10):951–6.

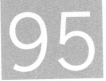

Pulmonary Emergencies: Asthma

Lawrence Lewis

GENERAL PRINCIPLES

Definition
- Asthma is characterized by chronic airway inflammation. It is defined by the history of respiratory symptoms such as wheeze, shortness of breath, chest tightness, and cough that vary over time and in intensity, together with variable expiratory airflow limitation.[1]

Epidemiology/Etiology
- The prevalence of asthma continues to rise and varies by age, race, income level, and ethnicity, being higher in those who are younger, female, living in poverty, and are multiracial, Puerto Rican, or African American.[1,2]
- Risk factors for asthma include genetics, environmental exposures (tobacco and other pollutants), infections, and other factors such as obesity and diet.[10]

Pathophysiology
- The physiologic response of the airways includes contraction at baseline and in response to external stimuli, increased mucous production, edema, and thickening of the bronchial wall with remodeling. The underlying cause of these changes is an aberrant inflammatory response to either allergen or irritant pollutant exposure or infection and involves circulating inflammatory cells and the epithelial cell itself.[3]
- Rarely, death from asthma can be sudden and unexpected, without obvious antecedent long-term deterioration of asthma control. Neutrophilic infiltration of the airways without significant mucous plugging is often the dominant feature in these patients.[4]

DIAGNOSIS

Clinical Presentation
- Patients with severely reduced air movement should be treated immediately.

History
- It is important to address the cause for the exacerbation (noncompliance, infection, weather change, allergen exposure) and to consider other possible causes of wheezing.
- The clinical presentation depends on the severity of the attack. There are a number of factors in the medical history (Table 95.1) as well as on physical examination (Table 95.2) that will help assess the current severity and the risk of an impending life-threatening attack.
- It is important to obtain a history of the present illness to include duration of the attack and what has been tried to alleviate the attack. Note other comorbidities, risk factors for asthma and other lung disease, and all medications, including reliever and controller medications. Any history of allergy or allergen exposure should be sought.

TABLE 95.1	Factors That Increase the Risk of Asthma-Related Death

- Previous severe exacerbation (intubation or ICU admission for asthma)
- ≥ 2 Hospitalization or ≥ 3 ED visits for asthma in the past year
- Hospitalization or ED visit for asthma in the past month
- Currently using or having recently stopped using oral corticosteroids
- Use of >2 canisters of SABAs monthly
- A history of psychiatric disease or psychosocial problems
- Low socioeconomic status or inner-city residence
- Comorbidities (cardiovascular, chronic lung disease, chronic psychiatric disease)
- Poor adherence with medications or poor adherence with a written asthma action plan
- Food allergy in a patient with asthma

Adapted from Camargo CA, Rachelefsky G, Schatz M. Managing asthma exacerbations in the emergency department. *Proc Am Thorac Soc* 2009;6:357–66 and EPR 3.

Physical Examination
- A rapid visual assessment of the patient to include level of consciousness, work of breathing, use of accessory muscles, and overall level of dyspnea should be performed.[5,7]
- A more focused exam should include an assessment of mental status, the upper airway, heart rate, volume and phase of wheezing, skin, and abdominal and extremity exam.

Differential Diagnosis
- Foreign body aspiration, vocal cord dysfunction, anaphylaxis, pneumonia, congestive heart failure (CHF), chronic obstructive pulmonary disease (COPD), pneumonitis, interstitial lung disease, or systemic vasculitis (Churg-Strauss)

Diagnostic Criteria and Testing
- In mild exacerbations that resolve quickly, no diagnostic testing is needed. In patients with more severe exacerbations that do not resolve over 1–2 hours, it is reasonable to perform further testing.

Laboratories
- A complete blood count may show eosinophilia and leukocytosis, but there are no specific laboratories that diagnose asthma.
- Arterial blood gas (ABG) analysis is not recommended routinely, but should be considered in severe asthma (forced expiratory volume in one second [FEV_1] < 50% predicted).[8]

Imaging
- A chest radiograph may help rule out alternative causes for the patient's symptoms or complicating factors.[8]

Diagnostic Procedures
- Bedside spirometry/peak flows may be used to track asthma and the response to treatment.

TABLE 95.2 Criteria for Categorizing Severity of Asthma Exacerbations in Adults and Children 6 Years and Older

Symptom/sign	Mild	Moderate	Severe	Imminent respiratory arrest
Breathlessness position	Not at rest	At rest	At rest	May be in tripod
	Can lie down	Prefers sitting	Sits upright	
Speech	Sentences	Phrases	Words	
Alertness	May be agitated	Usually agitated	Usually agitated	Drowsy or confused
Respiratory rate	Increased	Increased	Often >30/min	May be decreased
Accessory muscle use	Rarely	Often	Usually	Paradoxical thoracoabdominal movement
Wheeze	Moderate end expiratory	Loud throughout expiration	Loud inspiratory and expiratory	Usually absent
Pulse rate	<100	100–120	>120	Often bradycardic
Pulsus paradoxus	Absent (<10 mm Hg)	Often 10–25 mm Hg	>25 mm Hg (adult)	May be absent (respiratory fatigue)
ABG	Normal PaO_2[a]	$PaO_2 > 60$ Torr[a]	$PaO_2 < 60$ Torr	$PaO_2 < 60$ Torr[b]
	$PaCO_2 < 42$ Torr[a]	$PaCO_2 < 42$ Torr[a]	$PaCO_2 > 42$ Torr	$PaCO_2$ elevated[b]
SaO_2 (room air)	>95%	90–95%	<90%	<90%
PEF	>70%	40–69%	<40%	<25%[b]

[a]Suggests that this test is not usually necessary in the subcategory.

[b]Suggests that this test should not be performed before definitive treatment.

PaO_2, arterial oxygen pressure; PCO_2, partial pressure of carbon dioxide; PEF, peak expiratory flow; SaO_2, oxygen saturation.

The presence of several parameters, but not necessarily all, indicates the general classification of the exacerbation.

Many of these parameters have not been systematically studied, especially as they correlate with each other. Thus, they serve only as general guides.

Adapted from Camargo CA, Rachelefsky G, Schatz M. Managing asthma exacerbations in the emergency department. *Proc Am Thorac Soc* 2009;6:357–66, and Lim WJ, Mohammed Akram R, Carson KV, et al. Non-invasive positive pressure ventilation for treatment of respiratory failure due to severe acute exacerbations of asthma. *Cochrane Database Syst Rev* 2012;(12):CD004360 and the EPR 3.

TREATMENT

Medications

- The initial standard treatment for asthma exacerbations is an inhaled short-acting beta agonists (SABA), most often albuterol.
- Bronchodilators
  - Albuterol can be administered via a metered dose inhaler (with a spacer) as 4–8 puffs every 20 minutes up to 4 hours.[5,7]
  - Albuterol can also be administered via nebulization either intermittently (2.5–5 mg every 20–30 minutes for 3 doses) or continuously (10–15 mg over an hour).[5,7] Continuous administration of albuterol may be a better alternative in patients with worse lung function.[8]
  - During a severe acute exacerbation, some patients may be unable to use metered dose inhalers even with a spacer.
    - In this situation, subcutaneous administration of a beta agonist (e.g., terbutaline 0.25 mg or epinephrine 0.3 mg) is reasonable.[5,7]
    - Intravenous β-agonists are not recommended.[8] Intramuscular epinephrine (0.01 mg/kg up to 0.5 mg in adults) is only recommended if anaphylaxis or angioedema is suspected.[8]
- Corticosteroids (1 mg/kg prednisone in adults).
- Other medications.
  - Patients with severe exacerbations should also receive inhaled anticholinergics (ipratropium bromide). Oxygen supplementation should be used to maintain O_2 saturation 93–95% in adults.[8]
  - Magnesium sulfate (2 g infusion over 20 minutes) reduces hospital admissions in severe exacerbations.[7,8]

Other Nonpharmacologic Therapies

- Nonpharmacologic management of asthma includes fluid and electrolyte management and assisted ventilation.
- Both noninvasive positive pressure ventilation (NIPPV or NIV) and endotracheal intubation are mainstays of nonpharmacologic therapy in impending respiratory failure, but unlike COPD, the evidence for NIPPV in asthma is not as compelling.[6]

SPECIAL CONSIDERATIONS

Disposition

- Many patients with asthma exacerbation will improve over the course of 1–2 hours in the emergency department and be able to be discharged home. Discharge decisions are often based on improvement in clinical signs and symptoms.
  - Although bedside pulmonary function with peak flow or FEV_1 can help with disposition decision-making, patients can often be safely discharged even when these tests show persistent abnormalities.[9] Consensus recommendations from GINA (Global Initiative for Asthma) recommend hospitalization if pretreatment FEV_1 or peak expiratory flow (PEF) is <60–80% predicted or personal best.
- ICU admission is indicated for those with mental status changes, need for mechanical ventilation, hemodynamic instability, or other comorbid conditions, which would make them inappropriate for floor admission.

- Discharge planning.
  - Discharge medications should include a rapid-onset reliever medication (SABA), 5–7 days of an oral steroid (1 mg/kg up to 50 mg daily). Most patients should receive a controller medication (most commonly an inhaled corticosteroid).

REFERENCES

1. Lugogo NL, Kraft M. Epidemiology of asthma. *Clin Chest Med* 2006;27:1–15.
2. Fahy JV. Eosinophilic and neutrophilic inflammation in asthma: insights from clinical studies. *Proc Am Thorac Soc* 2009;6:256–9.
3. Chanez P, Bourdin A. Pathophysiology of Asthma. In: Castro M, Kraft M, eds. *Clinical Asthma*. 1st ed. Philadelphia: Mosby, 2008.
4. Papiris S, Kotanidou A, Malagari K, Roussos C. Clinical review: severe asthma. *Crit Care* 2002;6:30–44.
5. Camargo CA, Rachelefsky G, Schatz M. Managing asthma exacerbations in the emergency department. *Proc Am Thorac Soc* 2009;6:357–66.
6. Lim WJ, Mohammed Akram R, Carson KV, et al. Non-invasive positive pressure ventilation for treatment of respiratory failure due to severe acute exacerbations of asthma. *Cochrane Database Syst Rev* 2012;(12):CD004360.
7. US Department of Health and Human Services, National Institute of Health, National Heart, Lung, and Blood Institute. Expert Panel Report 3: guidelines for the diagnosis and management of asthma. Available at: http://www.nhlbi.nih.gov/guidelines/asthma/asthgdln.pdf (last accessed 2/3/2016).
8. Global Initiative for Asthma. Global Strategy for Asthma Management and Prevention. 2015. Available at: www.ginasthma.org.
9. Schneider JE, Lewis LM, Ferguson I, et al. Repeated dyspnea score and percent FEV_1 are modest predictors of hospitalization/relapse in patients with acute asthma exacerbation. *Respir Med* 2014;108:1284–91.
10. Strachan DP, Cook DG. Parental smoking and childhood asthma: longitudinal and case control studies. *Thorax* 1998;53:204–12.

96 Pulmonary Emergencies: Hemoptysis

Tanya Devnani and Christopher Holthaus

GENERAL PRINCIPLES

Definition

- Hemoptysis is defined as the expectoration of blood from the lower respiratory tract below the glottis (tracheobronchial tree and lungs).

Classification

- Massive hemoptysis
  - The definition of massive hemoptysis varies from >200 to >1000 mL of blood over a 24-hour period, but the commonly accepted definition is >600 mL over a 24-hour period or ≥100 mL/h.[1,2]
  - Massive hemoptysis has the potential to be acutely life threatening with 90% of cases arising from a bronchial artery.[2]
- Nonmassive hemoptysis
  - The definition of nonmassive hemoptysis is simply small volume expectoration of blood.
  - Even nonmassive hemoptysis can cause asphyxiation depending on the patient's underlying lung disease and ability to clear the blood.

Epidemiology/Etiology

- Hemoptysis is a common ED complaint, but only 1–5% of cases are massive or life threatening. In these cases, however, the mortality rate approaches nearly 80%.[3,4]
- Data to identify the most prevalent causes of hemoptysis are lacking, but some studies suggest that cancer, cystic fibrosis, arteriovenous malformations, and post-procedural complications play prominent roles in the developed world.[4]
- The various etiologies for hemoptysis include both pulmonary and systemic diseases. They are listed in Table 96.1.

Pathophysiology

- Hemoptysis is generally the result of inflammation, irritation, or laceration of the tissue or blood vessels of the lower respiratory tract.
- Blood flow to the lungs arises from pulmonary and bronchial arteries.[11]

DIAGNOSIS

Clinical Presentation

History

- Estimate the rate of bleeding and volume of expectorated blood while asking about general risk factors such as prior episodes of hemoptysis and known underlying lung disease.[5]
- Elicit symptoms specific to cardiopulmonary conditions such as congestive heart failure, malignancy, infection, vasculitides, coagulopathy, drug ingestions, and trauma or pulmonary procedures.

Physical Examination

- Examine the nares, oropharynx, and skin looking for active bleeding, dried blood, bruising, or petechiae.
- The lungs may have wheezing, rales, rhonchi, or decreased breath sounds from aspiration of blood or active bleeding in the lung parenchyma.

Differential Diagnosis

- Upper airway or gastrointestinal tract hemorrhage.
- See Table 96.1 for a list of potential causes of hemoptysis.

Diagnostic Criteria and Testing

Laboratories

- Initial studies include a complete blood count (CBC), comprehensive metabolic panel (CMP), coagulation studies, troponin, and urinalysis. Include a type and screen and an arterial blood gas (ABG) for more severe cases.

TABLE 96.1	Hemoptysis Etiologies
Class	**Disease**
Infectious	Acute bronchitis
	Acute pneumonia
	Tuberculosis
	Fungal disease (aspergilloma)
	Parasitic disease (paragonimiasis)
	Lung abscess
Toxic	Cocaine inhalation
	Nitrogen dioxide inhalation
	Bevacizumab treatment
Traumatic	Penetrating trauma
	Blunt trauma
Cardiovascular	Heart failure
	Mitral stenosis
	Pulmonary embolism
Neoplastic	Bronchogenic carcinoma
Structural	Arteriovenous malformation (hereditary hemorrhagic telangiectasia)
	Bronchiectasis (cystic fibrosis, chronic bronchitis)
	Fistula (tracheobronchial, aortobronchial)
Hematologic	Thrombocytopenia
	Disseminated intravascular coagulation
Inflammatory	Goodpasture syndrome
	ANCA+ vasculitis
	Systemic lupus erythematosus
	Behçet syndrome
	Idiopathic pulmonary hemosiderosis
Iatrogenic	Bronchoscopy
	Lung biopsy
	Pulmonary artery catheter
Other	Catamenial hemoptysis
	Foreign body

Imaging
- Chest plain radiograph can screen for various causes of hemoptysis. In the case of diffuse alveolar hemorrhage, the chest plain radiograph will reveal diffuse bilateral alveolar infiltrates.
- Chest CT is more sensitive for detection of causes of hemoptysis.
  - CT without contrast is sufficient to diagnose hemoptysis secondary to bronchiectasis, malignancy, and infection.[6]

○ Computed tomographic angiography (CTA) can be used to diagnose structural vascular abnormalities such as arteriovenous malformations.[6] CTA also helps to localize the source of bleeding.

Diagnostic Procedures
• Bronchoscopy can facilitate both localization of bleeding and therapeutic intervention.

TREATMENT

Medications

• In massive hemoptysis from an underlying coagulopathy, systemic procoagulants may be used.
  ○ Fresh frozen plasma should be administered in the setting of an elevated prothrombin time (PT) or partial thromboplastin time (PTT).
  ○ Platelet transfusion should be administered if the patient is on an antiplatelet agent or has thrombocytopenia.
  ○ Other options include recombinant factor VII and aminocaproic acid.

Other Nonpharmacologic Therapies

• For nonmassive hemoptysis, may treat conservatively addressing the underlying cause.
• For massive hemoptysis, focus on initial stabilization and rapid localization to target therapy.[3]
  ○ If the patient is not protecting the airway, have a low threshold for intubation.
  ○ A large diameter (8.0) endotracheal tube should be placed to facilitate bronchoscopy following intubation.
  ○ Consider mainstem intubation of the unaffected lung to facilitate selective ventilation of this lung.
  ○ Place the patient in the lateral decubitus position with the affected lung down to avoid blood entering into the unaffected lung.
  ○ Blood loss and hemodynamic instability should be managed with volume resuscitation and blood product administration.
• Bronchoscopy can facilitate both localization and therapeutic intervention through direct tamponade, balloon tamponade, thermocoagulation, and administration of hemostatic agents (epinephrine, vasopressin, thrombin).[3,7,8,13]
• Interventional angiography with bronchial artery embolization is an effective therapy in patients whom bronchoscopy has failed and whom cannot tolerate surgery.[6,9,10]

SPECIAL CONSIDERATIONS

Disposition

• Otherwise, healthy patients with nonmassive hemoptysis and stable vital signs can be discharged to follow up with a primary care doctor. They should be educated to return to the emergency department if symptoms are worsening.
• High-risk patients such as those with underlying lung disease with nonmassive hemoptysis should undergo brief hospitalization to an observation unit for monitoring.
• Any patient with massive hemoptysis should be admitted to an intensive care unit.

REFERENCES

1. Jean-Baptiste E. Clinical assessment and management of massive hemoptysis. *Crit Care Med* 2000;28(5):1642–7.
2. Weinberger S. Etiology and evaluation of hemoptysis in adults. *UpToDate*. Waltham: UpToDate (last accessed 2/27/16).
3. Lordan JL, Gascoigne A, Corris PA. The pulmonary physician in critical care * Illustrative case 7: assessment and management of massive haemoptysis. *Thorax* 2003;58(9):814–9.
4. Brown CA, Raja AS. Hemoptysis. In: Marx J, Hockeberger RS, Walls R, eds. *Rosen's Emergency Medicine: Concepts and Clinical Practice*. 8th ed. Saunders, Philadelphia 2014.
5. Bidwell JL, Pachner RW. Hemoptysis: diagnosis and management. *Am Fam Physician* 2005;72(7):1253–60.
6. Ketai LH, Mohammed TL, Kirsch J, et al. ACR appropriateness criteria(R) hemoptysis. *J Thorac Imaging* 2014;29(3):W19–22.
7. Morice RC, Ece T, Ece F, Keus L. Endobronchial argon plasma coagulation for treatment of hemoptysis and neoplastic airway obstruction. *Chest* 2001;119(3):781–7.
8. Tsukamoto T, Sasaki H, Nakamura H. Treatment of hemoptysis patients by thrombin and fibrinogen-thrombin infusion therapy using a fiberoptic bronchoscope. *Chest* 1989;96(3):473–6.
9. Chun JY, Morgan R, Belli AM. Radiological management of hemoptysis: a comprehensive review of diagnostic imaging and bronchial arterial embolization. *Cardiovasc Intervent Radiol* 2010;33(2):240–50.
10. Swanson KL, Johnson CM, Prakash UB, et al. Bronchial artery embolization: experience with 54 patients. *Chest* 2002;121(3):789–95.
11. Pump KK. Distribution of bronchial arteries in the human lung. *Chest* 1972;62(4):447–51.
12. Tsoumakidou M, Chrysofakis G, Tsiligianni I, et al. A prospective analysis of 184 hemoptysis cases: diagnostic impact of chest x-ray, computed tomography, bronchoscopy. *Respiration* 2006;73(6):808–14.

97

Pulmonary Emergencies: Lower Respiratory Tract Disease

Gregory Ratti

Pneumonia

GENERAL PRINCIPLES

Definition

- Pneumonia is defined as an infection of the lung parenchyma and is classified as community-acquired pneumonia (CAP) or health care–associated pneumonia (HCAP).

- HCAP pneumonia is defined as pneumonia in a patient who has been hospitalized for >48 hours, has been hospitalized for >2 days in the last 3 months, resides in a nursing home or extended care facility, has received antibiotics within the last 3 months, is on outpatient hemodialysis, has received home wound care, or has been in contact with anyone who has exposure to a multidrug-resistant organism.[1]

Epidemiology/Etiology

- The most common pathogen associated with CAP remains *Streptococcus pneumoniae*. HCAP may be associated with methicillin-resistant *Staphylococcus aureus* (MRSA) and *Pseudomonas*.
- Risk factors for pneumonia include increased age (>65), institutionalized patients, alcoholism, chronic obstructive pulmonary disease (COPD), cardiovascular disease, diabetes mellitus, renal failure, recent viral infection, aspiration, recent treatment with antibiotics, and immunosuppression.[2]

Pathophysiology

- Pneumonia occurs when microorganisms gain access to the lower respiratory tract, and a host's ability to fight invading microbial pathogens is compromised.

DIAGNOSIS

Clinical Presentation

History

- Patients often present with complaints of fever, dyspnea, cough, pleuritic chest pain, increased sputum production, or altered mentation in the elderly.
- History should focus on risk factors and possible exposures, which place them at risk for multidrug-resistant organisms.

Physical Examination

- Lung exam may reveal rales or rhonchi. In heavily consolidated areas, there may be associated dullness to percussion. Bronchial breath sounds may also be present.

Differential Diagnosis

- Aspiration pneumonitis, bronchitis, pulmonary edema, pulmonary embolism, bronchiolitis obliterans, malignancy, acute respiratory distress syndrome, alveolar hemorrhage, or vasculitis

Diagnostic Criteria and Testing

Laboratories

- Complete blood count (CBC) and basic metabolic panel (BMP) should be drawn.
- Arterial blood gas (ABG) should be performed in selected individuals to look for hypoxemia and acidosis.
- Pretreatment blood cultures should be drawn in any patient with a cavitary lesion, leukopenia, alcohol abuse, chronic liver disease, asplenia, pleural effusion, or those admitted to the ICU.[3,4] Sputum cultures are not recommended.

Imaging

- Upright PA and lateral chest plain radiograph are preferred.
- CT of the chest may be useful in determining the extent of lung consolidation as well as any associated lung pathology.

TREATMENT
- Patients should receive antibiotics within the first 4 hours of health care contact.

Medications
- For CAP, the patient may be discharged with a course of a macrolide such as azithromycin 500 mg for 1 day followed by 4 additional days at 250 mg/d.[3]
- For CAP inpatient treatment, patients should receive a fluoroquinolone such as moxifloxacin or levofloxacin or a beta-lactam such as amoxicillin plus a macrolide. An alternative treatment is with ceftriaxone as a single agent.[3]
- For patients presenting with HCAP and risk of multidrug-resistant organisms, an antipseudomonal cephalosporin, carbapenem, or a combination beta-lactam/lactamase inhibitor plus a respiratory fluoroquinolone or aminoglycoside plus vancomycin or linezolid is recommended.[5]

SPECIAL CONSIDERATIONS

Disposition
- There are several risk stratification tools available. Among these are the CURB-65 and the Pneumonia Severity Index.
- Patients who have a new oxygen requirement will require admission to the hospital, and those who are suffering from respiratory distress will need admission to the intensive care unit.

Bronchitis

GENERAL PRINCIPLES

Definition
- Bronchitis is an inflammatory condition involving the tracheobronchial tree.

Epidemiology/Etiology
- Viruses are thought to be the cause of acute bronchitis in >85% of cases.[6]
- Bronchitis affects ~5% of adults annually with the majority of cases occurring in the fall or winter.[4]
  - Most cases of bronchitis are self-limited, though patients with underlying lung disease such as COPD or bronchiectasis, congestive heart failure, or immune compromised are at high risk of complications.

Pathophysiology
- Cells lining the bronchi become irritated and membranes become hyperemic and edematous. The inflammation results in impaired mucociliary clearance and increased secretions causing cough.

DIAGNOSIS

Clinical Presentation
History
- Cough is the most common presenting symptom. Cough tends to begin within 2 days of exposure to infection.

- History should focus on exposure to viral or bacterial illnesses. History should also focus on past medical history and medication lists, which may suggest risk factors for complications.

Physical Examination
- May include increased sputum production, dyspnea, wheezing, pleuritic chest pain, fevers, hoarseness, malaise, rhonchi, or rales.

Differential Diagnosis

- Differential diagnosis includes asthma exacerbation, chronic bronchitis, COPD exacerbation, the common cold, congestive heart failure exacerbation, gastroesophageal reflux disease (GERD), pneumonia, postnasal drip, seasonal allergies, or sinusitis.
- Pertussis should be considered in any patient who has a known exposure or those individuals with a persistent cough who are not up to date on the vaccination.

Diagnostic Criteria and Testing

Laboratories
- There are no laboratory values that are specific for the diagnosis of bronchitis.[4]

Imaging
- A chest radiograph should be considered in anyone in whom pneumonia is suspected or in individuals who are at high risk if the diagnosis of pneumonia is delayed, such as the elderly.[7]

TREATMENT

Medications

- Beta agonists have been shown not to improve cough.[8,9] Treatment is directed at symptomatic management.
- Antibiotics are not recommended for treatment of bronchitis despite length of cough.[5]
- Patients with pertussis should be treated with azithromycin to reduce the risk of spread.

SPECIAL CONSIDERATIONS

Disposition

- Patients may be discharged for follow-up with their primary care doctor.

Tuberculosis

GENERAL PRINCIPLES

Definition

- Tuberculosis (TB) is the systemic disease caused by the bacterium, *Mycobacterium tuberculosis*.

Epidemiology/Etiology

- Most cases of active TB are the result of reactivation of prior TB exposure and will occur in 5–15% of patients with latent TB.[10]
- Those at high risk of reactivation include those who are malnourished or immunocompromised.

- Risk factors for TB include incarceration, homelessness, HIV, travel to or immigration from an area where TB is endemic, and IV drug use.

Pathophysiology

- TB occurs when *M. tuberculosis* is inhaled in droplet form and reaches the alveoli where it is ingested by macrophages, eventually rupturing them and spreading hematogenously.
- *M. tuberculosis* is extremely immunogenic and induces both cellular and humoral immunity within 2–4 weeks of infection. Eventually, granulomas form at the site of the primary lesion and any sites of dissemination.[6]

DIAGNOSIS

Clinical Presentation

- Primary disease may cause minimal symptoms and may include fever or pleuritic chest pain.
- In immunosuppressed individuals, primary disease can progress rapidly to significant clinical disease including effusions, cavitary lesions, and hematogenous spread (miliary TB).
- Reactivation TB usually presents with a more insidious onset, with symptoms including weight loss, anorexia, fever, night sweats, and malaise followed by cough and sputum production with blood streaks.

History

- Patients may complain of fever or pleuritic chest pain or give a history of hemoptysis.

Physical Examination

- With pulmonary TB, physical findings may include abnormal breath sounds, especially over the upper lobes or if there is an associated effusion. Rales or bronchial breath sounds may be present.
- Lymphadenopathy may be present within the bilateral anterior and posterior supraclavicular nodes.

Differential Diagnosis

- Differential diagnosis for TB includes fungal infections such as blastomycosis or histoplasma; bacteria such as tularemia and actinomycosis; other mycobacterial infections such as *Mycobacterium avium, M. chelonae, M. fortuitum,* and others; or squamous cell lung cancer.

Diagnostic Criteria and Testing

Laboratories

- Diagnosis is made by acid-fast or fluorochrome stain of sputum.
- Cultures and sensitivities should be sent for all new TB diagnosis but may take several weeks to grow; therefore, initial treatment is based on sputum stain and clinical suspicion.

Imaging

- Chest plain radiograph may show focal infiltrates, upper lobe cavitary lesions, miliary disease, or pleural effusions.

TREATMENT

- Place patient in a negative pressure isolation room.
- Anyone exposed to the patient should wear N95 mask to prevent spread of the disease.
- The patient should wear a simple face mask to contain the spread of airborne droplets.

Medications

- Initial therapy involves a four medication regimen consisting of isoniazid (5 mg/kg, max 300 mg/d), rifampin (10 mg/kg, max 600 mg/d), pyrazinamide (15–30 mg/kg, max 2 g/d), and ethambutol (15–25 mg/kg/d) with infectious disease consultation.[11]

SPECIAL CONSIDERATIONS

Disposition

- Patients do not need to be admitted for their full treatment course but should be admitted for initiation of therapy. While hospitalized, patients starting antituberculosis therapy should be placed in a negative pressure room.

Patient Education

- All patients should have follow-up arranged with the local health department. Patients should be enrolled in a directly observed therapy (DOT) program prior to discharge from the hospital.
- Patients must be educated about the importance of their disease and the need for isolation until they are no longer contagious, so as not to spread their disease.

Foreign Body Aspiration

GENERAL PRINCIPLES

Definition

- Foreign body aspiration (FBA) is classified as a potentially life-threatening event in which a foreign body blocks and obscures the airway.

Epidemiology/Etiology

- FBA often presents with delayed diagnosis.[12]

Pathophysiology

- Aspiration events may occur in the setting of loss of consciousness secondary to trauma, drug or alcohol abuse, anesthesia, or impaired swallow mechanism.
- If a pill, such as iron or potassium is aspirated, it may cause associated inflammation of the airway, but unless the object is sharp and causes direct trauma, there does not tend to be associated airway injury.

DIAGNOSIS

Clinical Presentation

History
- The most common symptoms include cough, which generally precedes tachypnea and stridor. It is important to note that just because coughing stops, this does not mean the event has resolved.
- Adults are often asymptomatic at the time of aspiration and tend to present later with a chronic cough, that may develop into pneumonia.
- In witnessed FBA, history should focus on the activities surrounding the event.
- If aspiration is not recalled, a high clinical suspicion must be maintained.

Physical Examination
- Tachycardia, tachypnea, and hypoxemia may indicate a need for emergent intervention.
- Cyanosis may be seen with high-grade proximal obstructions.
- Classic findings on the lung exam reveal a focal, wheeze, or regional variations in aeration. If the obstruction is proximal, breath sounds may be decreased over an area of the lungs.

Differential Diagnosis
- The differential diagnosis in adults presenting with delayed FBA may include asthma, COPD, pneumonia, TB, or aspiration pneumonitis.

Diagnostic Criteria and Testing
- Initial steps for management in a witnessed aspiration event where the patient is in extremis should include back blows or the Heimlich maneuver in an attempt to dislodge the obstruction.

Laboratories
- Laboratory values are not helpful in acute aspiration events.

Imaging
- CXR-associated findings may include lower airway hyperinflation in partial obstructions or atelectasis in complete obstructions. There may also be mediastinal shift. In delayed presentation, pneumonia may be present.[4,13]
- CT of the chest without contrast may be helpful if clinical suspicion remains high with a negative chest radiograph.

Diagnostic Procedures
- Fiber optic rigid or flexible bronchoscopy may be both diagnostic and therapeutic in moderate to high-grade obstructions.[14–17]

TREATMENT
- Early involvement of otolaryngology or thoracic surgery for extraction of the foreign body is the mainstay of therapy.

Medications
- There are no medications that will specifically treat an FBA.

Other Nonpharmacologic Therapies
- Bronchoscopy as noted above

SPECIAL CONSIDERATIONS

Disposition

• All patients who require intervention should be admitted to the hospital for observation.

Complications

• Delayed diagnosis may lead to acute and recurrent pneumonia, lung abscess, bronchiectasis, and hemoptysis.
• In more proximal airway obstructions, delay in diagnosis may result in significant morbidity such as anoxic brain injury or even death. Delay in diagnosis of distal obstructions, which is more common in the elderly presenting with atypical symptoms, may result in postobstructive pneumonia and damage to lung parenchyma.

REFERENCES

1. Longo DL, Fauci AS, Kasper DL, et al. Pneumonia, Bronchiectasis, and Lung Abscess. In: Longo DL, Fauci AS, Kasper DL, et al., eds. *Harrison's Manual of Medicine.* 18th ed. New York: McGraw-Hill, 2013.
2. Huchon G, Woodhead M, Gialdroni-Grassi G, et al. Guidelines for management of adult community-acquired lower respiratory tract infections. *Eur Respir J* 1998;11:986–91.
3. Mandell LA, Wunderink RG, Anzueto A, et al. Infectious Diseases Society of America/American Thoracic Society consensus guidelines on the management of community-acquired pneumonia in adults. *Clin Infect Dis* 2007;44:S27–72.
4. Braman SS. Chronic cough due to acute bronchitis: ACCP evidence-based clinical practice guidelines. *Chest* 2006;129:95S–103S.
5. Smith SM, Fahey T, Smucny J, Becker LA. Antibiotics for acute bronchitis. *Cochrane Database Syst Rev* 2014;(3):CD000245.
6. Longo DL, Fauci AS, Kasper DL, et al. Tuberculosis and Other Mycobacterial Infections. In: Longo DL, Fauci AS, Kasper DL, et al., eds. *Harrison's Manual of Medicine.* 18th ed. New York: McGraw-Hill, 2013.
7. Knutson D, Braun C. Diagnosis and management of acute bronchitis. *Am Fam Physician* 2002;65:2039–45.
8. Melbye H, Aasebo U, Straume B. Symptomatic effect of inhaled fenoterol in acute bronchitis: a placebo-controlled double-blind study. *Fam Pract* 1991;8:216–22.
9. Becker LA, Hom J, Villasis-Keever M, van der Wouden JC. Beta2-agonists for acute cough or a clinical diagnosis of acute bronchitis. *Cochrane Database Syst Rev* 2015;(6):CD001726.
10. Getahun H, Matteelli A, Chaisson RE, Raviglione M. Review article: latent *Mycobacterium tuberculosis* infection. *N Engl J Med* 2015;372:2127–35.
11. Horsburgh CR, Feldman S, Ridzon R. Practice guidelines for the treatment of tuberculosis. *Clin Infect Dis* 2000;31:633–9.
12. Committee on Injury, Violence, and Poison Prevention. Prevention of choking among children. *Pediatrics* 2010;125:601–7.
13. Jones BE, Jones J, Bewick T, et al. CURB-65 pneumonia severity assessment adapted for electronic decision support. *Chest* 2011;140:156–63.
14. Righini CA, Morel N, Karkas A, et al. What is the diagnostic value of flexible bronchoscopy in the initial investigation of children with suspected foreign body aspiration? *Int J Pediatr Otorhinolaryngol* 2007;71:1383–90.
15. Limper AH, Prakash UB. Tracheobronchial foreign bodies in adults. *Ann Inter Med* 1990;112:604–9.
16. Lan RS. Non-asphyxiating tracheobronchial foreign bodies in adults. *Eur Respir J* 1994;7:510–4.
17. Tang LF, Xu YC, Wang CF, et al. Airway foreign body removal by flexible bronchoscopy: experience with 1027 children during 2000-2008. *W J Pediatr* 2009;5:191–5.

Pulmonary Emergencies: Mediastinitis

Aimee Wendelsdorf

GENERAL PRINCIPLES

Definition

• Mediastinitis is the inflammation of the connective tissue filling the interpleural space and surrounding the organs of the mediastinum or middle thoracic cavity.

Epidemiology/Etiology

• Poststernotomy wound infections.
• Spread of descending head and neck infections into the thoracic cavity.
  ○ Common primary sources of descending infection include odontogenic sources, Ludwig's angina, pharyngeal/upper respiratory, cervical, infections of the salivary glands, and other head and neck infections such as epiglottitis.[1,2]
• Esophageal perforation.
  ○ 1% of perforations will progress to mediastinitis.[3] The majority of those patients who suffer esophageal perforations are between the age of 50 and 70 and are five times more commonly seen in men compared to women.[2]
  ○ Spontaneous occurrence or due to blunt or penetrating trauma or foreign body ingestion.[3]
  ○ Injury related to hyperemesis, also known as Boerhaave syndrome, and toxic ingestions are other less frequent causes of esophageal perforation.
• Chronic mediastinitis.
  ○ Histoplasmosis is the most common cause of chronic mediastinitis.[4]
  ○ Often asymptomatic but may result in clinically significant disease due to mass effect and obstruction of the airway or local vascular structures.[5]
  ○ Other potential less common causes of chronic mediastinitis are tuberculosis, sarcoidosis, coccidiomycosis, and syphilis.
• Risk factors for developing mediastinitis are advanced age, obesity, diabetes mellitus, oral glucocorticoid use, tobacco use, lower socioeconomic status, and poor dental hygiene.

Pathophysiology

Bacteria spreads from the head or neck into the thoracic cavity.

• Gases formed by the bacteria have the potential to further dissect between facial planes facilitating the spread of necrotizing infections.
  ○ The "danger space" lies directly behind the retropharyngeal space and plays the most clinical significance in descending neck infection allowing for mediastinal spread in 70% of cases.[1] Infection in this space develops from direct spread from the retropharyngeal, prevertebral, and parapharyngeal spaces.
  ○ Anaerobic bacteria are responsible for 41% of cases of acute mediastinitis with mixed aerobic–anaerobic bacteria accounting for another 41%.[3]

○ Diabetic patients are at a higher risk of *Klebsiella* and methicillin-resistant *Staphylococcus aureus* (MRSA) in intravenous drug users and the immunocompromised.[6]

DIAGNOSIS

Clinical Presentation

History
- Patients may report a history of recent upper respiratory infection, pharyngitis, or poor detention now complicated by shortness of breath, chest pain, or dysphagia.
- A history of recent endoscopic procedure or episodes of frequent emesis followed by fever, chest pain, and dysphagia may indicate esophageal injury complicated by mediastinitis. If patients present with chest pain and pleural effusion after a near-choking incident or foreign body ingestion, esophageal perforation is also a potential complication that may lead to mediastinal infection.
- Mediastinitis from sternal wound infections typically presents relatively late occurring weeks to months after surgery.

Physical Examination
- External signs of neck swelling may be appreciated in descending cervical neck infections but are not always seen when the deeper structures of the neck are affected.
- External signs of sternal wound infections such as tenderness, erythema, and sternal drainage may be seen in postoperative mediastinitis.[7]
- Signs and symptoms similar to superior vena cava (SVC) syndrome (cyanosis, facial swelling, dysphagia, dyspnea, congestion, headache, and dizziness) can be seen with severe progression of chronic mediastinitis.[8]

Differential Diagnosis
- Acute coronary syndrome, pulmonary embolism, thoracic aortic dissection, pleural effusion, pneumothorax, pneumonia, bronchitis, influenza, or pericarditis

Diagnostic Testing

Laboratories
- Initial laboratory studies should consist of a routine infectious workup including C-reactive protein and erythrocyte sedimentation rate (ESR).[6]

Imaging
- Chest radiography may show nonspecific mediastinal widening. Other findings suggestive of possible infection including subcutaneous gas and pleural effusions may also be identified.[3]
- CT scan of the neck and thorax may show a widened mediastinum, diffuse or focal gas bubbles within the mediastinum, air–fluid levels, or mediastinal soft tissue masses, all consistent with mediastinitis.[2,6,9]
- Gastrografin esophagram is an acceptable first-line form of imaging for the diagnosis of esophageal perforation and has a false-negative rate of 10%.[3]
  ○ Barium contrast should be avoided given risk of associated inflammation and injury if it were to contaminate the thoracic cavity.

TREATMENT

Medication

- Broad-spectrum antibiotics should be started as soon as mediastinitis is clinically suspected.
- Empiric antibiotics should not be delayed for fluid culture.
  - Vancomycin 15–20 mg/kg IV every 8–12 hours (max 2 g) or linezolid 600 mg orally or IV every 12 hours plus either piperacillin/tazobactam 3.375 g IV every 6 hours or cefepime 1 g IV every 8 hours plus clindamycin 600–900 mg IV every 8 hours.
  - If patient has a diagnosed severe penicillin allergy: vancomycin or linezolid plus ciprofloxacin 400 mg IV every 8 hours plus clindamycin 600–900 mg IV every 8 hours.
  - In diabetic patients who are at a higher risk of *Klebsiella pneumonia*, the addition of gentamicin should be considered given high rates of clindamycin resistance.[8]
- Antibiotic therapy alone is insufficient for the treatment of acute mediastinitis. Surgical drainage and attempted source control remain the gold standard therapy for acute mediastinitis.

Other Nonpharmacologic Therapies
- Patients with esophageal perforations may need surgery and should be NPO to limit further contamination of the mediastinum and will require parenteral nutrition until able to safely tolerate oral intake.[9]

SPECIAL CONSIDERATIONS

Disposition

- Patients with suspected acute mediastinitis should be admitted to the intensive care unit for close monitoring, aggressive resuscitation, and serial imaging to monitor for reaccumulation of infected fluid or further spread of infection.[1]

Complications

- The three most common complications following descending necrotizing mediastinitis are pleural effusions, pneumonia, and severe sepsis or septic shock.[13] The development of acute respiratory distress syndrome (ARDS) is not uncommon in acute mediastinitis.[1]

REFERENCES

1. Athanassiadi KA. Infections of the mediastinum. *Thorac Surg Clin* 2009;19:37–45.
2. Celakovsky P, Kalfert D, Tucek L, et al. Deep neck infections: risk factors for mediastinal spread. *Eur Arch Otorhinolaryngol* 2014;271:1679–83.
3. Cross MR, Greenwald MF, Dahhan A. Esophageal perforation and acute bacterial mediastinitis: other causes of chest pain that can be easily missed. *Medicine* 2015;94:1–4.
4. Marty-Ane CH, Berthet JP, Alric P, et al. Management of descending necrotizing mediastinitis: an aggressive treatment for an aggressive disease. *Ann Thorac Surg* 1999;69:212–7.
5. Strock SB, Gaudieri S, Mallal S, et al. Fibrosing mediastinitis complicating prior histoplasmosis is associated with human leukocyte antigen DQB1*04:02—a case control study. *BMC Infect Dis* 2015;15:206–10.
6. Solis-Suarez JA, Carillo-Munoz A. Deep Neck Infections. In: Dajer-Fadel WL, ed. *Mediastinal Infections: Clinical Diagnosis, Surgical and Alternative Treatments*. New York: Nova Science Publishers, 2015:17–33.

7. Vieira F, Allen SM, Stocks RM, Thompson JW. Deep neck infections. *Otolaryngology* 2008;41:458–83.
8. Dajer-Fadel WL. Chronic Mediastinitis. In: Dajer-Fadel WL, ed. *Mediastinal Infections: Clinical Diagnosis, Surgical and Alternative Treatments.* New York: Nova Science Publishers, 2015:175–82.
9. Nirula R. Esophageal perforation. *Surg Clin N Am* 2014;94:35–41.
10. Casillas-Enriquez JD, Dajer-Fadel WL. Medical Management for Descending Necrotizing Mediastinitis. In: Dajer-Fadel WL, ed. *Mediastinal Infections: Clinical Diagnosis, Surgical and Alternative Treatments.* New York: Nova Science Publishers, 2015:82–97.

Pulmonary Emergencies: Chronic Obstructive Pulmonary Disease

Lawrence Lewis

GENERAL PRINCIPLES

Definition

- Chronic obstructive pulmonary disease (COPD) is a disease characterized by airflow limitation that is not fully reversible. It is usually progressive and associated with an abnormal inflammatory response.[1] The diagnostic criterion is a postbronchodilator forced expiratory volume in one second (FEV_1)/forced vital capacity (FVC) ratio of <0.7.

Epidemiology

- COPD, including chronic bronchitis and emphysema, is currently the third leading cause of death in the United States[2] and is the third leading cause of death from noncommunicable diseases worldwide.[3]
- COPD has both environmental and genetic components that are associated with increased risk of disease.
  - Most sources still claim tobacco smoke to be the most common cause of COPD. However, air pollution, both in the form of particulates and noxious gases, has been shown to contribute significantly to the development of COPD in later life.[4]
- Genetic factors are also associated with risk for developing COPD.[5] Besides genetic susceptibility, there are specific genetic diseases that are well associated with COPD such as alpha-1 antitrypsin deficiency.

Pathophysiology

- The hallmark of COPD is chronic inflammation that affects the peripheral airways, the lung parenchyma, and the pulmonary vasculature.[6]
- Asthma and hyperreactive airway disease are risk factors for developing COPD, but the mechanisms involved in the inflammatory process differ.
  - Patients who develop COPD have increased numbers of CD8+ lymphocytes that, along with neutrophils and macrophages, release inflammatory mediators and enzymes that can destroy structural cells in the airways, parenchyma, and vascular bed. This can lead to the characteristic physiologic abnormalities and symptoms of COPD.[1]
  - This destruction, along with disruption in repair mechanisms, leads to further pathologic changes such as nonreversible airway fibrosis.
    - The peripheral airway changes result in obstruction to airflow, progressively trapping air during exhalation and resulting in hyperinflation. The hyperinflation reduces inspiratory capacity, particularly during exertion, and is one of the earliest causes of dyspnea in these patients.[7]
- Gas exchange is impaired in COPD as a result of V/Q mismatching, decreased alveolar surface area across which gases diffuse, and a decreased ventilation as a result of the increased work of breathing.[8]
- Many patients with COPD have an increased number of goblet cells and submucosal glands that result in mucous hypersecretion.

DIAGNOSIS

Clinical Presentation

History

- Patients with COPD can present with dyspnea, cough, and/or chest pain. It is important to recognize that other complaints such as headache, fatigue, or altered mental status may also be secondary to COPD.
- A medical history should include an assessment of risk factors for COPD or asthma (smoking, occupational); a past medical history of asthma, allergies, frequent respiratory infections, and other respiratory problems; and a pattern of symptom development over time to include dyspnea (especially on exertion), cough, colds, and bouts of respiratory illness requiring emergency department visits or hospitalizations. The number of times the patient has required hospitalization and whether the patient ever required mechanical ventilation can provide useful information regarding the severity of disease. One should also ask about a family history of asthma or COPD.
- Regarding the current exacerbation, it is important to note timing and precipitating factors.

Physical Examination

- Respiratory rate, use of accessory muscles, pursed lip breathing, and inability to speak a full sentence without taking additional breaths are easily recognized bedside clues.
- End tidal CO_2 and pulse oximetry should be evaluated early.
- The pulmonary exam will often demonstrate decreased breath sounds with a prolonged expiratory phase, and wheezing/rhonchi, which are initially heard in expiration but can be heard in both inspiration and expiration in more severe cases. Wheezing may not be heard at all in the most severe cases.
- A clear lung exam suggests and extrapulmonary cause.

TABLE 99.1	Management of Severe but Not Life-Threatening Exacerbations*
Assess severity of symptoms, blood gases, and chest radiograph	
Administer supplemental oxygen and obtain serial ABGs when indicated	
Increase doses and/or frequency of short-acting bronchodilators	
Combine short-acting beta-2 agonists and anticholinergics	
Use spacers or air-driven nebulizers	
Add oral or intravenous corticosteroids	
Consider antibiotics for signs of bacterial infection	
Consider noninvasive mechanical ventilation	
Monitor fluid balance and nutrition	
Consider subcutaneous heparin or low molecular weight heparin	
Identify and treat associated conditions (e.g., heart failure, arrhythmias)	
Closely monitor condition of the patient	

Adapted from the Global Strategy for the Diagnosis, Management and Prevention of COPD, Global Initiative for Chronic Obstructive Lung Disease (GOLD) 2016. Available from http://www.goldcopd.org.

Differential Diagnosis

- Congestive heart failure (CHF), asthma/chronic obstructive asthma, foreign body aspiration, bronchiolitis obliterans, bronchitis, pneumonia, PE, pneumothorax, and cancer

Diagnostic Testing

Laboratories

- A screening complete blood count (CBC) and basic metabolic panel (BMP) is recommended in patients unless their exacerbation is mild and improves quickly.
- Arterial blood gas (ABG) analysis is useful if considering the possibility of carbon dioxide retention or acidosis and is recommended in moderate to severe cases, especially when assisted ventilation is being considered or performed.[9]

Imaging

- A chest radiograph is more helpful in ruling out other conditions such as pneumonia, pleural effusion, or a pneumothorax and can also help distinguish pure COPD from CHF, or some combination thereof.

Diagnostic Procedures

- Bedside peak flow or percent forced expiratory volume in 1 second (% FEV_1) may be helpful.
- Spirometry is considered the gold standard for making the diagnosis, with a post-bronchodilator FEV_1/FVC ratio <0.70 being the diagnostic criterion.

TABLE 99.2	Criteria for NIPPV

Moderate to severe dyspnea with use of accessory muscles and paradoxical abdominal motion

Moderate to severe acidosis (pH 7.30–7.35) and hypercapnia ($PaCO_2$ 45–60 mm Hg)

Respiratory frequency >25 breaths/min

Adapted from the Global Strategy for the Diagnosis, Management and Prevention of COPD, Global Initiative for Chronic Obstructive Lung Disease (GOLD) 2016. Available from http://www.goldcopd.org.

TREATMENT

Medications
- Brochodilators
  - In the acute exacerbation of COPD, first-line medications include inhaled short-acting beta agonists (usually albuterol 5 mg) and anticholinergics (usually ipratropium 0.5 mg) using a spacer or nebulizer to improve delivery.
- Corticosteroids
  - Systemic steroids (a dose of prednisone 40 mg daily for 5 days is recommended) are another mainstay of treatment.
- Others
  - Supplemental oxygen should be administered to maintain an SpO_2 of 88–92%.[10]
  - There is some evidence that macrolide antibiotics such as azithromycin may also benefit patients through an immunomodulatory effect.[11]
  - A complete list of the many formulations of long-term and short-term beta agonists, anticholinergics, and inhaled corticosteroids can be found in the updated Global Strategy for the Diagnosis, Management, and Prevention of COPD.[12]

Nonpharmacologic Therapy
- Nonpharmacologic therapy in the management of acute exacerbations of COPD includes fluid balance and ventilatory support.
- Both noninvasive positive pressure ventilation (NIPPV or NIV) and endotracheal intubation are the mainstays of nonpharmacologic therapy.
  - In patients at risk for impending respiratory failure (Table 99.2), early initiation of NIPPV has been shown to reduce mortality, reduce the likelihood of endotracheal intubation, improve pH and PCO_2, and reduce length of stay in the hospital.[13]
  - Patients who are in respiratory extremis, have altered mental status, are moribund, or who are rapidly tiring, and would not likely benefit from NIPPV should be endotracheally intubated (Table 99.3). Early primary intubation in patients that are unlikely to benefit from NIPPV (i.e., will require rescue intubation) has been shown to reduce mortality among this cohort.[14]
    - The use of lower tidal volumes, lower pressures, longer expiratory times (increased expiratory to inspiratory time ratio), appropriate levels of positive end-expiratory pressure, and permissive hypercapnia are important principles to consider in these intubated patients.[15] Patients require sedation and often paralysis to decrease ventilator dyssynchrony and lessen the peak pressure required for adequate ventilation.[15]

TABLE 99.3	Indications for Endotracheal Intubation and Mechanical Ventilation

Severe dyspnea with use of accessory muscles and paradoxical abdominal motion

Respiratory frequency >35 breaths/min

Life-threatening hypoxemia (PaO_2 < 40 mm Hg or PaO_2/FIO_2, 200 mm Hg)

Severe acidosis (pH < 7.25) and hypercapnia ($PaCO_2$ > 60 mm Hg)

Respiratory arrest

Somnolence and impaired mental status

Cardiovascular complications (hypotension, shock, heart failure)

Other complications (metabolic abnormalities, sepsis, pneumonia, pulmonary embolism, barotrauma, massive pleural effusion)

NIPPV failure (or exclusion criteria)

Adapted from the Global Strategy for the Diagnosis, Management and Prevention of COPD, Global Initiative for Chronic Obstructive Lung Disease (GOLD) 2016. Available from http://www.goldcopd.org.

SPECIAL CONSIDERATIONS

Disposition

• Many patients with COPD exacerbation will improve with therapy and will be able to be discharged. The Global Initiative for Chronic Obstructive Lung Disease (GOLD) Workshop Summary has recommendations for when to consider admission to the general ward (Table 99.4) and when to consider admission to an intensive care unit (Table 99.5).[12]

TABLE 99.4	Indications for Hospital Admission for Acute Exacerbation of COPD

Marked increase in intensity of symptoms, such as sudden development of resting dyspnea

Severe background COPD

Onset of new physical signs (e.g., cyanosis, peripheral edema)

Failure of exacerbation to respond to initial medical management

Significant comorbidities

Newly occurring arrhythmias

Diagnostic uncertainty

Older age

Insufficient home support

Adapted from the Global Strategy for the Diagnosis, Management and Prevention of COPD, Global Initiative for Chronic Obstructive Lung Disease (GOLD) 2016. Available from http://www.goldcopd.org.

TABLE 99.5 Indications for ICU Admission

Severe dyspnea that responds inadequately to initial therapy

Confusion, lethargy, and coma

Placement on NIPPV or intubated patient

Persistent or worsening hypoxemia (PaO_2 < 50 mm Hg), or severe/worsening hypercapnia ($PaCO_2$ > 70 mm Hg), or severe/worsening respiratory acidosis (pH < 7.30) despite supplemental oxygen and NIPPV

Adapted from the Global Strategy for the Diagnosis, Management and Prevention of COPD, Global Initiative for Chronic Obstructive Lung Disease (GOLD) 2016. Available from http://www.goldcopd.org.

- Patients who have improved with therapy; who are able to ambulate short distances, eat, and rest without significant dyspnea; and who do not require bronchodilators more often than every 4 hours can be discharged home.

Complications
- Positive pressure ventilation may rupture blebs in the lung, causing pneumothorax or pneumomediastinum.

REFERENCES

1. Hogg JC, Chu F, Utokaparch S, et al. The nature of small-airway obstruction in chronic obstructive pulmonary disease. *N Engl J Med* 2004;350:2645–53.
2. Xu J, Kochanek KD, Murphy SL, Tejada-Vera B; National Vital Statistics System. *National Vital Statistics Reports*. From the Centers for Disease Control and Prevention, National Center for Health Statistics, Atlanta, 2010;58:1–19.
3. World Health Organization. *Global Health Observatory (GHO) Data: NCD Mortality and Morbidity*. Available at: http://www.who.int/gho/ncd/mortality_morbidity/en (last accessed 2/2/16).
4. Gauderman WJ, Avol E, Gilliland F, et al. The effect of air pollution on lung development from 10 to 18 years of age. *N Engl J Med* 2004;351:1057–67.
5. Kurzius-Spencer M, Sherrill DL, Holberg CJ, et al. Familial correlation in the decline of forced expiratory volume in one second. *Am J Respir Crit Care Med* 2001;164:1261–5.
6. Hogg C. Pathophysiology of airflow limitation in chronic obstructive pulmonary disease. *Lancet* 2004;364:709–21.
7. O'Donnell DE, Laveneziana P. Dyspnea and activity limitation in COPD: mechanical factors. *COPD* 2007;4:225–36.
8. Tuder RM, Petrache I. Review series: pathogenesis of chronic obstructive pulmonary disease. *J Clin Invest* 2012;122:2749–55.
9. Celli BR, MacNee W, Agusti A, et al. Standards for the diagnosis and treatment of patients with COPD: a summary of the ATS/ERS position paper. *Eur Respir J* 2004;23: 932–46.
10. Austin MA, Wills KE, Blizzard L, et al. Effect of high flow oxygen on mortality in chronic obstructive pulmonary disease patients in prehospital setting: randomised controlled trial. *BMJ* 2010;341:c5462.
11. Shinkai M, Henke MO, Rubin BK. Macrolide antibiotics as immunomodulatory medications: proposed mechanisms of action. *Pharmacol Ther* 2008;117:393–405.
12. From the Global Strategy for the Diagnosis, Management and Prevention of COPD, Global Initiative for Chronic Obstructive Lung Disease (GOLD). 2016. Available at: http://www.goldcopd.org

13. Lightowler JV, Wedzicha JA, Elliott MW, Ram FSF. Non-invasive positive pressure ventilation to treat respiratory failure resulting from exacerbations of chronic obstructive pulmonary disease: Cochrane systematic review and meta-analysis. *BMJ* 2003;326:1–5.
14. Chandra D, Stamm JA, Taylor B, et al. Outcomes of noninvasive ventilation for acute exacerbations of chronic obstructive pulmonary disease in the United States, 1998–2008. *Am J Respir Crit Care Med* 2012;185:152–9.
15. Mosier JM, Hypes C, Joshi R, et al. Ventilator strategies and rescue therapies for management of acute respiratory failure in the emergency department. *Ann Emerg Med* 2015;66:529–41.

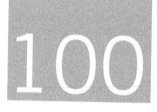

Pulmonary Emergencies: Pleural Disorders

Gregory Ratti

Pleural Effusions

GENERAL PRINCIPLES

Definition

- A pleural effusion is defined as the accumulation of fluid within the pleural space surrounding the lung.

Classification

- Pleural effusions are classified as either transudative or exudative based on Light's criteria (Table 100.1).[1]

TABLE 100.1	Light's Criteria	
Transudative	**Exudative—meets any one of the below criteria**
Fluid to serum protein ratio <0.5	Fluid to serum protein ratio >0.5
Fluid to serum LDH ratio <0.6	Fluid to serum LDH ratio >0.6
Pleural fluid LDH of <2/3 the upper limit of normal for serum LDH	Pleural fluid LDH of >2/3 the upper limit of normal for serum LDH

Pathophysiology

- Effusions result either when there is increased fluid formation by the lung interstitium, parietal pleura, or peritoneal cavity or if there is a decrease in drainage from the parietal pleura by the lymphatics from the parietal pleura.

DIAGNOSIS

Clinical Presentation

- The amount of fluid present tends to correlate poorly with a patient's symptoms and may be asymptomatic. Symptoms of dyspnea and hypoxia tend to develop when the effusion reaches 500–1000 mL.

History

- Most patients present with cough or dyspnea. These may be secondary to the effusion or the underlying disease that results in abnormal pulmonary mechanics.
- Patients may also complain of pleuritic chest pain that radiates to the back, chest, or neck.
- The history should include a survey for symptoms that may be associated with potential cause including infection, malignancy, or cardiovascular risk factors.

Physical Examination

- Chest exam may reveal dullness to percussion, decreased, breath sounds, egophony, and decreased tactile fremitus.

Differential Diagnosis

- Transudative effusions may be secondary to congestive heart failure (CHF), hepatic cirrhosis, nephrotic syndrome, superior vena cava (SVC) syndrome, hypoproteinemia, or malignancy.
- Exudative effusions may be secondary to infection, pneumonia, malignancy, pulmonary embolism, rheumatologic disease, pancreatitis, trauma, or surgery.

Diagnostic Criteria and Testing

Laboratories

- Pleural fluid should be sent for glucose, pH, protein, and lactate dehydrogenase (LDH). It may also be sent for amylase if pancreatitis or esophageal rupture is a concern.
- Cytology should be sent in any patient where there is a concern for malignancy.

Imaging

- Upright PA and lateral chest radiograph are useful in detecting pleural effusions.[2]
- Lateral decubitus plain radiograph may be useful in demonstrating fluidity of the effusions.
- Ultrasound has been shown to be useful in diagnosing and determining size of pleural effusions and loculations or complex architecture and guiding thoracentesis or thoracostomy tube placement.
- CT chest with contrast may identify any underlying pathology and is also helpful in determining the characteristics of an effusion.

Diagnostic Procedures

- Thoracentesis should be performed to improve respiratory status.
  - Prior to thoracentesis, patients should be off therapeutic anticoagulants, prothrombin time (PT)/partial thromboplastin time (PTT) should be <2 times the

upper limit of normal, platelets should be >25,000, and creatinine should be <6.[3] Exceptions can be made in the event of tension pathology.

○ Removal of up to 1.5 L of fluid is safe. Thoracentesis should be stopped if there is development of chest discomfort as this may serve as a surrogate for drop in intrathoracic pressure.[4] Re-expansion pulmonary edema is a very rare complication and may be overstated in the literature.[5]

TREATMENT

Medications

• In a patient with an effusion where infection is thought to be the cause, broad coverage antibiotics should be initiated.[6]

Other Nonpharmacologic Therapies

• Treatment should focus on the underlying cause and may require chest tube placement.[7]
• Patients with complex effusions (pleural thickening, fibrous organization, and multiple loculations) may require surgical consultation for decortication.

SPECIAL CONSIDERATIONS

Disposition

• If patients have known underlying disease, patients may be treated with observation alone and discharge to their outpatient specialist for follow-up.
• If the patient presents with symptoms requiring drainage, unknown etiology, or chest tube placement, admission will be necessary.

Pleurisy

GENERAL PRINCIPLES

Definition

• Inflammation of the parietal pleura of the lungs results in pain that is sharp, localized, and worse with inspiration or cough.

Pathophysiology

• The parietal pleura that lines the thoracic cavity is innervated by somatic nerves that sense pain when inflamed.[8]

DIAGNOSIS

Clinical Presentation

History

• Pain is typically localized to the area that is inflamed or along predictable referred pain pathways, such as inflammation of the diaphragm radiating to the shoulder. Pain is typically made worse with deep inspiration, talking, coughing, or sneezing. The pain is typically described as sharp in nature. Patients tend to assume a posture, which most limits motion of the inflamed area. Pleurisy may sometimes be associated with dyspnea as patient's inspiration is limited due to pain.

Physical Examination
- The classic physical exam finding for pleurisy is a friction rub during respiration.[8]

Differential Diagnosis
- The differential diagnosis may include acute myocardial infarction, pericarditis, pleural effusion, pneumonia, connective tissue disease such as rheumatoid arthritis or lupus, drug induced (bleomycin, amiodarone, minoxidil), tuberculosis, or familial Mediterranean fever.

Diagnostic Criteria and Testing
- Laboratory values, ECG, and imaging are nondiagnostic in pleurisy.[8]

TREATMENT

Medications
- The mainstay of treatment for pleurisy is NSAIDs such as indomethacin 50–100 mg tid.[9]
- Opioids have also been shown to improve pleuritic pain but may suppress cough and respiratory drive.
- Corticosteroids may be used in patients who cannot tolerate NSAIDs and may be most beneficial in pleuritic pain associated with rheumatologic conditions.

SPECIAL CONSIDERATIONS

Disposition
- Patients with simple pleurisy can be discharged from the emergency department.

REFERENCES

1. Light RW. *Pleural Diseases*. 4th ed. Baltimore: Lippincott Williams & Wilkins, 2001.
2. Blackmore CC, Black WC, Dallas RV, Crow HC. Pleural fluid volume estimation: a chest radiograph prediction rule. *Acad Radiol* 1996;3:103–9.
3. McVay PA, Toy PT. Lack of increased bleeding after paracentesis and thoracentesis in patients with mild coagulation abnormalities. *Transfusion* 1991;31:164–71.
4. Feller-Kopman D, Walkey A, Berkowitz D, Ernest A. The relationship of pleural pressure to symptom development during therapeutic thoracentesis. *Chest* 2006;129:1556–60.
5. Feller-Kopman D, Berkowitz D, Boiselle P, Ernest A. Large-volume thoracentesis and the risk of reexpansion pulmonary edema. *Ann Thorac Sur* 2007;84:1656–61.
6. Brook I, Frazier EH. Aerobic and anaerobic microbiology of empyema: a retrospective review in two military hospitals. *Chest* 1993;103:1502–7.
7. Colice GL, Curtis A, Deslauriers J, et al. Medical and surgical treatment of parapneumonic effusions. *Chest* 2000;118:1158–71.
8. Kass SM, Williams PM, Reamy B. Pleurisy. *Am J Fam Physician* 2007;75:1357–64.
9. Sacks PV, Kanarek D. Treatment of acute pleuritic pain: comparison between indomethacin and a placebo. *Am Rev Respir Dis* 1973;108:666–9.

101 Pulmonary Emergencies: Pneumothorax

Gregory Ratti

Pneumothorax

GENERAL PRINCIPLES

Definition

- A pneumothorax is an abnormal collection of air between the visceral and parietal pleura.

Classification

- Primary spontaneous pneumothorax is defined as a pneumothorax, which occurs without underlying disease or trauma.
- Secondary spontaneous pneumothorax occurs in the setting of underlying pulmonary disease, most commonly chronic obstructive pulmonary disease (COPD), interstitial lung disease, necrotizing pneumonia, tuberculosis, or cystic fibrosis.
- Traumatic pneumothorax may occur as a result of penetrating or blunt trauma.
- Iatrogenic pneumothorax occurs most often in the setting of medical procedures. Most commonly secondary to transthoracic needle biopsy in the outpatient setting.[1] It may also be seen after thoracentesis, central venous catheter placement, or secondary to barotrauma in the setting of mechanical ventilation.
- Tension pneumothorax is defined as a pneumothorax that causes cardiovascular instability.

Epidemiology/Etiology

- Risk factors for primary pneumothorax include male sex, tall stature, and smoking tobacco.[2] Smoking has been shown to increase the risk 20-fold over nonsmokers. Associated conditions for primary pneumothorax include Marfan syndrome, homocystinuria, and Birt-Hogg-Dube syndrome.
- Secondary spontaneous pneumothorax is more common in the older population. Average age is 60–65 years old. The most common comorbidity of patients developing a pneumothorax is COPD.
- Secondary pneumothoraces may also occur in the setting of mechanical ventilation, especially in patients who require high positive end-expiratory pressure (PEEP) or if tidal volumes >6–8 mL/kg are used.[3,4]
- Other risks factors for pneumothorax associated with barotrauma include asthma, COPD, interstitial lung disease, and marijuana use[9] acute respiratory distress syndrome.

Pathophysiology

- A pneumothorax occurs when there is a disruption of the lung parencyhma, which allows air to enter the thoracic cavity and disrupts the typical negative pressure cycle of respiration. The buildup of air and pressure in one hemithorax results in mediastinal shift and resulting compression of the contralateral lung, as well as impaired venous return to the heart. This results in impaired gas exchange, hypotension, and eventually, cardiovascular collapse.

DIAGNOSIS

Clinical Presentation

- Tension pneumothorax is a clinical diagnosis and should be considered in anyone presenting with hypoxia and hypotension after trauma to the chest. This is a life-threatening condition and should be treated promptly.
- Clinical features alone do not predict the relative size of the pneumothorax. More significant symptoms may be seen in patients with underlying disease or reduced lung reserve.

History

- Patients typically present with acute onset ipsilateral chest or shoulder pain. The pain is typically pleuritic in nature. Dyspnea tends to be a predominant feature.
- It is important to inquire about recent chest trauma or diagnostic procedures. Obtain a thorough past medical history looking for associated conditions.

Physical Examination

- With small pneumothoraces, the physical exam may be normal.
- Classically, on physical exam there will be decreased breath sounds, decreased tactile fremitus, and increased percussion on the effected side.
- Patients with tension pneumothorax may present in extremis with diaphoresis, severe dyspnea, cyanosis, hypoxia, and hypotension.
- With tension pneumothorax, as pressure builds within the chest, the trachea may be deviated to the contralateral side. These are late findings, which may suggest impending cardiovascular collapse.
- In pneumothoraces resulting from penetrating trauma, subcutaneous emphysema may be palpated.

Differential Diagnosis

- Asthma, COPD, pneumonia, costochondritis, diaphragmatic injury, esophageal spasm, mediastinitis, MI, myocarditis, pericarditis, tuberculosis,[5] or empyema

Diagnostic Criteria and Testing

Imaging

- A chest radiograph should be obtained. In patients who must remain supine, pneumothorax may be missed on AP films due to anterior layering of air. Pneumothorax may be seen as a deep costophrenic sulcus on the ipsilateral side.
- Ultrasound can be used as an adjunct to traditional radiographs, especially in patients who must remain supine or are unstable. Ultrasound can be used to examine for the lung sliding, which is seen when visceral and parietal pleura move along one another during normal inspiration. Lack of lung slide along with lack of "comet tails" on ultrasound has been shown to reliably predict presence of pneumothorax.[6]
- The gold standard for diagnosis of pneumothorax remains chest CT. It is also helpful in determining size and any underlying disease.

TREATMENT

- Primary spontaneous pneumothorax
  - A small pneumothorax, defined as <3 cm from the apex to the cupola, without evidence of further pleural leak may resolve spontaneously without need for

intervention.[7] Air is thought to be resorbed at a rate of 2.2% of hemithorax per day.[8]

- ○ Administration of 100% oxygenation can improve resorption in these patients.[7]
- ○ For larger pneumothorax >3 cm, simple aspiration of up to 2.5 L of air is a reasonable approach but may be unsuccessful in up to 50% of cases.[5]
- ○ Alternatively, a small bore (<14F) chest tube may be inserted via Seldinger technique and attached to a water seal or Heimlich device. Reliable patients with good follow-up may go home with a Heimlich device if follow-up can be arranged in <2 days.[5,7]
- Secondary spontaneous pneumothorax
  - ○ These patients often have persistent bronchopleural fistulas, which are unlikely to resolve spontaneously and will require further subsequent management.[5,7]
  - ○ All patients should be placed on supplemental oxygen.[5]
  - ○ All patients with secondary spontaneous pneumothorax will require insertion of a chest tube. Studies have shown equivalency between small bore and large bore chest tubes, which cause less discomfort for patients with small bore tubes. Although, patients who are unstable may require mechanical ventilation and may require larger bore tubes (22–24F) due to large air leaks.[7]
- Iatrogenic pneumothorax
  - ○ If the pneumothorax is small, this may be managed conservatively.
  - ○ If the pneumothorax is large, or the patient is symptomatic, simple aspiration or a small bore chest tube may be needed.
- Traumatic pneumothorax
  - ○ Any penetrating traumatic wounds that are sucking in nature should be covered with an occlusive dressing.
  - ○ Patients with otherwise no medical comorbidities may be managed similarly to primary spontaneous pneumothorax. Studies have shown that for occult pneumothoraces after trauma, there was no difference in morbidity and mortality between observation and insertion of a thoracostomy tube in small pneumothoraces.[8]
- Tension pneumothorax
  - ○ If there is clinical concern and physical exam supports this diagnosis, emergent decompression of the affected hemithorax may be accomplished by insertion of a 14-gauge needle into the second intercostal space at the midclavicular line. Release of air and immediate clinical improvement will confirm the diagnosis. The thoracostomy needle should be left in place until a thoracostomy tube can be placed to prevent reaccumulation of the tension.

SPECIAL CONSIDERATIONS

Disposition

- Disposition depends on the type and extent of the pneumothorax.
- Patients with poorly controlled symptoms should be admitted to the hospital for observation.
- Patients with secondary pneumothoraces, even if small, will need admission to the hospital for at least 24 hours for monitoring.
- In patients with small primary pneumothorax, a plain chest radiograph can be performed 6 hours after the first, and if stable, may be sent home, if they are asymptomatic. They should follow up in 2 days for repeat chest radiograph for resolution.
- Patients with a recent pneumothorax or who are discharged with a small pneumothorax still present should be discouraged from air travel or anything else that would decrease barometric pressure and therefore possibly make the pneumothorax worse.[5]

REFERENCES

1. Sassoon CS, Light RW, O'Hara VS, et al. Iatrogenic pneumothorax: etiology and morbidity. Results of a Department of Veterans Affairs Cooperative Study. *Respiration* 1992; 59:215–20.
2. Sahn SA, Heffner JE. Review article: spontaneous pneumothorax. *N Engl J Med* 2000; 342:868–74.
3. Anzueto A, Frutos-Vivar F, Esteban A. Incidence, risk factors and outcome of barotrauma in mechanically ventilated patients. *Intensive Care Med* 2004;30:612–9.
4. Noppen M. Spontaneous pneumothorax: epidemiology, pathophysiology and cause. *Eur Respir Rev* 2010;19:217–9.
5. MacDuff A, Arnold A, Harvey J. Management of spontaneous pneumothorax: British Thoracic Society pleural disease guideline 2010. *Thorax* 2010;65:ii18–31.
6. Rowan KR, Kirkpatrick AW, Liu D, et al. Traumatic pneumothorax detection with thoracic US: correlation with chest radiography and CT-initial experience. *Radiology* 2002;225:210–4.
7. Baumann MH, Strange C, Heffner JE, et al. Management of spontaneous pneumothorax: an American College of Chest Physicians Delphi consensus statement. *Chest* 2001;119: 590–602.
8. Yadav K, Jalili M, Zehtabchi S. Management of traumatic occult pneumothorax. *Resuscitation* 2010;81:1063–8.
9. Bintcliffe OJ, Hallifax RJ, Edey A, et al. Spontaneous pneumothorax: time to rethink management. *Lancet Respir Med* 2015;3:578–88.

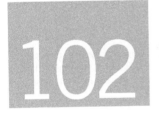

102 Pulmonary Emergencies: Pulmonary Embolism

Kevin M. Cullison and Christopher R. Carpenter

GENERAL PRINCIPLES

Definition

- A pulmonary embolism (PE) is defined as a mechanical obstruction in the pulmonary artery or once of its branches. The obstruction is most commonly a thrombus but may also be due to fat, air, or tumor.
- PE can also be classified according to temporal acuity, severity, and location:
  - Severity: defined by the presence or absence of hemodynamic instability
    - Massive PE is defined as the presence of hemodynamic instability or hypotension. Specifically, instability has been defined as systolic blood pressure <90 mm Hg for >15 minutes, hypotension requiring vasopressors, or other clinical signs of shock (i.e., not explained by hypovolemia, sepsis, or arrhythmia).[1]
    - Submassive PE occurs when patients have indirect signs of a significant PE burden (i.e., right ventricular dilatation, elevated troponin) in spite of being normotensive.

Epidemiology/Etiology

- Most PEs are believed to originate from deep veins in the proximal lower extremity (iliac, common femoral, deep femoral, and popliteal veins) although a small percentage of emboli may originate from the upper extremities.[2]
- ED-based epidemiologic studies characterized the following risk factors[3]:
  - Increased age[3]
  - Recent invasive surgery or trauma
  - Immobility: includes bed rest >72 hours, travel >6 hours
  - Malignancy
  - Indwelling catheters
  - Pregnancy: risk increases with trimester
  - Estrogen containing oral contraceptives
  - Lupus anticoagulant, Factor V Leiden, protein C and S, and antithrombin deficiency
  - History of prior PE

Pathophysiology

- Venous stasis with subsequent migration of the thrombosis to the lungs

DIAGNOSIS

Clinical Presentation

History

- Patients can present with dyspnea, pleuritic chest pain, cough, hemoptysis, or calf/thigh swelling.

Physical Examination

- The exam findings (in order of likelihood) are as follows: tachypnea, tachycardia, calf/thigh swelling/erythema/tenderness/palpable cords, rales, decreased breath sounds, jugular venous distension, accentuated pulmonic component of second heart sound, or fever.

Differential Diagnosis

- Acute coronary syndrome, aortic dissection, pneumonia, pneumothorax, pericarditis, or tamponade

Diagnostic Criteria and Testing

- There are many validated scoring methods that can be used to estimate pretest probability, including the Wells score, Pulmonary Embolism Rule-out Criteria (PERC) score, and the simplified Revised Geneva Score (Table 102.1). Importantly, gestalt estimation of pretest probability has been shown to have similar diagnostic performance characteristics to these structured scoring methods.

Pretest Probability

- **Low risk:** Wells score <2; actual prevalence of PE in this group is ~3%.[4] PE can be ruled out with either by application of the PERC rule or via a negative D-dimer. A positive D-dimer, however, would warrant further imaging to exclude PE.
- **Moderate risk:** Wells score 2–6; actual prevalence of PE in this group is 10–13%.[4] Patients with a moderate pretest probability require a negative D-dimer or advanced imaging to exclude PE.

TABLE 102.1   Prediction Rules for DVT and PE

Clinical variable	Points
Wells rule[13]	
Clinical signs and symptoms of deep vein thrombosis (minimum of leg swelling and pain with palpation in the deep veins)	3.0
Alternative diagnosis less likely than pulmonary embolism	3.0
Heart rate >100 beats/min	1.5
Immobilization (>3 d) or surgery in the previous 4 wk	1.5
Previous pulmonary embolism or deep vein thrombosis	1.5
Hemoptysis	1.0
Malignancy (receiving treatment, treated in the last 6 mo or palliative)	1.0
Clinical probability: low risk: <2; moderate risk: 2–4; high risk: >4	
Simplified, revised Geneva score for pulmonary embolism[14]	
Age >65 y	1
Previous DVT or PE	1
Surgery (under general anesthesia) or fracture (of lower limbs) within 1 mo	1
Active malignant condition (currently active or considered cured <1 y)	1
Unilateral lower-limb pain	1
Hemoptysis	1
Heart rate (beats/min)	1
75–94	1
≥95	
Pain on lower-limb deep venous palpation and unilateral edema	1
Clinical probability: low risk: <2; moderate risk: 2–4; high risk: >4	
PERC (Pulmonary Embolism Rule-out Criteria) Rule for patients with low* clinical suspicion for PE[15]	
Age <50 y	
Heart rate <100 beats/min during entire ED stay	
Pulse oximetry >94% on room air	
No hemoptysis	
No prior VTE history	
No surgery or trauma requiring endotracheal intubation or hospitalization within past 4 wk	
No estrogen use	
No unilateral leg swelling	

*Pretest probability of PE should be <15% based on gestalt estimation or by using validated scoring instrument.

- **High risk:** Wells score >6; actual prevalence of PE in this group is 33–36%.[4] A negative D-dimer in this subgroup of patients does not sufficiently reduce the posttest probability of PE.

Laboratories
- A complete blood count, basic metabolic panel, troponin, and a D-dimer (depending on the patient's pretest probability for PE)
  - Use of an age-adjusted D-dimer (age × 10 ng/mL for patients older than 50) is associated with a higher specificity for PE in older age groups.[5,6]
  - Troponin levels may be elevated in patients with an acute PE.[7]
  - BNP is elevated in more than half of patients with a PE.[8]

Electrocardiography (ECG)
- Sinus tachycardia is the most common finding. The $S_1Q_3T_3$ pattern is seen in <20% of patients with PE.[9,10] Complete or incomplete right bundle branch block, right ventricular strain pattern, right axis deviation, or right atrial enlargement can also be seen.

Imaging
- CT pulmonary angiography (CTPA) should be used as a first-line test in patients with a high pretest probability of PE.
- Ventilation–perfusion (V/Q) scans are considered advantageous over CTPA because of the smaller amount of associated radiation exposure and are therefore the imaging modality of choice in pregnant women. It is recommended that only patients with a normal chest radiograph undergo a V/Q scan.

TREATMENT

Medications
Anticoagulants
- Patients with acute PE should receive anticoagulation. If the patient is hospitalized, parenteral anticoagulation with unfractionated heparin (UFH), low molecular weight heparin (LMWH), or fondaparinux are appropriate to begin in the ED.
  - LMWH results in less thrombotic complications, less major hemorrhages, and a lower risk of heparin-induced thrombocytopenia than UFH.
  - UFH is often indicated in patients with renal impairment, obesity, or patients necessitating surgical intervention.
  - Novel oral anticoagulants (NOACs) not only have a similar efficacy in preventing recurrent venous thromboembolism (VTE) in comparison to warfarin but also have an improved safety profile.

Thrombolytics
- Massive PE—There are no major contraindications if a thrombolytic agent is given to a patient with suspected or known massive PE and hemodynamic instability.
- Submassive PE—There is currently insufficient evidence to support the use of systemic thrombolytics in patients with an acute PE who are hemodynamically stable but have evidence of RV dysfunction.
  - The use of thrombolytics should remain at the discretion of the treating physician and should probably be reserved for patients at lower risk for bleeding who fail to respond well to conventional treatment with UFH alone.[3]

Other Nonpharmacologic Therapies

- Pulmonary embolectomy requires consultation with cardiac surgery and should be considered in patients whom systemic thrombolysis has failed or is contraindicated.
- Percutaneous catheter-directed interventions require consultation with vascular surgery or interventional radiology and should be considered in patients with submassive or massive PE in whom systemic thrombolysis has failed or is contraindicated.
- Extracorporeal membrane oxygenation (ECMO) can be used as a bridging therapy to ensure adequate oxygenation and end-organ perfusion until definitive clot removal can occur.[11]

SPECIAL CONSIDERATIONS

Disposition

- evidence supporting outpatient treatment

Complications

Morbidity and mortality can be variable depending on the size and location of the PE and underlying comorbidities of the patient.

- Early complications include hemodynamic collapse, pulmonary infarction, and death.[12]
- Late complications include recurrent VTE, chronic thromboembolic pulmonary hypertension, or bleeding from anticoagulation.

REFERENCES

1. Kasper W, Konstantinides S, Geibel A, et al. Management strategies and determinants of outcome in acute major pulmonary embolism: results of a multicenter registry. *J Am Coll Cardiol* 1997;30(5):1165–73.
2. Tadlock MD, Chouliaras K, Kennedy M, et al. The origin of fatal pulmonary emboli: a postmortem analysis of 500 deaths from pulmonary embolism in trauma, surgical, and medical patients. *Am J Surg* 2015;209(6):959–68.
3. Konstantinides SV, Torbicki A, Agnelli G, et al. 2014 ESC guidelines on the diagnosis and management of acute pulmonary embolism. *Eur Heart J* 2014;35(43):3033–80.
4. Kabrhel C, Courtney DM, Camargo CA, et al. Potential impact of adjusting the threshold of the quantitative D-dimer based on pretest probability of acute pulmonary embolism. *Acad Emerg Med* 2009;16(4):325–32.
5. Schouten HJ, Geersing GJ, Koek HL, et al. Diagnostic accuracy of conventional or age adjusted D-dimer cut-off values in older patients with suspected venous thromboembolism: systematic review and meta-analysis. *BMJ* 2013;346(May):f2492.
6. Righini M, Van Es J, Den Exter PL, et al. Age-adjusted D-dimer cutoff levels to rule out pulmonary embolism: the ADJUST-PE study. *JAMA* 2014;311(11):1117–24.
7. Becattini C, Vedovati MC, Agnelli G. Prognostic value of troponins in acute pulmonary embolism: a meta-analysis. *Circulation* 2007;116(4):427–33.
8. Klok FA, Mos IC, Huisman MV. Brain-type natriuretic peptide levels in the prediction of adverse outcome in patients with pulmonary embolism: a systematic review and meta-analysis. *Am J Respir Crit Care Med* 2008;178(4):425–30.
9. Marchick MR, Courtney DM, Kabrhel C, et al. 12-Lead ECG findings of pulmonary hypertension occur more frequently in emergency department patients with pulmonary embolism than in patients without pulmonary embolism. *Ann Emerg Med* 2010;55(4):331–5.
10. Richman PB, Loutfi H, Lester SJ, et al. Electrocardiographic findings in emergency department patients with pulmonary embolism. *J Emerg Med* 2004;27(2):121–6.
11. Yusuff HO, Zochios V, Vuylsteke A. Extracorporeal membrane oxygenation in acute massive pulmonary embolism: a systematic review. *Perfusion* 2015;30(8):611–6.

12. Lin BW, Schreiber DH, Liu G, et al. Therapy and outcomes in massive pulmonary embolism from the emergency medicine pulmonary embolism in the real world registry. *Am J Emerg Med* 2012;30(9):1774–81.
13. Wells PS, Anderson DR, Rodger M, et al. Derivation of a simple clinical model to categorize patients probability of pulmonary embolism: Increasing the models utility with the SimpliRED D-dimer. *Thromb Haemost* 2000;83(3):416–20.
14. Klok FA, Mos ICM, Nijkeuter M, et al. Simplification of the revised Geneva score for assessing clinical probability of pulmonary embolism. *Arch Intern Med* 2008;168(19):2131–6.
15. Kline JA, Courtney DM, Kabrhel C, et al. Prospective multicenter evaluation of the pulmonary embolism rule-out criteria. *J Thromb Haemost* 2008;6(5):772–80.

103 Pulmonary Emergencies: Pulmonary Hypertension

Bob Cambridge and Niall Prendergast

GENERAL PRINCIPLES

Definition

- Pulmonary hypertension (PH) is defined as an increase in the blood pressure in the pulmonary vasculature, defined as a mean pulmonary arterial pressure ≥25 mm Hg.

Classification

- PH has a variety of causes divided into five groups by the WHO.[1]
  - Group 1: pulmonary arterial hypertension (PAH) (due to primary increases in peripheral vascular resistance (PVR))
  - Group 2: PH due to left heart disease
  - Group 3: PH due to lung disease
  - Group 4: chronic thromboembolic PH
  - Group 5: PH with unclear mechanisms

Epidemiology/Etiology

- Prevalence of PAH group 1 is rare and prevalence of group 2–5 PH is less well studied.
  - Group 1 causes: idiopathic, drugs and toxins, connective tissue disease, and HIV
  - Group 2 causes: left heart systolic/diastolic failure and mitral/aortic valve disease
  - Group 3 causes: chronic obstructive pulmonary disease (COPD), interstitial lung disease, chronic high-altitude exposure, and other pulmonary disorders

- ○ Group 4 causes: chronic pulmonary emboli
- ○ Group 5 causes: tumors, metabolic and endocrine disorders, sarcoidosis, histio-cytosis, hematologic diseases, fibrosing mediastinitis, and chronic kidney failure

Pathophysiology

- Progressive vascular remodeling with endothelial and smooth muscle proliferation, vasoconstriction, and arteriolar occlusion and/or thrombosis leads to an increase in PVR. This lowers cardiac output by the right heart, leading to increased afterload (from left heart strain) and decreased cardiac output and right heart failure.
- Group 1 PH is caused by progressive narrowing of blood vessels within the lungs with the increased resistance leading to right ventricular hypertrophy and eventual right heart failure.
- Group 2 PH is caused by failure of the left ventricle. As blood backs up in the system, it pools in the lungs. Pulmonary system pressure rises.
- Group 3 PH is caused by prolonged hypoxic states. The low oxygen level leads to pulmonary vasoconstriction and elevated pressures. Normally, this physiologic response occurs to shunt blood away from damaged lung to keep blood from being underoxygenated. When the lung injury is widespread, it causes a diffuse and chronic vasoconstriction.
- Group 4 PH is caused by the body's natural response to the presence of blood clots. Blocked vessels lead to increased resistance and increased pulmonary vasculature pressure.
- Group 5 PH is caused by mechanisms that are still unclear.

DIAGNOSIS

Clinical Presentation

History

- Patients with acute right ventricular (RV) failure can have multiple complaints, but more commonly report dyspnea, exercise intolerance, chest pain, palpitations, fatigue, leg swelling, and syncope.

Physical Examination

- PH can delay and accentuate pulmonic valve closure, giving a loud P2 and/or a split S2.
- Subsequent right ventricular hypertrophy and enlargement can cause a prominent wave in the jugular venous pulse, tricuspid regurgitation, right-sided S4, and/or parasternal/RV heave/lift.
- Decompensated right heart failure is marked by signs of peripheral volume overload, including peripheral edema, ascites, an enlarged or pulsatile liver, and/or pleural effusions.

Imaging

- Ultrasound
  - ○ At the bedside in the ED, RA and RV dilation (RV:LV ratio > 1), RV free wall thickening, and septal shifting toward the LV can be seen. Advanced operators can evaluate regurgitation across the tricuspid valve and can estimate pulmonary arterial pressures.
  - ○ Bedside ultrasound can also be useful for evaluation of volume status during treatment. PH patients, especially those in RV failure, tend to be volume overloaded with a large, noncollapsing inferior vena cava.

- Chest Plain Radiograph
  - Group 1 patients may show an enlarged right atrium and right heart border, an enlarged hilum, and/or venous congestion that tapers rapidly toward the periphery of the lung. Other patients may share the enlarged RA and right heart border, but will likely also have signs consistent with their underlying disease.[2]

Laboratories
- Troponin has been shown to be an independent predictor of mortality.
- B-type natriuretic peptide (BNP) has prognostic significance if the levels are over 180 pg/mL.

Electrocardiography
- When changes are seen, they are nonspecific and consistent with right-sided strain. Such changes include:
  - R wave > 7 mm in V_1 or V_2
  - Deep S wave in V_6 > 7 mm
  - Right axis deviation
  - ST depressions or T-wave inversions in V_1
- Changes of right atrial enlargement can also be seen:
  - Peaked P wave taller than 2.5 mm in lead II
  - P wave taller than 1.5 mm in V_1

TREATMENT

Medication

Inotropes
- Dobutamine, 2–20 µg/kg/min
- Milrinone, 0.1–0.75 µg/kg/min

Modifying RV Preload
- Diuresis
  - As the RV fails, diuretics may be given if the bedside echo shows massive RV dilation and pulmonary embolism (PE) has been ruled out.
- Fluid Therapy
  - In a patient with known PH but who is also in hypovolemic shock (as determined by bedside echo), fluids can be given but should be given at a slow rate.[3] After each bolus (preferably 250–500 mL), recheck RV function with a bedside ultrasound.

Modifying RV Afterload
- Systemic agents:
  - Initiation of systemic agents such as sildenafil, tadalafil, riociguat, bosentan, ambrisentan, macitentan, epoprostenol, treprostinil, iloprost, and selexipag should not be done without consultation with a PH specialist.
  - If a patient on such an agent presents to the emergency department, that agent should not be stopped.
- Inhaled epoprostenol
  - In the case of hypoxemia, inhaled epoprostenol (Flolan) can improve V/Q matching and decrease pulmonary vascular pressures.
- Hypercapnia and hypoxemia should be avoided.
- Limit noninvasive positive pressure ventilation (NIPPV) if possible (increases transpulmonary pressures) and only at the lowest level tolerated.

Vasopressors
- Norepinephrine (0.02–2 μg/kg/min)
- Epinephrine (0.02–0.2 μg/kg/min)

SPECIAL CONSIDERATIONS

Pulmonary vasodilators should never be stopped in a patient on established therapy. Doing so will lead to an acute increase in RV afterload and is likely to precipitate acute RV failure.

Disposition

Most patients with PH presenting with complaints related to their PH will be in some stage of RV failure and will require admission. Many patients will require continuous infusions of vasoactive medications and as such will require ICU admission.

REFERENCES

1. Vachiéry JL, Adir Y, Barberà JA, et al. Pulmonary hypertension due to left heart diseases. *J Am Coll Cardiol* 2013;62(25 Suppl):D100–8.
2. Sitbon O, Lascoux-Combe C, Delfraissy JF, et al. Prevalence of HIV-related pulmonary arterial hypertension in the current antiretroviral therapy era. *Am J Respir Crit Care Med* 2008;177(1):108.
3. Andersen KH, Iversen M, Kjaergaard J, et al. Prevalence, predictors, and survival in pulmonary hypertension related to end-stage chronic obstructive pulmonary disease. *J Heart Lung Transplant* 2012;31(4):373–80.

104 Pulmonary Emergencies: Restrictive Lung Disease

Lawrence Lewis

GENERAL PRINCIPLES

Definition

- Restrictive lung disease (RLD) is characterized by reduced lung volumes and is defined by a reduced total lung capacity, a reduced forced vital capacity (FVC < 80%), and a reduced forced expiratory volume in one second (FEV_1), but a preserved FEV_1 to FVC ratio ($FEV_1/FVC \geq 0.70$).[1]

Epidemiology

- The epidemiologic breakdown is gender specific, with occupational exposures being the leading cause among men, and pulmonary fibrosis, idiopathic pulmonary fibrosis, and connective tissue disease being the leading causes among women.[14]
- The causes of interstitial lung disease include infectious, idiopathic, occupational exposures (silica, asbestos, organic dust), malignancy, connective tissue diseases, medications (bleomycin, amiodarone), and primary diseases of the lung (sarcoidosis) reasons.[3]

Pathophysiology

- RLD can be due to pulmonary or extrapulmonary causes.[2]
  - Extrapulmonary causes include skeletal deformities (particularly chest wall or spinal), neuromuscular disease, and conditions that restrict diaphragmatic movement (obesity, pregnancy, ascites, phrenic nerve injury). These conditions can result in restriction of the lungs sufficient enough to cause symptoms and should be noted and considered in the differential diagnosis of RLD.
- There are a number of pathologic conditions of the lungs that can cause restrictive disease including pulmonary edema, acute respiratory distress syndrome, interstitial lung diseases, connective tissue diseases, atelectasis, vasculitis, granulomatous diseases, sarcoidosis, hypersensitivity pneumonitis, drug-related pulmonary fibrosis, radiation therapy, and lung resection.
- The pathogenesis of interstitial lung disease depends on the distinct causative entity and is either predominantly inflammatory or fibrotic.[4] The majority of these disorders are inflammatory and are precipitated by immunologic, environmental, or toxic factors. A minority appear to be infectious in origin.[3]
- Current research suggests that idiopathic interstitial pneumonia is a "two hit" disease, requiring both a genetic predisposition and environmental triggers.[1]

DIAGNOSIS

Clinical Presentation

History

- Patients with idiopathic lung disease (ILD) often have an insidious onset of cough and dyspnea, but certain conditions such as the interstitial pneumonias, hypersensitivity pneumonitis, and cryptogenic organizing pneumonia may manifest as acute or subacute disease. ILD should be suspected in patients with progressive dyspnea without another obvious cause.
  - A detailed occupational history and medical history can uncover risk factors such as occupational exposures, smoking, drug exposure, or evidence of connective tissue disease.
- Dry cough is common, but productive cough is unusual.
- Hemoptysis may occur in alveolar hemorrhagic syndromes and vasculitis.
  - Idiopathic pulmonary fibrosis (IPF) should be considered in patients over 50 years old with unexplained dyspnea, cough, bibasilar inspiratory crackles, and finger clubbing.[5]
- Inquire about a history of respiratory infections or other respiratory problems, and the pattern of symptom development over time include dyspnea (especially on exertion), cough, and colds. The number of hospitalizations, particularly over the past year or so, and whether the patient ever required mechanical ventilation can provide useful information regarding the severity of disease. One should ask about a family history of interstitial lung disease.

- Regarding the current exacerbation, one should note timing (days or weeks) and precipitating factors. Quantify worsening from baseline, increasing oxygen requirement, decreased exertional tolerance, worsening dyspnea, or recent evaluation by a health care provider (and what medication or treatments were provided).

Physical Examination
- The patient is often tachypneic and demonstrates increased work of breathing.
- Wheezing is not common but may occur in respiratory bronchiolitis, lymphangitic carcinomatosis, hypersensitivity pneumonitis, and chronic eosinophilic pneumonia. It may also be found in patients with coexisting chronic obstructive pulmonary disease (COPD) (which has been noted to coexist in up to 40% of patients with ILD).[6]
- Dry, fine rales may be present.
- There may be clues on physical exam to other extrapulmonary causes of RLD such as scoliosis and chest wall deformities. Neuromuscular disease will usually be documented in the history, but weakness of respiratory or skeletal muscles and a decreased negative inspiratory force (NIF) should help confirm the diagnosis.
- The pulmonary exam may suggest other pulmonary reasons such as pleural effusion, diaphragmatic paralysis, or pneumothorax. The extremity exam may show finger clubbing, which is often seen in IPF.

Differential Diagnosis
- Pneumonia (interstitial, hypersensitivity, cryptogenic organizing), alveolar hemorrhagic syndrome, interstitial pulmonary fibrosis, congestive heart failure (CHF), COPD, pulmonary embolism (PE), or neuromuscular disease

Diagnostic Testing
Laboratories
- Arterial blood gas testing can help to quantify the degree of hypoxemia and detect hypercapnia.
- Other laboratory tests are nonspecific.

Imaging
- In ILD, a chest CT can often be helpful. It is more sensitive than CXR and can identify other potential causes of dyspnea.
- CXR may show anything from interstitial infiltrate (honeycombing) to diffuse bilateral airspace opacification. A characteristic finding of peripheral distribution of opacities may be seen in eosinophilic pneumonia and cryptogenic pneumonia.[7]

TREATMENT

Medications
- Bronchodilators
  - Although bronchodilators are not effective in ILD, there is a significant percentage of patients with both obstructive and restrictive patterns, in whom bronchodilators may add benefit.[8]
- Corticosteroids
  - Many idiopathic interstitial pneumonias are steroid responsive, although IPF and acute interstitial pneumonia are not. If the diagnosis is not clear, then a trial of steroids is warranted.

TABLE 104.1	Indications for ICU Admission

Severe dyspnea that responds inadequately to initial therapy

Confusion, altered mental status

Placement on NIPPV or intubated patient

Persistent or worsening hypoxemia ($PaO_2 < 50$ mm Hg), or severe/worsening hypercapnia ($PaCO_2 > 70$ mm Hg), or severe/worsening respiratory acidosis (pH < 7.30) despite supplemental oxygen and treatment

- Patients with end-stage interstitial lung disease often are aware of their prognosis and may have specific wishes (advanced directives) as to how aggressively they want to be treated, including whether or not they want to be in an ICU.

Adjunct Therapy

- Adjunct therapy includes any medications for comorbid disease, proper positioning, and pulmonary toilet.

Nonpharmacologic Therapy

- Noninvasive positive pressure ventilation (NIPPV) in the acute setting has not been shown to improve outcomes of respiratory failure in RLD due to a pulmonary etiology.[6,9]
  ○ The primary problem in extrapulmonary RLD is ventilation, not gas exchange, thus mechanical ventilation (either noninvasive or invasive) may be effacacious in the chronic treatment of RLD of neuromuscular or skeletal origin.[10,11]
- In impending respiratory failure in the setting of RLD of neuromuscular or skeletal origin, NIPPV should be strongly considered if there are no contraindications. There is less information on the use of NIPPV in ILD, particularly in acute respiratory failure associated with IPF or the other interstitial pneumonias.
  ○ Clinical variables that favor early intubation include higher PCO_2, lower pH, higher APACHE II scores, and the presence of pneumonia.[12]
  ○ Clinical variables that favor NIPPV include a more rapid decrease in PCO_2, improvement in pH, and a more rapid improvement in dyspnea and tachypnea.[12,13]
  ○ Severe respiratory failure with refractory hypoxemia may occur in ILD, especially in IPF and some of the other interstitial pneumonias and is often due to progression of the disease, although other conditions such as superimposed pneumonia, CHF, or PE can also be the cause.[1]

SPECIAL CONSIDERATIONS

Disposition

- The majority of these patients will require admission, depending on the severity of their respiratory status, either to a medical floor or an intensive care unit. The criteria for ICU admission are similar to those in other causes of respiratory failure (Table 104.1).
- Those who do respond to therapy and are close enough to their baseline to be discharged, require close follow-up by an appropriate provider.

REFERENCES

1. Seibold MA, Wise AL, Speer MC, et al. A common MUC5B promoter polymorphism and pulmonary fibrosis. *N Engl J Med* 2011;362:1503–12.
2. Coultas DB, Zumwalt RE, Black WC, Sobonya RE. The epidemiology of interstitial lung diseases. *Am J Respir Crit Care Med* 1994;150:967–72.

3. Leslie KO. Pathology of interstitial lung disease. *Clin Chest Med* 2004;25:657–703.
4. Wells AU. Hirani N. Interstitial lung disease guideline: the British Thoracic Society in collaboration with the Thoracic Society of Australia and New Zealand and the Irish Thoracic Society. *Thorax* 2008;63(Suppl 5):1–58.
5. Raghu G, Collard HR, Egan JJ, et al. An official ATS/ERS/JRS/ALAT statement: idiopathic pulmonary fibrosis: evidence-based guidelines for diagnosis and treatment. *Am J Respir Crit Care Med* 2011;183:788–824.
6. Williams JW Jr, Cox CE, Hargett CW, et al. *Noninvasive Positive-Pressure Ventilation (NPPV) for Acute Respiratory Failure.* Comparative Effectiveness Review 68. AHRQ Publication No. 12-EHC089-EF. Rockville: Agency for Healthcare Research and Quality, 2012.
7. American Thoracic Society. Idiopathic pulmonary fibrosis: diagnosis and treatment. International consensus statement. *Am J Respir Crit Care Med* 2000;161:646–64.
8. Doherty MJ, Pearson MG, O'Grady EA, et al. Cryptogenic fibrosing alveolitis with preserved lung volumes. *Thorax* 1997;52:998–1002.
9. Lightowler JV, Wedzicha JA, Elliott MW, Ram FS. Non-invasive positive pressure ventilation to treat respiratory failure resulting from exacerbations of chronic obstructive pulmonary disease: cochrane systematic review and meta-analysis. *BMJ* 2003;326:1–5.
10. Mellies U, Ragette R, Schwake C, et al. Long-term noninvasive ventilation in children and adolescents with neuromuscular disorders. *Eur Respir J* 2003;22:631–6.
11. Simonds AK, Ward S, Heather S, et al. Outcome of paediatric domiciliary mask ventilation in neuromuscular and skeletal disease. *Eur Respir J* 2000;16:476–81.
12. Karnik AM. Noninvasive positive pressure ventilation: testing the bridge. *Chest* 2000;117:625–7.
13. Antón A, Güell R, Gómez J, et al. Predicting the result of noninvasive ventilation in severe acute exacerbations of patients with chronic airflow limitation. *Chest* 2000;117:828–33.
14. Saxena N. Restrictive Lung Disease. In: Jackson MB, et al., eds. *The Perioperative Medicine Consult Handbook.* Switzerland: Springer International Published, 2015.

105 Toxicology: General

David B. Liss and Anna Arroyo Plasencia

GENERAL PRINCIPLES

- When presented with an undifferentiated overdose patient, a full history and physical exam should be performed as certain physical exam and laboratory findings can give clues to the specific exposure.
- In addition to a complete history, each patient presenting following an unknown overdose should receive the following evaluation:
  - A complete physical examination including vital signs and temperature should be obtained, paying special attention for signs of a specific toxidrome.
  - An ECG to evaluate for cardiac effects of potential ingestants.
  - An acetaminophen concentration and aspartate transaminase (AST) to evaluate for acetaminophen toxicity.
  - Obtaining a serum salicylate concentration should also be considered.
  - The number used nationwide for contacting the local poison control center is 1-800-222-1222.

Aspirin Overdose

- A reported history of ingesting 150 mg/kg of body weight or 6.5 g of aspirin (whichever is less) is concerning for potential systemic toxicity.
- Abdominal pain, nausea, emesis, tinnitus, and lethargy are clinical characteristics of patients presenting with an aspirin overdose.
- Following ingestion, aspirin is rapidly hydrolyzed to salicylate. A serum salicylate concentration will guide treatment.
- A basic metabolic panel and anion gap, lactate concentration, arterial or venous blood gas determination, and serum or urine ketones may help to recognize an unrecognized aspirin overdose.
- Classically, salicylate poisoning is associated with a primary respiratory alkalosis and a primary metabolic acidosis resulting in net alkalemia.
- Salicylate concentrations need to be interpreted in the context of the reported units.
- Salicylate concentrations need to be repeated every 2–4 hours, with more frequent monitoring for cases of significant salicylate toxicity. Monitoring can stop once the salicylate concentration is clearly down-trending and <30 mg/dL (based on a minimum of two levels with one being done a minimum of 8 hours after the time of ingestion).
- Pharmacokinetics are altered in overdose, and consultation with a medical toxicologist or the local poison control center should be obtained in any patient with altered mental status attributable to aspirin, any detectable salicylate concentration, or an increasing serum salicylate concentration at or above 30 mg/dL.
- There is no antidote for aspirin; treatment for aspirin overdose is supportive and based on levels.
  - Following an acute aspirin overdose, sodium bicarbonate therapy, dosed as 150 mEq $NaHCO_3$ in 1 L of D5W with 40 mEq KCl added to each liter, should be started when the salicylate concentration is at or above 30 mg/dL.
  - Sodium bicarbonate administration is influenced by the acid–base status of the patient, but is generally initiated at a rate of 1.5–2 times maintenance to alkalinize the urine and aid in renal salicylate excretion. This is highly dependent on urine pH.[1] The goal urinary pH is 7.5–8, and pH should be checked every time the patient urinates.
  - Alkalemia is essential to preventing salicylate penetration into the central nervous system.
  - Caution should be used when administering sodium bicarbonate therapy in patients with congestive heart failure or any medical condition where they may experience difficulty with the volume of infusion. In these cases, the rate should be adjusted accordingly. Renal consultation for hemodialysis should be considered once the salicylate concentration reaches 80 mg/dL as this will allow setup of hemodialysis before the serum concentration reaches >90 mg/dL (an indication for dialysis in an acute overdose).

Acetaminophen Overdose

- After obtaining a complete history and physical, patients presenting following an acetaminophen overdose should undergo laboratory evaluation including an acetaminophen concentration and an AST.
- Patients reporting an acetaminophen ingestion of 150 mg/kg or greater are at risk for hepatic toxicity. However, overdose histories are not always accurate. An acetaminophen concentration is essential for evaluating potential toxicity risk.
- An acetaminophen concentration should be obtained at least 4 hours after the reported start time of their ingestion and as soon as possible if more than 4 hours have elapsed since their ingestion.

- Acetaminophen concentrations from patients presenting within 24 hours of their acute ingestion can be interpreted using the Rumack-Matthew nomogram[2] (Fig. 105.1) if their AST is normal.
- N-Acetylcysteine is the antidote used for patients at risk for possible or probable acetaminophen toxicity and should be started for anyone with a concentration of 150 μg/mL or higher at 4 hours following their ingestion. Table 105.1 lists acetaminophen

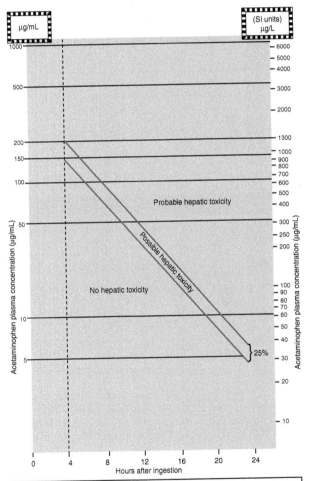

CAUTION FOR USE OF THIS CHART
1. The time coordinates refer to time of ingestion.
2. Serum levels drawn before 4 hours may not represent peak levels.
3. The graph should be used only in relation to a single acute ingestion.
4. The lower solid line is 25% below the standard nomogram and is included to allow for possible errors in acetaminophen plasma assays and estimated time from ingestion of an overdose.

Figure 105.1. Rumack-Matthew Nomogram. (Reprinted with permission from Rumack BH, Matthew H. Acetaminophen poisoning and toxicity. *Pediatrics* 1975;55:871–6.)

TABLE 105.1	Parameters for Initiation of *N*-acetylcysteine
Time since ingestion	Level at or above which acetylcysteine should be started
4 h	150 µg/mL
8 h	75 µg/mL
12 h	37.5 µg/mL
16 h	18.75 µg/mL
20 h	9.375 µg/mL

concentrations and the time following ingestion where *N*-acetylcysteine should be started, and Table 105.2 lists *N*-acetylcysteine dosing for patients presenting within 24 hours of their ingestion.

- A medical toxicologist or the local poison center should be contacted for any patient presenting 24 hours or more following their ingestion with a detectable acetaminophen level or an elevated AST or for any patient with an elevated AST following an acetaminophen overdose, regardless of their time of presentation.

Toxidromes

- Toxidromes are a pattern of symptoms and physical exam findings that can suggest a specific type of exposure.

THE ANTICHOLINERGIC (ANTIMUSCARINIC) TOXIDROME

- Signs and symptoms of the anticholinergic toxidrome include the following:
  - Mydriasis
  - Tachycardia
  - Anhidrosis
  - Hypoactive bowel sounds
  - Altered sensorium, hallucinations, psychosis, and delirium
  - Flushing
  - Urinary retention
- Treatment of patients presenting with signs of an anticholinergic toxidrome is mostly supportive, including IV fluids and benzodiazepines as needed for agitation.
- In selected cases of severe antimuscarinic toxicity consider physostigmine administration after consulting with a medical toxicologist or the local poison control center.

TABLE 105.2	*N*-Acetylcysteine Dosing for Patients Weighing >40 kg
Loading dose	150 mg/kg in 200 mL of diluent infused over 60 min
Dose 2	50 mg/kg in 500 mL of diluent infused over 4 h at a rate of 12.5 mg/kg/h
Dose 3	100 mg/kg in 1000 mL of diluent administered over 16 h at a rate of 6.25 mg/kg/h

THE CHOLINERGIC TOXIDROME

- Signs and symptoms of the cholinergic toxidrome include the following:
  - Diarrhea
  - Urination
  - Miosis
  - Bronchorrhea, bronchospasm, and bradycardia
  - Emesis
  - Lacrimation
  - Salivation
- Treatment is supportive.
  - Severe intoxication may require of atropine administration 2 mg IV with increasing doses every 5–10 minutes to an end point of improvement of bradycardia and reduction of respiratory secretions.
  - Seizures should be treated with IV/IM benzodiazepines.
  - If there is concern for organophosphate poisoning, a medical toxicologist or the local poison center should be consulted and pralidoxime administration should be considered.

THE SYMPATHOMIMETIC TOXIDROME

- Signs and symptoms of the sympathomimetic syndrome include the following:
  - Tachycardia
  - Hypertension
  - Hyperthermia
  - Diaphoresis
  - Mydriasis
  - Agitation
- Treatment is supportive and includes IV fluids; benzodiazepines IM, IV, or PO; and cooling if significantly hyperthermic.

THE SEDATIVE-HYPNOTIC TOXIDROME

- Signs and symptoms of the sedative-hypnotic syndrome include the following:
  - Somnolence
  - Coma
  - Slurred speech
  - Ataxia
  - Respiratory depression
- Treatment is supportive.
- Isolated oral benzodiazepine exposure is relatively safe even with substantial ingestion; however, coingestions may cause significant complications.
- It is not recommended to give the reversal agent flumazenil in a patient with unknown tolerance, with chronic benzodiazepine use, or with a mixed overdose.

Opioid Intoxication

- Signs and symptoms of opioid intoxication include the following:
  - Sedation and coma
  - Euphoria
  - Bradycardia and orthostatic hypotension
  - Respiratory depression

- ◦ Miosis
- ◦ Hypopnea or apnea
- ◦ Hypoactive bowel sounds
- ◦ Cyanosis
- ◦ Seizures (tramadol[3] and meperidine[4])
- • Laboratory evaluation should include basic serum electrolytes and glucose.
  - ◦ Opioid-intoxicated patients may be under the influence of other substances; frequently, a urine drug screen is sent on patients presenting with altered mental status. Results can suggest potential exposure but are not indicative of a level of intoxication.
  - ◦ An ECG is indicated in any patient with suspected methadone intoxication or overdose as methadone can prolong the QTc.
- • Treatment of opioid-intoxicated patients is primarily supportive. In addition to standard supportive measures of the airway, endotracheal intubation may be necessary.
  - ◦ Naloxone should be given to rapidly reverse the effects of opioid intoxication in any patient demonstrating significant respiratory depression.[5]
    - ▪ Caution should be used when administering naloxone to opioid-dependent patients as this can precipitate acute withdrawal. The goal of reversal of opioid intoxication is to reverse the respiratory depression.
    - ▪ In cases of opioid dependence, low-dose naloxone should be administered with dose titration as needed to reverse respiratory depression and prevent intubation.
    - ▪ For symptomatic respiratory depression, administer an initial dose of 0.4 mg naloxone and monitor until respiratory depression improves; additional doses may be given every 2 minutes.[6]
- • Some opioids are thought to be more resistant to naloxone (e.g., buprenorphine, codeine, fentanyl) and may require higher initial doses (10 mg) for full response.
  - ◦ Naloxone onset of action is ~2 minutes after intravenous administration.
- • Alternative routes of administration include intramuscular, subcutaneous, intranasal, and endotracheal routes. These offer different bioavailability and onset of action when compared to intravenous naloxone.[7]
  - ◦ The duration of action of naloxone is shorter than that of most opioid analgesics; be prepared to repeat the dose or begin a continuous naloxone infusion (two-thirds of the effective dose administered converted into an hourly rate).

REFERENCES

1. Prescott LF, Balali-Mood M, Critchley JA, et al. Diuresis or urinary alkalinisation for salicylate poisoning? *Br Med J (Clin Res Ed)* 1982;285:1383–6.
2. Rumack BH, Matthew H. Acetaminophen poisoning and toxicity. *Pediatrics* 1975;55:871–6.
3. *ULTRAM® (tramadol hydrochloride) Tablets [Prescribing Information]*. Gurabo, Puerto Rico: Janssen Ortho, LLC, 2008.
4. *DEMEROL® (meperidine hydrochloride, USP) [Prescribing Information]*. Bridgewater, NJ: Sanofi-Aventis U.S. LLC, 2014.
5. Kim HK, Nelson LS. Reducing the harm of opioid overdose with the safe use of naloxone: a pharmacologic review. *Expert Opin Drug Saf* 2015;14:1137–46.
6. Boyer EW. Management of opioid analgesic overdose. *N Engl J Med* 2012;367:146–55.
7. Dowling J, Isbister GK, Kirkpatrick CM, et al. Population pharmacokinetics of intravenous, intramuscular, and intranasal naloxone in human volunteers. *Ther Drug Monit* 2008;30:490–6.

106 Toxicology: Poisonous Plants

Steven Hung

GENERAL PRINCIPLES

- In addition to thorough history and physical, a picture or sample of the plant if possible should be obtained.
- Routine labs such as complete blood count, basic metabolic panel, hepatic function panel, and coagulation studies should be sent based on symptoms.
- Electrocardiogram should be obtained in plants thought to cause cardiac toxicity.

Clinical Presentation

- Anticholinergic toxidrome—belladonna, European or true mandrake, jimson weed, stramonium, henbane, and hyoscyamus
- Cardiac stimulant—ephedra, bala, and bitter orange
- Cardiac sodium channel blocker—rhododendron, azalea, yew, monkshood, hellebore, death camas
- Cholinergic toxidrome—Pilocarpus, Calabar bean, and ordeal bean
- Coagulopathy—Ginkgo
- Cyanide—pits and seeds of apricots, cherries, peach, plum pear, almond, apple, and cassava
- Digoxin toxicity—foxglove, lily of the valley, oleander, crown flower, and milkweed
- Gastrointestinal (GI) effects—pokeweed, nightshade
- Hepatic—thistle, kava kava, and pennyroyal
- Hypoglycemia—ackee fruit
- Mad honey disease (diaphragm or body paralysis)—Azalea and green tomatoes
- Multisystem organ failure—autumn crocus, Mayapple, and meadow saffron
- Pseudohypoaldosteronism—licorice
- Neuropathy and respiratory paralysis—blue–green algae and absinthe
- Nicotinic toxidrome—tobacco and poison hemlock
- Renal—licorice, snake root, water hemlock, and poison hemlock
- Respiratory paralysis—poison hemlock
- Seizures—water hemlock, ginkgo, Japanese star anise, bala, pennyroyal, and ackee fruit

TREATMENT

- Management can be determined by the primary effects of the plant and is mostly supportive care including airway support, intravenous fluids, and blood pressure support.
  - Anticholinergic—cooling, hydration, benzodiazepines, and physostigmine.
  - Cardiovascular—mainly from cardiac glycosides and digoxin antibody that may have some cross-reactivity.
  - Cholinergic crisis—atropine and bronchodilators.
  - Dermatologic reactions—cool compress, antihistamines, steroids, and epinephrine for anaphylaxis.
  - GI—hydration and antiemetics.

○ Hematologic—some may cause transient dysfunction of platelets and other clotting factors; treat only if a life-threatening bleed is suspected/occurs.
○ Hypoglycemia—glucose.
○ Metabolic effects—some cause cyanide toxicity and should be treated as such.
○ Nephrotoxicity—hydration.
○ Neurotoxicity—phenobarbital for seizures with water hemlock and benzodiazepines.

SUGGESTED READING

Kazzi ZN, Shih R. *Resident and Student Association Toxicology Handbook.* 2nd ed. AAEM.

107 Traumatic Emergencies: Evaluation

Mark D. Levine

GENERAL PRINCIPLES

Trauma is the leading cause of death in adults. Patients who are elderly, are obese, or have medical comorbidities have a higher incidence of poor outcome. There is an increase in mortality and morbidity in trauma patients with significant hemorrhage or a low GCS.

In the ideal scenario, emergency medical services (EMS) will provide advanced warning of a pending arrival of a trauma patient. This will allow the physician and team to designate roles in the resuscitation effort.

A thorough history should be taken by a member of the team and focus on the circumstances surrounding the injury. This may be obtained from the patient, a bystander, or a prehospital provider. In a motor vehicle accident, information about the condition of the car, location of the patient, airbag or seatbelt use, loss of consciousness, and whether extrication was required should be obtained. As with all other patients, past medical history, allergies, medications, etc. should also be obtained.

The usual approach to the physical examination of the trauma patient occurs according to advanced trauma life support protocols. Parts of the examination and resuscitation may be conducted simultaneously. Vital signs and adequate vascular access should be obtained during the primary survey.

The primary survey consists of:
A: Airway assessment and maintenance of the airway—this does not always mean immediate intubation of the patient.
B: Breathing and ventilation—oxygenate and ventilate the patient.
C: Circulation—control hemorrhage.

D: Disability—evaluate neurologic function and status.

E: Exposure—undress the patient and examine for hidden or occult injury but also protect against hypothermia.

Airway

Assessment of the airway may be done simply by asking the patient a question and seeing if there is a response. Airway obstruction can lead to hypoxia and death. Any debris or secretions should be suctioned away from the airway. Insertion of an oral or nasal airway may be performed if there is airway compromise. While maintaining in-line cervical spine stabilization, a jaw thrust maneuver may be performed to help open the airway. If the airway cannot be maintained by simple maneuvers, a definitive airway may need to be placed. Patients with significant facial trauma may require a surgical airway. Evaluation of the face and neck can be quickly done to look for signs of expanding hematoma, crepitus, or significant bleeding.

Breathing

Determination of adequate respiratory effort can be performed by evaluating the chest wall for symmetrical chest rise, accessory muscle use, abnormal respiratory patterns, and auscultation of the lung fields. The neck should be evaluated at this time for jugular venous distention and tracheal deviation. The chest wall should be examined for crepitus or a sucking chest wound. If there is question as to a pneumothorax, ultrasound may be used to aid in the diagnosis. If there are signs of tension pneumothorax, this should be treated emergently as it is a clinical diagnosis and a life threat. Patients who have had a needle decompression of the a will require a thoracostomy.

Circulation

Any obvious exsanguination needs should be controlled by direct pressure or application of a tourniquet. Central and peripheral pulses are evaluated for rate and intensity. Distended jugular veins combined with hypotension may also suggest pericardial tamponade. This can be evaluated by ultrasound and may require an emergent pericardiocentesis. Pregnant patients should be positioned by placing a roll under the right hip to alleviate inferior vena cava occlusion by the gravid uterus. Crystalloid IV solution should be started, and evaluation for blood products should be performed and administered if necessary.

Disability

A rapid evaluation of the patient's neurologic status should be performed including level of consciousness, GCS, pupillary size and response to light, and overall motor function. A GCS score below eight frequently requires airway management. Evaluation of rectal tone should be performed.

Exposure

The patient should be evaluated from head to toe and all clothing that may obscure visualization of any injury should be removed. Injuries can often be hidden in the axilla, back, perineum, gluteal cleft, and underneath the breasts. Special attention should be paid to these areas. Logroll the patient as a team in order to inspect the back, maintaining cervical spine precautions as necessary.

Secondary Survey

The secondary survey is a head to toe to evaluation of all body parts and organ systems. Plain radiography, ultrasonography, and computerized tomography may be ordered at this time. Evaluation of hemodynamic parameters and urinary output should be measured and resuscitation should be tapered or increased according to those findings. Disposition should be considered at this time, especially if the patient will need to be transferred to a trauma center. Tetanus status should be updated, antibiotics should be administered as necessary, splinting of fractures should be performed, and pain should be controlled. The patient should be kept comfortable with warm blankets.

SUGGESTED READING

Committee on Trauma, American College of Surgeons. *ATLS: Advanced Trauma Life Support Program for Doctors.* 8th ed. Chicago: American College of Surgeons, 2008.

108 Traumatic Emergencies: Blast Injuries

Bob Cambridge

GENERAL PRINCIPLES

Definition

• Anatomic and physiologic changes caused by an explosion or exacerbation of a chronic medical condition secondary to the explosion

Classification

• Primary blast injuries: these are only seen with high-order explosives such as TNT, dynamite, semtex, and C4 and occur as a direct effect of the blast pressure wave and its interaction as it moves through tissue. The pressure wave causes a shear effect on the organs, which is the greatest at air/tissue interfaces, but any location with density differentials can be affected. Any organ can be affected, but the ear, lung, and abdomen are particularly prone to primary blast injury. The farther the person is from the blast, the less damage will be done as the blast wave dissipates over distance.
• Secondary blast injuries: these occur as an effect of projectiles thrown by the blast or the blast wave and can cause penetrating or blunt injury. Secondary injuries are the leading cause of death in explosions (except in the case of major building collapse). Any wound on the skin should be evaluated for its depth and potential for retained foreign body. Any location of blunt force injury should be further evaluated.
• Tertiary blast injuries: these occur from the patient being thrown into something by the blast or by collapse of the structure the patient is in/near.

- Quaternary blast injuries: these are burns, inhalational injuries, or exacerbations of chronic conditions as a result of the blast.

Pathophysiology

- Blast waves from high-order explosives cause primary injury through rapid external loading on the body and organs. The force of the blast causes compression of the organs resulting in recoil and reexpansion as the blast wave exits. As the wave passes through the interface between two different densities, particles of the heavier tissue can be thrown into the lower density area through an effect called spalling. Spalling and rapid reexpansion lead to bleeding, tissue tearing, and other morbid conditions.
- Low-order (pipe bombs, gunpowder) explosives do not cause an overpressurization wave.

DIAGNOSIS

Clinical Presentation

History

- Patients may complain of tinnitus, bleeding from the ear, or vertigo. There may be transient hearing loss, although in up to 30% of patients the hearing loss may be permanent. Because of the utility of tympanic membrane (TM) rupture as a sensitive marker for other primary injuries, all blast injury patients need an otologic exam.
- Patients may also have complaints of dyspnea or chest pain from primary lung injury or exacerbation of underlying lung conditions.
- Patients with primary abdominal injuries can complain of a wide range of symptoms from vague abdominal pain, nausea and vomiting, hematemesis or hematochezia, rectal pain, testicular pain, and more.

Physical Examination

- A full physical exam should be performed on every patient, and immediate stabilization of life threats should occur.
- The ear is the organ most sensitive to the primary blast effect. 5 PSI is all that is needed to rupture the TM, and essentially, all patients with other primary blast injuries will have a ruptured TM.
- The lung is the second most susceptible organ after the ear; however, primary lung injury has the greatest morbidity and mortality and is the most common location for fatal primary blast injuries in patients who survive the initial blast.
  - Blast lung can lead to the severe clinical triad of dyspnea, bradycardia, and hypotension. It can manifest up to 48 hours after the blast and occurs due to the bronchial epithelium being stripped from the basal lamina. The air space fills with blood, fluid, and tissue.
- Blast waves can lead to globe rupture, retinitis, traumatic cataracts, and hyphema in the eyes. Patients can have traumatic brain injury (TBI) from the barotrauma of gas embolism. Consider TBI in any patient with headache, poor concentration, lethargy, or fatigue. Anxiety can also be a sign of TBI.
- The colon is the gas-filled abdominal organ most frequently affected. Solid organ injury is less common as the tissue density differentials throughout the organ are smaller.

Diagnostic Testing

Laboratories

- No specific blood work is diagnostic for a blast injury. Blood work may be useful in treatment and workup of the injured patient.

Imaging
- Any injured area should have further evaluation, either through direct visualization (wound exploration, surgical exploration) or through radiographic analysis.
  - Plain radiographs can be done to look for free air, chest injury (pneumothorax, pulmonary hemorrhage), or extremity/bony injuries.
  - Ultrasound exams can evaluate the abdomen for free fluid or the chest for pneumothorax.
  - CT scans of the head/neck/chest/abdomen/pelvis may be used as clinically indicated.

TREATMENT

- The treatment of any critically ill patient begins with the correction of the ABCs and stabilization of the patient.
  - If mechanical ventilation is needed, ventilate with a low positive end-expiratory pressure (PEEP) strategy according to the ARDSnet protocol. Positive pressure has been reported to increase mortality in blast injuries as it can exacerbate microtears and lead to increased air embolization.
  - Avoidance of high inspiratory pressures is recommended as well for the same reasons. Permissive hypercapnia can be pursued.
  - Managing blast lung injury requires judicious fluid use and administration, ensuring tissue perfusion without volume overload.
- Update the patient's tetanus immunization as necessary. It is recommended to give prophylactic antibiotics for all but the most trivial injuries.

Treatment of Air Embolism

- If an air embolism is found or suspected, place the patient in the left lateral recumbent position, apply 100% oxygen by nonrebreather, and make preparations to send the patient for hyperbaric therapy.
  - Aspirin can be considered as it can reduce inflammation-mediated injury in pulmonary barotrauma; however, its utility has to be weighed against any potential bleeding risk in the setting of acute trauma.

Treatment of Other Injuries

- The therapy will be based on the organ system injured and the degree of injury. Prompt evaluation of eye injuries by ophthalmology and ear injuries by otolaryngology is recommended.

SPECIAL CONSIDERATIONS

Disposition

- Low-risk patients can be discharged after 4 hours of observation.
  - These are patients exposed to an explosion in an open space, with no injury, normal vital signs, and a normal physical exam.
- Moderate-risk patients without significant injuries should be observed for longer periods of time to watch for delayed complications. Optimal observation time is unknown as there is limited data.
  - Moderate-risk factors include patients exposed to closed space explosions, underwater explosions (as the water transmits the blast wave with less degradation over distance than air), or patients with a TM rupture without other findings. After disposition, audiometry is recommended.

- High-risk patients should be admitted to the hospital.
  - High-risk factors include abnormal vital signs, abnormal physical exam findings especially lung/abdomen signs, persistent abdominal pain, penetrating injuries to the head/neck/torso, significant burns, suspected air embolisms, crush injuries, radiation exposure, or other concerning findings.

SUGGESTED READINGS

Arnold JL, Halperin P, Tsai MC, Smithline H. Mass casualty terrorist bombings: a comparison of outcomes by bombing type. *Ann Emerg Med* 2004;43:263–73.

Church EJ. Medical imaging of explosion injuries. *Radiol Technol* 2010;81:337–54.

DePalma RG, Burris DG, Champion HR, Hodgson MJ. Blast injuries. *N Engl J Med* 2005;352:1335–42.

Hogan DE, Waeckerle JF, Dire DJ, Lillebridge ST. Emergency department impact of the Oklahoma City terrorist bombing. *Ann Emerg Med* 1999;34:160–7.

Karmy-Jones R, Kissinger D, Golocovsky M, et al. Bombing related injuries. *Mil Med* 1994;159:536–9.

Leibovici D, Gofrit ON, Shapira SC. Eardrum perforation in explosion survivors: is it a marker of pulmonary blast injury? *Ann Emerg Med* 1999;34:168–72.

Leibovici D, Gofrit ON, Stein M, et al. Blast injuries: bus versus open-air bombings—a comparative study of injuries in survivors of open-air versus confined-space explosions pending. *J Trauma* 1996;41(6):1030–5.

Shaikh N, Ummunisa F. Acute management of vascular air embolism. *J Emerg Trauma Shock* 2009;2(3):180–5.

Spitz W. Medicolegal Investigation of Death. *Bannerstone House*, Charles C Thomas: Springfield IL, 1973.

Wightman JM, Gladish SL. Explosions and blast injuries. *Ann Emerg Med* 2001;37:664–78.

109 Traumatic Emergencies: Pregnancy

Mark D. Levine

GENERAL PRINCIPLES

Epidemiology

- The most common causes of trauma in pregnancy are from motor vehicle accidents and intimate partner violence.[1]

Pathophysiology

- Physiologic changes occur throughout the body and have multiple etiologies. These changes should be taken into account when evaluating the pregnant trauma patient.

- There is increased blood volume (50% by 30 weeks of pregnancy), decreased vascular resistance, and a 15–20-bpm increase in heart rate.[2,3]
- Hyperventilation and a chronic respiratory alkalosis cause an elevation in PaO_2. There is a decrease in functional residual capacity (FRC) due to displacement of the diaphragm during pregnancy after ~20 weeks.[4]
- A mild leukocytosis is frequently seen. There is a physiologic anemia of pregnancy (hemoglobin levels as low as 10–11 g/dL) throughout the pregnancy. Pregnancy leads to a procoagulant state.
- Due to an increased intra-abdominal pressure and a lower esophageal sphincter tone, pregnant patients are at a higher risk of gastric aspiration.
- The uterus is protected during the first 12 weeks of pregnancy by the bony pelvis. The pelvic vasculature is dilated during pregnancy and can lead to rapid hemorrhage. As the uterus enlarges, the bowel is displaced, increasing risk of bowel injury above the uterine fundus. Because uterine blood flow increases during the third trimester, a drop in maternal blood pressure can cause a significant decrease in blood flow to the uterus.[5]

DIAGNOSIS

Clinical Presentation

History

- A thorough history of the events surrounding the trauma as well as the patient's obstetrical history should be obtained.

Physical Examination

- The physical examination should occur in accordance to ATLS protocol. Gestational age should be determined by the use of dates or ultrasound but may also be determined by the fundal height (at the symphysis pubis at 12 weeks, at the umbilicus at 20 weeks, at the costal margin at 34 weeks).[6]
- Tenderness and rigidity of the uterus may indicate abruption or labor.
- A vaginal exam should be performed to assess for bleeding, fluid, or labor. Digital examination of the vagina should be avoided in pregnancies >20 weeks gestation until placenta previa can be excluded. A speculum can be used to look for bleeding. Bleeding can also be due to vaginal trauma, foreign bodies, or bone fragments from the pelvis.
- During trauma assessment and resuscitation, fetal heart rate and tocometric monitoring should be performed. The normal fetal heart rate is 100–160 bpm. The fetal heart rate pattern should be monitored by a clinician experienced in obstetrics and should be continued for a minimum of 4 hours.[7]

Diagnostic Criteria

Laboratories

- Laboratory values should be obtained as part of the normal trauma protocol. Rh status and a Kleihauer-Betke test should be obtained.

Imaging

- The risk–benefit of radiation exposure to the unborn child should be taken into consideration when evaluating a pregnant trauma patient. When possible, ultrasound or nonionizing radiation should be used.

TREATMENT

- The general approach to trauma in pregnancy is generally done in the same stepwise fashion as any other trauma evaluation. However, special attention should be paid to the fact that two patients are being treated at once and treatment of the mother usually influences fetal outcome.

- The obstetrical service should be consulted in conjunction with the trauma service especially in the event that an emergency cesarean section is necessary.
- In pregnant patients, the diaphragm may be elevated so a chest tube may need to be placed one or two intercostal spaces above the usual landmarks.[1]
- Pregnant patients who are at 20 weeks or above gestation should have the uterus displaced to the left to provide relief from impingement of the inferior vena cava. This is accomplished by placing the patient on her left side or placing a wedge under the right hip (or spine board if the patient needs to be immobilized on a backboard). Fluid replacement should be aggressive because changes in vital signs may not occur until 15–20% of the total blood volume has been lost.[8] Vasopressors may reduce uterine blood flow so it is important to give appropriate volume resuscitation. If blood products are necessary, O negative blood should be administered prior to type-specific blood availability.
- Abruptio placentae may occur due to sudden deceleration or direct trauma leading to a tearing at the uteroplacental border. Significant trauma uterine tenderness or vaginal bleeding warrants further monitoring and evaluation by an obstetrician.
- Uterine rupture may be secondary to either penetrating or blunt trauma, and it should be suspected with signs and symptoms of shock, fetal death, uterine tenderness, peritonitis, or vaginal bleeding. These patients need to be evaluated in the operating room.
- If cardiopulmonary resuscitation is necessary, emergent cesarean section may need to be performed to increase the effectiveness of cardiopulmonary resuscitation. Optimum survival of the newborn and mother is obtained when cesarean delivery is initiated within 4 minutes of loss of pulse.[9]

Medications

- Due to the possibility of fetal maternal bleeding, Rhogam (anti-D immunoglobulin) is frequently administered to females that are Rh positive.[10] The Kleihauer-Betke test may assist in determining the dose of Rhogam to be administered.

SPECIAL CONSIDERATIONS

Disposition

- The patient should have fetal heart monitoring for at least 4 hours if there is no obvious indication for trauma admission.[7]
- Stable patients may be admitted to the floor on either the surgical or obstetrical service, and unstable patients should be admitted to the intensive care unit.

Complications

- Maternal death, fetal injury or death, miscarriage, abruption, preterm delivery, premature rupture of membranes, or infection

REFERENCES

1. Mendez-Figueroa H, Dahlke JD, Vrees RA, et al. Trauma in pregnancy: an updated systematic review. *Am J Obstet Gynecol* 2013;209:1–10.
2. Shnider SM, Levinson G. *Anesthesia for Obstetrics*. 3rd ed. Baltimore: Williams and Wilkins.
3. Bonica JJ, McDonald JS. *Principle and Practice of Obstetric Analgesia and Anesthesia*. 2nd ed. Baltimore: Williams and Wilkins, 1994.

4. Prowse CM, Gaensler EA. Respiratory and acid-base changes during pregnancy. *Anesthesiology* 1965;26:381–92.
5. Stone IK. Trauma in the obstetric patient. *Obstet Gynecol Clin North Am* 1999;26:459–67.
6. Bickley LS, Szilagyi P. *Bates Guide to Physical Examination and History Taking.* 8th ed. Philadelphia: Lippincott Williams & Wilkins, 2003.
7. Connolly AM, Katz VL, Bash KL, et al. Trauma and pregnancy. *Am J Perinatol* 1997;14:331–6.
8. Brown HL. Trauma in pregnancy. *Obstet Gynecol* 2009;114:147–60.
9. Katz VL, Dotters DJ, Droegemueller W. Perimortem cesarean delivery. *Obset Gynecol* 1986;68: 571–6.
10. Barraco RD, Chiu WCX, Clancy TV, et al. Practice management guidelines for the diagnosis and management of injury in the pregnant patient: the EAST Practice Management Guidelines Work Group. *J Trauma* 2010;69:211–4.

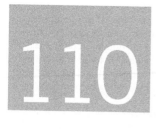

110 Traumatic Emergencies: Abdomen

Aldo Andino

GENERAL PRINCIPLES

Definition

- Blunt abdominal trauma
  - Trauma to the abdomen (direct blow, twisting/shearing or acceleration/deceleration forces) leading to injury of the abdominal or retroperitoneal organs.
- Penetrating abdominal trauma
  - Violation of the peritoneum due to any penetrating object

Epidemiology/Etiology

- Blunt
  - Accounts for majority of emergency department (ED) abdominal injuries (80%).[1]
  - The prevalence of intra-abdominal injury in blunt abdominal trauma is 13%.[1]
  - Most common trauma is due to motor vehicle collisions and pedestrians struck by automobiles (75%), direct blows to the abdomen (15%), and falls (6–10%).[2,3]
- Penetrating
  - Gunshot wounds are less common than stab wounds but have a greater mortality.[4]

Pathophysiology

- Blunt
  - Compression of the abdomen from an outward force can increase intra-abdominal pressure and rupture a hollow viscus or crush solid organs against spine/ribs

leading to a laceration (liver and spleen are the most commonly injured organs in blunt abdominal trauma).
   - Shearing forces from rapid deceleration (e.g., MVC) can lead to vascular tears.
- Penetrating
   - Any object that violates the peritoneum can injure organs, vascular structures, and bones depending on size and velocity.
   - Stab wounds will depend on the length/width of the weapon and the force used.
   - Hollow viscus organs are most commonly injured in penetrating wounds.

DIAGNOSIS

Clinical Presentation

History
- Information regarding the mechanism of injury should be obtained.
- Abdominal pain is highly sensitive, but not specific for intra-abdominal injury.

Physical Examination
- Examine the entire body including the perineum and gluteal folds for evidence of injury.
- Evaluation of the airway, breathing, circulation, and disability should occur in sequence, and life-threatening abnormalities addressed.

Differential Diagnosis
- Splenic, liver, kidney, bowel, diaphragm laceration or contusion, mesenteric shearing damage, or bladder rupture

Diagnostic Criteria and Testing
Laboratories
- Hematocrit on arrival may not reflect true blood loss in the acute setting.
- WBC may be elevated, but this finding is nonspecific and is more likely due to a stress response of the body.
- Elevated alanine transaminase (ALT) and aspartate transaminase (AST) may be suggestive of liver injury.[5]
- Acidosis with a base deficit less than −6 has been found to be associated with need for laparotomy and blood transfusions.[6]
- Urinalysis may identify renal, ureteral, or bladder injury.
- Elevated lactate may indicate a hypoperfusion state.

Imaging
- Ultrasound can be used to identify free fluid and pneumothoraces.[7]
   - Negative eFAST does not rule out intra-abdominal injury but simply suggests that there is no free fluid or pneumothorax present.
   - If positive, stability of the patient determines radiography or operative exploration.
- Chest and pelvis radiographs are indicated.
- A CT of the abdomen and pelvis with contrast is able to identify injuries that can be managed nonoperatively and provide details regarding injuries that do require surgery.
   - Limited in identifying injuries to the diaphragm, bowel, and pancreas.

Diagnostic Procedures
- In stable penetrating injuries, local wound exploration should be performed by a trauma surgeon.

TREATMENT

- Treatment is varied based on the hemodynamic state of the patient and the radio-graphic/ultrasonographic findings.
- If abdominal trauma is the suspected source of hemorrhage, vascular access should be obtained in the upper extremities or neck.

Medications

- Resuscitation of shock states from abdominal trauma should follow the general principles outlined in the resuscitation chapter (Chapter 130).
- Due to its favorable hemodynamic profile, fentanyl (1 μg/kg) should be used as a first-line agent for pain control.

Other Nonpharmacologic Therapies

Angiography

- Angiography can be used to control hemorrhage from bleeding pelvic vessels in an unstable pelvic fracture and/or abdominal organs.

Surgery

- Penetrating injuries or significant intra-abdominal injury necessitates emergent surgical consultation and intraoperative management.

SPECIAL CONSIDERATIONS

Disposition

- Patients in need of monitoring and ongoing resuscitation should be admitted to an ICU.
- If the patient has a positive focused assessment with sonography for trauma (FAST) exam and is unstable, they should be taken to the OR.
- In unstable penetrating abdominal trauma, the patient should be taken immediately to the OR.

Complications

- Infection, intra-abdominal abscess, and abdominal compartment syndrome

REFERENCES

1. Nishijima DK, Simel DL, Wisner DH, Holmes JF. Does this adult patient have a blunt intra-abdominal injury? *JAMA* 2012;307(14):1517–27.
2. Isenhour JL, Marx J. Advances in abdominal trauma. *Emerg Med Clin North Am* 2007;25(3):713–33.
3. Davis JJ, Cohn I Jr, Nance FC. Diagnosis and management of blunt abdominal trauma. *Ann Surg* 1976;183(6):672–8.
4. Zafar SN, Rushing A, Haut ER, et al. Outcome of selective non-operative management of penetrating abdominal injuries from the North American National Trauma Database. *Br J Surg* 2012;99(suppl 1):155–64.
5. Tan KK, Bang SL, Vijayan A, Chiu MT. Hepatic enzymes have a role in the diagnosis of hepatic injury after blunt abdominal trauma. *Injury* 2009;40(9):978–83.

6. Ibrahim I, Chor WP, Chue KM, et al. Is arterial base deficit still a useful prognostic marker in trauma? A systematic review. *Am J Emerg Med* 2016;34(3):626–35.
7. Cohen HL, Langer J, McGahan JP, et al.; American Institute of Ultrasound in Medicine; American College of Emergency Physicians. AIUM practice guideline for the performance of the focused assessment with sonography for trauma (FAST) examination. *J Ultrasound Med* 2014;33(11):2047–56.

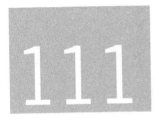

111 Traumatic Emergencies: Chest

Stephanie Charshafian and
Michael Willman

GENERAL PRINCIPLES

Traumatic Cardiac Arrest

- Causes can include tension pneumothorax (PTX), hemorrhage, cardiac tamponade, or severe traumatic brain injury.
- Chest compressions should be initiated, while the underlying cause is identified and treated.
- Standard advanced cardiac life support (ACLS) medications are ineffective in traumatic cardiac arrest.

Rib Fractures

GENERAL PRINCIPLES

- Rib fractures may indicate significant traumatic force and can injure underlying structures. Fractures of ribs 9–12 may be associated with abdominal injuries.[1]
- Rib fractures can be very painful, especially with inspiration. This can lead to shallow breathing, decreased clearance of secretions, and increased rates of pneumonia.
- Flail chest is defined as the fracture of three contiguous ribs at two sites creating a segment of the chest wall that paradoxically moves with inspiration and expiration.

DIAGNOSIS

- CXR will generally reveal significant rib fractures, but nondisplaced or occult fractures may be missed.
- A CT scan can help find occult fractures.

MANAGEMENT

- Most rib fractures require only supportive care, pain control, and pulmonary toilet to ensure adequate clearance of secretions.
- Patients with respiratory insufficiency due to flail chest, rib fractures, or pulmonary contusion may require supplemental oxygenation or mechanical ventilation.

Pneumothorax (see Chapter 101)

GENERAL PRINCIPLES

Tension Pneumothorax

- Tension physiology may be seen. Signs include shock, tracheal deviation, and distended jugular veins. This is a clinical diagnosis. If left untreated, can lead to cardiovascular collapse and death.

MANAGEMENT

- Needle decompression
  - Indicated for emergent treatment of suspected tension PTX. Do not wait for a chest plain radiograph for confirmation.
  - Insert a long (3.25 in.) 14–16-gauge angiocath in the 2nd intercostal space at the midclavicular line or the 5th intercostal space at the midaxillary line.
  - Use needle decompression as a bridge to placement of a chest tube.

Hemothorax

GENERAL PRINCIPLES

Definition

- Hemothorax is the accumulation of blood in the thorax, typically in between the visceral and parietal pleura. When a hemothorax presents in conjunction with free air, this is called a hemopneumothorax.

DIAGNOSIS

- Decreased or absent breath sounds may be appreciated on auscultation.
- An upright chest plain radiograph may reveal a collection of fluid blunting the costophrenic angle. A hemothorax is not detectable on chest plain radiograph until 200–300 mL of fluid accumulates in the chest cavity.
- As little as 20 mL of fluid in the pleural cavity can be detected by bedside ultrasound.
- A CT scan of the chest with contrast can better delineate the presence and amount of blood.

MANAGEMENT

- All hemothoraces should be considered for drainage.
- Initial treatment should be with tube thoracostomy.
- An initial output of more than 1000 mL of blood, output of 150-200 mL/hr for 2-4 hours, or the need for repeated blood transfusions should prompt consideration for operative management.
- Hemodynamic instability should prompt consideration for surgical intervention.

Cardiac Injury

GENERAL PRINCIPLES

- Blunt traumatic injury can lead to cardiac contusion and traumatic cardiac rupture.
- Penetrating injury can lead to penetrating cardiac injury, pericardial effusion, tamponade, and exsanguination.

Definition

- Cardiac contusion
  - Blunt traumatic force to the myocardium
- Commotio cordis
  - Cardiac arrest caused by blunt chest impact. Thought to arise from R-on-T phenomena precipitating ventricular tachycardia or fibrillation.
- Cardiac rupture
  - Blunt trauma to the chest leading to a rapid increase in pressure on the heart, causing an acute rupture of the myocardium, left ventricle (LV) free wall, right ventricle (RV) free wall, atria, or septum
- Penetrating cardiac injury
  - Penetrating injury into or through the myocardium
- Pericardial effusion
  - Fluid within the pericardium after traumatic injury of the myocardium
- Cardiac tamponade
  - A pericardial effusion resulting in diminished filling of the RV and hemodynamic instability.
  - Beck's triad includes hypotension, distended neck veins, and muffled heart sounds. This "classic" triad is only observed in 10% of patients with documented traumatic cardiac injury,[2] and a minority of patients with tamponade.

DIAGNOSIS

- Cardiac contusion
  - New ECG findings of ST- or T-wave changes anteriorly or elevation of troponin. Heart blocks, incomplete right bundle branch blocks, or q-waves may be present. Cardiac CT or MRI can be used to evaluate for blunt cardiac injury. Blunt cardiac injury can be ruled out in patients with normal ECG and troponin I level.[3]
- Cardiac rupture and penetrating cardiac injury
  - Patients often present with cardiovascular collapse or are pulseless. Bedside ultrasound can be useful in identifying pericardial effusion and tamponade physiology.
- Pericardial effusion and cardiac tamponade
  - Can be diagnosed by bedside ultrasound showing effusion and tamponade physiology

MANAGEMENT

- Cardiac contusion
  - Patients with blunt cardiac injury can be admitted for telemetry or observation.
- Cardiac rupture and penetrating cardiac injury
  - Thoracotomy may temporize myocardial injuries so that the patient can make it to the OR for definitive management.

- Pericardial effusion and cardiac tamponade
  - Pericardiocentesis, in contrast to nontraumatic pericardial effusions, often does not provide relief of tamponade due to the presence of clotted blood.
  - Thoracotomy is the treatment of choice for traumatic pericardial effusion and cardiac tamponade. Depending upon the stability of the patient, this may be performed in the emergency department or the operating room.

Great Vessel Injury

GENERAL PRINCIPLES

- Rapid deceleration can produce sudden shearing forces causing aortic injury or transection.
- Proximal clavicular fractures and/or fractures of the 1st and 2nd ribs are classically associated with higher risk for injury to the great vessels and their branches.

DIAGNOSIS

- A clinical history and mechanism of injury may be the only clue to injury to these vessels.
- CXR may show widening of the mediastinum, apical capping, deviation of the trachea or NG tube, depression of the left mainstem bronchus, or disruption of the calcium ring of the aortic knob.
- CT angiogram of the chest is the modality of choice.

MANAGEMENT

- Resuscitation is the mainstay of emergency department (ED) management of great vessel trauma.
- Correction of coagulopathies should be initiated immediately. This includes correction of hypothermia and acidosis.
- Vascular consultation is indicated.
- Hemodynamic instability is an indication for a thoracotomy.

REFERENCES

1. Shweiki E, Klena J, Wood GC, et al. Assessing the true risk of abdominal solid organ injury in hospitalized rib fracture patients. *J Trauma* 2000;50:684–8.
2. Brasel KJ, Moore EE, Albrecht RA, et al. Western trauma association critical decisions in trauma: Management of rib fractures. *J Trauma Acute Care Surg* 2016; 82(1): 200–3.
3. Clancy K, Velopulos C, Bilaniuk JW, et al. Screening for blunt cardiac injury: an eastern association for the surgery of trauma practice management guideline. *J Trauma Acute Care Surg* 2012;73(5 suppl 4):S301–6.

112 Traumatic Emergencies: Cutaneous and Soft Tissue

Deborah Shipley Kane

GENERAL PRINCIPLES

Definition

- Closed injuries are caused by blunt trauma and include contusions, hematoma, and crush injuries.
- Open injuries occur when there is a break in the skin, exposing underlying soft tissue to injury.
- Burns are characterized by the degree and amount of skin burned.
  - Superficial thickness—involves superficial layer only
  - Partial thickness—involves epidermis and dermis, often blisters
  - Full thickness—extends into the subcutaneous tissue, fat, and muscle

Epidemiology/Etiology

- Skin is the largest organ of the body and therefore is prone to being involved in trauma. Injuries related to skin and soft tissue account for 12% of emergency department (ED) visits.[1]

DIAGNOSIS

Clinical Presentation

History
- A full history should include timing of the incident (prolonged open wound time leads to more contamination), how injury occurred (animal bites, burns, and high-pressure injection injuries may require different treatments), comorbid conditions, and tetanus status.

Physical Examination
- Location, size, and type of wound should be noted.
- If deeper structures such as tendon, ligaments, or bone are involved, they should be fully assessed.
- Burns—estimate the size of the burn.
- High-pressure injection injuries may appear very small and have associated mild pain or swelling but have a high degree of morbidity if missed.[2]

Diagnostic Criteria and Testing

Imaging
- Plain radiograph may be helpful to look for foreign bodies (metal, glass), underlying bony injury, or gas.
- Ultrasound may be useful to evaluate for radiolucent foreign bodies.

TREATMENT

- Tetanus prophylaxis.
- Direct pressure to control hemorrhage.
- Decontamination and irrigation are essential to prevent infection.
- Antibiotic prophylaxis—usually not indicated in clean, simple wounds. It may be considered in certain conditions, including[3]:
  - Wound age—hand and foot wounds >8 hours old, facial wounds >24 hours old, and other sites >12 hours old
    - Cephalexin 500 mg PO qid can be prescribed.
    - Other antibiotics should be considered based upon the location of injury.
  - Wound condition—those that require extensive tissue debridement and revision
  - Contamination—soil and particulate matter
  - Animal bites—indicated in high-risk wounds including cat bites, puncture wounds, hand wounds, and delayed presentations.[4]
    - Ampicillin–sulbactam 1.5 g IV should be administered in the ED and amoxicillin-clavulanate 875 mg PO bid × 7–10 days should be started as outpatient therapy if no contraindications or allergies exist.
  - Wounds involving cartilage, tendon, bone, and joint
  - Immunocompromised patients (diabetes, HIV, chemotherapy, chronic steroids)
  - Burns[5]
  - Cardiac valvular disease
  - Orthopedic implants
- Wound repair should be performed as soon as possible.

SPECIAL CONSIDERATIONS

Disposition

- will be dependent on type of wound and possible complications. Full-thickness burns and high-pressure injection wounds require consultation and admission of the appropriate specialty.

Complications

- infection, bleeding, loss of vital tissue, and damage to underlying structures.

REFERENCES

1. CDC.gov. *Ambulatory Health Care Data.* National Center for Health Statistics, https://www.cdc.gov/nchs/ahcd/index.htm.
2. Verhoeven N, Hierner R. High-pressure injection injure of the hand: an often underestimated trauma: case report with study of the literature. *Strategies Trauma Limb Reconstr* 2008;3(1):27–33.
3. Trott AT. *Wounds and Lacerations: Emergency Care and Closure.* 3rd ed. Philadelphia: Mosby, 2005:P308.
4. Ellis R, Ellis C. Dog and cat bites. *Am Fam Physician* 2014;90(4):239–43.
5. Avni T, Levcovich A, Ad-El DD, et al. Prophylactic antibiotics for burn patients: systematic review and meta-analysis. *BMJ* 2010;340:c241.

113 | Traumatic Emergencies: Extremities

Kelly Counts and Kurt Eifling

GENERAL PRINCIPLES

Epidemiology/Etiology

- Falls are the most common cause of extremity trauma in the United States, causing 50–60% of lower extremity and 80% of upper extremity injuries.

Pathophysiology

- Force from penetrating or blunt trauma leads to tissue, bone, and vascular disruption. Disruption of the vascular system leads to tissue ischemia or hemorrhage.

DIAGNOSIS

Clinical Presentation

History
- The patient's mechanism of injury and sequelae offer clues about the nature of the injury.
- Patients may complain of pain, paresthesias, or paralysis. These may begin up to 48 hours after the initial insult.

Physical Examination
- Remove any clothing, jewelry, splints, or casts.
- Examine for wounds, deformity, length discrepancies, abnormal rotation or color, and necrotic tissue.
- Palpate to evaluate for crepitus, skin tenting, peripheral pulses, and tone of muscular compartments. Evaluate active and passive range of motion.
- Screen for neurologic injury using light touch and gross motor movements and compare two-point discrimination in the normal and injured extremity.
- One hard or two soft vascular signs suggest a vascular injury.
  - Hard signs of vascular injury include active hemorrhage, expanding or pulsatile hematoma, thrill or bruit over a wound, absence of distal pulses, and signs of extremity ischemia (pallor, pain, paralysis).
  - Soft signs of vascular injury include a small stable hematoma, nerve injury, unexplained hypotension, history of hemorrhage, or proximity to another concerning wound.

Differential Diagnosis

- Tendon rupture, dislocation, retained foreign body, neurovascular injury, fracture, crush injury, compartment syndrome, mononeuropathy

Diagnostic Criteria and Testing

Laboratories
- For evaluation of crush syndrome, a basic metabolic panel, calcium, phosphate, creatinine kinase, uric acid, and urine micro/macro should be checked and repeated every 2–4 hours for trending.

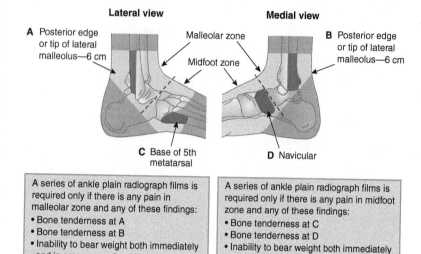

Figure 113.1. Ottawa Foot and Ankle Rules.

Imaging
- Evidence-based risk stratification may safely reduce the volume of radiographs in some injuries.
  - The Ottawa Foot and Ankle Rules (Fig. 113.1) are prospectively validated decision support tools that are 98% sensitive for radiographically significant injury in the foot and ankle.
  - The Ottawa Knee Rule (Fig. 113.2) is a prospectively validated decision support tool that is 98% sensitive for radiographically significant injury to the knee.
- Some injury patterns require recognition at the bedside and subsequent imaging.
  - Proximal fibular tenderness after ankle trauma is an indication for radiographs to diagnose a Maisonneuve fracture, which is associated with syndesmotic injury.
  - Anatomic snuffbox tenderness after wrist trauma is an indication for radiographs to diagnose a scaphoid bone fracture.
- CT imaging is used to evaluate complex or occult fractures, foreign bodies, or swelling.
- CT angiography is the test of choice for patients who are suspected to have occult vascular disruption or dissection.

Electrocardiography
- A screening ECG should be performed in patients at risk for crush syndrome.

Diagnostic Procedures
- The ankle–brachial index (ABI) is used as a screening tool for vascular injury (ABI < 0.9 suggests vascular disruption).
- Compartment pressures may be measured to evaluate for compartment syndrome (symptoms of pain, paresthesia, poikilothermia, pallor, paralysis, and pulselessness).
  - A compartment pressure of <30 mm Hg is considered normal.
  - The "delta pressure" is the systolic blood pressure minus compartment pressure. A value of <30 is suggestive of impending compartment syndrome.

ANTERIOR VIEW

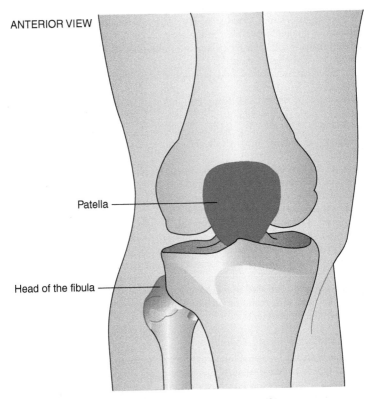

Patella

Head of the fibula

OTTAWA KNEE RULE (Demonstrated on the right leg)

Figure 113.2. Ottawa Knee Rule. In knee trauma, standard radiographs are indicated if the patient has any one of these factors: age 55 or older, tenderness at the fibular head, isolated patellar tenderness, inability to flex the knee >90 degrees, or inability to bear weight for four steps both immediately and in the emergency department. (Modified from Stiell IG, Wells GA, Hoag RH, et al. Implementation of the Ottawa Knee Rule for the use of radiography in acute knee injuries. *JAMA* 1997;278[23]:2075–9.)

TREATMENT

- Sprains and strains should be managed with rest, ice, compression, and elevation (RICE method) of the injured area.
- Vascular compromise should be treated as quickly as possible.
- For crush syndrome, aggressive IV fluid administration is the mainstay of therapy. Target a urine output of 3–4 mL/kg/h in most patients.
- Care of fractures and dislocations rely on restoring anatomic position through reduction of the injured structures.
  - Snuffbox tenderness is an indication for thumb spica splinting regardless of radiograph findings in the acute setting.
  - A Galeazzi fracture (fracture of the distal radius with distal radioulnar joint dislocation) requires operative fixation to avoid recurrent ulnar dislocation.

- ○ A Monteggia fracture (fracture of the forearm with proximal radioulnar joint dislocation) requires operative fixation to avoid chronic radial head complications.
- A sling is usually sufficient for treatment of traumatic neurapraxia (Saturday night palsy or brachial plexus "stinger").
- A shoulder immobilizer should be applied after the reduction of a shoulder dislocation.
- For most tendon or ligament disruptions, splinting or immobilization is sufficient.

Medications

- Analgesia and tetanus prophylaxis are expected in the routine care of trauma patients.
- Antibiotic administration for open fracture is standard of care.
  - ○ For unsoiled wounds, a first- or second-generation cephalosporin is adequate.
  - ○ Consider adding vancomycin if the patient is at risk for methicillin-resistant *Staphylococcus aureus* (MRSA) colonization.
  - ○ For soiled or extensive wounds at high risk for infection or involving lawnmowers, shoes, or vegetable matter, broaden coverage to include gram-negative bacteria and *Pseudomonas aeruginosa*; clindamycin and gentamicin are often used.
- In patients with crush syndrome, focus on treating electrolyte alterations and renal failure.
  - ○ No randomized controlled studies have been performed to compare IV fluid alone versus IV fluid with mannitol or bicarbonate. Aggressive fluid administration is the mainstay of treatment.

Other Nonpharmacologic Therapies

- Tourniquets are used over the humerus or femur to control massive hemorrhage. A windlass type is preferred, though a pneumatic cuff at a pressure of 300 mm Hg is also adequate. Often two windlass-type tourniquets are needed in series in patients with a large body habitus. Avoid tourniquet time of over 6 hours if limb salvage is planned.
- If a bleeding vessel is identified, it can be ligated and tagged with a large silk tie to be ultimately managed later in surgery.

SPECIAL CONSIDERATIONS

Disposition

- Intensive care is preferred for monitoring patients with compartment syndrome, crush syndrome, massive transfusion, or limb-salvaging vascular repairs. Most other extremity injuries can be managed on the hospital floor or at home with specialist follow-up.

Complications

- Knee dislocations may cause popliteal vascular injury.
- High-pressure injection injury may cause compartment syndrome.
- Humerus fracture may cause radial nerve palsy.
- Crush injury may cause compartment syndrome or crush syndrome.
- Long-term sequelae of compartment syndrome, crush injuries, nerve injuries, or unrepaired tendon or ligamentous injuries can have severe long-term impacts on function.

SUGGESTED READINGS

Gustilo R, Anderson J. Prevention of infection in the treatment of one thousand and twenty-five open fractures of long bones: retrospective and prospective analyses. *J Bone Joint Surg Am* 1976;58(4):453–8.

American College of Surgeons. *"Extremity Trauma" in Advanced Trauma Life Support.* 9th ed. Chicago, 2012:212.

Banerjee M, Bouillion B, Shafizadeh S, et al. Epidemiology of extremity injuries in multiple trauma patients. *Injury* 2012;44(8):1015–21.

American College of Surgeons. National Trauma Data Bank Annual Report. 2015. Available at: https://www.facs.org/~/media/files/quality%20programs/trauma/ntdb/ntdb%20annual%20 report%202015.ashx (last accessed 8/16/16).

Ritcey B, Pageau P, Woo M, Perry J. Regional nerve blocks For hip and femoral neck fractures in the emergency department: a systematic review. *CJEM* 2016;18(1):37–47.

Black K, Bevan C, Murphy N, Howard J. Nerve blocks for initial pain management of femoral fractures in children. *Cochrane Database Syst Rev* 2013;(12):CD009587.

Wheeless C. ed. *Wheeless' Textbook of Orthopedics.* Available at: http://www.wheelessonline.com/ (last accessed 1/14/17).

Chavez LO, Leon M, Einav S, Varon J. Beyond muscle destruction: a systematic review of rhabdomyolysis for clinical practice. *Crit Care* 2016;20(1):135.

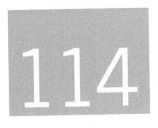

114 Traumatic Emergencies: Face Trauma

Mark D. Levine

GENERAL PRINCIPLES

Definition

- Blunt or penetrating injury to the soft tissues and bony structures of the face
- LeFort I fracture—a transverse fracture through the maxilla above the teeth
- LeFort II fracture—bilateral fractures that extend superiorly to the nasal bridge, maxilla, and orbital floor/rim
- LeFort III fracture—a fracture extending from the bridge of the nose to the floor and medial orbital walls and the zygomatic arch

Epidemiology/Etiology

- Mechanism varies greatly and can be secondary to blunt or penetrating trauma.

Pathophysiology

- In blunt trauma, energy is transmitted to the tissue, causing damage to the superficial and deeper structures.

- In penetrating trauma, there is a laceration or disruption of the tissue, leading to direct damage.

DIAGNOSIS

Clinical Presentation

History
- Unless there is a significant alteration in mentation, the patient will usually be able to describe the injury. Information may also come from bystanders or prehospital providers.
- Specific questions should cover respiratory compromise, visual disturbance, neurologic compromise, dental malocclusion, auditory compromise, and any history pertaining to prior medical/surgical treatment of problems.

Physical Examination
- Examination of the face should look for obvious injury and asymmetry of the facial structures. Cranial nerve function should also be tested.
- A full ocular exam should be performed, making sure that the eye has full range of motion and is not entrapped secondary to an orbital wall fracture. Evaluation for septal hematoma in the nose should not be overlooked. Any possible leakage of CSF from the nose or ears should be evaluated. Battle signs and raccoon eyes are highly suggestive for fracture.
- The midface should be examined for potential fractures. This includes numbness of any part of the face or teeth. Stability of the midface to evaluate for fractures should be evaluated.
- Any vocal change, stridor, or edema of the airway/mouth/larynx/mandible should raise concern for airway compromise and the need for airway control.
- Bruit, thrill, expanding hematoma, or lateralizing neurologic deficits should be noted and emergently evaluated and treated.

Differential Diagnosis
- Intoxication, CVA, metabolic disturbance, or preexisting conditions

Diagnostic Criteria and Testing

Laboratories
- There are no laboratory values that specifically diagnose facial trauma.

Imaging
- A CT scan will be able to evaluate bony and vascular abnormalities.
- Nasal bone films are not necessary unless there is a septal hematoma or there is significant difficulty breathing from each naris.
- A panorex is the most useful imaging modality for midline fractures in the area of the symphysis if CT is not available.

Diagnostic Procedures
- A "halo" test is often used to evaluate the presence of CSF dripping from the ear or nose.

TREATMENT

- Airway compromise from blood or debris should take precedence over further evaluation of trauma to the face.

- Bleeding can usually be controlled by direct pressure or suture placement but may need to be embolized emergently by radiology if it is not locally controlled. Blind clamping should not be performed.

Medications
- Antibiotic prophylaxis is administered on a case-by-case basis based on the type of injury and chance of wound infection, including bites, cartilage exposure, gross contamination, and open fractures.

Other Nonpharmacologic Therapies
- Wound closure should be performed within 24 hours.
- In the case of retro-orbital hematoma with an intraocular pressure (IOP) > 40, a marked difference in globe compressibility, proptosis, or decreased visual acuity, a lateral canthotomy may need to be performed.

SPECIAL CONSIDERATIONS

Disposition
- Patients with simple closed fractures or lacerations without evidence of neurologic complication may be discharged with close follow-up. Any patient with neurologic compromise, CSF leakage, complex facial/orbital wall fractures, or cause visual changes should be evaluated by a surgeon and admitted to the hospital.

Complications
- Disfigurement, disruption of visual or auditory abilities, and infection

Dental Injuries

GENERAL PRINCIPLES

Definition
- Ellis I—injury to the enamel only; pain is not necessarily present
- Ellis II—injury where the dentin is exposed and the tooth is painful and temperature sensitive
- Ellis III—injury where pulp is exposed and the tooth is painful and temperature sensitive
- Luxation injuries—injury where the peridontal ligament or alveolar bone is disrupted

Epidemiology/Etiology
- Similar to facial trauma

Pathophysiology
- Similar to facial trauma

DIAGNOSIS

Clinical Presentation
History
- The patient will report trauma and pain to palpation of the tooth, temperature/sensation sensitivity, and either loose teeth or malocclusion. Time of injury should be noted.

Physical Examination
• Examination of the buccal and lingual surface of the tooth should be evaluated, as well as the stability of the jaw and tooth.

Differential Diagnosis
• Trauma, dental infection, or decay/caries

Diagnostic Criteria and Testing

Imaging
• A panorex radiograph or CT scan of the face will assist in evaluating an alveolar ridge fracture.

TREATMENT

Medications
• Pain control and antibiotic therapy to cover oral flora is recommended such as penicillin or clindamycin.
• Chlorhexidine mouthwash should also be prescribed.

Other Nonpharmacologic Therapies
• Avulsed teeth should be placed in the socket as quickly as possible but may be stored in cold milk, culture medium, "Save-A-Tooth," or "Hank's Balanced Salt Solution" if unable to be reimplanted immediately. If none of these are available, then storage in a container of saliva is recommended. The tooth should not be cleaned or stripped of the ligament. The tooth should then be splinted in place.
• Teeth that are displaced laterally or extruded should be returned to their original position (local anesthesia may be necessary) and splinted in place.
• Intrusion injuries need emergent dental care.
• Ellis type II and III may need local pain control and occlusion of the exposed surface with commercially available dental fracture treatments.

SPECIAL CONSIDERATIONS

Disposition
• Most patients can be discharged home with dental or oral/maxillofacial surgery follow-up.

Complications
• Loss of tooth

SUGGESTED READINGS

Dula DJ, Fales W. The 'ring sign': is it a reliable indicator for cerebral spinal fluid? *Ann Emerg Med* 1993;22:718.
McInnes G, Howes DW. Lateral canthotomy and cantholysis: a simple, vision-saving procedure. *CJEM* 2002;4(1):49–52.

115

Traumatic Emergencies: Genitourinary

Aldo Andino

GENERAL PRINCIPLES

Epidemiology/Etiology

- Genitourinary (GU) tract injury occurs in 10% of cases of abdominal trauma.
- The kidney is the most commonly injured organ in the GU tract.[1,2]
- Ureteral injury is rare (1% of all injuries) and is usually due to iatrogenic injury from surgery.[2]
- Bladder injury is present in 1.6% of blunt trauma victims.[3]
- Urethral injury is divided into anterior and posterior injuries.
  ○ Posterior urethral injuries
    ▪ Located at or above the membranous urethra[4]
    ▪ Almost exclusively occur in association with a pelvic fracture[4]
  ○ Anterior urethral injuries
    ▪ Also known as the penile or bulbar urethra
    ▪ May be due to blunt trauma (e.g., straddle injuries) or penetrating trauma
  ○ Female urethral injuries
    ▪ Almost always associated with a pelvic fracture
- Genital injury (penis, testicle, vulva)
  ○ One-half to two-thirds of penetrating GU injuries involve the external genitalia.[5]
  ○ The most common injuries are penile fracture, testicular rupture, and penetrating penile injuries.

Pathophysiology

- Kidney
  ○ At risk of injury from a deceleration mechanism because it is a fixed structure.
- Ureteral
  ○ Usually iatrogenic, but may be due to penetrating trauma[4]
- Bladder rupture
  ○ Majority are associated with pelvic fractures and can be classified as extraperitoneal or intraperitoneal (may be both)[6]
- Urethral injury
  ○ Posterior is usually due to pelvic fractures.[4]
  ○ Anterior usually due to blunt or penetrating trauma in which the urethra is crushed between the pubic bones and another object (e.g., straddle injury).[4]
- Genital injury
  ○ Penile fracture
    ▪ Rupture of the tunica albuginea due to forceful bending of the erect penis with frequent associated urethral injury.[7]
  ○ Testicular rupture
    ▪ Rupture of the tunica albuginea[8,9]

○ Penile amputation
  ▪ Replantation is usually successful with timely microvascular repair.[10] Immediate urologic consultation is indicated.

DIAGNOSIS

Clinical Presentation

History

• A history of events surrounding the trauma should be obtained including mechanism, history of previous GU injuries, GU surgeries, or issues including anatomic variations.

Physical Examination

• Renal injuries: flank pain, ecchymosis, and rib fractures.
• Ureteral injuries: hematuria and peritonitis.
• Bladder injuries: gross hematuria.[11]
  ○ Urethral injuries: blood at the urethral meatus (classic, but not always present)[16], inability to urinate, perineal/genital edema and ecchymosis, high-riding prostate, and penile angulation
• Pelvic exam: look for labial swelling or blood in the vaginal vault.[4]

Diagnostic Testing

Laboratories

• Urinalysis (UA): gross and microscopic hematuria is considered suggestive of GU organ injury, but not severity.

Imaging

• Chest radiograph: lower rib fractures increase likelihood of renal injury.
• Pelvis radiograph: pelvic fractures can be associated with bladder injury.
• Ultrasound: may help identify penile fracture, testicular rupture, testicular torsion, and bladder rupture.
  ○ A CT scan with IV contrast can identify and stage renal injury as well as identify
  ○ extravasation in the collecting system.

Diagnostic Procedures

• Retrograde urethrogram
  ○ Contrast is injected into the urethra, and a KUB (single view abdominal film) or CT is obtained.
    ▪ Partial urethral disruption: contrast extravasates, but bladder filling is present
    ▪ Complete urethral disruption: contrast extravasates, and bladder filling is absent
• Retrograde cystogram
  ○ After a urethral injury is ruled out, a Foley catheter is advanced and placed in the bladder. Contrast is then injected to fill the bladder completely.
  ○ Obtain imaging with the bladder full (may be a KUB or a CT).
  ○ Drain the bladder completely and obtain postevacuation imaging.
    ▪ Contrast localized to the pelvis suggests extraperitoneal bladder rupture.
    ▪ Contrast outlining the bowel or intra-abdominal structures, suggests intraperitoneal bladder rupture.

TREATMENT

- Renal injury
  - Renal injuries are classified based on severity (Fig. 115.1) and may be managed conservatively if the patient is hemodynamically stable.[12]
  - Bed rest, hemodynamic monitoring, IVF, and pain control are recommended.
  - Higher-grade injuries may require surgery or embolization.
- Ureteral injury
  - Dependent on grade, usually supportive in the emergency department (ED) setting.
  - Urologic consultation should be obtained for nonemergent surgical planning.
- Bladder injury
  - Extraperitoneal bladder rupture is most commonly managed with Foley catheter placement and follow-up.
  - Repair may be indicated in intraperitoneal rupture or in those with injuries to surrounding vital structures.
- Urethral injury
  - Surgical repair may be indicated depending on the injury location and severity.[4]
  - Foley and supportive care may be an option.
- Penile fracture, scrotal rupture, and vaginal injuries typically require operative repair.[13]

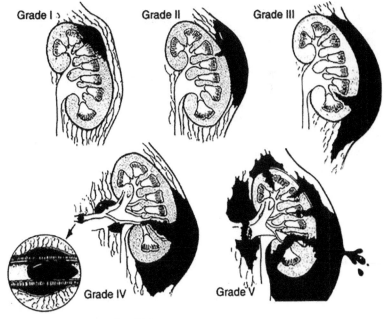

Figure 115.1. Grading of renal injury.

SPECIAL CONSIDERATIONS

Disposition

• Unless hemodynamically unstable and going to the ICU or operating room, nearly all patients should be admitted to the hospital.

Complications

• Renal injury: hypertension may develop in young patients.
• Bladder injuries: fistula formation.
• Urethral injuries: stricture formation, incontinence, and sexual dysfunction.
• Genital injury: infection, testicular atrophy, and sexual dysfunction.

REFERENCES

1. Meng MV, Brandes SB, McAninch JW. Renal trauma: indications and techniques for surgical exploration. *World J Urol* 1999;17:71–7.
2. Al-Awadi K, Kehinde EO, Al-Hunayan A, et al. Iatrogenic ureteric injuries: incidence, aetiological factors and the effect of early management on subsequent outcome. *Int Urol Nephrol* 2005;37:235–41.
3. Gomez RG, Ceballos L, Coburn M, et al. Consensus statement on bladder injuries. *BJU Int* 2004;94:27–32.
4. Morey AF, Brandes S, Dugi DD, et al. Urotrauma: AUA guideline. *J Urol* 2014;192:327–35.
5. Brandes SB, Buckman RF, Chelsky MJ, et al. External genitalia gunshot wounds: a ten-year experience with fifty-six cases. *J Trauma* 1995;39:266–71.
6. Brandes S, Borrelli J. Pelvic fracture and associated urologic injuries. *World J Surg* 2001;25:1578–87.
7. Tsang T, Demby AM. Penile fracture with urethral injury. *J Urol* 1992;147:466–8.
8. Cass AS, Luxenberg M. Testicular injuries. *Urology* 1991;37:528–30.
9. Phonsombat S, Master VA, McAninch JW. Penetrating external genital trauma: a 30-year single institution experience. *J Urol* 2008;180:192–5.
10. Jezior JR, Brady JD, Schlossberg SM. Management of penile amputation injuries. *World J Surg* 2001;25:1602–9.
11. Morey AF, Iverson AJ, Swan A. Bladder rupture after blunt trauma: guidelines for diagnostic imaging. *J Trauma* 2001;51:683–6.
12. Injury Scoring Scale: A Resource for Trauma Care Professionals. 2016. Available at: http://www.aast.org/library/traumatools/injuryscoringscales.aspx#kidney (last accessed 6/26/16).
13. Goldman HB, Idom CB Jr, Dmochowski RR. Traumatic injuries of the female external genitalia and their association with urological injuries. *J Urol* 1998;159(3):956–9.
14. Martinez-Pineiro L, Djakovic N, Plas E, et al. EAU guidelines on urethral trauma. *Eur Urol* 2010;57:791–803.

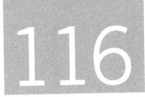

116 Traumatic Emergencies: Head

Daniel S. Greenstein

GENERAL PRINCIPLES

Definition

- Head trauma—blunt or penetrating trauma that causes intracranial or extracranial injury
- Subdural hematoma (SDH)—a layering of blood between the dura and arachnoid mater usually secondary to venous bleeding
- Epidural hematoma (EDH)—a layering of blood between the dura and the skull, usually secondary to arterial hemorrhage
- Traumatic subarachnoid hemorrhage (SAH)—bleeding in the subarachnoid space usually secondary to arterial bleeding between the arachnoid membrane and pia mater
- Intraparenchymal hemorrhage (IPH)—bleeding within the brain parenchyma
- Diffuse axonal injury (DAI)—widespread neuronal death from rotational, acceleration, or deceleration injury
- Traumatic brain injury (TBI)—brain dysfunction caused by an external force

Epidemiology/Etiology

- The most common causes of TBI are motor vehicle crashes, falls, workplace- and sports-related injuries, firearms, and assault.[1]
- SDH is the most common intracranial hemorrhages and is at risk for increased intracranial pressure (ICP), midline shift, cerebral vasoconstriction, cerebral ischemia, and seizures.
- An EDH is due to disruption of the middle meningeal artery and can rapidly expand.
- Traumatic SAH—secondary injury is common including hydrocephalus, increased ICP, cerebral vasospasm, and decreased cerebral perfusion.
- IPH—hematomas are likely to increase in size and can lead to increased ICP, midline shift, and eventual herniation.
- DAI are very susceptible to secondary injury from hypoxia and hypotension.[2]

Pathophysiology

- Primary brain injury occurs at the time of the initial insult and consists of the immediate and irreversible damage from direct impact, acceleration/deceleration, or penetrating trauma.
- Secondary injury occurs in the subsequent hours and days and can be caused by inflammation, electrolyte imbalances, hypoxia, and ischemia.

DIAGNOSIS

Clinical Presentation

History
- The patient will usually complain of a head injury. In the event of a severe injury that leads to altered mental status, corroborative information should be obtained.

Physical Examination
- A full physical examination (for trauma to the head and neck) should be performed with special attention paid to the mental status and neurologic exams.

Eye Opening	
Spontaneous	4
To speech	3
To pain	2
None	1
Verbal Response	
Oriented	5
Confused	4
Inappropriate words	3
Moans	2
None	1
Motor Response	
Follows commands	6
Localizes pain	5
Withdrawals	4
Decorticate (Flexion)	3
Decerebrate (Extension)	2
None	1

Figure 116.1. Glasgow Coma Scale.

Differential Diagnosis

- Intoxication, shock, hypoxia, stroke, metabolic derangement/hypoglycemia, central versus peripheral neuropathy, or psychogenic

Diagnostic Criteria and Testing

- TBI can be categorized by severity using the Glasgow coma scale (GCS) (Fig. 116.1).
  - ○ Mild—GCS score of 13–15
  - ○ Moderate—GCS score of 9–12
  - ○ Severe—GCS score of 8 or less
- Prognosis based on GCS alone can be misleading, as many factors can confound the score.

Laboratories
- There is no specific laboratory test to diagnose traumatic head injury.

Imaging
- Noncontrast head CT should be obtained for all patients with moderate to severe TBI. For mild TBI, the Canadian Head CT Rules or New Orleans Head CT Rules (Fig. 116.2 and Table 116.1) can be used to help guide decision-making for imaging.[3,4]

TREATMENT

- Patients who are not protecting their airway or are hypoxic should be intubated.

Medications

- Ketamine does not cause elevation of ICP and therefore is preferred for RSI.[5,6]
- IV fluids and vasopressors should be administered to keep the systolic BP above 90 mm Hg initially.[2]

High Risk (for Neurologic Intervention)
1. GCS score < 15 at 2 h after injury 2. Suspected open or depressed skull fracture 3. Any sign of basal skull fracture* 4. Vomiting ≥ two episodes 5. Age ≥ 65

Medium Risk (for Brain Injury on CT)
6. Amnesia before impact ≥ 30 min 7. Dangerous mechanism** (*pedestrian, occupant ejected, fall from elevation*)

*Signs of Basal Skull Fracture - hemotympanum, "raccoon" eyes, CSF otorrhea/rhinorrhea, Battle sign ****Dangerous Mechanism** - pedestrian struck by vehicle - occupant ejected from motor vehicle - fall from elevation ≥ 3 ft or five stairs	**Rule Not Applicable If:** - Nontrauma cases - GCS < 13 - Age < 16 - Coumadin or bleeding disorder - Obvious open skull fracture

Figure 116.2. Canadian Head CT rule.

- Adequate sedation and analgesia are critical, as agitation and pain can increase ICP.
- For signs of impending herniation (coma, pupillary dilation, miosis, lateral gaze palsy, hemiparesis, decerebrate posturing, or triad of hypertension/bradycardia/abnormal breathing), mannitol should be given as an IV bolus of 0.5–1 g/kg and can be repeated every 2–8 hours.[2]
- Phenytoin and levetiracetam have similar efficacy in decreasing the incidence of seizures in the first week postinjury.[7]

Other Nonpharmacologic Therapies

- The head of the bed should be elevated to 30 degrees.
- Mild hyperventilation can be used as a temporizing measure for acute herniation.[8]

TABLE 116.1	New Orleans Head CT Rule

Consider head CT if any of the follow is present in a patient with GCS 15 and blunt head trauma:

- Visible trauma above the clavicles
- Seizure
- Headache
- Vomiting
- Short-term memory loss
- Age > 60 years
- Drug or alcohol ingestion[4]

SPECIAL CONSIDERATIONS

Disposition

• Patients with signs of intracranial injury should be admitted to the hospital for a period of observation, and those with an intracranial hemorrhage may require admission to an intensive care unit.

Complications

• Seizure, respiratory compromise, neurologic disability, death

REFERENCES

1. Coronado VG, Xu L, Basavaraju SV, et al. Surveillance for traumatic brain injury-related deaths—United States, 1997–2007. *MMWR Surveill Summ* 2011;60(5):1–32.
2. Zammit C, Knight WA. Severe traumatic brain injury in adults. *Emerg Med Pract* 2013;15(3):1–28.
3. Stiell IG, Wells GA, Vandemheen K, et al. The Canadian CT head rule for patients with minor head injury. *Lancet* 2001;357(9266):1391–6.
4. Haydel MJ, Preston CA, Mills TJ, et al. Indications for computed tomography in patients with minor head injury. *N Engl J Med* 2000;343(2):100–5.
5. Bourgoin A, Albanèse J, Wereszczynski N, et al. Safety of sedation with ketamine in severe head injury patients: comparison with sufentanil. *Crit Care Med* 2003;31(3):711–7.
6. Schmittner MD, Vajkoczy SL, Horn P, et al. Effects of fentanyl and S(+)-ketamine on cerebral hemodynamics, gastrointestinal motility, and need of vasopressors in patients with intracranial pathologies: a pilot study. *J Neurosurg Anesthesiol* 2007;19(4):257–62.
7. Chesnut RM, Marshall LF, Klauber MR, et al. The role of secondary brain injury in determining outcome from severe head injury. *J Trauma* 1993;34(2):216–22.
8. Muizelaar JP, Marmarou A, Ward JD, et al. Adverse effects of prolonged hyperventilation in patients with severe head injury: a randomized clinical trial. *J Neurosurg* 1991;75(5):731–9.

117

Traumatic Emergencies: Neck

Al Lulla

GENERAL PRINCIPLES

Definition

• Penetrating neck trauma that violates the platysma.

Classification

• Zone 1: extends from the clavicles to the level of the cricoid cartilage
• Zone 2: extends from inferior margin of cricoid cartilage to the angle of the mandible
• Zone 3: extends between the angle of the mandible and the base of the skull[1,2]

Epidemiology/Etiology

- The common causes of penetrating neck trauma include firearm injury (45%), stab wounds (40%), and shotgun injuries (4%).[1]

Pathophysiology

- Injuries to the carotid may result from an expanding hematoma that may cause airway compromise.[2] Wounds which affect an artery may result in formation of a pseudoaneurysm and cause intimal injury, dissection, or formation of an arteriovenous fistula. Lacerations of the jugular vein may result in formation of air emboli.

DIAGNOSIS

Clinical Presentation

History

- The mechanism of injury and weapon(s) used should be obtained.
- The patient may report neurologic findings or presence of "whooshing" sound in the ears (referred to as pulsatile tinnitus [associated with carotid artery dissection]).
- Patients should also be asked about dysphagia or odynophagia.

Physical Examination

- Patients may present with "hard signs" (airway compromise, massive subcutaneous emphysema, air bubbling through penetrating wound, expanding or pulsatile hematoma, active bleeding, shock, neurologic deficit, hematemesis)[3,4] suggesting potential life-threatening injury.
- Radial or brachial pulse deficits may be an indicator of subclavian artery injury.
- Assess for the following: voice changes or hoarseness, dysphagia, or hemoptysis.[3,4]
- Vascular structures can be auscultated and palpated for presence of bruits or a thrill.
- The wound should be examined to assess for violation of the platysma.[2]
- A neurologic examination should be performed to assess for carotid artery injury, injury to spinal cord, or the brachial plexus.[2]

Differential Diagnosis

- Mass, spontaneous hemorrhage, pneumothorax, or hemoptysis

Diagnostic Criteria and Testing

Laboratories

- There are no specific laboratory tests that are diagnostic of traumatic neck injury.[2]

Imaging

- A plain chest radiograph is also indicated to evaluate for pneumothorax, hemothorax, mediastinal widening, and foreign body location. Zone 1 injuries are at particular high risk for thoracic injuries.[2]
- CT angiography should be used for the evaluation of penetrating neck trauma.[5]

TREATMENT

Other Nonpharmacologic Therapies

- Patients who have signs of significant airway swelling or expanding hematoma should have their airway emergently secured.

- Patients who are actively bleeding from a neck wound should have pressure applied to the site of injury until hemostasis is achieved or the wound is surgically repaired.

SPECIAL CONSIDERATIONS

Disposition

- Patients without violation of the platysma can undergo local wound repair and be discharged home.
- Patients who have hard signs of injury or violation of the platysma require surgical exploration and admission.

Complications

- Hemorrhage, death, or neurologic compromise

REFERENCES

1. Brywczynski JJ, Barrett TW, Lyon JA, Cotton BA. Management of penetrating neck injury in the emergency department: a structured literature review. *Emerg Med J* 2008;25: 711–5.
2. Schaider J, Bailitz J. Neck trauma: don't put your neck on the line. *Emerg Med Pract* 2003;5:1–28.
3. Sperry JL, Moore EE, Coimbra R, et al. Western Trauma Association critical decisions in trauma: penetrating neck trauma. *J Trauma Acute Care Surg* 2013;75:936–40.
4. Tisherman SA, Bokhari F, Collier B, et al. Clinical practice guideline: penetrating zone II neck trauma. *J Trauma* 2008;64:1392–405.
5. Rathlev NK, Medzon R, Bracken ME. Evaluation and management of neck trauma. *Emerg Med Clin North Am* 2007;25:679–94.

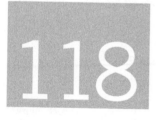

118 Traumatic Emergencies: Eye

Sahar Morkos El Hayek and Jason Wagner

GENERAL PRINCIPLES

Definitions

- Closed globe injuries describe traumatic injuries that preserve the integrity of the globe without penetration or perforation.
- Open globe injuries occur when globe integrity is violated.
- Ruptured globe injuries result from trauma that lead to prolapse and extrusion of intraocular contents.
- Blow-out fractures occur following direct trauma to the face, usually affecting the medial orbital wall and orbital floor.

Epidemiology
- The most common presentation is injury from foreign bodies, followed by falls and assaults.
- Risk factors that predispose to eye injury and worse outcome include:
  - Jobs involving tools and machinery, recreational sports, motor vehicle accidents, guns, and fireworks
  - Extremes of age, male gender, and low socioeconomic status
  - Previous eye surgeries, poor visual acuity prior to the accident, and history of wearing contact lenses

DIAGNOSIS
Clinical Presentation
History
- It is important to identify the mechanism of injury, the nature of the foreign object, if any, and any manipulation prior to arrival to the ED.
- A history of eye surgeries, visual acuity at baseline, and current or previous contact lens use should be documented.
- The patient may describe various symptoms including changes in vision, eye pain upon movement, foreign body sensation, double vision, floaters, or bleeding.

Physical Examination
- A complete ophthalmologic exam should be performed.
  - Strabismus or double vision indicates muscle entrapment.
- Examination may be difficult in the presence of periorbital swelling. Full eye exposure should be obtained nonetheless.

Differential Diagnosis
- The differential diagnosis includes open globe injuries, retrobulbar hematomas, traumatic hyphema, retinal detachment (RD), vitreous hemorrhage (VH), or ocular burns.

Diagnostic Testing
Laboratories
- Complete blood count (CBC) and coagulation studies are useful to rule out bleeding disorders in patients with hyphema.

Imaging
- CT scans of the orbit are indicated in cases where orbital hematomas, fractures, or globe rupture are suspected.
- Orbital ultrasound has high sensitivity and specificity in detecting orbital foreign bodies, lens dislocation, VH, RD, retrobulbar hematoma, papilledema, and globe rupture.

Diagnostic Procedures
- Intraocular pressure (IOP) should be measured in any patient following eye trauma, except in cases where an open globe is suspected. Normal eye pressures range between 10 and 20 mm Hg.
- Fundoscopy and a slit-lamp exam should be performed.

Eyelid Lacerations

GENERAL PRINCIPLES

Clinical Presentation

- Patients present with abrasions or lacerations, bleeding, and eyelid swelling. If the laceration is deep or transects the eyelid muscles, patients may present with the inability to open the eye.

Physical Examination

- Note should be taken of depth, location, proximity to the canalicular system, involvement of the tarsal muscles, and injury to the globe itself. Ptosis on exam indicates damage to the levator palpebrae and tarsal plates. Evaluation for foreign bodies should be performed.

TREATMENT

- All eyelid lacerations warrant an ophthalmology consult.

SPECIAL CONSIDERATIONS

- Patients can be discharged home with appropriate adequate follow-up with ophthalmology.

Corneal Abrasions

- See Eye Disorder chapter

Chemical Ocular Burns

GENERAL PRINCIPLES

- Exposure to acid or alkali solutions damages the surface epithelium of the eye. Acidic agents cause coagulative necrosis and eschar formation, while alkali agents cause liquefactive necrosis and damage deeper tissue.

Clinical Presentation

- Patients complain of severe pain and irritation and frequently present with inability to open eyes.

Physical Examination

- This is an emergent situation where treatment should precede physical exam.
- On exam, the cornea and superficial epithelium may exhibit burns ranging from abrasions to complete corneal opacification and perilimbal ischemia.

TREATMENT

- Immediate irrigation of the eye with normal saline, lactated Ringer's, or sterile water should be initiated prior to arrival to the ED if possible. At least 2 L of irrigating solution should be delivered either through a Morgan lens.
- Topical anesthetics are used for pain control during irrigation.
- The pH of the affected eye should be measured with pH paper within 10 minutes, and irrigation continued until pH is back to normal (7.4).

- Tetanus update is warranted.
- Artificial tears, oral or topical ascorbate, and topical steroids may also be prescribed.

SPECIAL CONSIDERATIONS

- Immediate ophthalmologic consultation is required for any chemical burn to the eye.
- High-grade chemical burns may progress to permanent vision loss, corneal scarring, cataract, and glaucoma.
- Re-epithelialization takes weeks.

Subconjunctival Hemorrhage

- See Eye Disorder chapter

Traumatic Iritis

GENERAL PRINCIPLES

- Traumatic iritis, a form of anterior uveitis, is the inflammation of the iris 2–3 days following blunt trauma due to irritation caused by dead cells.

Presentation

- Patients complain of pain, photophobia, and visual changes.

Physical Examination
- On gross inspection, patients will have perilimbic injection.
- Slit-lamp exam: cell and flare in the anterior chamber, with keratic precipitates accumulating on the cornea.
- More severe trauma can avulse the iris from the ciliary body, leading to pupillary irregularities known as iridodialysis.

TREATMENT

- Topical cycloplegics and close ophthalmology follow-up are recommended. Complete resolution of symptoms and findings is expected.

Lens Dislocation and Cataracts

GENERAL PRINCIPLES

- Cataracts occur with blunt trauma to the lens that leads to changes in the lens consistency and shape. The lens may also be dislocated from the zonular filaments into the anterior or posterior chambers.

Clinical Presentation

- Pain and visual changes are the major complaints when the lens is injured.

Physical Examination
- Cataracts appear as opacified lenses.
- A slit-lamp exam will show a dislocated lens lodged in the anterior chamber, free floating in the vitreous, or overlying the retina.

TREATMENT

- An ophthalmology consultation for surgical repair is indicated. The eye may be shielded in the meantime for protection.

Traumatic Hyphema

GENERAL PRINCIPLES

- Blunt trauma can shear the ciliary bodies, which causes pooling of blood in the anterior chamber. It can also occur spontaneously in patients with blood dyscrasias.

Clinical Presentation

- Patients present with ocular pain and various degrees of vision loss depending on the amount of blood in the anterior chamber obscuring the visual access.

Physical Examination
- Blood can be visualized as red shadowing with a penlight.
- Slit-lamp exam: blood pooling in the anterior chamber.
- IOP is normal to high on presentation and increases gradually if bleeding persists.

TREATMENT

- Head of bed elevation to 30–45 degrees, allowing blood cells to settle away from the visual axis.
- Topical miotics and cycloplegics are generally used but have not been shown to affect prognosis.
- Evaluation by an ophthalmologist is mandatory for hospital admission and adequate follow-up.

SPECIAL CONSIDERATIONS

- Delayed complications of traumatic hyphema are rebleeding 3–5 days after presentation, glaucoma, and corneal blood staining.
- Daily follow-up with an ophthalmologist should be set for the 5 days after injury.

Retinal Detachment (RD), Vitreous Hemorrhage (VH)

- See Eye Disorder chapter

Retrobulbar Hematoma

GENERAL PRINCIPLES

- Trauma to the face may result in retrobulbar hemorrhge that can lead to hematoma formation. This is a vision-threatening emergency because the hematoma can impinge on the blood supply to the retina and optic nerve, resulting in permanent vision loss as early as 90 minutes after complete ischemia.

- Retrobulbar hemorrhage is a clinical diagnosis but can also be seen on CT scan of the orbits or ocular ultrasound as a retro-orbital hypoechoic area with flattening of the posterior globe. However, imaging should not delay definitive treatment.

Clinical Presentation

- Patients usually complain of pain in the affected eye and progressive loss of vision. They may also present with proptosis and inability to move the globe as the hematoma enlarges.

Physical Examination

- Decreasing visual acuity in awake and cooperative patients raises concern for retrobulbar hematoma. Proptosis will be evident as the bleed expands. The affected eye will have an afferent pupillary defect.

TREATMENT

- Emergent lateral canthotomy and cantholysis should be performed in the ED to relieve the pressure caused by the hematoma (Fig. 118.1).

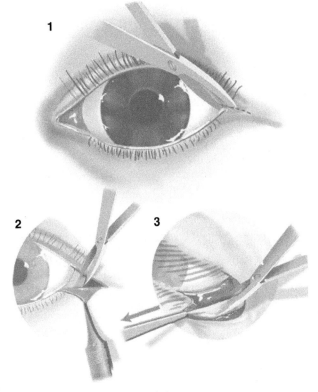

Figure 118.1. Lateral canthotomy and cantholysis.

- The lateral canthus is anesthetized and the lateral canthus skin is clamped for 1–2 minutes. The lateral canthus skin is incised, followed by inferior cantholysis (incision of the inferior crux).
- If proptosis persists after the procedure, attempt a superior cantholysis and if that does not relieve the pressure, the hematoma may be drained under ultrasound guidance for decompression of the retrobulbar space.

SPECIAL CONSIDERATIONS

- Proptosis in a trauma patient can be caused by retrobulbar hematoma, orbital fracture, or retrobulbar swelling. Distinction should be made since lateral canthotomy will be effective only in cases of retrobulbar hemorrhage.

Globe Rupture

GENERAL PRINCIPLES

- Forceful blunt or penetrating trauma can violate the globe integrity, leading to prolapse and possible extrusion of globe contents. It is a vision-threatening injury that should be recognized at presentation to prevent further ocular damage.
- Globe rupture can be diagnosed on physical exam, but CT of the orbit should be obtained to detect the severity of the injury, foreign body, or any associated orbital fractures. Suspected globe rupture is a relative contraindication to orbital ultrasound.

Clinical Presentation

- Patients present with painful loss of vision.

Physical Examination

- Visual acuity is usually reduced to light perception or hand motion. 360-degree subconjunctival hemorrhage, chemosis, and pupillary disruption usually in teardrop shape indicating complete avulsion may all be present.
- Seidel test: A large amount of fluorescein dye is instilled in the eye. The presence of a dark stream interrupting the dye indicates globe rupture.
- Slit-lamp exam findings: hyphema, anterior chamber distortion with lens dislocation, and extrusion of intraocular content.

TREATMENT

- Eye shield application is a vision-sparing procedure, as it prevents any added pressure on the globe that risks further extrusion of globe content.
- The patient should receive a tetanus update, antiemetics, and adequate pain control. Antibiotic prophylaxis with ceftazidime or vancomycin should be started in the ED to prevent posttraumatic endophthalmitis.
- If a foreign body has impaled the globe, it should not be removed but should be splinted in place with the other eye patched (to prevent movement with contralateral eye motion).
- An open globe warrants immediate ophthalmology consultation for surgical planning.

SPECIAL CONSIDERATIONS

- Open globe injuries are at high risk of permanent vision loss and posttraumatic endophthalmitis.

Orbital Fractures

GENERAL PRINCIPLES

- Orbital fractures result from blunt trauma to the eye, face, or head. They frequently occur at the inferior and medial walls of the orbit.
- CT scan of the orbit is the gold standard imaging technique to identify bony deformities, muscle entrapment, and hematomas.

Clinical Presentation

- Pain and periorbital swelling are the most common symptoms.
- Enophthalmos occurs if the globe sinks into the expanded space.
- Patients have diplopia on upward gaze occurs if the inferior rectus muscle is entrapped within the inferior wall fracture, causing the "white eye" finding.
- Patients may complain of infraorbital anesthesia if the fracture damages the infraorbital nerve.

Physical Examination

- Periocular swelling, ecchymosis, chemosis, subconjunctival hemorrhage, proptosis in the early posttraumatic period, and enophthalmos may be present. Globe injury should be ruled out.

TREATMENT

- Delayed surgical fracture repair is the mainstay of treatment unless there is persistent diplopia, enophthalmos of 3 mm or more, or involvement of more than 50% of the orbital floor.

SUGGESTED READINGS

Boyette JR, Pemberton JD, Bonilla-Velez J. Management of orbital fractures, challenges and solutions. *Clin Opthalmol* 2015;9:2127–37.

Barouch FC, Colby KA. Evaluation and Initial Management of Patients with Ocular and Adnexal Trauma. In: Barouch FC, Colb KA, eds. *Albert & Jakobiec's Principles & Practice of Ophthalmology.* 3rd ed. 1994 by W.B Saunders Company©, Elsevier Inc., 2008:5071–92.

Haring RS, Canner JK, Haider AH, Schneider EB. Ocular injury in the United States: emergency department visits from 2006–2011. *Injury* 2016;47:104–8.

Horowitz R, Bailits J. Ocular ultrasound-point of care imaging of the eye. *Clin Pediat Emerg Med* 2015;16(4):262–8.

Kilker BA, Holst JM, Hoffmann B. Bedside ocular ultrasound in the emergency department. *Eur J Emerg Med* 2014;21(4):246–53.

Messman AM. Ocular injuries: new strategies in emergency department management. *Emerg Med Pract* 2015;17(11):1–21. Available at: www.Ebmedicine.net.

Ocular Trauma. In: American College of Surgeons. *Advanced Trauma Life Support Student Course Manual.* 9th ed. Chicago: American College of Surgeons©, 2012:311–5.

Pargament JM, Armenia J, Nerad JA. Physical and chemical injuries to the eyes and eyelids. *Clin Dermatol* 2015;33:234–7.

Singh P, Tyagi M, Kumar Y, et al. Ocular chemical injuries and their management. *Oman J Ophthalmol* 2013;6:83–6.

Traumatic Emergencies: Spine

Emily Harkins

GENERAL PRINCIPLES

Classification

- Primary injury is irreversible damage to the nerve and is due to direct insult: compression, contusions, and shear injuries to the cord.
- Secondary injury is potentially preventable and/or reversible damage to the nearby tissue that is thought to be caused by decreased perfusion and inflammatory response.
- Complete cord injury: no sensation in levels below the injury, including S4–S5, and complete paralysis in distal myotomes.
- Incomplete cord injury includes central cord syndrome, anterior cord syndrome, and Brown-Sequard syndrome.

Epidemiology/Etiology

- The majority of new spinal cases annually result in incomplete tetraplegia.
  - Bimodal distribution with younger individuals affected by major trauma and older individuals affected by minor trauma.
  - Males are affected four times as often as females.
- Fifty percent of spinal cord injuries occur in the cervical spine due to motor vehicle accidents.

DIAGNOSIS

Clinical Presentation

History
- The awake patient will likely complain of pain at the site of an overlying spinal fracture. Patients with head or distracting injuries may not be able to report or localize spinal pain.

Physical Examination
- Provide in-line stabilization to prevent further damage to the spinal cord. If the patient needs to be rolled, use the log-roll technique and be sure that the patient has a cervical collar in place. Leaving the patient on the backboard is no longer recommended and may be harmful.
- Determine bilateral sensory levels and bilateral motor levels.
  - The neurologic level of injury is the most caudal segment of cord with intact sensation and motor function capable of resisting gravity.
  - Evaluate for sacral sparing and anal wink to determine if injury is complete or incomplete.
- Evaluate cranial nerve function and mental status.
- Patients in spinal shock will have an absent bulbocavernosus reflex.

- Assess for bladder distention.
- Assess deep tendon reflexes and examine for priapism.

Diagnostic Criteria

Laboratories
- There are no specific laboratory values that diagnose a spinal cord injury.

Imaging
- Use Canadian C-spine rules or NEXUS criteria (Fig. 119.1) to determine which patients do not require C-spine imaging; otherwise,
- A complete set of C-spine plain films should be obtained.
  - All cervical vertebrae must be visualized, as well as the top of T1 to be considered adequate.
- If the injury is to the thoracic or lumbar spine, obtain AP, lateral, and oblique films.
- A CT scan of the cervical spine with coronal and sagittal reconstructions may be undertaken in lieu of plain films.
- Patients may require an MRI, which provides better visualization of the spinal cord.

For Alert and Stable Trauma Patients

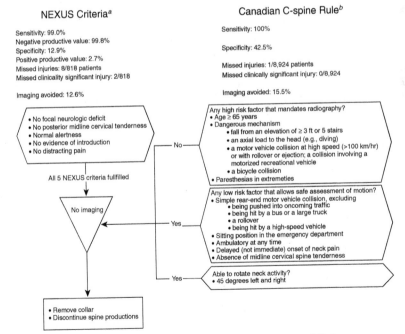

NEXUS Criteria[a]

Sensitivity: 99.0%
Negative productive value: 99.8%
Specificity: 12.9%
Positive productive value: 2.7%
Missed injuries: 8/818 patients
Missed clinicality significant injury: 2/818

Imaging avoided: 12.6%

- No focal neurologic deficit
- No posterior midline cervical tenderness
- Normal alertness
- No evidence of introduction
- No distracting pain

All 5 NEXUS criteria fullfilled

No imaging

Canadian C-spine Rule[b]

Sensitivity: 100%

Specificity: 42.5%

Missed injuries: 1/8,924 patients
Missed clinically significant injury: 0/8,924

Imaging avoided: 15.5%

Any high risk factor that mandates radiography?
- Age ≥ 65 years
- Dangerous mechanism
  - fall from an elevation of ≥ 3 ft or 5 stairs
  - an axial load to the head (e.g., diving)
  - a motor vehicle collision at high speed (>100 km/hr) or with rollover or ejection; a collision involving a motorized recreational vehicle
  - a bicycle collision
- Paresthesias in extremeties

Any low risk factor that allows safe assessment of motion?
- Simple rear-end motor vehicle collision, excluding
  - being pushed into oncoming traffic
  - being hit by a bus or a large truck
  - a rollover
  - being hit by a high-speed vehicle
- Sitting position in the emergency department
- Ambulatory at any time
- Delayed (not immediate) onset of neck pain
- Absence of midline cervical spine tenderness

Able to rotate neck activity?
- 45 degrees left and right

- Remove collar
- Discontinue spine productions

[a]Hoffman JR et al. Validity of a set of clinical criteria to rule cut injury to the cervical spine in patients with blunt trauma. National Emergency X-Radiography Utilization Study Group. *N Engl J Med* 2000;343.

[b]Stiet G et al. The Canadian C-spine rule for radiography in alert and stable trauma patients. *JAMA* 2001;286:1841.

Figure 119.1. C-spine clearance rules. (From Court-Brown CM, Heckman JD, McQueen MM, et al. *Rockwood and Green's Fractures in Adults, 8th ed.* Philadelphia, PA: Wolters Kluwer, 2015.)

TREATMENT

- Maintain manual in-line stabilization if intubation is necessary.
- Vasopressors and/or cardiac pacing may be needed to treat neurogenic shock.

Medications

- Current guidelines recommend maintaining a mean arterial pressure ≥85 mm.
  - Excessive fluid can contribute to spinal cord edema and worse outcomes.
- Glucocorticoids are not recommended in treatment of acute spinal cord injury.

SPECIAL CONSIDERATIONS

Disposition

- Any patient with unstable cervical spine injury will require ICU level monitoring.
- Neurosurgical intervention may be required, depending on the injury and spinal stability.

SUGGESTED READINGS

Antevil JL, Sise MJ, Sack DI, et al. Spiral computed tomography for the initial evaluation of spine trauma: a new standard of care? *J Trauma* 2006;61(2):382–7.

Daffner R, Sciulli R, Rodriguez A, Protetch J. Imaging for evaluation of suspected cervical spine trauma: a 2-year analysis. *Injury* 2006;37(7):652–8.

Jia X, Kowalski RG, Sciubba DM, Geocadin RG. Critical care of traumatic spinal cord injury. *J Intensive Care Med* 2013;28(1):12–23.

Kirshblum SC, Burns SP, Biering-Sorensen F, et al. International standards for neurological classification of spinal cord injury (revised 2011). *J Spinal Cord Med* 2011;34(6):535–46.

Moore D. Spinal cord injuries. Available at: http://www.orthobullets.com/spine/2006/spinal-cord-injuries (last accessed December 2016).

Pimentel L, Diegelmann L. Evaluation and management of acute cervical spine trauma. *Emerg Med Clin North Am* 2010;28(4):719–38.

Sekhon LH, Fehlings MG. Epidemiology, demographics, and pathophysiology of acute spinal cord injury. *Spine* 2001;26(24S):S2–12.

Stiell IG, Wells GA, Vandemheen KL, et al. The Canadian C-spine rule for radiography in alert and stable trauma patients. *JAMA* 2001;286(15):1841–8.

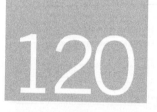

120 Airway Management

Bob Cambridge, Stephanie Charshafian, and Michael Willman

Oxygen Supplementation

INDICATIONS

Patients with hypoxia or a severe traumatic/medical condition will benefit from supplemental oxygen. It is generally indicated when hypoxia is present, with a $PaO_2 <$ 60 mm Hg, or with a pulse ox <90–92%. High-flow oxygen is indicated in carbon

TABLE 120.1	Common Oxygen Delivery Devices in the ED	
Device	Oxygen flow (L/min)	FiO$_2$ range
Nasal cannula	1–6	24–40%
High-flow NC	2–15	24–90%
Face mask	5–10	40–60%
Nonrebreather	6–15	60–90%
Venturi mask	15	24–100%[a]

[a]Venturi mask may differ by manufacturer, titrated using adjustable mixer valve at the base.

monoxide and cyanide poisoning (regardless of pulse ox reading). Some patients will need supplementation at high altitudes, especially if they have underlying lung disease.

CONTRAINDICATIONS

Use carefully with patients who have chronic obstructive pulmonary disease (COPD)/chronic lung disease. As the disease progresses, the respiratory drive changes from being controlled by CO_2 levels to being regulated by oxygen levels. Prolonged use of excessive supplemental oxygen (normally >24 hours) can result in an excess buildup of carbon dioxide leading to mental status changes and deterioration. This should not be a consideration in the acutely ill patient as normalizing oxygen levels can aid in stabilizing the underlying process.

LIMITATIONS

Do not use high levels of oxygen unnecessarily; dangers include cytotoxic injury and chronic effects of hyperoxygenation (Table 120.1).

AIRWAY ADJUNCTS

Nasopharyngeal Airway (NPA)

INDICATIONS

The NPA is used in situations where an artificial airway is indicated, but it is not possible to use an oropharyngeal airway (OPA) or other more invasive device. It can be used when a patient is conscious or when he or she has an intact gag reflex. It can help keep the tongue from relaxing too far against the back of the throat and causing obstruction.

CONTRAINDICATIONS

Avoid using the NPA in patients who have severe facial or head injuries or basilar skull fracture as this increases the risk of worsening facial fractures, bleeding, and injury to the cribriform plate.

METHODS

Measure the distance from the patient's nostril to tip of the earlobe and choose an NPA of the same length. The external circumference should be the same size as the nostril. Lubricate the device with a water-based lubricant. Insert the device with the bevel against the septum and parallel to the roof of the mouth, until the flared end comes in contact with the nostril.

Oropharyngeal Airway

INDICATIONS

The OPA is used to keep the tongue and oral airway structures from blocking the airway, or for an unresponsive patient with an absent gag reflex.

CONTRAINDICATIONS

Do not use with a patient who is awake, has an active gag reflex, or actively gags or vomits when the OPA is inserted.

METHODS

Measure the distance from the corner of the patient's mouth to the angle of the jaw and select a device that is the same length. Either the device can be placed upside down until it reaches the back of the oropharynx and then rotated 180 degrees, or the tongue can be depressed and the airway inserted until the flange rests against the teeth.

LIMITATIONS

This is not a definitive airway. The OPA can cause obstruction if not the proper size. In addition, it can cause aspiration or bleeding.

Bag Valve Mask (BVM) Ventilation

The BVM is an effective method of ventilation, but it requires practice and skill to do effectively. In order to get adequate tidal volume, the mask must have a tight seal against the face and frequently is used in conjunction with an NPA or OPA to maintain the airway.

INDICATIONS

To assist ventilations or to completely ventilate a patient.

CONTRAINDICATIONS

There are no absolute contraindications. Use caution with facial fractures. As this is not a definitive airway, this maneuver should be used as a bridge to obtaining definitive airway. Caution should also be used in patients with a full stomach or unknown last meal as air can be insufflated into the stomach and can cause vomiting and aspiration.

METHODS

There are clinical features that predict difficult ventilation using a BVM (Figure 129.1). Connect the BVM to an oxygen source. The mask should be sized to cover the nose and mouth but not extend beyond the chin or over the eyes. Place the patient in the sniffing position. If cervical spine precautions are in place, do not flex or extend the neck. If no cervical spine precautions are needed, the head can be positioned with gentle downward pressure on the forehead and upward pressure on the chin ("head tilt–chin lift"). Provide a jaw thrust by putting a finger behind the angle of the mandible on both sides and gently pulling forward. Place the mask over the nose and mouth. Maintain a tight seal with an "EC" hand grip, thumb and 2nd finger encircling the mask and 3rd, 4th, and 5th fingers along the mandible pulling the jaw up against the mask.

Once a seal is made, squeeze the bag every 4–6 seconds and keep it depressed for 1–2 seconds. The amount of squeeze on the bag should be regulated to an adequate chest rise.

This method is best performed with two people, one maintaining a seal on the mask and the other providing bag ventilations.

LIMITATIONS

BVM use can result in aspiration, gastric distention, emesis, inadequate oxygen delivery, or inadequate tidal volumes.

Supraglottic Airways

- Examples of supraglottic airways include the King, i-gel, and laryngeal mask airway (LMA).

INDICATIONS

Supraglottic airways are used when BVM is inadequate and endotracheal intubation would be problematic.

CONTRAINDICATIONS

Excessive secretions and active oropharyngeal bleeding are relative contraindications.

METHODS

Follow manufacturer's directions.

LIMITATIONS

Incorrect insertion angle causing inadequate seal with insufficient ventilation

Endotracheal Intubation

There are many methods for passing an endotracheal tube (ETT) through the vocal cords and into the trachea. They include direct or indirect laryngoscopy. There are also devices such as lighted stylet intubation, intubating LMAs, or other adjunctive devices. This section will focus on the standard procedure for direct laryngoscopy.

INDICATIONS

Endotracheal intubation is for patients who need definitive airway protection.

CONTRAINDICATIONS

If a less invasive method of respiratory support can be used, then intubation may not be indicated.

METHODS

There are clinical features that predict difficult intubation (Figure 129.1).
- Select the blade size:
  - The Macintosh blade is curved and inserted into the vallecula to apply pressure to the hyoepiglottic ligament and move the epiglottis out of the way in order to view the vocal cords.
  - The Miller blade is straight and mechanically lifts the epiglottis out of the way of the vocal cords.
- Blade sizes in adults are size three or four.
  - Three is a standard adult size.
  - Four is for large adults or those with long necks.
- Check that the blade and handle lock together securely and that the light is on and at full illumination. Assemble the other equipment:
- Ensure suction is on and working.
- The bag valve device should be connected to high-flow oxygen.
- Capnography should be ready for placement confirmation.
- Backup devices are ready at hand in case you encounter difficulties in placing the tube.
- A stylet can be used to give the ETT some rigidity.
- The ETT cuff should be tested for leaks.
- Preoxygenate the patient with 100% oxygenation for 2–3 minutes or 3–4 vital capacity breaths if time permits. In addition, a nasal cannula can be applied and remain on during intubation. After sedatives are given, nasal cannula oxygen can be turned up to 10–15 LPM to allow for passive oxygenation and delay potential desaturation.
- Stand at the head of the bed and have the stretcher raised to a position of comfort.
- Position the patient to best align the oropharyngeal axes; often, this is accomplished with a pad behind the occiput to place the patient in a sniffing position.
- Hold the laryngoscope in the left hand (regardless of operator hand dominance).
- Sedate and paralyze (if necessary) the patient.
- Open the mouth with the right hand, and insert the blade into the mouth along the right side and advance to the base of the tongue.
- Use the blade to sweep the tongue to the left as you continue to advance.
  - The Macintosh blade should follow the curvature of the anterior oropharynx until it seats into the vallecula.
  - The Miller blade continues directly down until it is just past the epiglottis.
- Apply traction along the axis of the laryngoscope handle (up and away), which should result in the lower jaw being lifted up. The handle should not be tilted back, and the teeth should not be used as a fulcrum as they can break.
- Once the vocal cords are visualized, have an assistant hand you the ETT and advance it through the cords under direct visualization. If no assistant is available, the ETT should be placed to your right during the preparation phase and immediately available to grab without taking your eyes off of the vocal cords.
- Once the cuff is through the cords, stop, remove the stylet, and inflate the balloon.
- Attach the capnography device and deliver breaths with the bag valve device.
- Once there is confirmation of proper positioning by confirming bilateral chest rise, auscultating breath sounds over both sides (at the axilla), visualizing mist in the

ETT, and recording CO_2 return with the capnography device, secure the ETT with tape or a commercial endotracheal tube holder.

POTENTIAL COMPLICATIONS

Endotracheal intubation can result in hypoxia, vagal-mediated bradycardia, cardiac decompensation from prolonged efforts, oropharyngeal and larynx trauma, teeth trauma, vomiting, aspiration, air leak, unrecognized esophageal intubation, endotracheal tube cuff leak, vocal cord damage, or tracheal stricture. In addition, neck movement may exacerbate any underlying fracture or spinal cord injury.

Cricothyroidotomy

INDICATIONS

An emergency cricothyroidotomy is used when the provider cannot oxygenate or cannot ventilate the patient, and other less invasive efforts have failed or are not possible.

CONTRAINDICATIONS

None, if the patient needs an airway

METHODS

There are clinical features that predict difficult cricothyroidotomy (Figure 129.1). The minimum equipment needed is a scalpel and a small (6.0 or 6.5) ETT. A bougie can be used as an adjunct to help guide the ETT in place in a Seldinger technique. A tracheal hook increases success rate and speed. There are many commercially available kits with equipment that typically includes a tracheostomy tube. Make sure you are familiar with the kits in your institution. The basic procedure is as follows:

- Stabilize the trachea with your nondominant hand.
- Locate the cricothyroid membrane. Make a vertical incision through the skin overlying the trachea centered on the cricothyroid membrane.
- Make a stab incision through the cricoid membrane with the blade in a horizontal orientation and then enlarge the hole by either twisting the blade or using the scalpel handle to bluntly dissect the membrane.
- Use the tracheal hook to provide caudal traction on the cricoid cartilage.
- Insert the tracheostomy tube or ETT, inflate the cuff, and ventilate the patient.

COMPLICATIONS

Can result in bleeding, incorrect tube placement, hematoma, subcutaneous emphysema, prolonged procedure time, aspiration, pneumothorax, or vocal cord injury.

SUGGESTED READING

Weiss A, Lutes M. *Focus On—Bag Valve Mask Ventilation*. ACEP News, September 2008.

Difficult Airway Society guidelines Flow-Chart 2004.

Reardon RF, McGill JW, and Clinton JE. Tracheal Intubation. In Roberts and Hedges Clinical Procedures in Emergency Medicine, Roberts JR, Custalow CB, Thomsen TW, eds. Elsevier-Saunders. Philadelphia. 2014. pp 62–106.

Hebert RB, Bose S, Mace SE. Cricothyrotomy and Translaryngeal Ventilation. In Roberts and Hedges Clinical Procedures in Emergency Medicine, Roberts JR, Custalow CB, Thomsen TW, eds. Elsevier-Saunders. Philadelphia. 2014. pp 120–133.

121 Analgesia

Christina Creel-Bulos

Pain

GENERAL PRINCIPLES

Definition

- Pain is a complex sensation involving multiple mediators, neurotransmitters, signaling pathways, and modulatory pathways.[1]

Pathophysiology

- Pain propagation begins with the activation of physiologic pain receptors (i.e., nociceptors) located throughout the body. These receptors correspond to free nerve endings associated with afferent nerve fibers that transmit signals to the spinal cord, brainstem, and diencephalon, including the hypothalamus, thalamus, amygdaloid complex, and medulla.[2]

Assessment

- Objective assessment of such a subjective sensation as pain can be challenging, particularly in the acutely or critically ill patient population.
- There are various methods of assessing pain in verbal patients. The numeric rating scale is most commonly employed and has been shown to be the most discriminative pain assessment tool when compared with other self-reports of pain.[3]
- Various pain assessment tools have been validated for use in nonverbal, critically ill patient populations.[4]

Analgesia

GENERAL PRINCIPLES

Definition

- Analgesia is the pharmacologic and neurologic state in which consciousness is preserved but painful stimuli is moderated, and it can be provided via local, regional, and systemic routes.[5]

Types of Analgesia

- Local analgesia involves administration of one or more analgesic agents via topical or infiltrative route for the purpose of inducing palliation of pain to a small, localized area of the body.
- Regional analgesia provides analgesia to a larger area of the body and is obtained by deposition of an analgesic agent via injection and infiltration of a more proximal nerve for the purpose of blocking innervation to the region it supplies.

- Systemic analgesia is obtained by administration of a systemic medication that targets different metabolic pathways to modulate and provide widespread relief from pain.

LOCAL ANALGESIA

Background

- Agents include esters and amides, respectively metabolized by plasma and hepatic enzymes. Both induce reversible sodium channel blockade along afferent nerve fibers, resulting in the disruption of nerve fiber depolarization. Common esters include tetracaine, benzocaine, and procaine. Common amides include lidocaine, bupivacaine, ropivacaine, and prilocaine.[6]
- Toxicity is rare but can occur locally due to direct injury or indirect induction of vasoconstriction, or systemically causing seizures, coma, and respiratory or cardiovascular collapse. Should severe toxicity occur, case studies have demonstrated the benefit of lipid emulsion boluses.[7,8]

TOPICAL ANALGESIA

- Topical analgesics may be applied to intact or open skin and to various mucous membranes.
- Topical agents come in spray, cream, gel, and liquid formulations and commonly contain medications such as lidocaine, tetracaine, epinephrine, ethyl chloride, etc. Commonly used formulation names are EMLA, LET, and LMX.

INFILTRATIVE ANALGESIA

- Agents may be infiltrated intradermally, subdermally, or via a combination of both techniques to provide local analgesia, after the area is properly cleansed (Table 121.1).
- Explain to patients that they will retain the sensation of pressure and movement, and test the area prior to starting the procedure to ensure that sharp and painful sensations are absent.
- Techniques to decrease pain include the following: use of a small gauge needle, slow injection, injection through wound margins instead of through intact skin, use of warmed or buffered solutions, and distracting a patient with conversation.[9–11]

REGIONAL ANALGESIA

Background

- Regional anesthesia can be used in the emergency department to facilitate complicated laceration repairs, the incision and drainage of abscesses, or reduction of orthopedic injuries.
- Regional analgesia can be administered using anatomical landmarks or ultrasonographic assistance.

Facial Nerve Blocks

- Useful for complex lacerations or in areas of the face that may be deformed by the infiltration of anesthesia (vermilion border).[13]
- Supraorbital nerve blockade provides analgesia to the forehead from the hairline to the bridge of the nose. Pertinent landmarks include the supraorbital foramen, with

TABLE 121.1	Common Agents[12]		
Agent	Maximum dose (mg/kg)	Onset (in min)	Duration (in min)
Lidocaine	4	5	30–60
Bupivacaine	3	10–15	200+
Procaine	7	15–20	40
Tetracaine	1.5	15	200

the injection starting point superior to the eyebrow near the superficial aspect of this structure.
- Infraorbital nerve blockade provides analgesia to the lower lid, medial cheek, ipsilateral nose, and upper lip. The nerve is anesthetized by placing the needle superior to the gingival reflection above the maxillary canine and by directing the needle superiorly toward the infraorbital foramen.
- Mental nerve blockade provides analgesia to the lower lip, gingiva, and chin. Pertinent landmarks include the mucosa inferior to the border of the canine and first molar.
- Inferior alveolar nerve blockade provides analgesia to the mandible from the angle posteriorly to the mental process anteriorly. Pertinent landmarks include the mucosa 1–2 cm superior to the last lower molar.
- Auricular nerve blockade provides analgesia to the entire ear through the anesthetization of the auriculotemporal, greater auricular, and lesser occipital nerve branches. Pertinent landmarks include the auricle of the ear—inferior to which bidirectional superioanterior and superioposterior injections are performed, and the superioanterior most aspect of the ear through which bidirectional inferioanterior and inferioposterior injections are performed.

Intercostal Nerve Block
- Intercostal nerve blockade provides analgesia along the superior and inferior portions of the entire blocked rib. It is used for rib fractures or thoracoabdominal procedures such as chest tubes.[14–16] Pertinent landmarks include the midaxillary or posterior axillary line and the inferior border of the selected rib.

Upper Extremity Nerve Blocks
- Shoulder and brachial plexus blocks are generally reserved for the operating room and postoperative areas.[17]
- Regional nerve blockade of the hand can be used in both the emergency department and operating room.[18]
- Median nerve blockade provides analgesia to the thumb, index, third digit, and one-half of the fourth digit of the hand. Pertinent landmarks include the palmaris longus and flexor carpi radialis tendons at the level of the most proximal palmar crease.
- Ulnar nerve blockade provides analgesia to the medial palm, wrist, fifth digit, and one-half of the fourth digit. Pertinent landmarks include the most distal wrist crease just above the extensor carpi ulnaris tendon.

- Radial nerve blockade provides analgesia to the dorsolateral half of the hand and thumb. Pertinent landmarks include the snuffbox and radial styloid process, which guide needle placement.

Lower Extremity Nerve Blocks

- The usage of femoral nerve blockade has recently been shown to assist with analgesic management in those suffering from femoral fractures and hip dislocations within the emergency department.[19,20] Femoral nerve blockade provides analgesia to the anterior aspect of the thigh but may extend to anesthetize regions innervated by the lateral cutaneous and obturator nerves. Pertinent landmarks include the inguinal ligament where injection is directed inferior to this crease and lateral to the femoral artery. Assistance through ultrasound guidance or peripheral nerve stimulation is recommended.

Foot Nerve Blocks

- Ankle and foot analgesia can be conveniently administered to regions of the foot to assist with rapid and easily accessible procedural analgesia.[21,22]
- Deep peroneal nerve blockade provides analgesia to the plantar aspect of the foot between the first and second toes. Pertinent landmarks include the extensor hallucis longus and tibialis anterior tendon at the level of the medial malleolus.
- Posterior tibial nerve blockade provides analgesia to the plantar aspect of the foot. Pertinent landmarks include the posterior tibial artery where injection is directed posteriorly from this site at the level of the medial malleolus.
- Superficial peroneal nerve blockade provides analgesia to the dorsolateral aspect of the foot. Pertinent landmarks include the superior aspect of the lateral malleolus near the tibialis anterior tendon.
- Sural nerve blockade provides analgesia to the lateral ankle. Pertinent landmarks include the superior aspect of the lateral malleolus near the Achilles tendon.
- Saphenous nerve blockade provides analgesia to the medial ankle. Pertinent landmarks include the superior aspect of the medial malleolus and the tibialis anterior tendon.

Digital Nerve Blocks

- Two general approaches to digital blocks exist, and both can be markedly useful in various situations.[23]
- Digital nerve blockade provides analgesia to the entire digit. Pertinent landmarks include the dorsolateral and dorsomedial aspects of the proximal phalanx of the digit of focus. Injection occurs at both points, with additional tracking across the dorsal aspect of the digit.
- Flexor tendon sheath blockade can provide analgesia to the entire digit but may occasionally spare the tip of the digit. Pertinent landmarks include the distal palmar crease of the digit of focus.

SYSTEMIC ANALGESIA

Introduction

- Multimodal analgesia can reduce medication-associated side effects and optimize pain control.[24]

ACUTE ANALGESIA

Nonopioid Analgesics: Concepts and Applications

- Acetaminophen is useful in managing pain in high-risk patient populations and in some studies has demonstrated a synergistic effect on pain when combined with other agents, such as nonsteroidal anti-inflammatory drugs (NSAIDs).[25,26]
- NSAID agents may be beneficial but should be used with caution in patients with existing gastrointestinal or renal insult.[27]
- Ketamine is a potent NMDA receptor channel antagonist that can reduce pain and opioid requirements.[28,29]
- The use of multimodal analgesia (including the use of gabapentinoids) has demonstrated promise, but use of these medications has not been formally evaluated in patients within the emergency department (Table 121.3).[30]

Opioid Analgesics: Concepts and Applications

- Opioid analgesics provide rapid relief for patients experiencing moderate to severe pain. Parenteral administration is employed when rapid onset is desired or the patient is unable to take them orally.
- Side effects include nausea, emesis, somnolence, hypotension, urinary retention, constipation, pruritus, bronchospasm, and respiratory depression.[33–35,41]
- Patients should be prescribed stool softeners with opiates and should be counseled on avoiding driving with use. Family members should be educated regarding signs of overdose in a loved one.

CHRONIC ANALGESIA

Chronic Pain: Concepts and Applications

- The management of chronic pain can be complex, due to the duration and associated comorbidities.
- Chronic pain is categorized as neuropathic or nociceptive, and opioids are ideally reserved as third-line treatment after alternative agents have been used.[36]

NEUROPATHIC PAIN: CONCEPTS AND APPLICATIONS

- Neuropathic pain is pain associated with damage or destruction of nervous tissue within either the central or peripheral nervous system. Antidepressants and anticonvulsants are used as first- or second-line adjuvant therapies; generally opioids are reserved as third-line agents if possible.[32,33]

Nociceptive Pain: Concepts and Applications

- No formal treatment guidelines exist, but recommendations suggest a stepwise approach using nonopioid analgesics as first-line agents, antidepressant therapy, and finally, the use of opioid analgesics.[36]

SPECIAL POPULATIONS

Maintenance Analgesia and Sedation in Intubated Patients

Approach and Considerations

- In the emergency department, intubated patients are typically managed with a combination of analgesic and sedating agents to maintain pain control and allow for

TABLE 121.2   Oral Nonopioid Regimens

Agent	Dosage	Frequency
Acetaminophen	325–1000 mg	q4–6h
Ibuprofen	400–800 mg	q6–8h
Clonidine	150–200 mcg	bid/daily
Gabapentin	300–1800 mg (3600 max)	Daily

adequate ventilatory support, with careful attention to underlying comorbidities or pathologies (Table 121.6 and table 121.7). Frequent reassessments are critical.[34,40]

Acute Pain in Chronic Opioid Users

General Approach

- As a result of independent and variable levels of tolerance, opioid requirements in this patient population may be high and unpredictable; thus, dosing regimens should be individualized and approached cautiously (Tables 121.2–121.5).

Considerations

- Guidelines dictating analgesia administration to patients experiencing acute pain within the context of a history of chronic opioid usage have been developed primarily based on studies of oncology patients. Recommendations include continuing patients' typical long-acting regimens and dosing as-needed short-acting analgesic medications to provide acute pain relief.
- Dosing breakthrough pain medications may be difficult; one point of reference is to calculate a patient's daily opioid requirement and begin by administering 10–20% of that as a first bolus.[36,37]

Analgesia in Pregnancy

- Despite the dramatic physiologic changes occur during pregnancy, the approach toward selection and dosing of analgesics is not typically affected.
- Exceptions include use of NSAIDs, which are associated with premature closure of the fetal ductus arteriosus and fetal renal injury, and opiates in the third trimester due to the risk of neonatal respiratory depression if delivery is imminent.[38–43]
- Maternal detoxification from chronic usage of opioids has been associated with increased risk of fetal loss, fetal distress, and neonatal abstinence syndrome, which can occur from 24 hours to 7 days after delivery.[45]

TABLE 121.3   Parenteral Nonopioid Regimens

Agent	Dosage	Frequency
Ketorolac	IM 30 mg	q6h
	IV 15–30 mg	q6h
Ketamine	0.2–0.8 mg/kg	Bolus

TABLE 121.4	Enteral Opioid Regimens	
Agent	Initial dosage	Frequency
Oxycodone	5–15 mg	q4–6h
Morphine	10–30 mg	q4h
Hydromorphone	2–4 mg	q4–6h
Percocet (oxycodone + acetaminophen)	Varying combinations	q4–6h
Norco/Lortab/Vicodin (hydrocodone + acetaminophen)	Varying combinations	q4–6h
Tylenol no. 3 (codeine + acetaminophen)	300 mg/30 mg	q4–6h

TABLE 121.5	Parenteral Opioid Regimens (intermittent dosing)		
Agent	Intravenous	IM	SQ
Morphine	2.5–5 mg Q3–4h	5–10 mg IM q3–4h	Not recommended
Hydromorphone	0.2–1 mg q2–3h	1–2 mg q2–3h	Not recommended
Fentanyl	0.35–0.5 mcg/kg q30–60 min	Not recommended	Not recommended

TABLE 121.6	Parenteral Opioid Regimens (PCA or infusion dosing)[40]			
Agent	Dosage: bolus	Dosage: infusion	Onset (min)	Duration (min)
Fentanyl	1–2 mcg/kg	0.7–1.0 mcg/kg/h	1–2	30–60
Hydromorphone	0.5–2 mg	0.5–3 mg/h	5–10	240–300
Morphine	2–10 mg	2–30 mg/h	5–10	240–300

TABLE 121.7	Sedation Agents[40]			
Agent	Dosage: bolus	Dosage: infusion	Onset (min)	Duration (min)
Propofol	Not recommended	5–50 mcg/kg/min	1–2	3–10
Ketamine	0.1–0.5 mg/kg	0.05–0.4 mg/kg/h	<1	10–15
Midazolam	0.01–0.05 mg/kg	0.02–0.1 mg/kg/h	2–5	30
Lorazepam	0.02–0.04 mg/kg	0.01–0.1 mg/kg/h	15–20	360–480

Renal Failure

- Patients with reduced glomerular filtration rate (GFR) or known chronic kidney disease are at increased risk for side effects related to analgesia.
- When possible, employing the short-acting, oral agents is ideal (Tables 121.6 and 121.7).
- Hydromorphone is better tolerated in this patient population; however, given its renal excretion, patients who receive this medication must be closely monitored.[48,49]
- Fentanyl is associated with fewer clinically significant accumulations and side effects; however, fentanyl has a propensity toward adipose deposition that may prolong its effects.[48]

Obesity

- Dosage calculators for more commonly used medications can be used as a reference. A general rule is to use lean body weight in one's calculations—unless the drug is very lipophilic, in which case calculating the dose based on total body weight is recommended.[49]

Geriatrics

- Increases in body fat combined with decreases in serum albumin levels, GFRs, total body water, and organ blood flow result in an overall increased susceptibility to the potency of opiates, resulting in more side effects at lower dosages.[50]
- Individual variability makes it difficult to provide generalized population recommendations, but one recommended approach is to start with a 50% dose reduction in this population and then titrate to the effect desired with unchanged interval frequency.[51]

REFERENCES

1. Argoff C. Mechanisms of pain transmission and pharmacologic management. *Curr Med Res Opin* 2011;27:2019–31.
2. Almeida T, Roizenblatt S, Tufik S. Afferent pain pathways: a neuroanatomical review. *Brain Res* 2004;1000:40–56.
3. Chanques G, Viel E, Constantin JM, et al. The measurement of pain in intensive care unit: comparison of 5 self-report intensity scales. *Pain* 2010;151:711–21.
4. Gélinas C, Puntillo KA, Joffe AM, et al. A validated approach to evaluating psychometric properties of pain assessment tools for use in nonverbal critically ill adults. *Semin Respir Crit Care Med* 2013;34:153–68.
5. Heavner JE. Local anesthetics. *Curr Opin Anaesthesiol* 2007;20:336–42.
6. Tetzlaff JE. The pharmacology of local anesthetics. *Anesthesiol Clin North Am* 2000;18:217.
7. Rosenblatt MA, Abel M, Fischer GW, et al. Successful use of a 20% lipid emulsion to resuscitate a patient after a presumed bupivacaine-related cardiac arrest. *Anesthesiology* 2006;105:217.
8. Weinberg G. Lipid rescue resuscitation from local anaesthetic cardiac toxicity. *Toxicol Rev* 2006;25:139.
9. Baibergenova A, Murray CA. Techniques to minimize the pain of injected local anesthetic. *J Cutan Med Surg* 2011;15:250.
10. Zilinsky I, Bar-Meir E, Zaslansky R, et al. Ten commandments for minimal pain during administration of local anesthetics. *J Drugs Dermatol* 2005;4:212.
11. Babamiri K, Nassab R. The evidence for reducing the pain of administration of local anesthesia and cosmetic injectables. *J Cosmet Dermatol* 2010;9:242.
12. Dillon DC, Gibbs MA. Local and Regional Anesthesia. In: Tintinalli JE, Stapczynski J, Ma O, Yealy DM, Meckler GD, Cline DM. eds. *Tintinalli's Emergency Medicine: A Comprehensive Study Guide, 8e* New York, NY: McGraw-Hill; 2016.
13. Lacroix G, Meaudre E, Prunet B, et al. Appreciation of the role of regional anesthesia in managing facial wounds in the emergency unit. *Ann Fr Anesth Reanim* 2010;29:3.

14. Kopacz DJ, Thompson GE. Intercostal blocks for thoracic and abdominal surgery. *Tech Reg Anesth Pain Manage* 1998;2:25.

15. Roué C, Wallaert M, Kacha M, Havet E. Intercostal/paraspinal nerve block for thoracic nerve block for thoracic surgery. *Anaesthesia* 2016;71(1):112–3.

16. Karmakar MK, Ho AM. Acute pain management of patients with multiple fractured ribs. *J Trauma* 2003;54:615–25.

17. Fredrickson MJ, Krishnan S, Chen CY. Postoperative analgesia for shoulder surgery: a critical appraisal and review of current techniques. *Anesthesia* 2010;65:608.

18. Thompson WL, Malchow RJ. Peripheral nerve blocks and anesthesia of the hand. *Mil Med* 2002;167:478–82.

19. Paul JE, Arya A, Hurlburt L, et al. Femoral nerve block improves analgesia outcomes after total knee arthroplasty: a meta-analysis of randomized controlled trials. *Anesthesiology* 2010;113:1144.

20. Dickman E, Pushkar I, Likourezos A, et al. Ultrasound-guided nerve blocks for intracapsular and extracapsular hip fractures. *Am J Emerg Med* 2016;34(3):586–9.

21. Ferrera PC, Chandler R. Anesthesia in the emergency setting: part I. Hand and foot injuries. *Am Fam Physician* 1994;50:569–73.

22. Whiteley B, Rees S. A randomized controlled trial to compare two techniques for partial digital local anesthetic blocks. *J Foot Ankle Surg* 2010;49:143.

23. Hill RG Jr, Patterson JW, Parker JC, et al. Comparison of transthecal digital block and traditional digital block for anesthesia of the finger. *Ann Emerg Med* 1995;25:604.

24. Costantini R, Affaitati G, Fabrizio A, Giamberardino MA. Controlling pain in the postoperative setting. *Int J Clin Pharmacol Ther* 2011;49:116–27.

25. Ong CK, Seymour RA, Lirk P, Merry AF. Combining paracetamol (acetaminophen) with nonsteroidal antiinflammatory drugs: a qualitative systematic review of analgesic efficacy for acute postoperative pain. *Anesth Analg* 2010;110:1170.

26. Hyllested M, Jones S, Pedersen JL, Kehlet H. Comparative effect of paracetamol, NSAIDs or their combination in postoperative pain management: a qualitative review. *Br J Anaesth* 2002;88:199–214.

27. Antman EM, Bennett JS, Daugherty A, Furberg C. Use of nonsteroidal antiinflammatory drugs: an update for clinicians: a scientific statement from the American Heart Association. *Circulation* 2007;115:1634.

28. Quibell R, Prommer EE, Mihalyo M, et al. Ketamine. *J Pain Symptom Manage* 2011;41:640–9.

29. Subramaniam K, Subramaniam B, Steinbrook R. Ketamine as adjuvant analgesic to opioids: a quantitative and qualitative systematic review. *Anesth Analg* 2004;99:482–95.

30. Dauri M, Faria S, Gatti A, Celidonio L, et al. Gabapentin and pregabalin for the acute postoperative pain management. A systematic-narrative review of the recent clinical evidences. *Curr Drug Targets* 2009;10:716.

31. Lexicomp Online. Copyright © 1978–2016 Lexicomp, Inc. All Rights Reserved.

32. Ghuran A, Nolan J. Recreational drug misuse: issues for the cardiologist. *Heart* 2000;83:627.

33. Clemens KE, Klaschik E. Management of constipation in palliative care patients. *Curr Opin Support Palliat Care* 2008;2:22.

34. Quigley C. Opioids in people with cancer-related pain. *BMJ Clin Evid* 2008;2008. pii: 2408.

35. Aronoff GM. What do we know about the pathophysiology of chronic pain? *Med Clin North Am* 2016;100:31–42.

36. Dworkin RH, O'Connor AB, Backonja M, Farrar JT. Pharmacologic management of neuropathic pain: evidence-based recommendations. *Pain* 2007;132:237.

37. Dobecki DA, Schocket SM, Wallace MS. Update on pharmacotherapy guidelines for the treatment of neuropathic pain. *Curr Pain Headache Rep* 2006;10:185.

38. Shruti B, Patell J, Kressl P. Sedation and analgesia in the mechanically ventilated patient. *Am J Respir Crit Care Med* 2012;185:486–97.

39. Barr J, Fraser GL, Puntillo K, et al. Clinical practice guidelines for the management of pain, agitation, and delirium in adult patients in the intensive care unit. *Crit Care Med* 2013;41:263.

40. Walsh D, Rivera NI, Davis MP, et al. Strategies for pain management: Cleveland Clinic Foundation guidelines for opioid dosing for cancer pain. *Support Cancer Ther* 2004;1(3):157.

41. Moryl N, Coyle N, Foley KM. Managing an acute pain crisis in a patient with advanced cancer: "this is as much of a crisis as a code". *JAMA* 2008;299(12):1457.
42. Koren G, Florescu A, Costei AM, et al. Nonsteroidal antiinflammatory drugs during third trimester and the risk of premature closure of the ductus arteriosus: a meta-analysis. *Ann Pharmacother* 2006;40:824.
43. Hudak ML, Tan RC. Neonatal drug withdrawal. *Pediatrics* 2012;129:540–60.
44. Babul N, Darke AC, Hagen N. Hydromorphone metabolite accumulation in renal failure. *J Pain Symptom Manage* 1995;10:184.
45. Davison SN, Mayo PR. Pain management in chronic kidney disease: the pharmacokinetics and pharmacodynamics of hydromorphone and hydromorphone-3-glucuronide in hemodialysis patients. *J Opioid Manag* 2008;4:335.
46. McClain DA, Hug CC Jr. Intravenous fentanyl kinetics. *Clin Pharmacol Ther* 1980;28:106.
47. Hanley MJ, Abernethy DR, Greenblatt DJ. Effect of obesity on the pharmacokinetics of drugs in humans. *Clin Pharmacokinet* 2010;49:71.
48. Spanjer MR, Bakker NA, Absalon AR. Pharmacology in the elderly and newer anaesthesia drugs. *Best Pract Res Clin Anaesthesiol* 2011;25:355–265.
49. Gupta DK, Avram MJ. Rational opioid dosing in the elderly: dose and dosing interval when initiating opioid therapy. *Clin Pharmacol Ther* 2012;91:339–43.

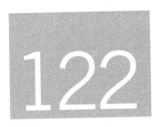

122 Procedures: Arthrocentesis

Steven Hung and Michael Willman

GENERAL PRINCIPLES

- Joint aspiration is performed in the emergency department to obtain synovial fluid to diagnose septic or inflammatory conditions.
- Therapeutic injections of local anesthetic or steroids can be done; however, this is not typically performed in the emergency department.

Indications

- The indications for an arthrocentesis is to assist in the diagnosis of a septic joint, or crystal arthropathy.

Contraindications

- Absolute: Cellulitis overlying the area of needle insertion
- Relative: Bleeding diathesis
  - Patients on therapeutic warfarin appear to tolerate arthrocentesis without bleeding complications.[1] These data have been used to support arthrocentesis for patients on aspirin and clopidogrel.
    - It is advised that the smallest possible needle is used.
- Joint prosthesis—should consult orthopedic surgery

PROCEDURE

Preparation

- A time out should be performed.
- Position the patient so that the joint of interest is easily accessible and at a height that is comfortable.
- Identify appropriate landmarks and mark the planned insertion site.
- *Knee Joint*
  - Position: Patient is supine. Knee is flexed between 15 and 30 degrees. Place a towel under the knee to keep the quadriceps loose.
  - Landmark: Midpoint of the medial (or lateral) patellar ridge.
  - Insertion site: Approximately 1 cm medial (or lateral) to the patellar ridge, aiming between the posterior surface of the patella and the intercondylar femoral notch.
- *Tibiotalar Joint (Ankle)*
  - Position: Patient is supine. Plantar-flex the foot.
  - Landmarks: Identify the anterior border of medial malleolus and the tibialis anterior tendon (identified with active dorsiflexion).
  - Insertion site: Medial to the tibialis anterior tendon, directed posteriorly and inferiorly toward the joint space.
- *Metatarsophalangeal Joint (Great Toe)*
  - Position: Patient is supine. Flex toe slightly. Apply gentle traction.
  - Landmarks: Distal metatarsal head and proximal base of first phalanx.
  - Insertion site: On the dorsal aspect, just medial or lateral to extensor tendon.
- *Radiohumeral Joint (Elbow)*
  - Position: Elbow flexed to 90 degrees. Pronate the forearm with hand flat on table.
  - Landmarks: Radial head and lateral epicondyle of the humerus. More easily identified by palpation with the elbow fully extended.
  - Insertion site: Lateral approach only. Just distal to the lateral epicondyle, directed medially.
- *Radiocarpal Joint (Wrist)*
  - Position: Hand is prone with slight flexion and ulnar deviation. Apply gentle traction.
  - Landmarks: The dorsal radial tubercle, ulnar side of extensor pollicis longus, and radial side of common extensor tendon.
  - Insertion site: Just distal to the radial tubercle on the ulnar side of the extensor pollicis longus, aimed perpendicular to the plane of the hand.

Equipment

- Syringes: 30 or 60 mL (for aspiration), 5 mL (for lidocaine)
- Needles: 18 or 22 gauge (for aspiration), 25 or 27 gauge (for lidocaine)
- Chlorhexidine or povidone–iodine antiseptic solution
- Sterile gloves
- Lidocaine 1%

Procedure

- Use sterile technique, including universal precautions for the entire procedure.
- Prep the area with chlorhexidine or povidone–iodine.
- Anesthetize the skin at the insertion site with lidocaine using a 25- or 27-gauge needle.

- Refrigerant spray can be used instead of lidocaine injection.
- Insert 18- or 22-gauge needle attached to a 30- or 60-mL syringe at the marked site.
- Gently aspirate while advancing slowly until there is fluid return.
- Once you enter the joint space, aspirate as much fluid as possible.
- Withdraw the needle and apply light pressure with clean dressing.
- Send the fluid for cell count and differential, culture, and crystal analysis.[2,3]

SPECIAL CONSIDERATIONS

- Shoulder and hip arthrocentesis can be more difficult, sometimes done under ultrasound guidance, and may require radiology or orthopedic consultation.
- Patients should be instructed to keep the insertion site clean and dry.

COMPICATIONS

- Pain, infection, bleeding, injury to nerve/vessels/tendons

ADDITIONAL RESOURCES

Thomsen TW, Shen S, Shaffer RW, Setnik GS. Videos in clinical medicine. Arthrocentesis of the knee. *N Engl J Med* 2006;354(19):e19.

REFERENCES

1. Ahmed I, Gertner E. Safety of arthrocentesis and joint injection in patients receiving anticoagulation at therapeutic levels. *Am J Med* 2012;125(3):265–9.
2. Shmerling RH, Delbanco TL, Tosteson AN, Trentham DE. Synovial fluid tests. What should be ordered? *JAMA* 1990;264(8):1009–14.
3. Margaretten ME, Kohlwes J, Moore D, Bent S. Does this adult patient have septic arthritis? *JAMA* 2007;297(13):1478–88.
4. Mathews CJ, Coakley G. Septic arthritis: current diagnostic and therapeutic algorithm. *Curr Opin Rheumatol* 2008;20(4):457–62.

123 Procedures: Epistaxis Treatment

Mark D. Levine

GENERAL PRINCIPLES

- The nasal mucosa is supplied by branches from the internal and external carotid arteries.
- The majority of nosebleeds are anterior in nature and are secondary to trauma, drying of the mucosa, irritants, vascular issues/hypertension, or foreign bodies.

- Most minor nosebleeds can be treated with direct pressure (squeezing of the nasal ala) for ~10 minutes.
- Anterior epistaxis
  ◦ Easily identified by direct visualization
- Posterior epistaxis
  ◦ Identified by nasal hemorrhage that flows posteriorly into the oropharynx.
  ◦ Bleeding may occur posterior to the anterior packing.
  ◦ Not amenable to direct pressure.

Indications

- Anterior nosebleed that does not stop with simple direct pressure
- Posterior epistaxis

PROCEDURE

Preparation

- Adjust the height of the bed to a level comfortable to perform the procedure.
- Place the patient in the sitting position and remove clots with a suction catheter or have the patient expel (gently) any blood clots by blowing the nose.
- Instill topical vasoconstrictors (one inhalation of oxymetazoline is usually recommended; however, topical cocaine or other vasoconstrictor may be used). This may be all that is necessary for hemostasis.

Procedure

Anterior Epistaxis

- For an anterior source that can be visualized, a silver nitrate stick can be used, starting in concentric circles away from the site so as to cauterize the vessels supplying the site of injury. The stick should be placed for 5–10 seconds, turning the end of the stick. The mucosa will turn a gray-black color.
- There are many packing materials available:
  ◦ Vaseline gauze strips can be inserted in an accordion fashion along the base of the nose and continued in a superior fashion.
  ◦ A Rhino Rocket may also be used. Use according to the manufacturer's instructions.
  ◦ FloSeal has also been shown to be effective for hemostasis in anterior nosebleeds.

Posterior Epistaxis

- A Foley catheter may be passed into the nasopharynx, past the site of bleeding; inflated; and then pulled back to tamponade the bleed. Anterior packing should also be placed around the catheter.
- After local anesthesia, a rubber catheter may be passed through the nares to the oropharynx, where it is grasped by a Magill forceps and pulled anteriorly out the mouth. A folded gauze pad can then be secured to the distal end of the catheter with silk ties or umbilical tape, and the proximal end of the catheter can then be backed out of the nares until the packing lodges in the posterior nasopharynx.
- Commercial products like a balloon tamponade device or a Rhino Rocket may also be used per manufacturer's guidelines.
- There is some evidence that patients with posterior packing should receive prophylactic antibiotics.

SPECIAL CONSIDERATIONS

Disposition

• Patients who have a posterior packing placed should be admitted to an intensive care unit to be monitored and in the event that the packing comes loose and lodges in the airway.
• Patients with anterior packing may be discharged to follow up with their primary physician or otolaryngologist within 48 hours. Antibiotics are not indicated as prophylaxis.

Complications

• Continued bleeding may require arterial ligation by otolaryngology.
• Loss of airway if posterior packing comes loose and lodges in the airway.
• Infection.

SUGGESTED READINGS

Riviello RJ. Otolaryngologic Procedures. In Roberts JR, Custalow CB, ThomsenTW, eds. Roberts and Hedges Clinical Procedures in Emergency Medicine, 6th ed. Elselvier-Saunders. Philadelphia. 2014.
Derkay CS, Hirsch BE, Johnson JT, et al. Posterior nasal packing: are antibiotics really necessary? *Arch Otolaryngol Head Neck Surg* 1989;115(4):439–41.
Pepper C, Lo S, Toma A. Prospective study of the risk of not using prophylactic antibiotics in nasal packing for epistaxis. *J Laryngol Otol* 2012;126(3):257–9.
Wakelam OC, Dimitriadis PA, Stephens J. The use of FloSeal haemostatic sealant in the management of epistaxis: a prospective clinical study and literature review. *Ann R Coll Sug Engl* 2016;4:1–3.

124

Procedures: Intraosseous Access

Steven Hung and Michael Willman

GENERAL PRINCIPLES

• Intraosseous (IO) access can quickly and reliably be started when normal intravenous (IV) access cannot be obtained due to patient age, time, or patient condition.[1-3]
• IO infusion is possible due to venous drainage from the marrow of long bones, a noncompressible source of infusion that is easily accessible regardless of the patient's volume status.
• All medications and fluids that can be delivered through a peripheral or central venous catheter can be given through an IO line with a similar onset of action to those medications administered through the IV route.

- Types of IO needles include manual (Jamshidi, Sur-Fast, modified Dieckmann), impact driven (FAST1, BIG), and power driven (EZ-IO).

Indications
- Need to obtain IV access quickly

Contraindications
Absolute
- Fracture proximal to IO site
- Previously placed IO site in the same bone (fluids can extravasate through prior access)
- Proximal vascular injury

Relative
- Burn or infection involving site of access

PROCEDURE

Preparation
- Clean site with antiseptic solution.

Equipment
- Personal protective equipment
- Antiseptic solution (alcohol, povidone–iodine, chlorhexidine)
- Syringe, saline flush
- Stabilizing device (there are some specific to IO needles)

Procedure
- Use universal precautions. This is an aseptic procedure.
- Palpate for landmarks, and clean the area with antiseptic solution.
- Position the needle perpendicular to the skin, insert the needle down to the bone, and then place per manufacturer instructions.
- The needle should sink into the bone and feel stable.
- Hook up IV tubing to needle and infuse per manufacturer's instructions.
- In the awake patient, slowly infuse 40 mg preservative-free lidocaine (cardiac lidocaine) through the IO over 120 seconds. Allow it to dwell in the space for 60 seconds, and then forcefully flush with 5–10mL of normal saline.

SPECIAL CONSIDERATIONS
- Monitor for bleeding, infection, swelling, and extravasation.
- IO needles are not MRI compatible.
- IO access needs to be removed within 24 hours of insertion.

Complications
- Extravasation, compartment syndrome, fracture, skin necrosis, osteomyelitis or other infection/abscess, fat embolus[5]

REFERENCES

1. Reades R, Studnek JR, Vandeventer S, Garrett J. Intraosseous versus intravenous vascular access during out-of-hospital cardiac arrest: a randomized controlled trial. *Ann Emerg Med* 2011;58(6):509–16.

2. Levitan RM, Bortle CD, Snyder TA, et al. Use of a battery-operated needle driver for intraosseous access by novice users: skill acquisition with cadavers. *Ann Emerg Med* 2009;54(5):692–4.
3. Rosetti VA, Thompson BM, Miller J, et al. Intraosseous infusion: an alternative route of pediatric intravascular access. *Ann Emerg Med* 1985;14(9):885–8.
4. Hasan MY, Kissoon N, Khan TM, et al. Intraosseous infusion and pulmonary fat embolism. *Pediatr Crit Care Med* 2001;2:133–8.

125

Procedures: Incision and Drainage

Michael Willman and Steven Hung

GENERAL PRINCIPLES

- Skin and soft tissue infections (SSTI) account for 3.2% of emergency department visits, with nearly a quarter of those requiring incision and drainage (I&D).[1]
- The increasing number of SSTIs requiring I&D is driven by the rising incidence of methicillin-resistant *Staphylococcus aureus* (MRSA), accounting for nearly two-thirds of all SSTIs in some areas of the United States.[2]
- Abscesses will usually present with an area of increasing swelling, pain, erythema, and/or spontaneous drainage.
- History should focus on injury, immunosuppression, and IV drug use.
- Use of a high-frequency, linear ultrasound probe may help locate pockets of purulent material.
- Plain radiograph of the affected area should be obtained if a foreign body is suspected.

Indications

- Abscess

Contraindications

- Near vital structures or major vessels.
- Specialist consultation should be considered for abscesses in the hand, breast, genital, or perianal/perirectal abscesses.

PROCEDURE

Equipment

- Clean (nonsterile) gloves, mask with face shield (or goggles)
- Povidone–iodine or chlorhexidine antiseptic solution

- Local anesthetic (e.g., 1% lidocaine)
- #11 blade scalpel
- Hemostat or needle driver
- Culture swab
- Packing material (e.g., plain or iodoform gauze)

Preparation

- A time out should be performed.
- Adjust the height of the bed to a level comfortable to perform the procedure.
- If necessary, pain medication, anxiolytics, or procedural sedation should be administered to the patient prior to the procedure.
- Prep the area with iodine or chlorhexidine solution.
- Anesthetize the area:
  ○ Infiltrate the lidocaine in a ringlike pattern around the abscess and superficially at the site of incision.
  ○ Consider using the lidocaine to perform a regional/nerve block for better analgesia.

Procedure

- Using a scalpel, incise the area of greatest fluctuance and extend the incision. Make it large enough to allow complete drainage, exploration, and placement of packing.
  ○ A common mistake is making too small an incision.
- Obtain a culture of the purulent material if present.
- Using a hemostat or needle driver, break up any loculations.
  ○ Insert instrument in the closed position, open, and then withdraw; repeat process in all directions.
- Applying pressure around the wound will help "milk" the abscess.
- Recent studies suggest that irrigation/packing does not improve outcome.
- Dress the wound.

SPECIAL CONSIDERATIONS

Complications

- Pain, bleeding, spread of infection, injury to underlying structure (use of ultrasound beforehand can assist in identifying these structures)

Disposition

- Consult the appropriate surgeon if complicated abscess (e.g., on hand, breast, perianal/perirectal).
- Return for follow-up if there is increased redness, swelling, pain, or new fever over the next week.
- Remove the packing in 24–48 hours (at home).
- Wash the area with soap and water daily after the packing is removed.
- Can tell them to take a shower and use the showerhead to rinse it inside and out.
- Avoid long soaking of wound.

REFERENCES

1. Pallin DJ, Camargo CA, Schuur JD. Skin infections and antibiotic stewardship: analysis of emergency department prescribing practices, 2007–2010. *West J Emerg Med* 2014;15(3):282–9.
2. Talan DA, Krishnadasan A, Gorwitz RJ, et al. Comparison of *Staphylococcus aureus* from skin and soft-tissue infections in US emergency department patients, 2004 and 2008. *Clin Infect Dis* 2011;53:144–9.

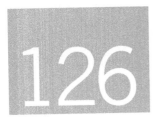

126 Procedures: Lumbar Puncture

Steven Hung and Michael Willman

GENERAL PRINCIPLES

- A lumbar puncture (LP) is both a diagnostic and therapeutic procedure. It can be used to identify central nervous system infections, noninfectious pathology (e.g., subarachnoid hemorrhage [SAH]), measurement of opening pressure, and to reduce intracranial pressure by removing CSF.

Indications
- Suspected meningitis.
- Suspected SAH with a negative head CT.
  - The sensitivity for SAH in patients presenting within 6 hours of symptoms is high enough with the new CT scanners that an LP is no longer required.
- Headache as a result of pseudotumor cerebri.

Contraindications
Absolute
- Increased intracranial pressure (risk of herniation).
  - A head CT should be performed prior to LP to rule out increased intracranial pressure in patients with altered mental status, focal neurologic deficits, papilledema, seizures, impaired cellular immunity, or likely mass effect.[2]
- Suspected spinal epidural abscess.
- Clinical instability.
- Infection overlying area of LP.
- Bleeding diathesis (risk of epidural hematoma).
  - It is recommended that patients have a platelet count above 50,000/μL.[3]
  - Defer LP in patients with and INR >1.4 until it is corrected.
  - Delay systemic anticoagulation for 1 hour after an LP is performed.
  - Aspirin and other antiplatelet agents do not raise the risk of epidural hematoma.[4]

Relative
- Lumbar spinal fusion or laminectomy.
- Intrathecal pump (e.g., baclofen pump).
  - Intrathecal pumps can sometimes be accessed to retrieve CSF. Consult neurosurgery for this.
- Spinal hardware.
- Uncooperative patient (may need sedation prior to procedure).

PROCEDURE

- There are two common positions to perform an LP:
  - Sitting—opens up the intervertebral spaces and is generally easier
  - Lateral recumbent/fetal position—allows accurate measurement of the opening pressure
  - Ultrasound or fluoroscopic guidance may help reduce the number of failed attempts.[5]

Equipment
- Povidone–iodine or chlorhexidine antiseptic solution
- Face mask, sterile gloves, gown
- LP kit/tray

Preparation
- A time out should be performed.
- Raise the bed to a height that is comfortable for the person performing the procedure.
- Palpate the highest points of the iliac crests. Midline to this should be the L3–L4 or L4–L5 interspace, which is below the termination of the spinal cord.
  - Mark the area of insertion by indenting the skin (i.e., pressing firmly with a red cap, syringe cap, needle cap, or sterile surgical marker).
- Sterilize the area with antiseptic solution in three concentric outward circles.
- Drape using sterile technique including face mask, gown, and gloves.
- Open the kit and unscrew the specimen vials.
- Place the fenestrated drape on the patient, centered over the insertion site. A second drape should be placed on the stretcher underneath the first to expand the sterile field.
- Create a wheal of lidocaine in the skin at insertion site and inject more along the anticipated needle tract.

Procedure
- Insert spinal needle with stylet in, aimed toward the patient's umbilicus.
  - If bone is encountered, withdraw the needle most of the way and change the angles of insertion.
  - Sometimes, multiple small pops are felt as the ligaments are penetrated and the dural space is entered.
  - Remove the stylet periodically to check for CSF flow and reinsert if the needle is going to be advanced.

○ Optional: Opening pressure (in lateral recumbent position only)
  ▪ Once the CSF is flowing freely, attach the manometer and stopcock.
  ▪ Open the stopcock toward the manometer to measure the pressure.
  ▪ Once the opening pressure is obtained, open the stopcock and collect CSF.
○ Collect the CSF serially in numbered tubes, at least 1–2 mL in each tube (more, if extensive testing is anticipated).
○ Replace stylet and withdraw needle, apply dressing.
○ Send tubes for testing:
  ▪ Tubes 1 and 4—cell count and differential
  ▪ Tube 2—protein and glucose
  ▪ Tube 3—Gram stain, culture/sensitivity
  ▪ Tube 4—saved for future studies

SPECIAL CONSIDERATIONS

- Fluoroscopic guidance may be necessary if the patient is morbidly obese, if there have been multiple unsuccessful attempts, or if the anatomy is distorted (extreme kyphosis/scoliosis).
- Previously, patients were instructed to have strict bed rest after for at least an hour after LP; however, recent literature has demonstrated that patients do not need strict bed rest.[7]

Complications
- Post-LP headache
- Infection including epidural abscess
- Bleeding—epidural hematoma
- Cerebral herniation
- Back pain, radicular pain, or numbness

ADDITIONAL RESOURCE

Ellenby MS, Tegtmeyer K, Lai S, Braner DAV. Lumbar puncture. *N Engl J Med* 2006;355:e12.

REFERENCES

1. Perry JJ, Stiell IG, Sivilotti ML, et al. Sensitivity of computed tomography performed within six hours of onset of headache for diagnosis of subarachnoid haemorrhage: prospective cohort study. *BMJ* 2011;343:d4277.
2. Hasbun R, Abrahams J, Jekel J, Quagliarello VJ. Computed tomography of the head before lumbar puncture in adults with suspected meningitis. *N Engl J Med* 2001;345(24):1727.
3. Wolfe KS, Kress JP. Risk of procedural hemorrhage. *Chest* 2016;150(1):237–46.
4. Horlocker TT, Wedel DJ, Schroeder DR, et al. Preoperative antiplatelet therapy does not increase the risk of spinal hematoma associated with regional anesthesia. *Anesth Analg* 1995;80(2):303.
5. Shaikh F, Brzezinski J, Alexander S, et al. Ultrasound imaging for lumbar punctures and epidural catheterisations: systematic review and meta-analysis. *BMJ* 2013;346:f1720.
6. Sviggum HP, Jacob AK, Arendt KW, et al. Neurologic complications after chlorhexidine antisepsis for spinal anesthesia. *Reg Anesth Pain Med* 2012;37:139–44.
7. Arevalo-Rodriguez I, Ciapponi A, Munoz L, et al. Posture and fluids for preventing postdural puncture headache. *Cochrane Database Syst Rev* 2013;7:CD009199.

127 Procedures: Diagnostic Paracentesis

Steven Hung and Michael Willman

GENERAL PRINCIPLES

- Diagnostic paracentesis is most commonly performed for the diagnosis of spontaneous bacterial peritonitis (SBP).
- Performing a diagnostic paracentesis on patients admitted with ascites or hepatic encephalopathy has been shown to reduce overall in-hospital mortality.[1]
- While the principles of a large volume (or therapeutic) paracentesis are similar, they are rarely needed in an emergent condition.
- Paracentesis can be performed safely without the need for transfusion of blood products even in patients with a slightly elevated INR or slightly decreased platelet count.[2,3]

Indications

- Patients with ascites and the presence of abdominal pain and/or signs of infection

Contraindications

- Extreme hypercoagulability (e.g., disseminated intravascular coagulation [DIC])
- Lack of adequately sized fluid collection distal to bowel, vessels, or other organs.

PROCEDURE

Preparation

- A time out should be performed.
- Adjust the height of the bed to a level comfortable to perform the procedure.
- Position the patient lying supine with the head of the bed at a slight incline.
- Assess what labs are needed:
  ○ Infectious workup—cell count and differential, aerobic and anaerobic culture
- Use universal precautions.
- Use ultrasound to identify an adequate fluid collection (at least 2–3 cm of fluid without loops of bowel), usually in the right or left (preferred) lower quadrant.
- If it is difficult to find an adequate pocket of fluid away from loops of bowel, try rotating the patient slightly to the left or right side.
  ○ Ascites will appear anechoic (black) on US.
  ○ A linear probe can be used to identify underlying vessels to avoid vascular injury.[4]
  ○ Mark the site with a surgical marker, or use a needle cap to press into the skin to leave an indentation.
  ○ Keep the patient immobile once the site is marked to avoid shifting of fluid or bowel.

- Sterilize a wide area around the site with chlorhexidine or povidone–iodine and drape in the usual sterile fashion.
- Make a wheal of lidocaine in the skin at the entry site and deep to the peritoneum. Remember to always aspirate while advancing the needle to make sure that a vessel is not entered.

Procedure

- Use a 30-mL syringe attached to an 18-g needle (use a spinal needle without a stylet for morbidly obese patients).
  - While aspirating, slowly advance the needle along the same tract until there is a return of ascetic fluid.
    - Pull the skin caudad or cephalad by 2 cm before inserting the needle, so that the resulting tract will be less likely to leak fluid after the procedure.
    - Alternatively, the "Z" technique can be used to help limit postparacentesis leak. This is done by inserting the needle halfway at an angle, then reangling it and advancing it the rest of the way to make a "Z"-like tract that will decrease a postprocedural leak of fluid (because the needle follows a nonlinear tract).
- Once the peritoneal cavity is entered, start drawing back ascitic fluid. Stop advancing the needle to avoid nicking the bowel.
- Remove the required sample fluid, and then withdraw the needle.
- Cover the insertion site with a sterile pressure dressing. Alternatively, if a significant leak continues, attach an ostomy bag to the site to catch the leaking ascetic fluid or place a figure-of-eight suture to close the site.

SPECIAL CONSIDERATIONS

- Keep the site clean and dry once completed.
- Monitor the patient after the procedure for hemodynamic instability; consider complications related to the procedure (e.g., vascular injury).
- Patients with concern for SBP require admission and IV antibiotics.
- If there is a large amount of ascites causing discomfort or difficulty breathing, the patient may require a large-volume paracentesis.

Complications

- Infection
- Vascular injury and bleeding
- Bowel perforation
- Continued ascites leak at site

REFERENCES

1. Orman ES, Hayashi PH, Bataller R, Barritt AS. Paracentesis is associated with reduced mortality in patients hospitalized with cirrhosis and ascites. *Clin Gastroenterol Hepatol* 2014;12(3):496.
2. Grabau CM, Crago SF, Hoff LK, et al. Performance standards for therapeutic abdominal paracentesis. *Hepatology* 2004;40(2):484.
3. McVay PA, Toy PT. Lack of increased bleeding after paracentesis and thoracentesis in patients with mild coagulation abnormalities. *Transfusion* 1991;31(2):164.
4. Stone JC, Moak JH. Feasibility of sonographic localization of the inferior epigastric artery before ultrasound-guided paracentesis. *Am J Emerg Med* 2015;33(12):1795–8.

128 Procedures: Pericardiocentesis

Mark D. Levine

GENERAL PRINCIPLES

- An emergent pericardiocentesis should be performed in the event of pericardial tamponade.
- Classically, patients will report severe dyspnea and anxiety.
- Hypotension, tachycardia, distended neck veins, muffled heart sounds, and pulsus paradoxus are often seen on physical examination.
- Transthoracic echocardiography is usually the initial diagnostic test of choice.
- As little as 50 mL of blood may cause tamponade.
- The patient in cardiac arrest from pericardial tamponade may present with pulseless electrical activity.

PROCEDURE

Preparation

- A time out should be performed.
- Adjust the height of the bed to a level comfortable to perform the procedure.
- Place the patient in the sitting position with the head elevated ~45 degrees.
- The patient should be on a cardiac monitor.
- Prep and drape the chest in the usual sterile fashion.
- The ultrasound view should be in the standard parasternal long axis or subxiphoid view.
- Local anesthetic should be infiltrated along the site of the planned needle entry, both superficial and deep to the skin surface, just above the rib (avoiding the neurovascular bundle).
- Attach a syringe (10 mL) to an 18- or 20-g needle at least 1½ inch long (or use the needle provided in a pericardiocentesis kit).

Procedure

- The best approach should aim for the region of maximal effusion with the fewest intervening structures.
- Aspirate as the needle is advanced until fluid is drawn back. The fluid should be nonclotting.
- Removal of 5–10 mL can improve cardiac output and blood pressure.
- If ultrasound is not available, this can be performed as a blind procedure. Enter the skin at a 45-degree angle at the xiphoid process, aiming toward the left scapular tip. It is recommended that continuous ECG monitoring be performed, and the V5 lead should be attached to the proximal end of the needle. As the needle touches the epicardium, there will be transmission of a current with an injury pattern (ST elevation or PVC). This monitoring is performed to prevent ventricular puncture.

SPECIAL CONSIDERATIONS

Disposition

- These patients should be admitted to the hospital for a pericardial window or definitive treatment of the pericardial effusion.

Complications

- Pneumothorax, myocardial injury, arrhythmia, cardiac arrest, RV damage, coronary artery damage, or liver injury

SUGGESTED READINGS

Mallemat MJ, Tewelde SZ. Pericardiocentesis. In Roberts JR, Custalow CB, Thomsen TW, eds. *Roberts and Hedges Clinical Procedures in Emergency Medicine*. Elselvier-Saunders. Philadelphia. 2014.

Chest Trauma. In: Jenkins JL, Loscalzo J, Braen GR, eds. *Manual of Emergency Medicine*. Little Brown and Company, NY: 1995:44–5.

Synovitz CK, Brown EJ. Pericardiocentesis. In: Tintinalli JE, Stapczynski J, Ma O, Yealy DM, Meckler GD, Cline DM. eds.Tintinalli's Emergency Medicine: A Comprehensive Study Guide, 8e New York, NY: McGraw-Hill.

129 Procedural Sedation

Louis Jamtgaard

GENERAL PRINCIPLES

- Procedural sedation is the technique of administering sedatives or dissociative agents with or without analgesia to induced altered consciousness that allows patients to tolerate unpleasant procedures, while preserving cardiorespiratory function.[1]

Levels of Sedation

- Minimal sedation: a drug-induced state with near-baseline level of alertness, with normal response to verbal commands. Cognitive function and coordination may be minimally impaired. Cardiorespiratory function is not compromised.[2]
- Moderate: a drug-induced state with depressed consciousness in which patients respond purposefully to verbal commands, either alone or with light tactile stimulation. Cardiorespiratory function is usually maintained.[3]
- Deep: a drug-induced state with depressed consciousness in which the patient cannot be easily aroused but responds purposefully to repeated painful stimulation. Cardiorespiratory function may be impaired.[3]

TABLE 129.1	American Society of Anesthesiologists (ASA) Physical Status Classification[12]
Status	Disease state
ASA class 1	No organic, physiologic, biochemical, or psychiatric disturbance
ASA class 2	Mild to moderate systemic disturbance that may not be related to the reason for surgery
ASA class 3	Severe systemic disturbance that may or may not be related to the reason for surgery
ASA class 4	Severe systemic disturbance that is life threatening with or without surgery
ASA class 5	Moribund patient who has little chance of survival but is submitted to surgery as a last resort (resuscitative effort)
Emergency operation (E)	

- Dissociative: A trancelike cataleptic state characterized by profound analgesia and amnesia, with retention of protective airway reflexes, spontaneous respirations, and cardiopulmonary stability.[4]
- *General anesthesia*: a drug-induced state with loss of consciousness in which patients are not arousable, even by painful stimulation. Independent cardiorespiratory function is often impaired. Patients may require assisted ventilation.[3]

Preprocedural Assessment

- Preprocedural sedation assessment should at minimum include evaluation of physical status, difficult airway features, prior anesthesia history, current medications, and any known allergies.
- Patients with poor physical status combined with associated difficult airway features should be considered for alternatives to ED procedural sedation, such as regional nerve blocks or the OR.
- Physical assessment should include evaluation of cardiorespiratory impairments and conditions that could potentially affect drug metabolism. The most accepted assessment of physical status continues to be the American Society of Anesthesiologist (ASA) physical classification system (Table 129.1). Increased adverse rates occur with ASA PS III or greater.[5] Consultation with anesthesiology should be considered in patients having an ASA PS IV.
- Airway Assessment
  - Sedation providers should be prepared to manage the patient's airway if airway control becomes necessary.
  - Airway evaluation should include assessment for difficult airway features, potential for difficult bag valve mask ventilation, laryngoscopy, and even rescue surgical airway.
  - Increasing Mallampati scale does predict difficulty laryngoscopy, and most features of the "MOANS" mnemonic have been correlated with difficult bag valve mask ventilation[6] (Fig. 129.1).

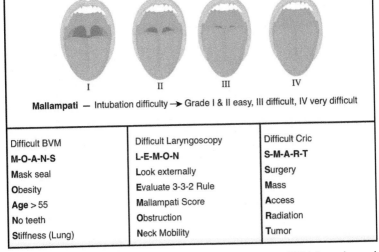

Mallampati — Intubation difficulty → Grade I & II easy, III difficult, IV very difficult

Difficult BVM	Difficult Laryngoscopy	Difficult Cric
M-O-A-N-S	**L-E-M-O-N**	**S-M-A-R-T**
Mask seal	Look externally	Surgery
Obesity	Evaluate 3-3-2 Rule	Mass
Age > 55	Mallampati Score	Access
No teeth	Obstruction	Radiation
Stiffness (Lung)	Neck Mobility	Tumor

Figure 129.1. Clinical predictors for difficult airway management. BVM, bag valve mask. (Modified from Walls RM. The Emergency Airway Algorithms. In: Walls RM, Murphy MF, eds. *Manual of Emergency Airway Management.* 4th ed. Philadelphia: Lippincott Williams and Wilkins, 2012:24, and Mallampati score by Jmarchn, used under CC BY-SA 3.0 via Wikimedia Commons. January 11, 2011.)

Set Up

- Perform informed consent for the sedation and planned procedure.
- Document weight (in kilograms) and last oral intake. Consult your hospital's NPO recommendations. Fasting for any time has not shown to reduce the risk of aspiration. Current recommendations are not to delay emergent procedures based on fasting times.[2]
- The patient should be monitored carefully using cardiac, NIBP, pulse oximetry, and continuous end tidal capnography monitoring.
- Current ASA guidelines recommend supplemental oxygen for all deep sedations unless contraindicated.[7]
- Have the bag valve mask (BVM), suction, nasal airway, and rescue airway equipment at bedside.
- Draw up and label syringes (including concentrations) of selected sedative and reversal agents.

Sedating Agents

- Select a sedative agent based on the patient's risk factors, the depth desired sedation, and length of the planned procedure (Table 129.2).

Postsedation Assessment

- Patients are still at risk for developing complications after their procedure is completed. This is most commonly from decreased procedural stimulation but may also result from delayed drug absorption and elimination. The following recommendations may reduce the risk of post procedural complications.

TABLE 129.2	Sedative Agents, Dosing, and Duration of Action		
Agent	Adult dose[8]	Duration	Comments
Ketamine	IV: 1–2 mg/kg over 30–60 s, then repeat half dose prn	10–15 min IV 30–60 min	Ideal for longer procedures. Avoid in HTN or Tachy pts. Common: emergence phenomenon, nausea
			Rare: laryngospasm
Propofol	IV: 0.5–1 mg/kg then 0.5 mg/kg q1–2min prn	3–10 min	Rapid onset and recovery. Ideal for muscle relaxation. Common: hypotension and apnea
Ketofol	IV: Mix 1:1 ratio, 1 mg/kg Propofol and ketamine. Give in 0.5 mg/kg increments[8]	15–30 min	Counterbalance hypotension and tachycardia. Analgesia and amnesia properties
Etomidate	IV: 0.1 mg/kg then 0.05 mg/kg q2–3 min prn	3–5 min	Hemodynamically stable. Myoclonus common
Midazolam	IV: 1–2 mg or 0.05 mg/kg then prn q2–3min	30–60 min	Respiratory depression and hypotension when rapidly administered
Fentanyl	IV: 1–2 mcg/kg, then 1 mcg/kg q3–5min prn	30–60 min	Minimal cardiovascular depression. Rare chest wall rigidity
Nitrous oxide	Same as peds	<5 min after discontinued	Needs cooperative patient. Contraindicated in pregnancy, Meal < 1h. Causes nausea, vomiting
Reversal agents			
Naloxone	IV: 0.01–0.1 mg/kg IV or IM typical dose 0.4 mg (max 2 mg)	20–40 min	Can precipitate opioid withdrawal
Flumazenil	0.01 mg/kg IV typical dose 0.2 mg	20–40 min	Use only in benzodiazepine naive patient

Adapted and modified from Reichman EF, Simon RR. *Emergency Medicine Procedures.* New York: McGraw-Hill, 2004:1006–8. Table 109-4.[8]

○ Consider keeping MD or RN at bedside until the patient is responding to voice.
○ Cardiac monitoring, $EtCO_2$, SpO_2 until the patient is responding to questions appropriately.
○ If reversal agent or multiple medications during the sedation are administered, observe for a minimum of 2 hours after the patient is able to answer questions appropriately.
○ Prior to discharge, preprocedural level of consciousness and mental status must be present. Ability to ambulate safely and tolerate oral fluids should be documented.[9]

Troubleshooting

- Serious adverse events during procedural sedation requiring medical intervention are rare.
  - Detectable respiratory events such as hypoxia and apnea may be precursors to more serious adverse events (respiratory failure, intubation, laryngospasm).[10]
  - Use of continuous end tidal CO_2 monitoring may detect unrecognized hypoventilation.
  - If hypoventilation is detected:
    - Stop administering the medication.
    - Position the patient, provide jaw thrust, and proceed to nasal airway placement and slow bag mask ventilation if there are still inadequate ventilations.
    - Consider reversal agents and advanced airway maneuvers (supraglottic airway, endotracheal intubation) if the above measures fail.

REFERENCES

1. Godwin SA, Caro DA, Wolf SJ, et al.; American College of Emergency Physicians. ACEP clinical policy: procedural sedation and analgesia in the emergency department. *Ann Emerg Med* 2005;45:177–96.
2. Godwin SA, Burton JH, Gerardo CJ, et al.; American College of Emergency Physicians. ACEP clinical policy: procedural sedation and analgesia in the emergency department. *Ann Emerg Med* 2014;63:247–58.
3. Centers for Medicare & Medicaid Services (CMS). Revised Appendix A, Interpretive Guidelines for Hospitals—State Operations Manual, Anesthesia Services. Effective December 2, 2011. Available at: http://www.cms.gov/Regulations-and-Guidance/Guidance/Transmittals/ downloads/R74SOMA.pdf (last accessed April 2016).
4. Green SM, Roback MG, Kennedy RM, Krauss B. Clinical practice guideline for emergency department ketamine dissociative sedation: 2011 update. *Ann Emerg Med* 2011;57:449–61.
5. Miller MA. Procedural sedation and analgesia in the emergency department: what are the risks? *Emerg Med Clin North Am* 2005;23(2):551–72.
6. Walls RM. The Emergency Airway Algorithms. In: Walls RM, Murphy MF, eds. *Manual of Emergency Airway Management.* 4th ed. Philadelphia: Lippincott Williams & Wilkins, 2012:24.
7. American Society of Anesthesiologists Task Force on Sedation and Analgesia by Non-Anesthesiologists. Practice guidelines for sedation and analgesia by non-anesthesiologists. *Anesthesiology* 2002;96:1004–17.
8. Reichman EF, Simon RR. *Emergency Medicine Procedures.* New York: McGraw-Hill, 2004:1006–8. Table 109-4.
9. Strayer R, Andrus P. Emergency Department Procedural Sedation and Analgesia Physician checklist. Available at: http://emupdates.com/2013/11/28/emergency-department-procedural-sedation-checklist-v2 (last accessed April 2016).
10. Bellolio MF, Gilani WI, Barrionuevo P, et al. Incidence of adverse events in adults undergoing procedural sedation in the emergency department: a systematic review and meta-analysis. *Acad Emerg Med* 2016;23:119–34.
11. American Society of Anesthesiologists. ASA Physical Status Classification System. October 15, 2014. Available at: https://www.asahq.org/resources/clinical-information/asa-physical-status-classification-system (last accessed April 2016).

130

Procedures: Resuscitation

Christina Creel-Bulos, Jacob Keeperman, and Christopher Holthaus

GENERAL PRINCIPLES

Definition

- Conventionally, resuscitation is used to denote interventions aimed at reversing shock or restoring life during prearrest or arrest conditions.
- Resuscitation, regardless of etiology, is fundamentally the act of restoring homeostasis to prevent irreversible deterioration and death.

Stress and Communication

- Resuscitations can be physically and emotionally stressful for all those involved.
- Training, effective communication skills, and debriefing can help to improve stress inoculation and interdisciplinary team dynamics when managing patients in extremis.

Crisis Management

- Crisis resource management is based on the principles of teamwork and establishment of a team leader.
- Development of standardized medical and traumatic resuscitation algorithms has facilitated organization and pattern recognition during intensely demanding times, optimizing provider performance and enhancing the provision of resuscitative care.[1,2]

Initial First Steps

- Prior to or upon entering the room, don personal protective gear and request IV placement, O_2 application, monitoring, advanced airway equipment, and ultrasound to the bedside.
- Check pulse and breathing, vital signs, "ABCD" (airway–breathing–circulation–disability) assessment.
- Intervene as indicated.
- Obtain blood sugar, case-specific labs, ECG, bedside ultrasound (FAST or RUSH exam to narrow potential shock etiologies), chest plain radiograph, and CTs as indicated.

Prearrest Care

AIRWAY COMPROMISE

Background

- The primary objective of performing an airway assessment is to evaluate a patient's ability to immediately maintain and ensure airway patency to allow adequate oxygenation and ventilation.

- Airway maintenance describes the ability to maintain airway patency and tone. Airway maintenance can be compromised by obstruction, malignancy, infection, inflammation, stenosis, sedation, or exogenous factors such as foreign body or trauma.[3]
- Airway protection refers to the ability to sense and protect against aspiration.[4-6] Loss of protective abilities is typically a result of neurocognitive impairment.

Assessment

- Symptoms of present or impending airway compromise depend on the degree of compromise but may include dyspnea, cough, chest tightness, chest pain, hoarseness, wheezing, hemoptysis, weakness, or light-headedness.[4]
- Observe for evidence of trauma, angioedema, or anxiety and distress (commonly manifested by tachypnea, hypopnea, tachycardia, accessory muscle use, drooling or inability to properly tolerate secretions, abnormal posturing, atypical respiratory rate, depth, and pattern, and cyanosis).
- Listening to the patient's vocalization can reveal hoarseness, stridor, gurgling, grunting, snorting, or wheezing.
- Eliciting a gag reflex has been used historically to denote an ability to protect the airway; however, the gag reflex can be absent up to 37% of the time in adults without airway compromise.[7] A patient's ability to phonate and handle his or her secretions has been shown to be more useful in assessing the need for protective intubation, and thus, the gag reflex testing should not be used in isolation.

Diagnostics and Monitoring

- While diagnostic adjuncts assist in the evaluation of a patient's ability to oxygenate, ventilate, and maintain his or her airway, they should not replace clinical assessment or supersede decisions made based on clinical assessment of decompensation.
- Methods of external monitoring and evaluation of oxygenation and ventilation may include pulse oximetry (POx) and end-tidal carbon dioxide ($EtCO_2$) monitoring.
- Although identification of airway compromise is rarely diagnosed via imaging modalities, radiography and computed tomography (CT) can demonstrate tracheal deviation or show evidence of dynamic airway or parenchymal collapse.[3]
- Methods of direct visual evaluation including video, fiberoptic, or direct laryngoscopy are useful in assessing and intervening in airway compromise.

Therapeutic Interventions

- Basic positional maneuvers (head-tilt, jaw-thrust) can be used to improve airflow and airway patency.
- Airway adjuncts such as nasopharyngeal and oropharyngeal airways may be used to assist with patency.
- Bag mask ventilation may be used while facilitating or preparing for a definitive airway in a patient who does not respond to the above maneuvers or adjuncts or is apneic or in cardiopulmonary arrest.
- Validated predictors of difficult ventilation are described in the "MOANS" acronym (see figure 129.1).[8,9]

BREATHING OR RESPIRATORY COMPROMISE

Background

- Cerebral regulation of respiratory muscle coordination and breathing occurs through signal intake from various centrally and peripherally based neural and chemical receptors throughout the body.[10]
- Isolated hypoxic respiratory failure is the result of impaired oxygenation and can improve with oxygen administration.
- Hypercapnic respiratory failure is the result of impaired ventilation and often requires an improvement in minute ventilation (tidal volume × respiratory rate).

Assessment

- Patients suffering from impending respiratory failure may report anxiety, agitation, dyspnea, confusion, cough, chest tightness, pain, wheezing, weakness, fatigue, or light-headedness.
- Clinical signs of respiratory compromise may include decreased or absent aeration, hypoxia, hypercarbia, tachypnea, hypopnea, tachycardia, accessory muscle use, abnormal posturing, atypical respiratory rate, depth, and pattern, anxiety, confusion, apnea, cyanosis, and arrest.
- It is important to assess for both hypoxia and hypercapnia since both can present similarly with restlessness, agitation, mental status changes, and cyanosis.

Diagnostics and Monitoring

- Pulse oximetry may affected by motion artifact, hypotension, vasoconstriction, anemia, carboxyhemoglobinemia, or methemoglobinemia. Additionally, the delay time associated with continuous oxygen saturation monitoring can postpone detection (20- to 90-second) of a hypoxic event.[1]
- Capnography can be useful in assessing respiratory illness and ventilation adequacy in obtunded patients or patients undergoing procedural sedation. In intubated patients, capnography can be used to confirm and monitor endotracheal tube placement.[2]

Therapeutic Interventions

- Oxygen administration via low-flow oxygen is typically an initial intervention.[11,12]
- Noninvasive positive pressure ventilation (NIPPV) may benefit atraumatic, conscious, and hemodynamically stable patients suffering from hypercapnic respiratory failure.[13,14]
- NIPPV has been shown to lower intubation rates in patients suffering from acute COPD exacerbations and cardiogenic pulmonary edema.[15]
- BiPAP provides bilevel inspiratory pressure to decrease the work of breathing with inspiration as well as positive end-expiratory pressure to maintain optimal alveolar recruitment and may be better than CPAP in cardiogenic pulmonary edema.
- When NIPPV fails to improve or correct a patient's ability to oxygenate or ventilate, a definitive airway must be established.

CARDIOVASCULAR COMPROMISE

Background

- Shock etiologies are generally classified into groups: hypovolemic, distributive, cardiogenic, or obstructive.
  - Hypovolemic shock can be hemorrhagic or nonhemorrhagic (i.e., vomiting, diarrhea, osmotic or diuretic-induced diuresis, third spacing/capillary leak).

○ Distributive shock can have an infectious or noninfectious etiology (i.e., neurogenic, anaphylaxis, endocrine, pancreatitis, drugs).
○ Cardiogenic shock arises from cardiac etiologies.
○ Obstructive shock is caused by vascular or mechanical obstruction.

Assessment

- Symptoms associated with shock can include anxiety, confusion, syncope, lightheadedness, dyspnea, and diaphoresis.
- Systemic and organ-based signs of shock include ill appearance, altered mentation, pallor, diaphoresis, grunting, tachypnea, hypoxia, abnormal breath sounds, tachycardia, hypotension, jugular venous distension, decreased heart sounds, decreased capillary refill, cold or warm skin, distended abdomen, GI bleeding, and decreased urine output.
- Classifications include compensated (normotensive), uncompensated, and irreversible multisystem organ failure.

Diagnostics and Monitoring

- Initial workup, laboratory values, and imaging may offer further insight as to the etiology and extent of shock. Serum lactate levels can assist with early recognition and assessment of systemic perfusion.[16]
- The "RUSH" ultrasound exam is extremely useful in rapidly ruling in or out shock etiologies at the bedside.
- Noninvasive methods for monitoring end-organ perfusion include trending of hourly urine output (goal ≥ 0.5 mL/kg/h), heart rate, and systolic and mean arterial pressures (goal MAP ≥ 40 mm Hg in active traumatic hemorrhage; MAP ≥ 65 mm Hg in other forms of shock).[17,18]
- Methods of invasive hemodynamic monitoring include central venous oxygen saturation, central venous and arterial pressure measurements.

Therapeutic Interventions

- Obtain adequate vascular access with two large-bore peripheral IVs, intraosseous access, or central venous access.
- Begin isotonic intravenous fluid resuscitation.
- When large volume resuscitation is anticipated, consider a "balanced" or "chloride-restrictive" crystalloid solution (i.e., lactated Ringer's or PlasmaLyte).[19–21]
- Vasopressors, inotropic therapy, or a combination of both is indicated if hypotension persists despite adequate intravascular volume repletion or if volume administration is met without a response (Tables 130.1 and 130.2).

INTRA-ARREST CARE

Basic Life Support

- Basic life support (BLS) aims to achieve rapid return of spontaneous circulation by providing high-quality, minimally interrupted chest compressions and early defibrillation.
- Compressions should be administered with the patient's body against a firm surface, at a rate of at 100–120 beats/min with an associated depth of 2–2.4 inches.[22]

TABLE 130.1	Commonly Used Vasopressors	
Medication	Dosage	Mechanism of action: receptor agonism
Dopamine	2–20 mcg/kg/min	Alpha, beta, and dopaminergic
Epinephrine	0.05–0.5 mcg/kg/min	Alpha and beta
Norepinephrine	0.02–2 mcg/kg/min	Alpha and beta
Phenylephrine	0.02–2 mcg/kg/min	Alpha
Vasopressin	0.01–0.04 units/min	V1

- Continuous capnography is useful in determining the adequacy of compressions (indicated by $PETCO_2 > 10$ mm Hg) and in observing for return of spontaneous circulation (indicated by $PETCO_2 > 40$ mm Hg).[23,24]

Advanced Cardiac Life Support

- Advanced cardiac life support (ACLS) aims to provide rapid intervention for non-perfusing rhythms or severely impaired perfusion. While specific guidelines are updated regularly, it is important to always provide high-quality compressions and cardiopulmonary resuscitation (Table 130.3).
- During asystolic and pulseless electrical arrests, electrical intervention is ineffective, and resuscitation efforts are centered on provision of high-quality BLS maneuvers, administration of epinephrine, and identification of potential reversible etiologies for arrest.[24]
- Ventricular arrests employ both electrical and chemical interventions, including early defibrillation, administration of epinephrine, and (if indicated) additional administration of amiodarone, lidocaine, or magnesium.[25]
- Interventions for symptomatic bradycardia with concomitant evidence of inadequate tissue perfusion include administration of atropine, transcutaneous or transvenous pacing, and administration of chronotropic agents (e.g., epinephrine or dopamine) if refractory bradycardia persists.[24,26]
- The treatment of severely symptomatic tachycardia is based on two factors: the hemodynamic stability of the patient and the observed duration of the QRS complex. Hemodynamic stability may commence with chemical intervention, while instability requires immediate electrical cardioversion.

TABLE 130.2	Commonly Used Inotropes	
Medication	Dosage	Mechanism of action
Dobutamine	2–20 mcg/kg/min	Beta
Milrinone	0.25–0.75 mcg/kg/min	Phosphodiesterase inhibition

TABLE 130.3 Advanced Cardiac Life Support Medications Reference[40]

Medication	Initial intravenous dosing	Subsequent intravenous dosing
Nonperfusing rhythms		
Epinephrine	1 mg	Repeat every 3–5 min
Amiodarone	300 mg	150 mg
Lidocaine	1–1.5 mg/kg	0.5–0.75 mg/kg every 5–10 min
Magnesium sulfate	2 g	3–20 mg/min infusion
Rhythms of impaired perfusion		
Bradyarrhythmias		
Atropine	0.5 mg	Repeat every 3–5 min for maximum 3 mg
Dopamine infusion	2–20 mcg/kg/min	—
Epinephrine infusion	2–10 mcg/min	—
Tachyarrhythmias		
Adenosine	6 mg	May repeat additional two doses of 12 mg
Diltiazem	15–20 mg	5–10 mg/h infusion
Metoprolol	5 mg	Repeat every 2–5 min for maximum 15 mg
Amiodarone	150 mg over 10 min	0.5 mg/min infusion
Procainamide	15–17 mg/kg over 30 min	20–50 mg/min infusion

- Narrow QRS (<0.12 seconds) complex tachycardias may benefit from adenosine, calcium channel blockade, or beta blockade; wide QRS (>0.12 seconds) complex tachycardias traditionally respond to agents such as amiodarone, sotalol, or procainamide.[24,26]

POSTARREST CARE

Background

- The goals of postarrest resuscitative care include optimization of cardiopulmonary function and vital organ perfusion, identification and treatment of the precipitating cause of the arrest, prevention of recurrent arrest, controlling body temperature to optimize neurologic recovery, identification and treatment of ACS, optimizing mechanical ventilation to minimize lung injury, and reducing the risk of multiorgan injury and supporting organ function as required.[15]

Therapeutics

- Hemodynamic support and optimization aims to prevent secondary injury and additional ischemic insult; thus, regulation and management of cerebral and end-organ perfusion are crucial.
  - Cerebral autoregulation may be impaired in postarrest patient populations; thus, higher MAP goals should be set (minimum ≥65 mm Hg; 80–100 mm Hg to optimize cerebral perfusion).[27–30]
  - Fluid, vasopressor, and inotropic therapy should be individually tailored.
  - Consideration of the potential need for revascularization should be given regarding patients with persistent cardiovascular shock.
- Respiratory support and optimization centers on the avoidance of extremes of carbon dioxide and oxygenation. Current recommendations exist to guide postarrest goals as follows: $PaCO_2$ (35–45 mm Hg), $EtCO_2$ (30–40 mm Hg), and POx (94%).[24,31–33,48]
- Targeted Temperature Management (32–36°C)[15,50]: Fever and hyperthermia should be avoided in postarrest patients.
- Glycemic Control—is controversial although the avoidance of hyper- or hypoglycemia through liberal glycemic control may be beneficial in postarrest patients.
- Prophylaxis—patients with prolonged ED stays and without contraindications should receive standard ICU measures for venous thromboembolism, head-of-bed elevation, and stress ulcer prophylaxis.

ADVANCED RESUSCITATION

Extracorporeal Membrane Oxygenation

- Extracorporeal membrane oxygenation (ECMO) provides cardiopulmonary support to patients with severe, but reversible, respiratory or cardiovascular failure unresponsive to conventional methods.[34,35]
- E-CPR is the term given to ECMO performed during or immediately following cardiac arrest.
- Indications include hypoxemic respiratory failure with a PaO_2/FiO_2 ratio of <100 mm Hg despite ventilator optimization; hypercapnic respiratory failure with an arterial pH < 7.20; and refractory cardiogenic shock and cardiac arrest.
- Contraindications include inability to anticoagulate the patient.[36,37]
- Complications include bleeding secondary to platelet dysfunction and continuous heparin infusion, thromboembolism, heparin-induced thrombocytopenia, and cannulation complications such as vessel perforation, hemorrhage, dissection, and subsequent ischemia.[38]

REFERENCES

1. Meyers CW, Scott. Respiratory monitoring in the emergency department. *J Emerg Crit Care* 2011;1(1):12. Available at: http://www.ebmedicine.net/topics.php?paction=showTopic&topic_id=264 (last accessed 4/11/16).
2. Nagler J, Krauss B. Capnography: a valuable tool for airway management. *Emerg Med Clin North Am* 2008;26(4):881–97, vii.
3. Ernst A, Feller-Kopman D, Becker HD, Mehta AC. Central airway obstruction. *Am J Respir Crit Care Med* 2004;169:1278.

4. Shorten GD, Opie NJ,Graziotti P, et al. Assessment of upper airway anatomy in awake, sedated and anaesthetised patients using magnetic resonance imaging. *Anaesth Intensive Care* 1994;22:165.

5. Reza Shariatzadeh M, Huang JQ, Marrie TJ. Differences in the features of aspiration pneumonia according to site of acquisition: community or continuing care facility. *J Am Geriatr Soc* 2006;54:296.

6. Christ A, Arranto CA, Schindler C, et al. Incidence, risk factors, and outcome of aspiration pneumonitis in ICU overdose patients. *Intensive Care Med* 2006;32:1423.

7. Davies AE, Kidd D, Stone SP, MacMahon J. Pharyngeal sensation and gag reflex in healthy subjects. *Lancet* 1995;345(8948):487–8.

8. Langeron O, Masso E, Huraux C, et al. Prediction of difficult mask ventilation. *Anesthesiology* 2000;92:1229–36.

9. Kheterpal S, Han R, Tremper K, et al. Incidence and predictors of difficult and impossible mask ventilation. *Anesthesiology* 2006;105:885–91.

10. Horner RL, Bradley TD. Update in sleep and control of ventilation 2006. *Am J Respir Crit Care Med* 2007;175(5):426–31.

11. Bateman NT, Leach RM. Acute oxygen therapy. *BMJ* 1998;317(7161):798–801.

12. Frat JP, Thille AW, Mercat A, et al. High-flow oxygen through nasal cannula in acute hypoxemic respiratory failure. *N Engl J Med* 2015;372:2185.

13. Lenique F, Habis M, Lofaso F, et al. Ventilatory and hemodynamic effects of continuous positive airway pressure in left heart failure. *Am J Respir Crit Care Med* 1997;155:500–5.

14. Celikel T, Sungur M, Ceyhan B, Karakurt S. Comparison of noninvasive positive pressure ventilation with standard medical therapy in hypercapnic acute respiratory failure. *Chest* 1998;114:1636.

15. Callaway CW, Donnino MW, Fink EL, et al. Part 8: post-cardiac arrest care: 2015 American Heart Association guidelines update for cardiopulmonary resuscitation and emergency cardiovascular care. *Circulation* 2015;132(18 Suppl 2):S465–82.

16. Junhasavasdikul D, Theerawit P, Ingsathit A, Kiatboonsri S. Lactate and combined parameters for triaging sepsis patients into intensive care facilities. *J Crit Care* 2016;33:71–7.

17. Asfar P Meziani F, Hamel JF, et al. High versus low blood-pressure target in patients with septic shock. *N Engl J Med* 2014;370:1583.

18. Antonelli M, Levy M, Andrews PJ, et al. Hemodynamic monitoring in shock and implications for management. International Consensus Conference, Paris, France, 27–28 April 2006. *Intensive Care Med* 2007;33(4):575–90.

19. Yunos N, Bellomo R, Hegarty C, et al. Association between a chloride-liberal vs chloride-restrictive intravenous fluid administration strategy and kidney injury in critically ill adults. *JAMA* 2012;308(15):1566–72.

20. Raghunathan K, Shaw A, Nathanson B, et al. Association between the choice of IV crystalloid and in-hospital mortality among critically ill adults with sepsis. *Crit Care Med* 2014;42(7):1585–91.

21. Raghunathan K, Bonavia A, Nathanson BH, et al. Association between initial fluid choice and subsequent in-hospital mortality during the resuscitation of adults with septic shock. *Anesthesiology* 2015;123(6):1385–93.

22. Kleinman ME, Brennan EE, Goldberger ZD, et al. Part 5: adult basic life support and cardiopulmonary resuscitation quality: 2015 American Heart Association guidelines update for cardiopulmonary resuscitation and emergency cardiovascular care. *Circulation* 2015;132:414–35.

23. Falk JL, Racknow EC, Weil MH. End-tidal carbon dioxide concentration during cardiopulmonary resuscitation. *N Engl J Med* 1988;318:607.

24. Link MS, Berkow LC, Kudenchuk PJ, et al. Part 7: adult advanced cardiovascular life support: 2015 American Heart Association guidelines update for cardiopulmonary resuscitation and emergency cardiovascular care. *Circulation* 2015;132:444–64.

25. Brady WJ, Laughrey TS, Ghaemmaghami CA. Cardiac Rhythm Disturbances. In: Tintinalli JE, Stapczynski JS, Ma OJ, et al., eds. *Tintinalli's Emergency Medicine: A Comprehensive Study Guide.* 8th ed. New York: McGraw-Hill Education, 2016.

26. Neumar RW, Otto CW, Link MS, et al. Part 8: adult advanced cardiovascular life support: 2010 American Heart Association guidelines for cardiopulmonary resuscitation and emergency cardiovascular care. *Circulation* 2010;122:729.

27. Spaulding CM, Joly LM, Rosenberg A, et al. Immediate coronary angiography in survivors of out-of-hospital cardiac arrest. *N Engl J Med* 1997;336:1629.

28. Sundgreen C, Larsen FS, Herzog TM, et al. Autoregulation of cerebral blood flow in patients resuscitated from cardiac arrest. *Stroke* 2001;32:128.

29. Donnino MW, Rittenberger JC, Gaieski D, et al. The development and implementation of cardiac arrest centers. *Resuscitation* 2011;82:974.

30. Gaieski DF, Band RA, Abella BS, et al. Early goal-directed hemodynamic optimization combined with therapeutic hypothermia in comatose survivors of out-of-hospital cardiac arrest. *Resuscitation* 2009;80:418.

31. Wang CH, Chang WT, Huang CH, et al. The effect of hyperoxia on survival following adult cardiac arrest: a systematic review and meta-analysis of observational studies. *Resuscitation* 2014;85:1142–8.

32. Damiani E, Adrario E, Girardis M, et al. Arterial hyperoxia and mortality in critically ill patients: a systematic review and meta-analysis. *Crit Care* 2014;18:711.

33. Zeiner A, Holzer M, Sterz F, et al. Hyperthermia after cardiac arrest is associated with an unfavorable neurologic outcome. *Arch Intern Med* 2001;161:2007.

34. ELSO Guidelines for Cardiopulmonary Extracorporeal Life Support. Extracorporeal Life Support Organization. 2013. Available at: www.elsonet.org (last accessed 4/14/16).

35. Tsai HC, Chang CH, Tsai FC, et al. Acute respiratory distress syndrome with and without extracorporeal membrane oxygenation: a score matched study. *Ann Thorac Surg* 2015;100:458–64.

36. Hemmila MR, Rowe SA, Boules TN, et al. Extracorporeal life support for severe acute respiratory distress syndrome in adults. *Ann Surg* 2004;240:595.

37. Peek GJ, Moore HM, Moore N, et al. Extracorporeal membrane oxygenation for adult respiratory failure. *Chest* 1997;112:759.

38. Wilson JM, Bower LL, Fackler JC, et al. Aminocaproic acid decreases the incidence of intracranial hemorrhage and other hemorrhagic complications of ECMO. *J Pediatr Surg* 1993;28:536.

39. Perera P, Mailhot T, Riley D, Mandavia D. The RUSH exam: rapid ultrasound in shock in the evaluation of the critically Ill. *Emerg Med Clin North Am* 2010;28(1):29–56, vii.

40. Link MS, Atkins DL, Passman RS, et al. Part 6: electrical therapies: automated external defibrillators, defibrillation, cardioversion, and pacing: 2010 American Heart Association guidelines for cardiopulmonary resuscitation and emergency cardiovascular care. *Circulation* 2010(122):S706.

41. Aufderheide TP, Lurie KG. Death by hyperventilation: a common and life-threatening problem during cardiopulmonary resuscitation. *Crit Care Med* 2004;32(9 Suppl):S345–51.

42. Suffoletto B, Peberdy MA, van der Hoek T, Callaway C. Body temperature changes are associated with outcomes following in-hospital cardiac arrest and return of spontaneous circulation. *Resuscitation* 2009;80:1365.

131 Procedures: Splinting

Steven Hung

GENERAL PRINCIPLES

- Splinting decreases pain and prevents further injury and is sometimes a definitive treatment for some injuries.
- Splinting, in contrast to circumferential casting, allows for swelling of the extremity.

TREATMENT

- Splinting is often done with plaster.
  - When plaster comes in contact with water, it will harden over 2–8 minutes in an exothermic reaction, gaining full strength in about 24 hours.
  - Hotter water allows for faster setting time, but it also generates more heat due to the exothermic reaction and may injure the patient.
- Other methods of splinting include but are not limited to preformed plaster, fiberglass, air splints, aluminum, and preformed plastic splints.

Indications

- Fracture

Contraindications

- There are no absolute contraindications to splinting.
- Relative contraindications include injuries that need immediate definitive management such as open fractures, fracture with compartment syndrome, or neurovascular compromise.

PROCEDURE

Preparation

- Expose the injured extremity, examine neurovascular status, and examine for other wounds, dressing skin abrasions with petroleum-impregnated gauze prior to placing splint over them.
- Position the extremity in position of function.

Equipment

- Cotton padding
- plaster
- room temperature water
- stockinette
- elastic compression bandage

Procedure

- Provide adequate pain control with analgesics and/or procedural sedation.

- Measure out the plaster. It should extend to the joint above and below the site of injury when possible and should cover the width of the extremity.
  - Cut/tear off 10 layers.
- Use a stockinette to cover the area to be splinted.
- Wrap the area smoothly with cotton padding and use extra padding over bony prominences to prevent skin breakdown.
  - Avoid wrinkles on the skin side of the plaster as these can cause pressure points.
- Immerse the plaster in water and wring out.
- Smooth out to remove excess water until the layers are indistinguishable.
  - Grip plaster between thumb and index and run the length of plaster, stripping it to remove excess water and place on towel and smooth the plaster out.
- Apply the plaster to the extremity, molding it to place. Do not place the plaster circumferentially around the extremity.
- (Optional) Place additional layer of cotton padding over the plaster to prevent the elastic bandage from sticking to the plaster.
- Wrap the extremity firmly but not tightly in an elastic bandage.
- Mold the plaster into the desired position; hold until the plaster starts to set.
- Evaluate neurovascular status after splint placement.
- Obtain postsplint plain radiographs if needed.
- Upper extremity splints
  - Sugar-tong splints—arm held flexed at 90 degrees at the elbow, forearm in neutral
    - Proximal sugar-tong splint—humeral fractures
      □ Apply plaster from axilla, around the elbow, and back up the arm on the other side
    - Distal sugar-tong splint—wrist and distal forearm fractures
      □ Apply plaster from the metacarpophalangeal joints, around the elbow, and back up to midpalm
    - Double sugar-tong splint—elbow and forearm fractures
      □ Combination of proximal and distal sugar-tong splint
    - Reverse sugar-tong splint—Colles fracture
      □ Cut the plaster partially transversely around the midpoint, leaving a small strip the length of the web space between the thumb and index finger. Apply the plaster at that web space, wrapping along each side of the forearm and wrapping around the elbow.
  - Long arm splint (posterior splint)—arm held flexed at 90 degrees at the elbow, forearm in neutral
    - Injuries of the elbow (e.g., supracondylar fracture)
      □ Apply the plaster along the posterior of the arm, elbow, and forearm up to the wrist.
  - Dorsal/volar splint
    - Carpal tunnel syndrome, fractures of the wrist
      □ Apply plaster from midpalm to almost the elbow, on either the dorsal or volar side.
  - Gutter splint
    - Phalangeal and metacarpal fractures
      □ Extend from the proximal forearm beyond the distal interphalangeal joint, on either the radial or ulnar surface; the splint needs to be wide enough to surround both fingers and the wrist.
    - Cut a hole for the thumb before applying the radial gutter splint.
  - Thumb spica splint
    - Scaphoid fractures, injury of ulnar collateral ligament
      □ Apply on the radial aspect of the forearm, wrapping the thumb up to the distal interphalangeal joint.

- Lower extremity splints
  - Short leg splint
    - Distal leg, ankle, tarsal, and metatarsal fractures
      - Apply plaster along the midposterior calf down to the foot.
      - Apply plaster in a stirrup/sugar-tong fashion around the ankle; alternatively can have a strip of plaster wrap around from the calf around ankle on each side, ending just superior to the contralateral ankle.
      - Do not compress the fibular head as this can affect the peroneal nerve.
  - Long leg splint
    - Used to stabilize distal femur and proximal tibia/fibula fracture
      - Apply plaster along posterior leg from proximal hip to foot, having the knee flexed about 15 degrees with the leg propped on pillows

SPECIAL CONSIDERATIONS

Complications
- Pain from increased swelling—The first step should be to loosen the elastic bandage; if this does not resolve the pain, remove the splint and create a new one.
- Skin breakdown
- Infection

Patient Education
- Keep the splint clean and dry.
- Return for increasing pain, numbness, or tingling.
- Give patient sling or crutches based upon weight-bearing status.

SUGGESTED READINGS

Fitch MT, Nicks BA, Pariyadath M, et al. Videos in clinical medicine. Basic splinting techniques. *N Engl J Med* 2008;359(26):e32.

Menkes JS. Initial Evaluation and Management of Orthopedic Injuries. In: Tintinalli JE, Stapczynski J, Ma O, et al., eds. *Tintinalli's Emergency Medicine: A Comprehensive Study Guide.* 8th ed. New York: McGraw-Hill, 2016.

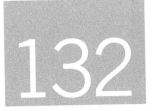

132 Procedures: Suturing

Steven Hung and Michael Willman

GENERAL PRINCIPLES

- Laceration closure can be performed with the use of sutures, adhesive bandages, staples, and/or tissue glue.
- The goal of wound repair is to decrease the tension on the wound to promote cosmesis, prevent wound infection, and increase hemostasis.

- A history and examination should be performed, taking into consideration:
  - Mechanism
    - Bites are at the highest risk of infection and generally should not be closed.
    - Stab wounds are at higher risk of injuring deep structures.
    - Contamination.
  - Time since injury
    - There are no well-defined studies; however, it is generally agreed that lacerations repaired earlier, usually within 24 hours, heal better.
  - Extent
    - Examine for nerve, vascular, bony, and tendon injury.
    - When examining for tendon injury, make sure the area injured is moved through its entire range of motion and the tendon is visualized through that range, if the wound is open.
  - Foreign bodies left in wounds will delay healing and increase risk of infection.
    - Most foreign bodies should be removed. However, nonirritating material, such as metal (e.g., bullet fragments) or glass, can be safely left in place if not near a vital structure (e.g., major vessel, joint space).
    - Wound inspection may reveal a foreign body; however, puncture wounds may leave foreign bodies in a deep position that are difficult to palpate.
    - Plain radiographs may be helpful in identifying radiopaque objects.
    - Ultrasound may be able to identify nonradiopaque objects.
  - Cosmetic importance—Location and cosmesis will help determine the type of closure used.

Indications
- Uncomplicated wounds that present within 18 hours of injury (up to 24 hours for facial injuries)

Contraindications
Relative
- Significantly delayed presentation
- Heavy contamination, bite wounds, retained foreign body
  - Exception—Bite wounds to face can often be closed due to its extensive vascularity.
- Deep puncture wounds
- Superficial wounds (such as abrasions) that would be expected to heal well on their own
- Disease processes that may lead to poor wound healing
  - May be candidates for delayed primary closure

PROCEDURE

Preparation
- Position the injured area to allow for easy wound closure and patient comfort.
- Raise bed to a position for operator comfort.
- Irrigation—most important intervention to decrease risk of infection.
  - Normal saline is most commonly used. However, tap water can also be used with no clinically significant difference in outcome.[1,2]
  - Should be of sufficient pressure to dislodge bacteria—such pressure (2–3 lb/in²) can be obtained by attaching an 18-gauge catheter to a syringe.
  - Should be of sufficient volume, ranging from 100 to 1000 mL depending on the location and contamination of the wound.
  - When irrigating, use a spray shield or face mask to prevent exposure.

- Hair
  - Shaving of hair can cause increased infection rate.
  - Use antibiotic ointment to hold the hair out of the field.
  - Some scalp lacerations are amendable to repair with hair tying.
- Debridement
  - Remove devitalized tissue to help prevent infection or wound dehiscence.
- Remove any foreign bodies.

Equipment

- Suture
  - Size—Suture size is inversely proportional to the number.
    - 1-0 and 2-0: for deep wounds with high tension
    - 3-0: for moderate tension
    - 4-0: for minimal tension (most commonly used)
    - 5-0 and 6-0: for facial wounds
  - Type
    - Monofilament—less reactive to tissue but requires more knots to hold
    - Braided—fewer knots needed
  - Material—no significant difference in cosmetic result between absorbable and nonabsorbable sutures[3]
    - Absorbable—does not require removal but has decreased tensile strength
    - Nonabsorbable—higher tensile strength, requires follow-up and removal
- Needle holder, forceps, scissors
- Antiseptic solution, drape, dressing, gauze
- Lidocaine, syringe, needles
- Sterile/nonsterile gloves
  - There is no significant difference in infection risk between sterile and nonsterile gloves (for uncomplicated wounds in immunocompetent patients with normal wound healing).[4]

Procedure

- Use universal precautions. This is an aseptic procedure.
- Anesthetize the wound.
  - Local anesthesia with lidocaine is appropriate. Allow the medicine to take effect prior to suturing the skin. Be aware of total lidocaine dose administered to the patient. There is potential for toxicity with total doses >4.5 mg/kg of 1% lidocaine (or ~0.5 mL/kg).
- Irrigate the wound, and after irrigation, clean the wound edges (not inside) with iodine antiseptic solution. Apply clean drapes around the wound as appropriate.
- Deep "buried" sutures (Fig. 132.1)
  - Placed when there is a large wound and high tension is expected with the percutaneous sutures, or to help approximate the wound edges for improved cosmesis.
  - Absorbable sutures must be used for deep sutures, as these will not be removed.
  - The needle is introduced in the dermis, directed toward the skin surface, and then inserted on opposite side at the dermal–epidermal junction and directed into the dermis (deep–superficial then superficial–deep). The knot is then tied and buried in the dermis.
- Simple interrupted sutures (Fig. 132.2A)
  - The needle is introduced at 90-degree angle to the skin surface and pushed through by turning the wrist. Introduce the needle to the opposing side at the same depth to ensure proper cosmesis.

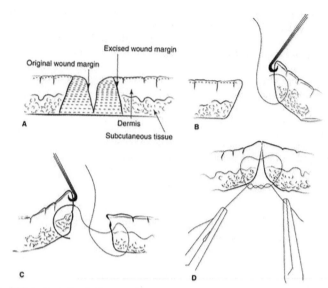

Figure 132.1. Deep "buried" suture placement.

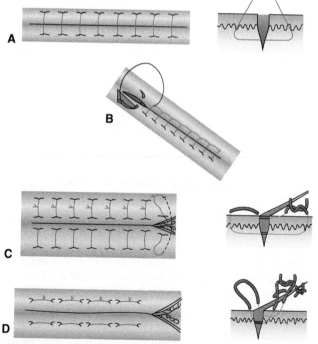

Figure 132.2. Simple, horizontal mattress, and vertical mattress suture placement.

- The distance from the wound edge and depth of insertion should be similar to the thickness of the dermis of the wound location.
- Distance between sutures should be roughly similar to distance between entry point and exit point of the sutures, but this may vary depending on the wound. The goal is to minimize and close any gaps in the wound.
- Skin eversion (outward) is recommended to provide good cosmesis.
- The number of ties will depend on the suture type, typically 6 ties (3 complete knots) for braided suture and 8 ties (4 complete knots) for monofilament.
- Running sutures (Fig. 132.2B)
  - Rapid closure applying even tension along the length of the wound. However, if the suture breaks at one point, the whole repair becomes undone.
  - Started similar to simple interrupted, without cutting the first knot, it is continued through the length of the wound with the last bite left as a loose loop to act as the free end to tie the knot.
- Vertical mattress sutures (Fig. 132.2C)
  - Used for wounds with high tension
  - Insert the needle at a distance from the wound edge, going deep through the dermis and exiting at an equal distance on the other side of the wound ("far–far").
  - Reinsert the needle closer to the wound edge on the same side and exit on the opposite side at the same distance (near–near).
  - The knot is then tied with the tail of the suture from the initial step.
- Horizontal mattress sutures (Fig. 132.2D)
  - Used for wounds with high tension
  - The suture is started like a simple interrupted. However, instead of tying a knot, the needle is reinserted at a distance of a short distance from the exit site along the wound and finished up back on the other side (like performing a simple interrupted in the other direction).
  - This exit site is then tied with the tail of the entry site.

POTENTIAL COMPLICATIONS

- Infection
- Wound dehiscence
- Poor cosmetic result

SPECIAL CONSIDERATIONS

- Consider specialist consultation if the wounds involve the eye, genitalia, hands, joint spaces, vascular, nerve, or tendon injuries. High-pressure or severely contaminated wounds may also need operative washout.
- Antibiotic ointment can be applied to wound if nonabsorbable suture was used.
- Patients can shower; however, patients should not soak the wound (e.g., no baths or swimming) and should dab the wound dry (instead of rubbing).
- Advise all patients there will be a scar. To improve cosmesis, they should use sunscreen when out in the sun and that final scar formation could take up to 1 year to take final form.
- Prophylactic antibiotics are not needed for minor wounds in healthy patients. Bite wounds, however, may require antibiotics.
- Suture removal will depend on the site.
  - Eyelids: 3 days
  - Neck: 3–4 days

- ○ Face: 5 days
- ○ Trunk and upper extremities: 7 days
- ○ Scalp: 7–14 days
- ○ Lower extremities: 8–10 days

REFERENCES

1. Fernandez R, Griffiths R. Water for wound cleansing. *Cochrane Database Syst Rev* 2008;(1):CD003861. doi: 10.1002/14651858.CD003861.pub2.
2. Moscati RM, Mayrose J, Reardon RF, et al. A multicenter comparison of tap water versus sterile saline for wound irrigation. *Acad Emerg Med* 2007;14(5):404–9.
3. Karounis H, Gouin S, Eisman H, et al. A randomized, controlled trial comparing long-term cosmetic outcomes of traumatic pediatric lacerations repaired with absorbable plain gut versus non-absorbable nylon sutures. *Acad Emerg Med* 2004;11(7):730–5.
4. Perelman VS, Francis GJ, Rutledge T, et al. Sterile versus nonsterile gloves for repair of uncomplicated lacerations in the emergency department: a randomized controlled trial. *Ann Emerg Med* 2004;43(3):362–70.
5. Mansouri M, Tidley M, Sanati KA, Roberts C. Comparison of blood transmission through latex and nitrile glove materials. *Occup Med (Lond)* 2010;60(3):205–10. doi: 10.1093/occmed/kqp196.
6. Cummings P, Del Beccaro MA. Antibiotics to prevent infection of simple wounds: a meta-analysis of randomized studies. *Am J Emerg Med* 1995;13(4):396.

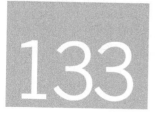

133

Procedures: Thoracostomy

Michael Willman and Nathan Woltman

GENERAL PRINCIPLES

- A tube thoracostomy (i.e., chest tube) is performed to treat an abnormal accumulation of air or fluid in the pleural space (e.g., pneumothorax, hemothorax, empyema).
- Open thoracostomies are more commonly performed than closed (percutaneous) types in the ED. Controversy exists over the appropriate size of chest tube for traumatic hemothorax. Some early data suggest that using smaller (thus better tolerated) tubes may not change outcome.[1,2]
- Local anesthesia with lidocaine is appropriate. Allow the medicine to take effect prior to incising the skin, unless tension physiology is present. There is a potential for toxicity with total doses >4.5 mg/kg of 1% lidocaine (or ~0.5 mL/kg).
- Indications:
  - ○ Pneumothorax (PTX)—especially tension PTX
  - ○ Hemothorax
  - ○ Relative: hepatic hydrothorax, chylothorax, empyema, malignant effusion

PROCEDURE

Preparation

- Perform a time out.
- Adjust the height of the bed to a level comfortable to perform the procedure.
- Place the patient in the supine position with adequate exposure of the axilla and surrounding landmarks. If the patient can tolerate it, secure his/her arm above the head using tape or a soft arm restraint. Position the bed to a comfortable height for the provider.
- Palpate the ribs and mark the appropriate insertion site at the 4th or 5th intercostal space. The nipple (in men) or inframammary crease (in women) are useful landmarks.
- Scrub a very wide area with chlorhexidine for 30 seconds. Be sure to include appropriate landmarks (e.g., nipple, inframammary crease) so that they can be seen within the sterile field.
- This is a sterile procedure. A sterile gown, gloves, cap, and mask should be worn.
  - It is a good idea to wear two pairs of gloves to prevent infection in the case of a glove tear. The bottom set should be indicator gloves (darker color) to aid in detecting a torn glove.
- Anesthetize the insertion site.
  - Instill lidocaine in the skin at the incision site using a 25 or 27 g needle to anesthetize the whole incision length.
  - Anesthetize the pleura by inserting the needle directly into the site, in while aspirating. Slowly advance until air or blood returns. Then slowly retract the needle, just beyond where no aspirate is returned. This is directly over the parietal pleura and will provide significant analgesia.

Procedure

- Make the incision.
  - Using a #10 scalpel, make an incision parallel and directly over lower rib.
  - The incision should be long enough to fit your finger and the chest tube with clamps.
- Enter the pleural space.
  - Using a clamp, bluntly dissect the surrounding tissue down to the superior aspect of the lower rib. Insert the clamp in the closed position, open it to dissect, and withdraw.
  - Once at the intercostal muscles, use the clamps to push through them directly above the rib and into the pleural space. Do this with one hand grasping the clamp in the middle, which will also serve to prevent the clamp from going in too far and causing injury to the underlying lung.
    - A rush of air or blood will signify the correct space.
  - Separate the muscle by opening the clamp and retracting it.
  - Use your finger to ensure you are in the pleural space and that there are no adhesions.
- Insert the chest tube using the clamp or your finger as a guide.
  - Insert the clamp and tube aiming posteriorly. Use your finger to verify that the tube is in the pleural space before advancing.
  - Once in, aim the clamp curve superiorly and posteriorly and advance the tube along the posterior aspect of the chest wall. Release the clamp and withdraw it while continuing to advance the tube. Spinning the tube while advancing will

help it stay out of the lung fissure (counterclockwise if on the patient's left side and clockwise on the right).
  - For most adult patients (without a lot of subcutaneous tissue), the tube should be inserted to about 14–16 cm at the skin.
  - Attach the chest tube to a water-seal or triple-chamber chest drain system. This can be done before or after securing the chest tube.
- Secure the chest tube.
  - Silk suture, sized either 0-0 or 2-0, is commonly used.
    - Place a simple interrupted suture above and below the chest tube, tied down to the skin. The tails are then wrapped around the tube repeatedly and again tied down to secure them around the tube.
    - Or tie a purse-string suture, similar to a horizontal mattress with the tails wrapped around the tube. Doing this allows the purse string to be tightened down later when pulling the chest tube and closing the incision.
- Dress the chest tube.
  - Petroleum-impregnated gauze should be wrapped around the base of the chest tube to create an airtight seal.
  - Clean gauze should be folded in half and put on the inferior aspect of chest tube before it is tapped down. This will give it a more perpendicular path near the ribs and be more comfortable for the patient.
  - More clean gauze should be used to cover the entire chest tube insertion site and taped down to the skin.
- Always verify chest tube placement with chest plain radiograph.
- Monitor output in traumatic hemothorax.

SPECIAL CONSIDERATIONS

Complications

- Pain, bleeding, injury to the neurovascular bundle beneath the ribs, infection, or empyema
- Entry into liver, spleen, or heart, or placement outside the pleural space
- Injury to provider (broken ribs/bones and foreign bodies may lacerate the provider's fingers)

Referral

- Thoracic surgery consultation may be required for patients who have had recent thoracic surgery, VATS (video-assisted thorascopic surgery), or thoracostomy at the same site.

SUGGESTED READINGS

Dev SP, Nascimiento B, Simone C, Chien V. Chest-tube insertion. *N Engl J Med* 2007;357:e15. Available at: http://www.nejm.org/doi/full/10.1056/nejmvcm071974.

REFERENCES

1. Penrose N. BET 4: does size matter? Chest drains in haemothorax following trauma. *Emerg Med J* 2013;30(11):965–7.
2. Russo RM, Zakaluzny SA, Neff LP, et al. A pilot study of chest tube versus pigtail catheter drainage of acute hemothorax in swine. *J Trauma Acute Care Surg* 2015;79(6):1038–43.

134

Procedures: Thoracotomy

Michael Willman and Stephanie Charshafian

GENERAL PRINCIPLES

- Emergency thoracotomy may be indicated when a trauma patient experiences cardiovascular collapse or has a recent loss of pulse.

Indications

- East Guidelines: strongly recommend thoracotomy for patients who present pulseless with signs of life (pupillary response, spontaneous ventilation or movement, or cardiac electrical activity) after penetrating thoracic injury.
- West Guidelines: patients undergoing CPR or profound refractory shock with no signs of life, penetrating trauma patients with no signs of life and CPR time <15 minutes, and blunt trauma patients with no signs of life and CPR time <10 minutes.

Contraindications

- No signs of life on arrival, severe traumatic brain injury, or most likely extrathoracic cause of circulatory collapse/pulselessness without signs of life after blunt injury

PROCEDURE

- Always start with a left-sided thoracotomy, which can be immediately extended into a clamshell thoracotomy for suspected right chest exsanguinating injury.
- Raise the left arm above the head. The incision starts at sternum and is directed transversely in the inframammary fold curving toward the axilla. This incision is repeated on the right side with division of the sternum if a clamshell thoracotomy is performed.
- The pericardium is opened from the apex extending toward the aortic root above the phrenic nerve. Care should be taken to identify and avoid the phrenic nerve. Opening the pericardium will relieve tamponade and expose the heart for repair of cardiac injuries.
  - This allows for open cardiac massage, intracardiac epinephrine injection, and internal defibrillation.
  - Patients in asystole without cardiac tamponade can be declared dead.
- Cross-clamp the descending aorta. (This should be performed first in extrathoracic exsanguination.)
- If other thoracic hemorrhage is identified, obtain direct control of the site of bleeding. For pulmonary hemorrhage, cross-clamping the hilar vessels is potentially indicated.
- If a bronchovenous air embolism is suspected, cross-clamp the pulmonary hilum; place the patient in Trendelenburg position, trapping air in the LV apex; needle aspirate the intracardiac air; and consider needle aspiration of the aortic root and right coronary artery. Vigorous cardiac massage can help dissolution of air trapped within the coronaries.

SPECIAL CONSIDERATIONS

- Emergency department thoracotomy should only be performed in a trauma center with immediate availability of either trauma or cardiothoracic surgery.
- Even with timely thoracotomy, survival remains low.
- This is a procedure with significant risk to providers (i.e., blood-borne pathogen exposure, bone fragment, or shrapnel injury).

135

Procedures: Ultrasound

Alicia Oberle, Enyo Ablordeppey, Daniel Theodoro, Michael Willman, Steven Hung, Deborah Shipley Kane, and Nicholas Renz

GENERAL PRINCIPLES

- Ultrasound (US) utilizes high-frequency sound waves to measure distances and detect objects. The US machine measures the amplitude of returning echoes and uses the intensity of the wave to generate an image on the screen.
- High-frequency sound waves create better resolution pictures, but are not able to penetrate the body deeply, limiting them to superficial structures.
- Hyperechoic images appear bright or white on the screen, indicating strong returning echoes.
- Hypoechoic images appear gray or weaker in intensity.
- Anechoic images are black indicating no returning echo.

Probe Selection

- Probes come in different frequencies and sizes to best capture objects found at different depths and densities.
- All probes have a marker or indicator on one side to correlate with probe marker on the screen. In all studies with the exception of cardiac examinations, the indicator should always be toward the patient's right or toward the patient's head.
  - The curvilinear probe is a lower-frequency probe best used for looking at deep structures.
  - Linear and intercavitary probes are high frequency and best used for evaluating at superficial structures.
  - Phased array probes are similar to curvilinear probes but have a smaller footprint to allow for visualization of objects in small space (between the rib spaces).

Image Optimization

- Adjust the depth of the screen to insure the tissue or object of interest is included on the screen. Adjusting depth improves the focus of the image as the US beam is narrowed at that point.
- Gain refers to the intensity of returned echoes displayed on the screen. Increasing gain brightens the screen; decreasing gain darkens the screen. Increasing gain does not improve the quality of the image.
- Artifact can lead to image misinterpretation and is important to recognize.
  - Acoustic shadowing occurs when beams encounter a highly reflective surface and are unable to pass through, creating anechoic area behind the structure.
  - Air will distort an image by scattering beams.

Abdominal Aortic Aneurysm Examination

GENERAL PRINCIPLES

- An abdominal aortic aneurysm (AAA) exam can quickly diagnose this life-threatening condition.
- Use the curvilinear probe to evaluate the entire aorta and the iliac arteries.

DIAGNOSIS

- A complete AAA exam consists of five views: transverse view of the proximal aorta, transverse view of the midaorta, transverse view of the distal aorta, transverse view of the iliac bifurcation, and a longitudinal view of the aorta.
- Views are best obtained with steady pressure to displace bowel gas, with the probe depth set as deep as the vertebral shadow, and with the IVC visualized next to the aorta.
- The aortic diameter should be measured from outer wall to outer wall to include any echogenic material or clot. The normal aortic diameter is <3 cm. At the bifurcation of the iliacs, a diameter of <1.5 cm is considered normal.
- If the diameter of the aorta is normal over the entire aorta, there is 100% negative predictive value for a ruptured AAA.

Transverse View of the Proximal Aorta

- Begin in the epigastrium with the probe perpendicular (transverse) to the patient. This most proximal view begins at the celiac trunk, creating a view called the "seagull's sign" as the celiac trunk enters the abdominal aorta.
- The superior mesenteric artery (SMA) should be visualized anterior to the aorta, just caudal to the celiac trunk, with the splenic vein passing anterior to the SMA.

Transverse View of the Midaorta

- Move the probe caudally along the aorta to the midaorta. There are no landmarks at the midaorta.
- Since most AAAs are infrarenal, they are commonly identified in this view.

Transverse View of the Distal Aorta

- Move the probe caudally to the level of the umbilicus or the L4 level. The bifurcation of the iliacs should be visualized.
- Measure the aortic diameter just proximal to the bifurcation of the iliacs.

Transverse View of the Bifurcation of the Iliacs

- This is the same view as the distal aorta. Measure both iliac arteries at the level of the bifurcation.
- The iliac artery diameter should be <1.5 cm.

Longitudinal View of the Proximal Aorta

- This view should be obtained at the proximal to midaorta level. Rotate the probe 90 degrees from the initial transverse view with the indicator now pointing to the patient's head.
- You may need to rock the probe slightly side to side to find the midline of the vessel. Measure the diameter of the vessel in this plane.
- This view is best for evaluating for outpouchings of the aortic wall.

Echocardiography Examination

GENERAL PRINCIPLES

- A bedside echocardiography exam is useful for assessing cardiac activity, pericardial effusions, and global cardiac function. It is not meant to replace a comprehensive assessment interpreted by a cardiologist.
- Presence of cardiac activity and identification of a pericardial effusion can rapidly impact care.
- In all views, evaluate for cardiac activity, pericardial effusion, left cardiac function, and right cardiac function.
- A lower-frequency (2–5 MHz), phased array (cardiac) probe is used to assess four cardiac windows.
- A curvilinear probe can be used alternatively to obtain the left parasternal view or the subcostal/subxiphoid view.
- Placing the patient in left lateral decubitus position can bring the heart closer to the chest wall and reduces lung artifact to aid in optimizing cardiac views.
- Cardiac images can be obtained in either the cardiac orientation (screen indicator to the right of the monitor) or abdominal orientation (screen indicator to the left of the monitor). These orientations are mirror images (180-degree orientation).

DIAGNOSIS

- A basic echocardiography exam consists of four views: subcostal/subxiphoid, left parasternal long, left parasternal short, and an apical four-chamber view.
- Contractility and evidence of effusion should be assessed first to rule out life-threatening tamponade.

Subcostal/Subxiphoid View

- Use the phased array probe or the curvilinear probe.
- Begin in the subxiphoid space, with the phased array probe, pointing the probe indicator to the patient's left (probe indicator should be pointed toward patient's right when using the curvilinear probe) and aiming the probe toward the left shoulder, using the liver as an acoustic window. The probe will be nearly flat on the abdomen, angled at a 15-degree angle toward the head. Adjust the depth as needed, typically 15–20 cm.
- Given the heart's position in the chest, the right ventricle will be closest to the probe regardless of the probe or orientation used.

- This is the most common view used to evaluate for a pericardial effusion. The pericardium appears bright white adjacent to the gray myocardium.
- A pericardial effusion should appear as anechoic fluid between the white pericardium and the gray myocardium.

Left Parasternal Long Axis View

- Place the probe in the 3rd or 4th intercostal space, just left of the sternum. The probe indicator should be toward the patient's right shoulder (cardiac orientation) or left hip (abdominal orientation) to create the view.
- The right ventricle will be closest to the probe, and a pericardial effusion can be identified.
- In this view, one can assess the global function of the left ventricle by looking at the overall contraction of the left ventricle and with E-point septal separation (EPSS) (below), as well as assessment of the size of the right ventricle.

Left Parasternal Short Axis View

- From the long axis view, rotate the probe 90 degrees clockwise to capture the short axis view. The probe indication will be pointed either toward the left shoulder (cardiac orientation) or toward the right hip (abdominal orientation).
- In this view, one can evaluate the left and right ventricles at the level of the mitral valve, through the papillary muscles and to the apex.
- This view will predominately show the left ventricle where one can assess the left ventricular overall contraction at the midpapillary level.
- Normally, the left ventricle is circular in the view. Flattening of the intraventricular septum in this view creates an image that appears like the letter D (the "D sign,") and indicates an overfilled right ventricle.

Apical Four-Chamber View

- Turning the patient onto their left hip can optimize the image quality in this view.
- Place the probe over the patient's point of maximal impulse with the probe orientation either toward the left shoulder (cardiac orientation) or toward the right shoulder (abdominal orientation). This is typically near the 5th intercostal space at the T4/T5 level near the nipple line.
- In this view, all four chambers as well as the tricuspid and mitral valves can be visualized.
- The right ventricular size can be evaluated in this view and should be two-thirds the size of the left ventricle.

Pericardial Effusion and Tamponade

- The pericardium is a fibrous sac and will appear hyperechogenic surrounding the heart both anteriorly and posteriorly. Pericardial effusions will appear as fluid that separates the pericardium from the myocardium. Clot or fibrin can appear in the fluid collection.
- Effusions up to 50 mL can be physiologic and usually occur posteriorly and inferiorly.
- Moderate-sized effusions measure 10–20 mm during diastole and large effusions >20 mm during diastole.
- Pericardial fat pads, found anterior to the right ventricle, can be confused for an effusion.
- Tamponade is a clinical diagnosis.

- US can aid in tamponade diagnosis by identifying:
  - Right heart "scalloping"—diastolic collapse of the right ventricle or right atrium
  - A dilated IVC that does not change with inspiration
  - A heart swinging in a circumferential effusion

Pulseless Electrical Activity

- Visualization should be sufficient to determine activity; however, if there is uncertainty, place the US in M-mode across the left ventricular wall to assess for cardiac contractions (waveforms on M-mode) versus cardiac standstill (flat line).

E-Point Septal Separation

- EPSS can help assess global cardiac function by estimating the left ventricular ejection function.
- In diastole, the anterior leaflet of the mitral valve should touch or approach the septum. The amount of separation between the septum and the anterior leaflet is the EPSS. EPSS > 7 mm suggests decreased left ventricular function.
- The EPSS can be visualized or calculated in the left parasternal long axis view. To calculate EPSS, place the US in M-mode with the cursor crossing the septum and the most distal segment of the anterior leaflet of the mitral valve. The M-mode tracing should be measured for the distance from the E-point to the septum.

Extended Focused Abdominal Sonography in Trauma Examination

GENERAL PRINCIPLES

- The extended focused abdominal sonography in trauma (eFAST) exam can accurately detect fluid in the peritoneal, pleural, and pericardial cavities as well as air in the pleural cavity and is more reliable than physical exam.
- Use of bedside US in trauma can expedite time to definitive care, determine whether a lifesaving intervention is warranted.
- Allows for repeated noninvasive examinations.

DIAGNOSIS

- A complete eFAST exam consists of four views of the traditional FAST exam: right upper quadrant, left upper quadrant, suprapubic and subxiphoid, and additional right and left anterior thoracic lung windows.
- Generally, the FAST views are performed with either a curvilinear or phased array probe while the lung windows are viewed with a linear probe.
- Free fluid appears black or anechoic on US.
- Limitations to the eFAST include an unreliable assessment of the retroperitoneum for hemorrhage and further is not able to account of extremity injuries or blood lost on scene in trauma patients; furthermore, it does not identify the source of bleeding when present.
- The lung US is more sensitive than a plain chest radiograph for pneumothorax and will pick up even small insignificant pneumothorax—not all of which will require a thoracotomy. Clinical criteria make this determination.

VIEWS

Right Upper Quadrant View

- Probe placement on the right lateral upper abdomen with indicator directed cephalad.
- The view should include the diaphragm, liver, and hepatorenal space (Morison's pouch) and continue down to the inferior pole of the right kidney.
- The pleural space should be evaluated for fluid—fluid appears black on the US. A mirror image artifact (recreation of the liver above the diaphragm) indicates no free fluid in the dependent portion of the lung, while black fluid indicates a hemothorax.
- The potential space surrounding the liver, in the hepatorenal space (Morison's pouch), and down to the inferior pole of the right kidney, should be assessed for free fluid.

Left Upper Quadrant View

- Probe placement on the left lateral upper abdomen with the indicator directed cephalad—this is more posterior and superior to the right upper quadrant, owing to the relative size of the spleen in most patients.
- The view should include the diaphragm, spleen, and splenorenal space, and continue down to the inferior pole of the left kidney.
- The pleural space should be evaluated for fluid. A mirror image artifact (recreation of the spleen above the diaphragm) indicates no free fluid in the dependent portion of the lung, while black fluid indicates a hemothorax.
- The potential space surrounding the spleen, in the splenorenal space and down to the inferior pole of the right kidney, should be assessed for free fluid.

Suprapubic View

- Two views of the suprapubic space are required: transverse and long axis.
- Transverse view—the probe is placed just above the pubic symphysis in the midline with the indicator directed to the patient's right; evaluation should be done while fanning from the lower portion of the bladder up to the head and should include the edges of the uterus in females.
- Long axis view—the probe is placed just above the pubic symphysis in the midline with indicator directed cephalic; evaluation should be done while fanning from the right side to the left side of the abdomen.
- Free fluid in the suprapubic space presents as fluid outside the bladder and uterus and often creates a "double-wall sign" on the bladder, as the outer wall of the bladder should not be easily distinguished when free fluid is not present.

Subxiphoid View

- Probe placement is on the subxiphoid space, with the indicator to the patient's right and the probe directed cephalic and toward the left clavicle.
- The heart is identified and the pericardium is assessed for free fluid (a black line outlining the heart).
- If the subxiphoid image in unobtainable, the parasternal long view may provide better visualization (see Echocardiography Exam).

Lung Windows

- Use the linear or phased array probe on the right and left anterior chest wall, at the second intercostal space in the midclavicular line.

- Identify the pleural line and observe for lung sliding (normal lung), lung pulse sign (atelectasis), and lung point sign (definitive pneumothorax).
- Consider verification with M-mode observing for sky–ocean–beach phenomenon (normal lung) versus bar code sign (pneumothorax).

Renal and Bladder

GENERAL PRINCIPLES

- Ureteral nephroliths are not commonly visualized on US.
- Hydronephrosis can be a sign of obstructing nephrolithiasis. Visualization of ureteral jets in the bladder (or lack thereof) can help confirm or exclude obstruction of the ureters on a specific side.

Renal Windows

- Place the phased array or curvilinear probe, with the indicator toward the patient's head, along the midaxillary line near the inferior costal margin. Slide the probe inferiorly until the kidney is located. Note that the kidney is more superior and posterior on the left than on the right.
- Once located, scan anterior to posterior and visualize the entire kidney to obtain a longitudinal view. Rotate the probe 90 degrees and scan superior to inferior to obtain a transverse view of the kidney.
- In mild hydronephrosis, the proximal ureter and renal pelvis will be dilated. In moderate disease, the calyces will become distended, but the papillae are still easily visualized. In severe disease, the calyces will be severely distended with obliteration of the papillae.

Bladder Windows

- Place the curvilinear or phased array probe just superior to the pubis symphysis, with the indicator to the patient's right. Scan inferiorly to locate the bladder. Note that it can be difficult to locate the bladder if the patient has recently (and completely) voided or if there is a Foley catheter in place. Once located, scan superior to inferior (up and down) to obtain a transverse view of the bladder. Rotate the probe 90 degrees and scan left to right to obtain a longitudinal view.
- Use color Doppler at the base of the trigone of the bladder to assess for the presence of periodic ureteral jets.
- Measure the volume of the bladder by taking three measurements. Start with the transverse view and find the largest area, and then measure the widest portions vertically and horizontally. Next, find the longitudinal view of the bladder and measure the widest horizontal portion for the third measurement. Some machines have a built-in calculator to estimate the bladder volume based on these measurements.

Right Upper Quadrant

GENERAL PRINCIPLES

- This approach is used primarily in the workup of abdominal symptoms suggestive of gallbladder disease.

DIAGNOSIS

- The gallbladder normally lies on the visceral surface of the liver between the right and quadrate hepatic lobes. It has a fundus, body, and neck (which continues to become the cystic duct, which then connects with the common bile duct [CBD]).
- Gallstones will appear as hyperechoic with a distal acoustic shadow.
- The gallbladder wall should measure <3 mm.
- The CBD can range in size from 4 to 10 mm, enlarging with age and postcholecystectomy.

View of the Gallbladder and Common Bile Duct

- The gallbladder is found with several possible approaches.
  - Subcostal sweep—The probe is in a longitudinal orientation with indicator toward the patient's head and sweep along the subcostal margin laterally.
  - Find the xiphoid process and move laterally to patient's right about 7 cm and visualize the gallbladder through the ribs.
  - In some patients, it may be easier to visualize the gallbladder with the patient lying in the left lateral decubitus position and positioning the probe either to the side or to the back.
- The gallbladder will appear like a fluid-filled structure with hyperechoic walls surrounding a hypoechoic interior.
  - In long axis, the gallbladder will appear like an exclamation point or pear shape.
  - In short axis, the gallbladder will appear circular.
- The entire gallbladder should be scanned to look for abnormalities and stones.
- Gallbladder wall—measure the most narrow point of the anterior gallbladder wall; it is important to be perpendicular to the gallbladder to avoid a falsely enlarged gallbladder wall due to measuring it at an oblique angle.
- The CBD is found by first finding the portal vein, a circular structure most easily found in long axis as the point of the exclamation mark.
- The portal vein, hepatic artery, and CBD form a face that is common called the "Mickey Mouse" sign with the portal vein acting as the head and the hepatic artery and CBD as the ears.
  - With the indicator toward the patient's right, the right ear is the CBD and the left ear is the hepatic artery; using color flow, there will be no discernible flow in the CBD.
- With the triad in short axis, rotate the probe 90 degrees to view it on long axis; there will appear to be three echogenic lines across the screen, forming two tubes.
  - The closest line to the probe will be the anterior wall of the CBD.
  - The middle line is the shared wall of the CBD and portal vein.

Pelvic Ultrasound

GENERAL PRINCIPLES

- US is utilized in the emergency department for pregnant patients with pelvic complaints to confirm intrauterine pregnancy (IUP) or for the diagnosis of an ectopic pregnancy in a patient with pain and/or vaginal bleeding.
- There are two approaches, transabdominal (curvilinear probe) and transvaginal (endocavitary probe).

- Supine positioning is the best position for the exam.
  - Transabdominal US is best performed with a full bladder.
  - Transvaginal US is best performed with an empty bladder.

DIAGNOSIS

- An IUP should be able to be visualized at least on transvaginal US when the serum beta hCG level is between 1000 and 2000 mIU/mL.
- A thin-walled sac within the uterus is not a definitive sign of IUP because it can represent a pseudogestational sac.
- In order to be considered an IUP, a gestational sac containing a yolk sac in the uterus must be visualized. This occurs around 5 weeks of gestation.
  - A gestational sac will appear as an anechoic space surrounded by a hyperechoic rim embedded in the endometrium of the uterus.
  - A yolk sac will appear in the gestational sac as a circular thick-walled echogenic structure with an anechoic center.
  - A fetal pole is thickening of yolk sac and when it measures >7 mm, a fetal heartbeat should be detected.
- In the rare case of heterotopic pregnancy, an ectopic pregnancy with a visualized IUP may still be possible. The incidence ranges from 1 in 30,000 to 1.5 in 1000 with risk increasing with the use of assisted reproduction techniques.
- Ectopic pregnancy
  - The most common site is within the fallopian tubes.
  - To definitively diagnose an ectopic pregnancy, an extrauterine pregnancy must be visualized, although failure to visualize an IUP should raise suspicion.
  - A tubal ring is an anechoic sac surrounded by thick, echogenic wall separate from the ovary; it is suspicious for ectopic pregnancy.
  - A complex adnexal mass in the setting of a positive pregnancy test is also suspicious for ectopic pregnancy.

Transabdominal Pelvic US

- Position the probe in the suprapubic area and scan both transversely and longitudinally through the uterus (positioned posterior to bladder) looking for an IUP.
- Examine for free pelvic fluid before focusing on the IUP; it will appear as anechoic material outside the structures that normally contain fluid (i.e., bladder).
- Once an IUP is found, can perform several measurements.
  - Fetal heart rate can be measured starting around 6 weeks gestation; it is measured by using M-mode, positioning the line through the fetal heart and using included calculators to measure from one peak to the next.
  - Other included calculators can measure approximate gestational age.
- The ovaries are generally better visualized transvaginally.

Transvaginal Pelvic US

- Using a clean endocavitary probe, place some gel on the probe before covering with a clean rubber protective cover, and then place sterile lubricant on the covered probe.
- Insert the probe with the indicator pointing to the ceiling.
  - With the indicator up, the uterus will be visualized in the longitudinal axis.
  - Move the probe laterally to visualize the entire uterus.

- Rotate the probe 90 degrees counterclockwise so that the indicator is now pointing to patient's right.
  - The uterus will now be viewed in the transverse axis.
  - Move the probe up and down to visualize the entire uterus.
- Scan through the uterus in each view, looking for an IUP as well as free fluid.
- With the probe still held in the transverse axis, examine each ovary.
  - Aim the probe to either the RLQ or LLQ, keeping part of the uterus in view.
  - The ovaries can be identified by the presence of follicles.
  - One hand can be used to provide external compression to bring the adnexal structures into view.

Ultrasound-Guided Intravenous Access

GENERAL PRINCIPLES

- US-guided intravenous (IV) catheters are often needed when attempts at peripheral IV access has failed.
- US-guided IV access is usually aimed toward deep veins that are usually not visible/palpable superficially.

Indications

- A need for and inability to obtain peripheral IV access in a noncritically ill patient

Contraindications

- Infection, burn, or injury at the selected site
- Fistula in the arm or mastectomy on the site of the IV
- Need for more emergent access due to time constraint (e.g., cardiac arrest)

PROCEDURE

- The patient should be laying supine with the arm outstretched on a padded mayo stand.
- The US machine should be placed in a position so that the operator can see the selected site and machine at the same time.
- Assess what size access is needed.
  - If contrast CT scans are needed, specific catheter size and placement are required.
- Use universal precautions.
- Apply tourniquet.
- Clean and prep the area.
- Use the high-frequency probe to locate the desired vessel.
  - Decrease the depth to the lowest level that the vessel is still visible.
- Find the potential vein.
  - It will appear as an easily compressible circular structure with dark anechoic center.
  - The areas to start looking are in the AC and the area medial and proximal to the elbow (brachial vein).
- Trace the vessel to see which way it runs.
  - Rotate the probe to keep the vessel in the middle of the screen.
  - Tracing the vessel allows for determination of direction of insertion of the IV.

- Choose the insertion point distal to the probe.
- Wipe off the excess gel and clean again.
- Use lidocaine to anesthetize the area since deep vessels require some probing.
- While holding the probe in your nondominant hand, insert the angiocatheter 5–10 mm distal to the vein.
  - Do not move the US probe; instead, tilt it away from you to visualize the tip of the angiocatheter as it is advanced.
  - Insert the needle with the bevel up, to enter the skin with the sharpest point.
  - Try to be as parallel to the skin as the angiocatheter length and depth of the vessel will allow.
- As you near the vessel, you will start to see the needle tent the vessel.
  - Do not put too much pressure on the vessel with the probe as this will compress the tissue around the vessel. Also, once you enter the vessel and release the US probe to advance the catheter, the tissue may spring back and likely displace your catheter resulting in a failed attempt.
- Once the needle tip appears in the middle of the vessel, there should be a flash of blood in the angiocatheter.
- Advance the entire angiocatheter slightly forward.
- Without moving the needle, advance the catheter off of the needle and into the vessel.
- Secure the catheter, release the tourniquet, and flush the IV.

SUGGESTED READINGS

Arntfield RT, Millington SJ. Point of care cardiac ultrasound applications in the emergency department and intensive care unit—a review. *Curr Cardiol Rev* 2012;8(2):98–108.

Dalziel PJ, Noble VE. Bedside ultrasound and the assessment of renal colic: a review. *Emerg Med J* 2013;30:3–8.

Dogra V, Paspulati RM, Bhatt S. First trimester bleeding evaluation. *Ultrasound Q* 2005;21(2):69–85.

Kirk E, Bourne T. Diagnosis of ectopic pregnancy with ultrasound. *Best Pract Res Clin Obstet Gynaecol* 2009;23(4):501–8.

Lichtenstein DA, Menu Y. A bedside ultrasound sign ruling out pneumothorax in the critically ill: lung sliding. *Chest* 1995;108(5):1345.

McKaigney CJ, Krantz MH, La Rocque CL, et al. E-point septal separation: a bedside tool for emergency physician assessment of left ventricular ejection fraction. *Am J Emerg Med* 2014;32(6):493–7.

Moylan M, Newgard CD, Ma OJ, et al. Association between a positive FAST examination and therapeutic laparotomy in normotensive blunt trauma patients. *J Emerg Med* 2007;33(3): 265–71.

Nishijima DK, Simel DL, Wisner DH, et al. Does this adult trauma patient have blunt intra-abdominal injury? *JAMA* 2012;307(14):1517–27. Available at: http://pmid.us/22496266.

Noble VE, Nelson B, Sutingo AN. *Manual of Emergency and Critical Care Ultrasound.* New York: Cambridge University Press, 2007.

Plummer D. Abdominal Aortic Aneurysm. In: Ma OJ, Mateer Jr, eds. *Emergency Ultrasound.* New York: McGraw-Hill, 2003:129–43.

Plummer D, Clinton J, Matthew B. Emergency department ultrasound improves time to diagnosis and survival in ruptured abdominal aortic aneurysm. *Acad Emerg Med* 1998;5:417.

Shea JA, Berline JA, Escarce JJ, et al. Revised estimates of diagnostic test sensitivity and specificity in suspected biliary tract disease. *Arch Intern Med* 1994;154(22):2573.

136 Procedures: Central Venous Catheter Placement

Michael Willman and Steven Hung

GENERAL PRINCIPLES

- Central venous catheters (CVCs) are inserted into large central veins to provide specific therapies (administration of vasopressors, monitoring of central hemodynamics, hemodialysis, etc.).
- The use of ultrasound to insert a CVC into the internal jugular (IJ) or femoral vein has improved the safety of and time needed to place central lines.[1]

Indications

- Unable to obtain peripheral intravenous (IV) access or need for more access
- Administration of vasopressors
  - Peripheral administration of vasopressors may be safer than previously thought,[2] and can be considered while awaiting central access if necessary. Standard of care still requires central access for prolonged administration of vasopressors.
- Emergent hemodialysis or plasmapheresis
- Transvenous pacing
- Hemodynamic monitoring (e.g., central venous saturation)
- Administration of medications caustic to peripheral vasculature

Contraindications

- As most central lines are placed into critically ill patients, contraindications are relative to the benefit of the line versus the risk of placing the line. These include but are not limited to:
  - Infection at site
  - Distorted anatomy or previous surgery in the area of placement
  - Proximal vascular injury (e.g., placing a femoral line in patient with an inferior vena cava injury)
  - Uncooperative patient
  - Bleeding diathesis
  - Other indwelling intravascular device (e.g., other catheter, pacemaker, hemodialysis catheter)
- If there is concern for injury to the femoral, iliac, or intra-abdominal vessels (e.g., penetrating abdominal injury, pelvic fracture, etc.), a femoral CVC should be avoided. Consider internal jugular (IJ) or subclavian (SC) line placement instead.

PROCEDURE

Preparation

- Perform a time out.
- Adjust the height of the bed so that you have comfortable access to the insertion site.

591

- Best patient position is determined by the CVC being placed:
  ○ IJ—Position the patient supine and in Trendelenburg position to increase venous pressure and distend the veins.
  ○ SC—Position the patient supine. Ensure that the ipsilateral arm is adducted and pulled inferiorly, so that the shoulder and clavicle are in neutral anatomic position (not drawn superiorly, distorting the angle of the clavicle).
  ○ Femoral—Position the patient supine with the ipsilateral leg slightly abducted.
- Use the US to find the desired vein, which should be patent and compressible. Locate the associated artery, which is circular and more difficult to compress, to help prevent accidental arterial cannulation.

Equipment

- Ultrasound with high-frequency probe (e.g., linear probe)
- Sterile probe cover and ultrasound gel (if not included in kit)
- Sterile gloves and gown. Cap and face mask (if not included in kit)
- CVC (e.g., triple lumen, cordis, introducer)
- CVC kit (will vary based on manufacturer):
  ○ Chlorhexidine
  ○ Fenestrated drape
  ○ Ultrasound cover, sterile ultrasound gel
  ○ Various syringes, needles, filter needle, lidocaine
  ○ Introducer ("finder") needle, Angiocath needle
  ○ Guidewire, dilator, scalpel
  ○ Sterile saline flushes, Luer locks (IV caps)
  ○ Suture, needle driver, scissors
  ○ Sterile gauze and dressing

Procedure

- Use universal precautions and perform a time-out.
- Clean area with chlorhexidine, a larger area than you think you need. If doing an IJ or SC, clean both of these sites on the same side to facilitate changing to the other if the first results in a failed attempt.
- Place ultrasound gel on the high-frequency probe (so that there is gel inside sterile cover).
- Use sterile technique for all remaining steps.
- Open the kit, and place the CVC and sterile saline flushes on the field. Don sterile gown and gloves.
- Set up:
  ○ Apply drape over the patient, with the fenestration centered over the insertion site.
  ○ Apply the US probe cover over the high-frequency probe and secure with the rubber band(s).
    ▪ When placing the probe on the sterile drape, be careful the probe cover does not drag against nonsterile areas.
    ▪ A set of needle drivers can clamp the drape and probe cover together to help prevent the probe from sliding off of the field. Just unclamp the needle drivers when ready for use.
  ○ Apply the Luer locks and flush all the lines/ports of the CVC, and leave the cap off the line through which the guidewire will pass.

- ○ Lay out all the equipment in an easily accessible area and preferentially in the order of use (guidewire, scalpel, dilator, CVC).
- • Finding the vein:

For an IJ:

- ○ Using the US, locate the left or right IJ vein *and center* it on *the screen*. Find a view where the artery is lateral, not inferior to the vein. This will help prevent accidental arterial cannulation.
- ○ Use lidocaine to anesthetize the skin at the insertion site.
- ○ Attach the introducer needle to a "slip tip" syringe (one without a Luer lock). Insert the needle, bevel up, about 1–2 cm cephalad to the vessel at a 45-degree angle. Slowly advance the needle while gently aspirating.
- ○ Follow the needle tip with the US as it tracks down to the vessel. Do not advance if you cannot locate the needle tip.
- ○ As you near the vessel, you will start to see the tenting of the vessel on the ultrasound image (consider switching to a longitudinal view).
  - ■ Do not put too much pressure on the vessel with the US probe as this will compress the vessel and surrounding tissue. This may cause visual or physical occlusion of the vessel. Once you enter the vessel and release the ultrasound probe, the tissue may spring back and displace your needle resulting in a failed attempt.
- ○ Once you enter the vessel, dark venous blood should be easily drawn into the syringe.
- ○ Note: A landmark approach can be done for an IJ line. Insert the needle in between the junction of the sternal and clavicular heads of the sternocleidomastoid muscle, aiming at the ipsilateral nipple. The landmark approach is not as common given the increased safety and widespread availability of ultrasound.

For a SC:

- ○ Use your nondominant hand to palpate landmarks through the drape. Place your middle and index fingers just superior to the suprasternal notch. Place your thumb on the clavicle at the junction between the medial and middle portions (where it curves). Keep your hand in this position to ensure location of landmarks until the vein is found. The needle insertion site is approximately 1cm lateral and slightly inferior to your thumb.
- ○ Use lidocaine to anesthetize the skin at the insertion site. Then advance the needle until it hits the clavicle and instill more lidocaine there.
- ○ Attach the introducer needle to a "slip tip" syringe (one without a Luer lock). Insert the needle, bevel up, aiming at your top finger in the suprasternal notch. As soon as the bevel is completely in the skin, level out the needle, parallel to the floor. Maintaining this angle will help prevent entering the thoracic cavity and causing a pneumothorax. Instead of angling the needle, you will need to use the thumb on your nondominant hand to push the needle deep while advancing.
- ○ Slowly advance the needle while gently aspirating. If you hit the clavicle, withdraw the needle most of the way and push it deeper with your nondominant thumb until you are able to get beneath the clavicle. Avoid "walking the needle" down the clavicle without first withdrawing it to avoid making sweeping motions with the needle tip and causing unseen injury.
- ○ Once under the clavicle, advance the needle while gently aspirating until venous blood returns. If advancing all the way without a return of blood, withdraw the needle and redirect it before advancing again.

- Once you enter the vessel, dark venous blood should be easily drawn into the syringe.
- Note: Ultrasound-guided SC lines can be done but require more advanced training.

For a femoral:

- Palpate the femoral artery. Make sure you are at least two fingerbreadths below the inguinal ligament to avoid accidentally entering the peritoneum. The femoral vein will be located ~1 cm medial to the artery.
- Alternatively, landmarks can be used if unable to palpate a pulse (as in an obese or hypotensive patient). The femoral vein is typically found 1/3 of the way along a line drawn from the pubic symphysis to the anterior superior iliac spine. Place the needle in the groove between your thumb and index finger, aiming at the contralateral nipple. The femoral vein will be encountered deep to this tract.
- Insert the needle at a 45-degree angle. Advance slowly while gently aspirating.
- Once you enter the vessel, dark venous blood should be easily drawn into the syringe.
- Note: Ultrasound-guided femoral lines can be done using a similar method as the IJ approach. Place the probe 2–3 cm below the inguinal ligament. Locate the femora vein and advance the needle as done with the IJ.

- Placing the CVC
  - Remove the syringe without moving the needle (slow venous bleeding should come from the needle). Feed the guidewire through the needle, while aiming the "J" curve in the direction of the heart.
  - Advance the guidewire to about 20 cm (there should be dark hash marks on the guidewire, advance to the point with hash marks indicating 20 cm).
    - The guidewire should advance easily. Do not force it. If it does not advance easily, you may have lost access. Remove the guidewire and attach the syringe, and adjust the needle under ultrasound guidance.
    - Always keep a hand on the guidewire so that it is not does not come out (and lose access) or advance too far (and damage tissue).
  - Remove the needle, leaving the guidewire in place.
  - Confirm placement in the vein prior to dilation with ultrasound or transduction.
    - Visualize the guidewire in a compressible vessel in both the transverse and longitudinal view on US.
  - Load the dilator on the guidewire and advance it to skin level.
  - Place the scalpel along the guidewire and make a small stab incision into the skin. Ensure that the incision is continuous with the guidewire access site.
  - Advance the dilator, using a corkscrew-type motion through the skin, subcutaneous tissue, and into the vessel.
  - Remove the dilator, leaving the guidewire in place. There will be some bleeding, which can be controlled with gauze.
  - Load the CVC onto the guidewire.
  - Advance the CVC into the vein and secure it at an appropriate distance:
    - Femoral veins—20 cm
    - Right IJ—14–15 cm
    - Left IJ—17–20 cm
    - Right SC—15–16 cm
    - Left SC—16–18 cm

○ Remove the guidewire; attach Luer lock; make sure all the lines draw and flush all the lines.

○ Secure the line with suture and dressing.

○ Confirm IJ or SC CVC placement with a chest plain radiograph; femoral vein CVC placement generally does not require verification by plain radiograph.

POTENTIAL COMPLICATIONS

• Complications vary by site, but all include infection, arterial injury, hematoma, and/or nerve injury.

• SC lines may be associated with fewer CVC-related bloodstream infections overall. Lines placed under emergent conditions (nonsterile) should be removed within 24 hours or as soon as possible.[3]

• IJ and SC lines risk possible pneumothorax, so confirmation of proper placement should be visualized with a plain chest radiograph.

SPECIAL CONSIDERATIONS

• If placing an SC line in a penetrating torso injury, consider placing it on the ipsilateral side unless there is concern for SC vessel injury. This will minimize the risk for an additional pneumothorax.

• If arterial blood is encountered with the needle, withdraw immediately and apply pressure.

• When using ultrasound, always make sure that the tip is visualized before advancing to avoid passing through the back end of a vessel and puncturing nonvenous structures.

• When placing SC or IJ central lines, place the patient on a monitor. If the guidewire advances into the right atrium, it may cause ectopic beats, which will signify that the wire is touching the myocardium (and should not be advanced any further). Withdraw the wire about 1–2 cm and place the central line as indicated.[4]

• Accidental arterial dilation or cannulation requires vascular surgery consultation.

SUGGESTED READINGS

Graham AS, Ozment C, Tegtmeyer K, et al. Central venous catheterization. *N Engl J Med* 2007;356:e21.

REFERENCES

1. Shekelle PG, Dallas P. Use of Real-Time Ultrasound Guidance During Central Line Insertion: Brief Update Review. In: *Making Health Care Safer II: An Updated Critical Analysis of the Evidence for Patient Safety Practices*. Rockville: Agency for Healthcare Research and Quality (US), 2013. (Evidence Reports/Technology Assessments, No. 211.) Chapter 18.

2. Loubani OM, Green RS. A systematic review of extravasation and local tissue injury from administration of vasopressors through peripheral intravenous catheters and central venous catheters. *J Crit Care* 2015;30:653.e9–17.

3. Marik PE, Flemmer M, Harrison W. The risk of catheter-related bloodstream infection with femoral venous catheters as compared to subclavian and internal jugular venous catheters: a systematic review of the literature and meta-analysis. *Crit Care Med* 2012;40(8):2479–85.

4. Parienti JJ, Mongardon N, Megarbane B, et al. Intravascular complications of central venous catheterization by insertion site. *N Engl J Med* 2015;373:1220–9.

137 Procedures: Ventilator Management

Bob Cambridge, Michael Willman, and Brian T. Wessman

GENERAL PRINCIPLES

Reasons for endotracheal intubation include:
- Hypoxemia (Type I respiratory failure); $PaO_2 < 55$
- Hypercarbia (Type II respiratory failure); $PaCO_2 > 50$
- Airway protection
- Metabolic demand

Correcting hypoxemia is the most urgent concern after intubation. All modes of advanced mechanical ventilation are designed to increase the mean airway pressure (MAP) with the goal of supporting oxygenation (even with sacrificing ventilation, i.e., permissive hypercapnia).

A typical human tidal volume (TV) is ~6–8 mL/kg of ideal body weight (Fig. 137.1).

Normal inspiration is completed through a negative pressure system. Expiration is a passive process. A normal inspiratory to expiratory (I:E) ratio is 1:2 or 1:3 (expiratory phase becomes prolonged in obstructive lung pathology). Mechanical ventilation, both invasive (being intubated) and noninvasive, use positive pressure to support inspiration.

Once intubated, the patient is usually placed on a ventilator. It is key to understand the potential physiologic damage that occurs as mechanical ventilation is initiated and if a ventilator is set incorrectly.

Ventilators can cause four types of damage, or trauma:
- Barotrauma: excessive pressures (i.e., pneumothorax)
- Volutrauma: over distention of the lung (i.e., lung stretch)

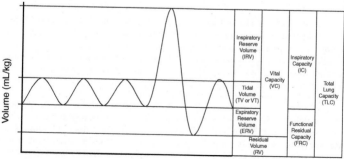

Figure 137.1. Lung volumes and capacities.

- Atelectrauma: shear force stress (i.e., repetitive open/closing of alveoli)
- Oxygen toxicity: overexposure to the drug oxygen

Recommendations from the Acute Respiratory Distress Syndrome research group (ARDSnet) to limit ventilator-induced damage include:

- Maintain plateau pressures <30 mm Hg
- Use TVs of 6–8 mL/kg of ideal body weight (IBW; based on a patient's height)
- Use positive end-expiratory pressure (PEEP) appropriately to support type 1 respiratory failure
- Diuresis as needed to keep lungs dry
- Minimize oxygen support; goal PaO_2 55–80

The ventilator controls respiration through trigger (initiate inspiration period), cycle (switch over from inspiration to expiration), and limits (pressure, time, flow, volume). The lungs interact with the ventilator based on their compliance (ability to stretch to accommodate a volume).

Adjustable Parameters

- Respiratory rate (RR): the minimum number of times per minute the ventilator will deliver a fully supported breath.
- Tidal volume (TV): the desired size of each breath in volume control mode. This parameter is not set in pressure control mode.
- Peak inspiratory pressure (PIP): the maximum pressure level the ventilator will deliver in pressure control mode. This parameter is not set in volume control mode.
- Fractional Percent of Oxygen (FiO_2): the percentage of oxygen in the delivered air.
- Positive end expiratory pressure (PEEP): the level of airway pressure above atmospheric pressure maintained in the circuit at the end of exhalation.
- Trigger: the method by which the ventilator senses patient effort and initiates a breath. The trigger can be a set change in pressure or a set amount of flow in the circuit. In the absence of a trigger, an elapsed amount of time will cause the ventilator to deliver a breath.

Modes of Ventilation

Pressure Control

- In pressure control mode, a PIP is set. When the ventilator is triggered, the PIP is applied. The lungs inflate until the PIP is achieved at which time the ventilator cycles off and passive exhalation occurs. Inspiratory time is set directly, and a prolonged inspiratory time can result in a period of time with no flow (as the PIP would have been achieved in the lungs) (Table 137.1).
- Peak and Plateau pressures: basically equitable, set by the clinician.
- Advantages: barotrauma can be avoided. The inspiratory flow can taper as the peak pressure is achieved in order to allow for more uniform distribution of air and pressure throughout the lungs. No studies have proven a definite benefit in lungs with heterogenous parenchyma.
- Disadvantages: as lung compliance changes, the delivered volume can change over time. Minute ventilation (MV) is not assured. If increases in airway resistance develop or if lung compliance worsens, the result is a lower volume delivered and worsened ventilation.

TABLE 137.1	Modes of Ventilation
Basic modes of ventilation	**Variations of control**
• Controlled mechanical ventilation (CMV)	• Volume control (VC) • Pressure control (PC)
• Assist control (A/C)	• Volume control (A/C-VC) • Pressure control (A/C-PC) • Pressure-regulated volume control (PRVC, A/C-VC+)
• Synchronized intermittent ventilation (SIMV)	• Volume control • Pressure control • Pressure-regulated volume control (PRVC, VC+)
• Pressure support ventilation (PSV)	

Volume Control
- In volume control mode, a desired volume is set and the machine delivers the volume at a set flow rate. Inspiratory time is determined by the desired volume and flow rate; as flow rate is increased, inspiratory time decreases.
- Peak pressure: determined by airway resistance and is measured when there is airflow in the circuit.
- Plateau pressure: determined by lung compliance and is measured when there is no airflow in the circuit (inspiratory hold/pause).
- Advantages: assured minimum MV.
- Disadvantages: as lung compliance increases, the peak pressure and plateau pressures can rise. Close monitoring of airway pressures should be done while in this mode.

Pressure-Regulated Volume Control (PRVC/VC+)
- In a pressure-regulated volume control mode, a desired TV is set and the machine uses varying pressures to meet this goal. The ventilator will evaluate each returning TV breath and subsequently adjust the pressure to obtain the set goal.
- Advantages: assured minimum MV while automatically adjusting airway pressures; improved patient comfort due to flow control.
- Disadvantages: as lung compliance changes to the extremes, the ventilator may not deliver the requested breath (due to set pressure limits).

Types of Support
Control Mode versus Support Mode
- Control Mode: Each breath is fully supported. Once a breath has been triggered, the machine delivers a full breath as determined by the settings. The volume/pressure characteristics of each breath are intended to be the same.
- Support Mode: The patient gets assistance from the machine in the form of increased pressure (pressure support) during the breath, but the flow rate and total volume are determined by the patient's effort and lung compliance. This assistive pressure support is additive to the set PEEP.

Assist Control Mode (A/C)
- Every trigger results in a fully supported breath. If the patient breathes above the set rate (i.e., triggers the ventilator above the set rate), each of those breaths are fully supported as well.

Synchronous Intermittent Mandatory Ventilation (SIMV)
- A set number of fully supported breaths are given. Between fully supported breaths, the patient can trigger the ventilator to take assisted breaths. The machine synchronizes the fully supported breaths to the patient effort to avoid barotrauma caused by delivering a fully supported breath on top of an assisted breath. The additional assisted breaths receive only pressure support (not the full TV or pressure of the fully supported breaths) that is set.

Pressure Support Ventilation (PSV)
- A level of support pressure is set, and the resultant volume and flow are determined by patient effort. The patient must trigger all of the breaths. Airway pressure support is maintained until flow falls below a preset amount at which time the machine cycles back to only maintaining PEEP, which allows for exhalation. This mode is similar to BiPAP in nonintubated patients.

Initial Settings
- The choice of initial settings depends on the specific clinical scenario.
- Cycle: The choice of volume versus pressure is somewhat practitioner dependent. However in the emergency department (ED), where knowledge of the patient's underlying lung conditions are often not known, volume cycled is often a good starting point because MV can be assured. If adequate volume cannot be achieved without dangerously high pressures (i.e., plateau pressures >30), change to pressure-cycled ventilation.
- Mode: Assist control is a good mode to start with, as most intubated patients are initially given paralytics. The machine will assure set ventilation while the patient is still under the effect of the paralytics, and can ensure MV.
- TV: Recommendations are for a goal TV equal to 6–8 mL/kg of ideal body weight. The patient's height can be used to estimate this value when intubation is done under emergent circumstances (Table 137.2). Adjust the TV to keep plateau pressures under 30 cm H_2O.
- RR: A normal MV is 5–8 liters; however, patients requiring mechanical ventilation will often have higher physiologic needs (septic patient will need a higher MV to compensate for their metabolic acidosis). A RR of 18–22 is a good starting point. Asthmatics or other air-trapping conditions will need a lower rate to allow more time in exhalation. Aspirin overdoses and other metabolic conditions with profound acidosis will need a faster rate (i.e., 26–30) to maintain the appropriate respiratory compensation.
- Inspiratory:Expiratory Ratio (I:E): Some machines allow this to be set directly, others infer it from a combination of other factors. If it can be set directly, start with a normal ratio of 1:2, then adjust as necessary. In the air-trapping conditions

TABLE 137.2	Ideal Body Weight Calculator	
	First 5 feet	Additional inches
Male	50 kg	2.3 kg/inch
Female	45.5 kg	2.3 kg/inch

mentioned above, that can be expanded to 1:4 or more. In profound hypoxemia, an inverse ratio can be employed (2:1, 3:1, etc.) as needed.

- PEEP: Start at 5 and adjust as needed for hypoxemia according to ARDSnet PEEP tables. The initial goal of PEEP is to prevent end-expiratory alveolar collapse.
- Oxygen (FiO_2): immediately post intubation and during a reasonable ED stay, most patients can be set on an FiO_2 of 0.4–0.6. After an ABG shows a $PaO_2 > 55$, the FiO_2 can be down titrated. FiO_2 can also be weaned to keep an SaO_2 above 90%.

TROUBLESHOOTING PEARLS

- All patients who are receiving mechanical ventilation should be continuously monitored with end-tidal capnography ($EtCO_2$), pulse oximetry (SpO_2), and continued appropriate cardiovascular monitoring.
- A nice acronym for ventilator alarms is DOPE (displacement, obstruction, pneumothorax, equipment failure). Upon entering the room, review the appropriate monitor waveforms.
  - Lack of $EtCO_2$ should immediately signal that the endotracheal tube has been displaced.
  - Auscultate the patient (or consider bedside ultrasound to evaluate for lung slide).
  - Disconnect the patient from the ventilator and provide several manual breaths via bagging the patient to evaluate compliance.
  - If indicated, a suction catheter or a bougie can be passed down the internal lumen of the endotracheal tube to dislodge secretion plugs.
- It is NOT necessary to repeat multiple arterial blood gasses (ABG) when making ventilator adjustments. However, it is ideal to correlate an initial ABG with monitoring devices and then use $EtCO_2$ and SpO_2 to monitor adequate ventilation and oxygenation.
- Problems with oxygenation: the modifiable parameters to improve oxygenation are FiO_2 and PEEP. ARDSnet has a recommended FiO_2/PEEP ramp up table (Table 137.3) for patients with difficulty oxygenating.
  - PEEP is what provides the long-term support to help with oxygen exchange. This is reflected in the mean airway pressure. Initially placing the patient on 100%

TABLE 137.3	ARDSnet PEEP Table

Lower PEEP/higher FiO_2 strategy

	Start here	If still not adequately oxygenating, increase to the next setting combination ⟶											
FiO_2	0.3	0.4	0.4	0.5	0.5	0.6	0.7	0.7	0.7	0.8	0.9	0.9	0.9	1
PEEP	5	5	8	8	10	10	10	12	14	14	14	16	18	18–24

Higher PEEP/lower FiO_2 strategy

	Start here	If still not adequately oxygenating, increase to the next setting combination ⟶											
FiO_2	0.3	0.3	0.3	0.3	0.3	0.4	0.4	0.5	0.5	0.5–0.8	0.8	0.9	1	1
PEEP	5	8	10	12	14	14	16	16	18	20	22	22	22	24

FiO$_2$ (most ventilators have an "emergent 2-minute 100% FiO$_2$ button"), should only be a temporizing maneuver while PEEP parameters are adjusted.
- Problems with ventilation: the modifiable parameters to improve ventilation are TV and RR.
  - Changes in MV lead to changes in PaCO$_2$ and therefore pH.
- If the plateau pressures get too high as a result of worsening compliance, decrease the TV by 1 mL/kg increments until a minimum of 4 mL/kg is reached.
- If hypotension develops during mechanical ventilation and it is suspected to be directly caused by ventilation, decrease PEEP or TV to reduce intrathoracic pressure.
  - Intrathoracic pressure can theoretically decrease preload.

COMMON VENTILATOR ALARMS

- High-pressure alarm: Acute changes in peak/plateau pressures can help narrow down the cause for increased or elevated pressures.
  - Elevated peak pressures (plateau pressures remain unchanged): reflects a resistance to airflow (plugged ET tube, bronchospasm, secretions).
  - Both peak and plateau pressures rise: reflects a worsening lung compliance (pneumothorax, auto-PEEP, pulmonary edema, abdominal distension, ARDS, main-stemmed ETT).
- Low-pressure alarm or low-exhaled TV: occurs when the ventilator does not reach the expected inhalation pressure or measured a smaller returned volume than expected.
  - This occurs when there is a leak in the circuit (hole in the tubing, deflated ETT cuff).
- Apnea alarm: if the ventilator does not have an apnea backup setting, this signals that the patient is not breathing. In most machines, it signals that the tubing has become disconnected.

138 Consent and Capacity

Laura Ruble

GENERAL PRINCIPLES

Definitions

- Consent: A permissive decision made by a person with capacity. Consent is "informed" if given after being told the risks, benefits, and alternatives to the intervention.
- Capacity: The ability to make a specific decision in one's own best interest in a particular circumstance.
- Competence: The ability to make decisions in one's own best interest in many or all circumstances. This is a legal determination.

- Autonomy: The right of an individual to govern their own actions and the actions performed upon them.

A physician can legally perform or authorize interventions that are invasive to the patient's privacy and bodily integrity. The physician should always perform these interventions in pursuit of the patient's well-being, but there are circumstances in which they may be done in the absence of the patient's consent. These circumstances include obtundation, true emergency, or even cases of refusal in a person with impaired cognition or judgment.

Obtundation

If the patient has a significantly decreased global awareness due to metabolic encephalopathy or coma, every effort should be made to find the patient's health care proxy to obtain consent. Variably known as a proxy, a health care power of attorney, or a surrogate decision-maker, this person is entrusted to making decisions and giving consent for the patient based on what he or she thinks would be the wishes of the patient.

True Emergency

Some procedures are so emergent that there is no time to obtain informed consent from the patient or a proxy. These procedures are undertaken to avert life- or limb-threatening events, and consent is implied rather than explicit in these circumstances. Examples include emergent intubation, cricothyrotomy, or massive blood transfusion.

Impaired Capacity

Most often encountered in patients with psychiatric complaints, intoxicant ingestion, dementia, and delirium, the presentation of impaired capacity can cause patients to make decisions that are, in the physician's assessment, not in the patient's best interest. If possible, interventions should be postponed until underlying causes of impaired capacity have been resolved. If unable to do so, the physician should attempt to find a surrogate decision-maker to obtain consent.

In the event of being unable to find a surrogate decision-maker, the physician can act as a proxy to make decisions in the patient's best interest until legal guardianship proceedings can be completed.

SUGGESTED READINGS

Chaet DH. The AMA Code of Medical Ethics' opinions on patient decision-making capacity and competence and surrogate decision-making. *AMA J Ethics* 2016;18(6):601–3.

Riddick FA. The Code of Ethics of the American Medical Association. *Oschner J.* 2003 Spring 5(2):6–10.

Lai JM, Gill TM, Cooney LM, et al. Everyday decision-making ability in older persons with cognitive impairment. *Am J Geriatr Psychiatry* 2008;16(8):693–6.

139

Cultural Awareness: Providing Culturally Appropriate Care

Douglas Char

GENERAL PRINCIPLES

Culture

- Culture may be defined as the learned and shared beliefs, behaviors, and attitudes by members of a group defined by socioeconomic characteristics. Culture guides thinking, actions, behaviors, and emotional reactions to daily living. Cultural awareness is the ability of the health care provider to understand and respond to the unique cultural needs brought by the patient to the health care encounter.[1]
- Emergency physicians should consider the patient's culture as it relates to the patient's history and presenting symptoms. Do not assume that the patient wants to be treated the same way you want to be treated.
- Language barriers, economic hardships, differences in held values, and cultural practices all may serve as obstacles to excellent care.[2]
- Culture shapes our patients' confidence in and view of modern medicine and health care professionals. It colors self-assessment of their own illness and willingness to comply with medical advice and treatments. Cultural differences affect how health information and health care services are received, understood, and acted upon.

Health Care Disparities

- African Americans, Hispanics, and immigrant populations often receive a lower quality of care throughout the health care system. Disparities are likely to be similar or greater for smaller minority populations. Disparities contribute to decreased life expectancy and increased disease-specific morbidity and mortality.[3]
- There is a belief that minority and immigrant groups use the emergency department more frequently. Poor access to care, lack of insurance coverage, and regulatory barriers contribute to disparate levels of care for underserved, minority, and immigrant populations.[4]
- Patient factors impact health care seeking, disease understanding, treatment decisions, and health care utilization (compliance). They may be related to family roles and structure, rituals, opposition to acculturation, and perceived response of the majority culture.

Cultural Awareness

- Health care provider factors impact one's willingness to be open to alternative or complementary health care, incorporation of traditional medical practices, appreciation of systemic barriers to access, and medications, priority setting that the patient is facing.
- Risk factors for not having a cultural awareness of patients include language barriers (including visually and hearing-impaired patients and family members), not accounting for the patients' beliefs in the supernatural (in health or role of healing traditions), or not ascertaining the value of involving the entire family in decision making.

- Increased cultural awareness leads to better patient–doctor relationships and communication related to diagnosis and in treatment planning. This may in turn reduce health care disparities by reducing biases and ensuring quality care across racial and cultural groups. It also reduces clinical uncertainty related to caring for patients from unfamiliar backgrounds.[2]

Strategies to Improve Cultural Awareness

- Improving cross-cultural communication skills so that providers ascertain and understand the patient's values will enhance patient–provider trust and satisfaction. The physician will be better equipped to negotiate medical interventions.
- Language is a frequent barrier to culturally appropriate emergency care.[5] Routine use of translators and communication devices (including those for visual- and hearing-impaired patients) should be made available around the clock.
- Watch for verbal and nonverbal cues (body language).
  - Reserve judgment about patient and family personal behavior.
- Learn about acceptable social behaviors for groups of patients you may be called upon to care for frequently.
- "Do no harm" can only occur if we understand, appreciate, and honor the patient's needs and desires as informed by their cultural framework.
- Not all individuals from a given cultural group will assimilate their culture to the same extent, so while generalities may provide a starting point, they should not be relied upon or else the provider risks stereotyping the patient based on group affiliation.
- The U.S. health care system has its own beliefs, values, and practices that may not be shared by all patients (illness as having a physical cause, patient deference to physicians, expectations about promptness, timeliness, and role of one's family).
- Despite emergency medicine's historical commitment to provide access to all those needing medical care, research show that we are not immune from providing culturally inappropriate care and continue to provide disparate care to certain populations of patients.[4]
- Providers must recognize that they bring their own culture and implicit biases to the clinical setting during each and every patient–provider interaction—culture is not something that only belongs to the patient.
- Strategies to reduce health care disparities and increase cultural competence within emergency medicine include the following[2]:
  - Reducing provider bias and increasing cultural awareness training (being aware of one's implicit bias will not alone change behavior) will improve attitudes toward minority patients and enhance cross-cultural communication.
  - Clinically accommodate patients—create a clinical setting that fully utilizes a health care team approach to address a variety of cultural norms.
  - Promote workforce diversity—culturally appropriate care is more likely to occur when the health care team more closely resembles the patient population.
- Three models to enhance cultural awareness, knowledge, and skills[6] (training programs often utilize components of all three):
  - Cultural competence: The level of a provider's knowledge, attitude, and skills about cultural values and health-related beliefs, disease incidence and prevalence, and treatment efficacy for diverse cultural groups.
  - Cross-cultural efficacy: Providers learn how their own culture and behaviors can impact others of different cultures and understand how patient's culturally based behaviors may impact the provider.
  - Cultural humility: Provider engages in regular self-evaluation and self-critique. The goal is to develop power-balanced relationships with patients of different cultures.

- Take a flexible patient-centered approach: This allows ascertainment of the patient's perception of medicine as well as communication and negotiation related to diagnosis and treatment.[7]
- Becoming cultural aware and competent is not a simple or straightforward process. It occurs slowly over time. First attempts are often awkward and unsatisfactory, but it is only through continued ongoing patient–provider encounters that one becomes more comfortable and natural looking for and making use of cultural cues and opportunities.
- Culturally sensitive care requires accommodating patient needs and modifying provider expectations, practices, and behaviors based on patient values. Patients must be empowered to negotiate clinical interventions informed by their cultural values. This often means that providers must compromise with patients to identify optimal outcomes.

REFERENCES

1. ACEP Policy Statement: Cultural Awareness and Emergency Care. 2014. Available at: https://www.acep.org/Clinical—Practice-Management/Cultural-Awareness-and-Emergency-Care.
2. Padela A, Punekar I. Emergency medicine practice: advancing cultural competence and reducing health care disparities. *Acad Emerg Med* 2009;16:69–75.
3. Institute of Medicine (US) Committee on Understanding and Eliminating Racial and Ethnic Disparities in Health Care. Smedley BD, Stith AY, Nelson AR eds.; *Unequal Treatment: Confronting Racial and Ethnic Disparities in Health Care*. Washington: National Academies Press, 2003.
4. Heron SL, Stettner E, Haley LL Jr. Racial and ethnic disparities in the emergency department: a public health perspective. *Emerg Med Clin North Am* 2006;24:905–23.
5. Dees L. Culturally competent care in the emergency medical services. *Texas EMS Mag* 2007;34–8.
6. Robertson P, Zeh, D. Cross-Cultural Issues in Integrated Care. In: Curtis R, Christian E, eds. *Integrated Care: Applying Theory to Practice*. New York: Routledge, 2012.
7. Levin SJ, Like RC, Gottlieb JE. ETHNIC: a framework for culturally competent clinical practice. *Patient Care* 2000;9(special issue):188.

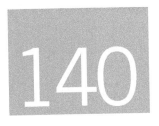

140 Delivering Bad News

Sonya Naganathan

GENERAL PRINCIPLES

- Delivering bad news is a frequent occurrence, and bad news may manifest itself in many forms including new diagnoses, death, or an otherwise unexpected outcome of a patient's visit.[1,2]

- Death in the ED is often due to unexpected and traumatic circumstances. This often does not leave loved ones the time to anticipate their grief.
- Similarly, patients receiving an unexpected diagnosis, need for emergency surgery, or admission to the hospital are also caught off guard.

APPROACH

SPIKES

- This approach was originally tailored toward the field of oncology. The goal of this method is to create an organized approach to delivering bad news. (Table 140.1)[3]

TABLE 140.1	SPIKES Approach
Setting up the interview	• Facilitate a private environment • Ask the patient if they would like anyone else in the room with them • Sit down in order to relax the patient • Attempt to limit amount of interruptions during the discussion
Assessing patient **P**erception	• Ask the patient what they understand of the current situation
Obtain patient's **I**nvitation	• How much does the patient want to know about the situation/illness? • Is there any information they would rather wait to hear, or not hear at all?
Giving **K**nowledge and information to the patient	• Use both nonverbal and verbal cues to warn the patient of impending bad news • Use layman's terms whenever possible • It is important to be direct, yet not overtly blunt
Addressing patient's **E**motions with empathic responses	• Allow for some time for the patient to process what they have just heard • Allow the patient to initiate a response and express their emotions • If the patient remains silent, use an open-ended question to attempt to understand the underlying emotion • Respond to a patient's emotions with an empathic response (e.g., "I know this is not what you were expecting to hear.") and/or a validating response (e.g., "It is very common for others to also feel this way.")
Strategy and **S**ummary	• Evaluate the patient's readiness to discuss the next steps • Summarize the plan of care and address patient goals as much as possible

TABLE 140.2	GRIEV_ING Approach
Gather	Gather family members
Resources	Resources geared toward grief support—clergy, family, hospital chaplain, etc.
Identify	Identify (1) yourself, (2) the patient, (3) the relationship of the family members to the patient, and (4) what information the family had prior to patient's presentation to the ED
Educate	Educate the patient's loved ones as to the events that occurred in the ED and the current state of the situation
Verify	Verify to the family that the patient has died. Be direct, and make sure to use the word "death" or "died"
_	Give the family space to process the loss
Inquire	Ask if family members have questions; answer questions
Nuts and bolts	Inquire about the following: funeral home services, patient's personal belongings, and organ donation
Give	Give the family your contact information and state your availability to answer questions at a later time if necessary

GRIEV_ING

- This approach was designed specifically to educate EM residents on the process of death notification and assess their ability to deliver death notifications in a controlled setting (Table 140.2).[4]

SPECIAL CONSIDERATIONS

- Adult resuscitation attempts
  - Most of the readily available literature describes positive effects on the families of the deceased when they were present during resuscitative efforts.
  - The ED team should use a family-centered and team-based approach.
    - This will ensure required steps following death such as offering the family an autopsy, notifying law enforcement if necessary, notifying the patient's primary care provider of the patient's death, and organ donation are taken.

REFERENCES

1. Shoenberger JM, Yeghiazarian S, Rios C, Henderson SO. Death notification in the emergency department: survivors and physicians. *West J Emerg Med* 2013;14:181–5.
2. Park I, Gupta A, Mandani K, et al. Breaking bad news education for emergency medicine residents: a novel training module using simulation with the SPIKES protocol. *J Emerg Trauma Shock* 2010;3:385–8.
3. Baile WF, Buckman R, Lenzi R, et al. SPIKES—a six-step protocol for delivering bad news: application to the patient with cancer. *Oncologist* 2000;5:302–11.
4. Hobgood C, Harward D, Newton K. The educational intervention "GRIEV_ING" improves the death notification skills of residents. *Acad Emerg Med* 2005;12:296–301.

Evidence-Based Medicine

Gary M. Gaddis

GENERAL PRINCIPLES

- Evidence-based medicine (EBM) is defined as the integration of best research evidence with clinical expertise and patient values.[1]
- It is important to differentiate testing and treating to attempt to meet patient expectations and increase satisfaction from the true practice of EBM, while being mindful of patient values.
- In one example, the Ottawa Ankle Rules[3,4] determine when no foot or ankle radiographs are required. However, the patient may request, or even demand a plain radiographs which is non–evidence-based care. Unfortunately, the time it takes to explain why no radiograph is needed often far exceeds the time and effort required to simply cave into the patient's non–evidence-based expectations and obtain the film that will be negative.
- On the other hand, consider a patient with advanced lung cancer, who now has pneumonia. The patient may decide near the end of life not to allow the doctor to administer antibiotics, despite that the medical evidence suggests that it may be possible to successfully treat the patient's pneumonia with the right antibiotics. To withhold antibiotics for this patient, who is content to forego treatment even if this shortens their life, is to provide evidence-based care, mindful of the patient's values and preferences.
- The bottom line: Do not confuse the obtaining of non–evidence-based testing and treatments to enhance patient satisfaction with the provision of care that is mindful of the patient's values and preferences.

HIERARCHY OF EVIDENCE

Evidence Pyramid

- Figure 141.1 is an example of the recognized hierarchy of evidence.
- The "Evidence Pyramid" conceptualizes levels and quality of evidence, from least useful for the practice of EBM to the most useful. At the bottom of the pyramid are "Expert Opinion" and "Case Series/Reports." Sometimes, this level of evidence is sufficient to validate our practice. However, for most medical matters, a series of prospective, randomized controlled trials (which may have been synthesized into a Critically Appraised Topic or Systematic Review) are required to change practice.

Practice-Changing Manuscripts

- An example of a series of practice-changing manuscripts are the ProCESS,[5] ARISE,[6] and PROMISE[7] trials. These quickly changed emergency practice, without a systematic review having been published. These trials were highly concordant. They showed that the monitoring of mixed central venous oxygen saturation was not associated with any measurable improvement in mortality compared to standard sepsis care without central mixed venous oxygen saturation monitoring. Based on these articles, the National Quality Forum changed its recommendation for emergency

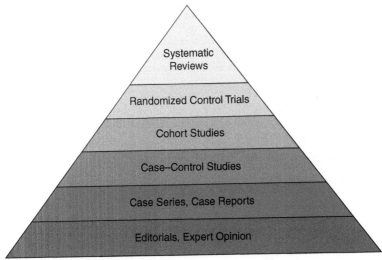

Figure 141.1. The evidence pyramid. (Adapted from Sackett DL, Straus SE, Richardson WS, et al. *Evidence-Based Medicine: How to Practice and Teach EBM, 2nd ed.* Edinburgh: Churchill Livingstone, 2000, with permission.)

department care of patients with severe sepsis and septic shock based solely upon these manuscripts.
- The five manuscripts that appeared in the *New England Journal of Medicine* in 2015 regarding endovascular treatment of large vessel acute ischemic strokes represent another example where new, concordant evidence from several similar trials immediately changed medical practice via the new evidence they conveyed.
- However, for most medical matters, a thorough systematic review is required to change medical practice. For example, in the mid 1990s, only after the National Institutes of Health convened a conference to develop a consensus, the use of antibiotics to treat gastritis due to *Helicobacter pylori* became widespread (despite that prior dogma held that microbes could not live in the gut).[9] As is the case for most EBM matters, a synthesis of available information was necessary before dogma was overturned and new, correct evidence would be widely implemented.
- Sometimes a group of concordant, practice-changing manuscripts will appear nearly simultaneously in the medical literature. However, usually, what is accepted widely as sufficient evidence to change practice emerges only after a synthesis of all available evidence.

SPECIAL CONSIDERATIONS

Barriers to Implementation of EBM
- It has been recognized for over a decade that various barriers exist to the widespread deployment of EBM.
- It is not sufficient for knowledge just to be available. Clinicians must become aware of the evidence and must accept it as true. It is then deemed applicable to

the appropriate clinical context. These are the steps needed to bring evidence to the bedside. Next, the medical care team needs to be able to act on the evidence. This is done through the Quality Improvement process. Finally, clinicians must agree with and comply with the evidence in their provision of care. This can be enhanced via clinical decision aids, patient educational materials.

Implementation at the Bedside

- There are frequently updated, curated sources such as UpToDate, MDCalc.com, and TheNNT.com that can often provide qualitative and quantitative data to assist the bedside implementation of EBM.

REFERENCES

1. Straus SE, Glasziou P, Richardson WS, Haynes RB. *Evidence-Based Medicine. How to Practice and Teach It.* Edinburgh: Elsevier Churchill Livingstone. 2011 ISBN 9 780 70203 1274.
2. Steill IG, Greenburg GH, McKnight RD, et al. Decision rules for the use of radiography in acute ankle injuries. Refinement and prospective validation. *JAMA* 1993;269: 1127–32.
3. Available at: http://www.mdcalc.com/ottawa-ankle-rule/ (last accessed 20/12/16).
4. ProCESS Investigators. A randomized trial of protocol-based care for early septic shock. *N Engl J Med* 2014;370:1683–93.
5. The ARISE Investigators. Goal-directed resuscitation for patients with early septic shock. *N Engl J Med* 2014;371:1496–506.
6. Mouncey PR, Osborn TM, Power GS, et al. Trial of early, goal-directed resuscitation for septic shock. *N Engl J Med* 2014;327:1301–11.
7. Gaddis GM. Chapter 18: How to Design a Study That Everyone Will Believe: Prospective Studies. In: Wilson MP, Guluma KZ, Hayden SR, eds. *Doing Research in Emergency and Acute Care. Making Order out of Chaos.* 2015. Wiley and Sons. Oxford ISBN 978-1-118-64348-8.
8. Glasziou P, Haynes B. Get title. *Evidence Based Med* 2005;10:4–7.

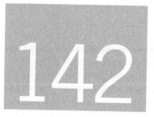

142 Burnout and Fatigue
Sonya Naganathan and Randall A. Howell

GENERAL PRINCIPLES

- Variations in work hours, physical exhaustion, challenging patients, and high-stress situations are considered to be major contributions to burnout among physicians.
- As a result, increasing rates of substance abuse, depression, anxiety, and suicide are seen in this population.
- Approximately 400 physicians commit suicide annually.

- Stress reduction techniques such as mindfulness meditation have come to the forefront as a means of preventing burnout.

Definition

- Burnout, though recognized in our society as a mental health issue, is not considered to be an official condition—it is not characterized in the *Diagnostic and Statistical Manual of Mental Disorders*. Multiple definitions exist, though it is generally characterized by "emotional exhaustion, depersonalization, and reduced personal accomplishment."
- Burnout is described in the context of a job or other occupational stressors. It is a chronic process, occurring over weeks to years.

Epidemiology

- The rate of burnout among emergency medicine physicians on a 2012 national study of all physicians was between 65% and 70%.
- A 57.1% burnout rate was noted in both residents and attending physicians in a recent study held at academic emergency medicine programs.

Risk Factors

- Differing levels of autonomy, marital statuses, depression, hours worked, uncertainty related to patient outcomes are all factors that have been correlated with burnout in various studies.

Prevention

- Preventing burnout is ideal, though recognition of its symptoms can sometimes be difficult.
- Coping methods such as mindfulness meditation, exercise, and having a good network of friends and family have been shown to prevent these symptoms from developing.

DIAGNOSIS

- Burnout is not well understood; thus, controversy still exists as to whether it is a true, diagnosable condition. It is not currently included in the *Diagnostic and Statistical Manual of Mental Disorders*, Fifth Edition.
- The Maslach Burnout Inventory (MBI) has long since been used to measure the amount of burnout in an individual. This survey measures responses to questions on three scales: emotional exhaustion, depersonalization, and personal accomplishment. A higher score in the former two sections and a lower score on the last section are linked with burnout.

Clinical Presentation

- There is no classic presentation for burnout, though characteristics of each of the three measures of burnout may point to underlying burnout.
  - Emotional exhaustion is typified by wholly negative attitudes, cynicism, and bitterness toward those individuals who are at the receiving end of the service (e.g., "Will this even matter?").
  - Depersonalization refers to feelings of detachment from the outcome (e.g., "That patient is back again complaining of the same knee pain—he obviously won't listen to anything we say.").

○ Loss of personal accomplishment described by a low sense of achievement (e.g., "I can't seem to do anything right.").
- Symptoms of depression may be concomitant with burnout.
- Poor coping methods have led to an increase in substance abuse to deal with daily stresses. A 2006 survey among EM residents shows an increasing trend in daily alcohol use.
- When surveyed, residents and physicians have admitted to providing a lower quality of patient care due to burnout.

TREATMENT

- Once the symptoms of burnout have been recognized, steps must be taken to address the symptoms on a short-term basis. Additionally, it is important to establish preventative strategies to prevent future burnout.

Mindfulness

- The concept of mindfulness is described as the act of focusing on the present moment.
- The mindfulness-based stress reduction (MBSR) method developed by Dr. Jon Kabat-Zinn in 1979 has been shown in the literature to have a positive effect on anxiety, depression, and stress.
- Studies conducted with health care providers in the last decade have shown a decrease in the indices for burnout as indicated by the MBI.

TABLE 142.1	Stressors and Coping Mechanisms
Issues	**Ways to address**
Substance abuse	Maintain close support system
	Utilize community resource programs
	Encourage culture of self-reporting
Sleep deprivation	Regular exercise
	Circadian shift scheduling
	Limit caffeine and alcohol
Negative outcomes in the workplace	Postdeath debriefing
	Close support system
	Accepting death as normal, and at times unavoidable, in this line of work
Maintaining healthy lifestyle	Schedule a time for exercise
	Keep healthy snacks both at work and at home
	Rotate both food and exercise so you do not tire of routine

Adapted from Schmitz GR, Clark M, Heron S, et al. Strategies for coping with stress in emergency medicine: early education is vital. *J Emerg Trauma Shock* 2012;5:64–9.

SUGGESTED READINGS

Beach MC, Roter D, Korthuis PT, et al. A multicenter study of physician mindfulness and health care quality. *Ann Fam Med* 2013;11:421–8.

Fortney L, Luchterhand C, Zakletskaia L, et al. Abbreviated mindfulness intervention for job satisfaction, quality of life, and compassion in primary care clinicians: a pilot study. *Ann Fam Med* 2013;11:412–20.

Goodman MJ, Schorling JB. A mindfulness course decreases burnout and improves well-being among healthcare providers. *Int J Psychiatry Med* 2012;43:119–28.

Lu D, Dresden S, McCloskey C, et al. The impact of burnout on patient care among emergency physicians. *Ann Emerg Med* 2014;64:S43–4.

Maslach C, Jackson SE. The measurement of experienced burnout. *J Organ Behav* 1981;2: 99–113.

Physician and Medical Student Depression and Suicide Prevention. 2016. Available at: http://afsp.org/our-work/education/physician-medical-student-depression-suicide-prevention (last accessed 4/29/16).

Takayesu JK, Ramoska EA, Clark TR, et al. Factors associated with burnout during emergency medicine residency. *Acad Emerg Med* 2014;21:1031–5.

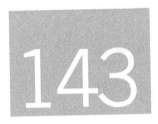

143 Federal Laws Affecting Provision of Emergency Care: EMTALA

Randy Jotte

GENERAL PRINCIPLES

- The Emergency Medical Treatment and Labor Act (EMTALA), passed by the U.S. Congress in 1986, assures access to emergency care and prohibits the practice of patient transfer from private to public facilities for financial reasons.
- EMTALA has three principle components:
  - Medical screening requirement
  - Stabilization of emergency medical condition and labor
  - Restriction of transfer until patient stabilization

Impact on Emergency Care

Each component of EMTALA significantly regulates emergency physicians, hospitals, and consultants in order to assure access to emergency care.

- Under EMTALA, each hospital must provide an appropriate medical screening exam within the capabilities of the hospital's emergency department.
  - Definition of the location of a hospital's emergency department is broad: "the entire main hospital campus…including the parking lot, sidewalk and driveway or hospital departments, including any buildings owned by the hospital that are within 250 yards of the hospital."[1]
  - In addition, request for examination and treatment of an emergency condition can be specifically requested by a patient or presumed to be desired based on a perception of "suffering from an emergency medical condition by a prudent layperson."[2]
  - Hospital-owned or hospital-operated ambulance services are considered part of the ED.
  - EMTALA does not specify the nature and extent of the screening exam. It requires that a hospital emergency department apply whatever resources are available and appropriate. In addition, such a level of screening must be performed uniformly to all patients presenting with substantially similar complaints.[3]
- Transfer to another hospital with appropriate facilities can follow best efforts at stabilization.
  - The receiving hospital must report any above-noted refusing on-call physicians to the federal Health Care and Financing Administration, HCFA.[4]
- Transfers can occur:
  - When an informed patient requests transfer
  - When a physician verifies that the benefits of transfer outweigh the risks
  - When the transferring hospital minimizes the risks of transfer to the best of its ability
  - When the receiving hospital has adequate space and personnel
  - When the receiving hospital accepts the patient
  - When the transferring hospital sends all records
  - When the patient is transferred with qualified personnel
- Failure to comply with EMTALA risks civil monetary penalties to the hospital and physician.

REFERENCES

1. CMSManualSystem.Pub.100-07,StateOperationsProvider Certification, Transmittal 46, Interpretive Guidelines for §489.24(a)(1)(i) May 29, 2009. Available at: http://www.cms.gov/Regulations- and- Guidance/Guidance/Transmittals/downloads/R46SOMA.pdf (last accessed 1/20/5).
2. CMSManualSystem.Pub.100-07,StateOperationsProvider Certification, Transmittal 46, Interpretive Guidelines for §489.24(a)(1)(i) May 29, 2009. Available at: http://www.cms.gov/Regulations- and- Guidance/Guidance/Transmittals/downloads/R46SOMA.pdf (last accessed 1/20/15).
3. Correa v. Hospital San Francisco, 69 F.3d 1184 (1st Cir. 1995).
4. 42 US Code§1395dd - Examination and treatment for emergency medical conditions and women in labor.

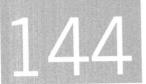

Goals of Care Communication, End-of-Life Care, and Palliative Care

Brian T. Wessman

GENERAL PRINCIPLES

Despite individuals' stated preference to die at home, the majority of people die in institutions (hospital or nursing homes). Medicare data shows that over one-third of patients who die receive medical care in the ED and ICU during their last 6 months of life. At the end of life (EOL), patients will often find themselves struggling with their need for critical care medical expertise versus their desire to avoid invasive procedures. EOL discussions have been shown to reduce both the incidence of aggressive interventions and the subsequent psychological stress among surviving family members. Helping patients and families delineate life values, and preferred care outcomes have been shown to reduce medical provider stress.

Medical Ethics

The four traditional pillars of medical ethics are autonomy, beneficence, nonmaleficence, and justice:

Autonomy: patients are the best arbiters of which medical options promote their self-interest and values. Therefore, physicians should help patients come to their own decision by providing full information about treatment options and potential outcomes.

Physicians should uphold a competent adult patient's decision, even if it appears medically wrong (and it doesn't impact the other three pillars of medical ethics).

Beneficence: the general moral principle of doing what is best for the patient. This idea may originate from the physician's professional judgment or the patient's wishes. At the heart of beneficence is the idea of "quality of life" and how the patient defines and values this. At times, beneficence may even imply not intervening in cases where the benefit of therapy would be minimal.

Nonmaleficence: the moral principle of "first, do no harm." All therapies involve some degree of risk or have side effects. The physician should always consider the risk of doing harm to a patient, especially when the specific disease process cannot be cured.

Justice: allocate medical care fairly and equally to all patients in similar situations.

Establishing Goals of Care

A goal of care (GOC) is not a code status. A GOC is a patient-centered value such as "returning home to resume my gardening" or "being able to independently attend a baseball game." The medical team should then subsequently help the patient or family match an appropriate patient-centered medical code status to this expressed personal quality of life goal.

For a critically ill patient arriving to the ED, the physician should ascertain whether a patient has previously appointed a Durable Power of Attorney for Health Care and/or completed an Advance Directive. If so, these documents should be obtained, and if possible, the contents of them should be discussed with the patients and family. Realistically, an Advanced Directive without in-depth communication about what intensity of medical care each individual desires does little to guide medical decision making.

Unfortunately, the majority of patients have neither document. Despite the presence of life-limiting illness, many patients will have not discussed EOL care with either their personal physician or family members, and this may occur for the first time in the ED setting. Discussions to establish goals of care should include the patient if he/she is capable of participating and should be shared with the patient's family and loved ones, as directed by the patient. If the patient is not decisional either due to the acute condition or previous underlying disease, the discussion should be held with an appropriate surrogate. For patients who are unstable on arrival, the EM physician should act in accordance with his/her best judgment; often, the default is to attempt to stabilize the patient to provide the benefit of time and further discussions.

The purpose of the initial GOC discussion is to ascertain what the patient and family's expectations are for the acute hospitalization as well as for the underlying disease process. In addition, the EM physician should elicit the values, preferences, and wishes of the patient with respect to what they view as an acceptable outcome for their hospital stay, anywhere from a hope for cure to a desire for a pain free death. Often, patients have multiple seemingly contradictory goals, in which case the physician should take time to help in clarification and prioritization. It is equally important for the physician to provide adequate prognostic information and advise the patient/family as to what can reasonably be expected during this hospitalization. These conversations should be chronicled in the medical record.

When establishing goals of care, employ positive phrases. For example, during a family conversation, list the things you *will* do and not what you *will not* do: WILL provide comfort, WILL provide pain medications, WILL provide dignity, WILL respect the patient's autonomy, and WILL "allow natural death" (instead of the commonly employed "do not resuscitate [DNR]"). This change in terminology ultimately changes the code status mentality as the medical team is allowing the natural progression of life into death and not withholding therapies or treatment.

Poignant phrases have impact and remove any false hope that a family may be harboring. If clinically indicated, make sure to simply use the word "*death*" instead of other euphemistic terms. Phrases such as "Your loved one will not return to the way they were previously..." and "I wish (we could cure the cancer)..." help to convey clear meaning and show empathy. It is not fair to "request a decision" from a family as no one wants to be burdened with the choice to end their loved one's life. Instead, focus on specific patient-centered values and goals. Encourage the family to act as the voice of the patient. The goal is to communicate and develop a medical plan that best respects patient/family values in light of what is medically achievable.

Shared Decision Making and Surrogate Decision Making

Shared decision making (SDM) is of utmost importance when approaching a GOC discussion and also for EOL decisions. Physician input should include information about the disease state(s), current treatments, realistic medical feasibility, and prognosis. Patient/surrogate input should include information about the patient's values, quality of life, and treatment preferences. This should lead to the joint deliberation and decision stage where both sides focus on the best available options for the patient.

Patients in extremis are often unable to participate in decision making due to either their acute illness or underlying disease process. In these instances, appropriate surrogates must be identified. If the patient has appointed a specific individual as Durable Power of Attorney for Health Care, that individual should serve as the primary decision maker. Many but not all states have a legal order of surrogacy established (i.e., spouse or offspring) if an individual is not specified. One should be familiar with the relevant laws of their state. A valid surrogate can be defined as an individual that can faithfully represent the goals, values, and wishes of the patient and act accordingly and in the patient's best interest. However, this is often a difficult task and is almost always colored by the surrogates own values and preferences.

Typically, both surrogates and caregivers underestimate the willingness of patients to undergo aggressive interventions and underestimate the quality of life that patients deem to be acceptable. The physician plays an active role in this process of arriving at a consensus medical plan as part of SDM.

Withdrawing and Withholding Life-Sustaining Treatments

EM physicians may be faced with decisions to limit life-sustaining treatments as patients face EOL decisions. These decisions can be a source of distress and conflict for health care providers as well as patients and families.

The autonomous patient or their surrogate may make an informed decision to refuse any proposed treatment, even if the physician believes that such a decision is not in their best interest. From this, it follows directly that patients or their surrogates may opt to discontinue any treatment once initiated. If this were not the case, many patients might be reluctant to initiate potentially beneficial therapies for fear they would not be permitted to stop at a later time.

Most commonly, withdrawal of life-sustaining treatments is equated with discontinuation of mechanical ventilation. However, discontinuation of hemodynamic support, hemodialysis, enteral nutrition, transfusions, or other interventions also should be considered in this context. One published strategy is that of "stuttered withdrawal" or the staggered removal of life-sustaining treatments (i.e., stopping enteral nutrition, followed by stopping renal replacement therapy at a subsequent time interval, followed by stopping vent support at another time interval). Another strategy is that of a "time-limited trial of therapy" (i.e., trial of renal replacement therapy for 3 days to see if there is renal recovery). Published data with this strategy highlights the importance of explaining to families what to expect at the EOL. The decision to withdraw life-sustaining treatments should be approached in a manner similar to all other treatment decisions. While neither of these strategies are congruent with typical ED timelines of patient care, it his helpful for the EM physician to be aware of these EOL options as they engage families in discussions. Ultimately, the goal of withdrawal of life-sustaining interventions is to remove treatments that are no longer congruent with the patient's goals and values and are therefore no longer appropriate.

TABLE 144.1	The Principle of Double Effect

An action with two possible consequences, one good and one bad, is morally permissible if the action:

1. Is not in itself immoral.
2. Is undertaken only with the intention of achieving the possible good effect, without intending the possible bad effect, even though the bad effect may be foreseen.
3. The action does not bring about the good effect solely by means of the bad effect.
4. Is undertaken for a proportionately grave reason.

Attention to the patient's comfort is paramount during the process of withdrawal of life-sustaining treatments. Reluctance to administer adequate doses of analgesics and sedatives can result in undue and unacceptable levels of suffering to both the patient and surviving family members. There is ethical and legal consensus that although respiratory depression or hypotension may be a foreseeable consequence of these medications, if the intent is to relieve specific symptoms such as pain or dyspnea, it is essential to treat in adequate doses despite the possibility that death may be hastened. Ethically, the justification for this has been termed the principle of "double effect" (Table 144.1).

Palliative sedation is the goal of providing vigorous pre-emptive deep sedation to avoid patient suffering when death is imminent. Studies have repeatedly shown that there is no relationship with palliative sedation and "hastening of death." Most commonly, narcotics are given in combination with a benzodiazepine. The medications should be liberally administered initially as a bolus followed by continuous infusion to allow for a rapid achievement of steady-state levels. It is paramount to confirm patient comfort prior to proceeding with withdrawal of mechanical ventilation. The synthetic anticholinergic glycopyrrolate can be considered to reduce oral secretions associated with a terminal extubation. Neuromuscular blocking agents should never be used as they do not provide any palliative effect to the patient and make assessment of comfort impossible.

There should be frequent reassessment by the nursing and medical staff for comfort as a patient approaches the EOL. Family members can be given the option of being present during the extubation, depending solely on their personal preference. If possible, the monitor screen in the patient's room should be turned off to allow the family to focus on the patient without distraction.

Futility

There remains no clear consensus on an approach to futility. The vast majority of clinical situations in which these conflicts arise can be favorably resolved by improved communication between the physician, the various consulting services, and the family.

There are three specific conditions that define interventions that are futile in the strictest sense: the intervention has no pathophysiologic rationale; cardiac arrest occurs due to refractory hypotension or hypoxemia despite maximal supportive therapy (performance of CPR in such a circumstance will be ineffective in restoring circulation); and the intervention has been tried and already failed in the patient. Treatments that meet these strict criteria do not need to be provided.

It is advisable to employ a strategy that focuses on process and conflict resolution rather than on absolute definitions. Ultimately, it is the process of increased communication between the health care providers and family members that leads to the satisfactory resolution of these difficult situations.

SUGGESTED READINGS

Berlinger N, Jennings B, Wolf S. *The Hastings Center Guidelines for Decisions on Life-sustaining Treatment and Care Near the End of Life.* Oxford University Press, Oxford 2013.

Blinderman CD, Krakauer EL, Solomon MZ. Time to revise the approach to determining cardiopulmonary resuscitation status. *JAMA* 2012;307(9):917–8.

Chan JD, Treece PD, Engelberg RA, et al. Narcotic and benzodiazepine use after withdrawal of life support. *Chest* 2004;126(1):286–93.

Cook D, Rocker G, Marshall J, et al. Understanding the treatment preferences of seriously ill patients. *N Engl J Med* 2002;346:1061–6.

Cook D, Rocker G, Marshall J, et al. Withdrawal of mechanical ventilation in anticipation of death in the intensive care unit. *N Engl J Med* 2003;349:1123–32.

Curtis J, Engelberg RA. What is the "right" intensity of care at the end of life and how do we get there? *Ann Intern Med* 2011;154(4):283–4.

Curtis JR, Tonelli MR. Shared decision-making in the ICU: value, challenges, and limitations. *Am J Respir Crit Care Med* 2011;183(7):840–1.

de Graeff AQ, Dean M. Palliative sedation therapy in the last weeks of life: a literature review and recommendations for standards. *J Palliat Med* 2007;10(1):67–85.

Elpern EH, Patterson PA, Gloskey D, Bone RC. Patients' preferences for intensive care. *Crit Care Med* 1992;20:43–47.

Halevy A, Brody BA. A multi-institution collaborative policy on medical futility. *JAMA* 1996;276:571–4.

Hua M, Wunsch W. Integrating palliative care in the ICU. *CO Crit Care* 2014;20(6):673–80.

Lo B. *Resolving Ethical Dilemmas: A guide for Clinicians.* Philadelphia: Lippincott Williams & Wilkins, 2005.

Nelson JE, Azoulay E, Curtis JR, et al. Palliative Care in the ICU. *J Palliat Med* 2012;15(2):168–74.

Quill TE, Arnold R, Back AL. Discussing treatment preferences with patients who want everything. *Ann Intern Med* 2009;151(5):345–9.

Quill CM, Ratcliffe SJ, Harhay MO, Halpern SD. Variation on decisions to forgo life-sustaining therapies in US ICUs. *Chest* 2014;146(3):573–82.

Scheunemann LP, Cunningham TV, Arnold RM, et al. How clinicians discuss critically ill patients' preferences and values with surrogates: an empirical analysis. *Crit Care Med* 2015;43(4):757–64.

Thompson BT, Cox PN, Antonelli M, et al. Challenges in end-of-life care in the ICU: statement of the 5th International Consensus Conference in Critical Care: Brussels, Belgium, April 2003: executive summary. *Crit Care Med* 2004;32:1781.

Sheridan SL, Harris RP, Woolf SH. Shared decision making about screening and chemoprevention. A suggested approach from the U.S. Preventive Services Task Forces. *Am J Prev Med* 2004;26:56–66.

Support Principal Investigators. A controlled trial to improve care for seriously ill hospitalized patients. The study to understand prognoses and preferences for outcomes and risks of treatments (SUPPORT). *JAMA* 1995;274:1591–8.

The Concept of Futility. SCCM consensus statement. *Crit Care Med* 1997;25:887–91.

Truog RD, Cist AF, Brackett SE, et al. Recommendations for end-of-life care in the intensive care unit: the Ethics Committee of the Society of Critical Care Medicine. *Crit Care Med* 2001;29(12):2332–48.

Wessman B, Sona C, Schallom M. Improving caregivers' perceptions regarding patient goals of care/end-of-life issues for the multidisciplinary critical care team. *J Intensive Care Med* 2015;32(1):68–76.

145 Physician Impairment

Douglas Char and Aldo Andino

GENERAL PRINCIPLES

- Physician impairment occurs due to a health problem that may be a result of physical or mental illness, substance abuse, burnout, and/or several other conditions.[1]
- Suicide rates are higher among physicians than in the general public, and depression is likely underreported due to the stigma associated with the diagnosis.[2]

Definition of Physician Impairment

- Per ACEP's policy statement, physician impairment "exists when a physician becomes unable to practice medicine with reasonable skill and safety because of personal health problems or other stressors."[1]
- The presence of a health problem in a physician is not synonymous with occupational impairment.[1]
- Impairment is thought to be a self-limited state that is amenable to intervention, assistance, recovery, and/or resolution.[1]

Causes of Physician Impairment

In JAMA in July 2010, 17% of nearly 1900 responding physicians reported having had direct personal knowledge of an impaired or incompetent physician in their hospital, group, or practice in the 3 preceding years. Of those, one-third did not report the individual. Those who kept silent said they believed someone else was taking care of the problem (19%), did not think reporting the problem would make a difference (15%), feared retribution (12%), felt it was not their responsibility to report (10%), or worried that the physician would be excessively punished (9%).[3]

Substance Abuse

- The incidence of alcoholism and drug addiction in physicians is 10%, which is the same as that observed in the general population.[4]
- Alcohol is the most common drug used by physicians.[4]
- A longitudinal cohort study from 1995 to 2001 of physicians enrolled in a Physician Health Program (PHP) found that emergency physicians (EPs) had a higher rate of substance use disorders.[5]
- EPs most commonly abused alcohol, followed by opioids and stimulants.[19]

Depression

- Estimated to be as common in physicians as in the general population affecting 12% of males and 15% of females.[6]
- Likely, depression is underreported due to associated stigma.
- A high professional burden may lead to social isolation.
- Physicians are more likely to become depressed with adverse life events (death of a family member, divorce).[7]

Divorce
- Marital issues are more common in physician marriages due to a tendency to delay addressing issues.[8]
- Divorce rates are thought to be higher in physicians than in the general population, but the true incidence is unknown.

Risk Factors
- Litigation stress[9]
- Burnout
- Social isolation
- Personal medical illness

DIAGNOSIS

- While physician impairment is well defined, there are no concrete diagnostic criteria due to the several possible underlying etiologies of impairment.

Clinical Presentation
- In 2005, a survey study was performed of the then 49 state PHPs with an 86% response rate.
- The major sources of referrals were as follows[10]:
  - Self-referrals (26%)
  - Clinical colleagues (20%)
  - State licensing board (21%)
  - Hospital medical staff (14%)
  - Other referral sources (17%)
    - Treatment providers, medical schools, law enforcement officials, family members, attorneys, and other PHPs
- Warning signs of impairment include the following[11]:
  - Deterioration in performance
    - Inconsistent work quality and lowered productivity
    - Spasmodic work pace leading to altered concentration
    - Signs of fatigue
    - Increased mistakes, carelessness, and errors in judgment
  - Poor attendance and absenteeism
    - Absenteeism and lateness increase in frequency, particularly before and after weekends.
    - Often will complain of vaguely defined illnesses, such as flu, upset stomach, sore throat, and headache.
  - Changes in attitude and physical appearance
    - Inattention to details; assignments are handled in a disorganized manner.
    - Others are blamed for the individual's own shortcomings.
    - Colleagues and supervisors are often deliberately avoided.
    - Personal appearance and ability to get along with others deteriorate.
    - Colleagues may show signs of poor morale and reduced productivity, often because of the time spent "covering up" for the impaired physician.
  - Increase in health and safety hazards
    - Higher than average accident rate emerges.
    - Machinery and equipment are handled carelessly.
    - Increased risk-taking behavior to compensate for periods of low achievement.

- Decreased regard for the safety of colleagues.
  ○ Emergence of domestic problems
  - Issues at home and with family increase.
  - Separation and divorce may occur.
  - Delinquent behavior in children is reported.
  - Financial problems recur with frequency.

It is impossible to note all the behavioral symptoms that may occur in this process of deterioration or to define precisely their sequence and severity. They may appear single or in combination, and they may very well signify problems other than substance abuse.[11]

- Areas where physician impairment may become apparent[11]:
  ○ Work–life balance
  ○ Clinical interactions/patient relationships
  ○ Chemical dependency
  ○ Obesity or lack of attention to personal fitness/health issues
  ○ Depression and other mental health issues
  ○ Loss of previously employed coping skills

TREATMENT

Physician Health Programs

- Present in 47 states except California, Nebraska, and Wisconsin.[12]
- Depending on the state, there are broad forms of rehabilitation available for a variety of conditions (e.g., drug addiction, depression).
- Both intensive outpatient and inpatient (from 1 to 3 months) treatment exists, with individual and group therapy available.[10]
- Physicians in treatment for substance abuse are protected by Title 42 in the Code of Federal Regulations (42 CFR) in addition to the Health Insurance Portability and Accountability Act (HIPAA) and do not need to disclose their addiction to colleagues or Medical Boards.[13]
- Physicians are typically monitored for 5 years after initiation of treatment and are subject to drug testing 5–7 days a week.[10]
- A retrospective cohort of 16 PHPs with 904 impaired physicians found a relapse of rate of drug/alcohol use of 19%. Of these physicians, 26% had a second positive test result.[14]
- Positive test results were monitored with more intensive therapy and more frequent testing.[10]

PHYSICIAN SUICIDE

- Physicians have a suicide rate that is 1.4–2.3 times the general population.[15]
- Female physicians attempt suicide less often, but complete suicide at an equal rate as male MDs, and therefore have a suicide rate of 2.3–4 times the general population.[15,16]
- The most common diagnoses in physicians that commit suicide are depression and bipolar disorder, alcoholism, and polysubstance abuse.[17]
- The most common means of suicide are prescription medication overdoses and firearms.[17]

OUTCOME/PROGNOSIS

- Incidence of physician self-reporting is increasing.[18]
- Of 904 physicians admitted to PHPs from 1995 to 2001, at 5-year follow up, 631 (78.7%) were licensed and working, 87 (10.8%) had their license revoked, 28 (3.5%) had retired, 30 (3.7%) had died, and 26 (3.2%) had unknown status.[14]

REFERENCES

1. ACEP Policy Statements: Physician Impairment. 2013. Available at: https://www.acep.org/Clinical—Practice-Management/Physician-Impairment/ (last accessed 4/10/16)
2. Andrew L, Brenner B. Physician Suicide. 2015. Available at: emedicine.medscape.com/article/806779-overview#a1
3. DesRoches CM, Rao SR, Fromson JA, et al. Physicians' perceptions, preparedness for reporting, and experiences related to impaired and incompetent colleagues. *JAMA* 2010; 304:187–93.
4. Earley PH. Physician health programs and addiction among physicians. In: Ries RK, ed. *The ASAM Principles of Addiction Medicine.* 5th ed. Philadelphia: Wolters Kluwer, 2014.
5. Rose J, Campbell M, Skipper G. Prognosis for emergency physician with substance abuse recovery: 5-year outcome study. *West J Emerg Med* 2014;15(1). doi: 10.5811/westjem.2013.7.17871. uciem_westjem_17871. Available at: http://escholarship.org/uc/item/6m2122s7
6. Rose J, Campbell M, Skipper G. Prognosis for emergency physicians with substance abuse recovery: 5-year outcome study. *West J Emerg Med* 2014;15(1). doi: 10.5811/westjem.2013.7.17871. uciem_westjem_17871. Available at: http://escholarship.org/uc/item/6m2122s7
7. Schernhammer E. Taking their own lives—the high rate of physician suicide. *N Engl J Med* 2005;352(24):2473–6.
8. Myers M. *Doctors' Marriages: A Look at the Problems and Their Solutions.* 2nd ed. New York: Springer, 1994.
9. Charles SC, Frisch PR. *Adverse Events, Stress, and Litigation: A Physician's Guide.* New York: Oxford University Press, 2005.
10. DuPont RL, McLellan AT, Carr G, et al. How are addicted physicians treated? A national survey of Physician Health Programs. *J Subst Abuse Treat* 2009;37:1–7.
11. Char D. *ACEP Physician Wellness Handbook.*
12. Federation of State Physician Heath Programs. Available at: http://fsphp.org/ (last accessed 30/12/14).
13. Reese S. Drug Abuse Among Doctors: Easy, Tempting, and Not Uncommon. Medscape Business of Medicine. Available at: http://www.medscape.com/viewarticle/819223_2
14. McLellan AT, Skipper GS, Campbell M, DuPont RL. Five year outcomes in a cohort study of physicians treated for substance use disorders in the United States. *BMJ* 2008;337:a2038.
15. Schernhammer ES, Colditz GA. Suicide rates among physicians: a quantitative and gender assessment (meta-analysis). *Am J Psychiatry* 2004;161(12):2295–302.
16. Frank E, Dingle AD. Self-reported depression and suicide attempts among U.S. women physicians. *Am J Psychiatry* 1999;156(12):1887–9.
17. Austin AE, van den Heuvel C, Byard RW. Physician suicide. *J Forensic Sci* 2013;58 (Suppl 1):S91–3.
18. Chesanow N. Impairment Among Physicians is Growing: Why? The Impaired Physician. Medscape Business of Medicine. Available at: http://www.medscape.com/viewarticle/840110
19. Merlo LJ, Singhakant S, Cummings SM, Cottler LB. Reasons for misuse of prescription medication among physicians undergoing monitoring by a physician health program. *J Addict Med* 2013;7:349–53.

146

EMS: Emergency Medical Services

Jeffrey Siegler and Vincent Boston

GENERAL PRINCIPLES

- Emergency medical services (EMS) is a growing part of the health care system that responds to medical emergencies and assists in the management of chronic medical conditions.
- EMS began as a "transport-only" system and has now evolved into a field that includes research and evidence-based care.
- When appropriate, EMS professionals may provide out-of-hospital medical care to patients in situations that do not require transport to an emergency department.

Definition

- EMS is evolving into a "community-based health management that is fully integrated with the overall health care system. It has the ability to identify and modify illness and injury risks, provide acute illness and injury care and follow-up, and contribute to treatment of chronic conditions and community health monitoring."[1]

CLASSIFICATION

EMS can be classified by several schemes. One of the schemes for classification looks at the funding stream for the EMS system, and another classifies EMS systems by the level of care or service that is provided.

Classification by Funding Source

Fire-Based EMS
- Fire-based EMS provides first-responder and transport services primarily via the 9-1-1 system and is a division within the local fire department.

Private EMS
- An EMS system that operates privately on a for-profit basis that provides both emergent and nonemergent transport

Hospital-Based EMS
- An EMS system that is operated by a hospital or hospital system that provides both emergent and nonemergent transport

Public Utility Model
- An EMS system in which a public agency purchases all components from a private EMS provider

Third Service EMS
- A government-run EMS system that is separate and distinct from other public service agencies such as police and fire

Volunteer EMS
- Volunteer EMS services depend on volunteers who are first responders or emergency medical technicians (EMTs) of varying levels.

Classification Based on Level of Care
Basic Life Support
- The BLS level provides basic emergency medical care and transportation for critical and emergent patients who access the emergency medical system. This level of care is normally provided by EMTs.

Advanced Life Support
- The ALS level provides advanced emergency medical care and transportation for critical and emergent patients who access the emergency medical system. This level of care is normally provided by at least one paramedic.

Critical Care Transport
- The critical care transport provides advanced emergency medical care and transportation for critical patients who are being transferred to between hospitals. At least one Critical Care Paramedic or RN normally provides this level of care. This level of care is most commonly encountered in the setting of air medical ambulances such as helicopters and fixed wing aircraft.

Components of an EMS System
An EMS system is comprised of several distinct components. According to the 1996 EMS Agenda for the Future, these components included the following:

- Integration of health services, EMS research, legislation and regulation, system finance, human resources, medical direction, education systems, public education, prevention, public access, communication systems, clinical care, information systems, and evaluation

Out-of-Hospital Providers
Emergency Medical Technician
- This individual possesses the basic knowledge and skills necessary to provide patient care and transportation. EMTs function as part of a comprehensive EMS response, under medical oversight. EMTs perform interventions with the basic equipment typically found on an ambulance.[2]
- Skills—simple oxygen delivery devices, airway adjuncts, manual ventilation, assisting patients with his/her own medications, administration of oral glucose and aspirin, splinting, hemorrhage control, and AED use.

Advanced Emergency Medical Technician
- This individual possesses the basic knowledge and skills necessary to provide patient care and transportation with a more fundamental knowledge base in caring for critical patients. Advanced Emergency Medical Technicians (AEMTs) also function as part of a comprehensive EMS response under medical oversight. AEMTs perform interventions with the basic and advanced equipment typically found on an ambulance.[2]
- Skills—all the skills of the EMT plus supraglottic airways, blood glucose monitoring, peripheral IV insertion, IV fluid administration, pediatric IO placement, administration of nitroglycerin, epinephrine for anaphylaxis, glucagon, dextrose, inhaled beta agonists, and narcotic antagonists.

TABLE 146.1	Hours of Training per Provider Level
Provider	**Hours of training**
Emergency first responder	40
Emergency medical technician	100–150
Advanced emergency medical technician	300–400
Paramedic	1000–1200

Paramedic
- This individual possesses the complex knowledge and skills necessary to provide patient care and transportation. Paramedics function as part of a comprehensive EMS response, under medical oversight. Paramedics perform interventions with the basic and advanced equipment typically found on an ambulance.[2]
- Skills—all the skills of the AEMT plus BiPAP, CPAP, needle decompression, orotracheal intubation, percutaneous cricothyroidotomy, capnography, EKG interpretation, blood chemistry analysis, central line monitoring, IO placement, administration of physician-approved medications, maintenance of blood administration, and thrombolytic initiation.

There are additional certifications available based on the work environment. These include Tactical Medic, Haz-Medic, Community Paramedic, Fight Paramedic, and Critical Care Paramedic. However, all of these individuals are licensed by the state as a paramedic.

Training

The time spent training varies depending on the classification of provider, as seen in Table 146.1.

INTERFACILITY TRANSPORT

- Arranged between the sending facility and the transport service.
- Must have an accepting physician.
- May be emergent or nonemergent.
- EMTALA applies here.

Modes of Transportation
- Ground ambulance
  - Staffed by two out-of-hospital providers
- Rotor wing (helicopter)
  - Most common staffing is one paramedic and one RN.
  - May use other medical providers like respiratory therapists, perfusionists, or physicians.
  - Limited by distance and weather. Extra time needed for patient packaging and engine warm-up/shutdown.[3]
  - Always approach a helicopter from the side or from downhill and only when cleared by the pilot.[3]
- Fixed wing
  - Has the ability to transport multiple patients.

○ Crew includes some complement of physicians, nurses, paramedics, respiratory therapists, or perfusionists.
○ Able to travel or fly farther distances, higher altitudes, and in inclement weather.
○ Requires a dedicated landing strip and transport to and from the airport to the hospital.

MEDICAL CONTROL/OVERSIGHT

• Advice and direction provided by a physician to out-of-hospital care providers who are providing medical care to a patient
• Direct medical control—the medical control that is provided while the out-of-hospital providers are actively caring for a patient
  ○ EMS physician on scene with the EMS providers.
  ○ ED physician communicating with the EMS providers via radio, cell phone, or video.
  ○ Patients can refuse transport if they demonstrate decision-making capacity and after risks and benefits have been discussed. Refusals must often be approved by a physician providing direct medical control.
• Indirect (off-line) medical control—any medical direction or oversight that is provided to out-of-hospital providers when not caring for a patient
  ○ Prospective: Protocol development and training, which are developed under a license from the medical director.
  ○ Retrospective: EMS chart review, QA/QI. Call reports are reviewed to assess whether treatment protocols were followed.

REFERENCES

1. Emergency Medical Services Agenda for the Future. US Department of Transportation, National Highway Traffic Association. 1996. Available at: www.ems.gov/pdf/2010/EMSA-gendaWeb_7-06-10.pdf
2. National EMS Scope of Practice Model. US Department of Transportation, National Highway Traffic Association. 2007. Available at: www.ems.gov/pdf/education/EMS-Education-for-the-Future-A-Systems-Approach/National_EMS_Scope_Practice_Model.pdf
3. Available at: https://www.nwmedstar.org/Helicopter-Safety/

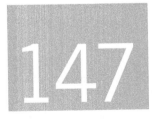

147 Coding and Documentation

David Seltzer

GENERAL PRINCIPLES

It is only through the written medical record that others can obtain the information of the patient encounter. It is important not only for medical personnel involved in the patient's care but also for collection of data for research and education, utilization review and quality of care evaluations, billing, and medical–legal situations. It is through careful and complete documentation that Coders are able to bill for services.

Basic evaluation and management codes (E/M codes) are based on documentation element of your history, exam, and medical decision making (MDM).

HISTORY

Chief Complaint

A concise statement, often in a patient's own words, of the reason the patient presents to the emergency department. This must be included in all records.

History of Present Illness

The history of present illness (HPI) is a chronologic description of the patient's present illness from its onset to the present. It includes eight elements: location, quality, severity, duration, timing, context, modifying factors, and associated signs/symptoms. A brief HPI describes one to three elements; an extended HPI contains at least four elements.

Review of Systems

The review of systems (ROS) is an inventory of body systems to identify signs/symptoms the patient has or had in the past. It is obtained by a series of questions. There are 14 systems recognized: constitutional symptoms (eyes; ears, nose, mouth, and throat), cardiovascular; respiratory; gastrointestinal; genitourinary; musculoskeletal; integumentary (skin and/or breast), neurologic, psychiatric, endocrine, hematologic and lymphatic, allergic, and immunologic. A problem-pertinent ROS reviews the system directly related to the chief complaint. An extended ROS includes 2–9 systems. A complete ROS includes 10–14 systems. It is permissible to individually document only the positive and pertinent negative responses with a notation indicating all other systems are negative if the patient was asked about 10 organ systems.

Past, Family, and Social History

The past history includes past illnesses, surgeries, injuries, and treatments. Family history reviews medical illnesses in close relatives that are hereditary or place the patient at medical risk. Social history reviews past and current activities including use of tobacco, alcohol and drugs. A pertinent past, family, and social history (PFSH) includes at least one item from any of the three history areas. A complete PFSH includes at least one item from at least two of the three PSFH areas.

PHYSICAL EXAMINATION

The exam consists of 14 organ systems: constitutional; eyes; ears, nose, mouth, and throat; neck; cardiovascular; respiratory; chest/breast; gastrointestinal; genitourinary; musculoskeletal; skin; neurologic; psychiatric; and lymphatic. There are defined elements within each organ system (Table 147.1). For a problem-focused exam, you must perform and document 1–5 defined elements in one or more organ systems. An expanded problem-focused exam should include exam and documentation of at least 6 defined elements in one or more organ systems. A detailed exam requires examination and documentation of at least 6 organ systems with at least 2 defined elements in each organ system or exam and documentation of at least 12 defined elements from 2 or more organ systems. A comprehensive exam will include at least

TABLE 147.1 Elements of the Physical Examination

Constitutional	• Measure any three of seven vital signs: blood pressure (sitting or standing, supine), pulse rate and regularity, respiration, temperature, height, weight • General appearance
Eyes	• Conjunctiva and lids • Pupils and irises • Ophthalmoscopic exam
Ears, nose, mouth, and throat	• External ear and nose • Otoscopic exam • Assess hearing • Inspect nasal mucosa, septum, turbinates • Inspection of lips, teeth, and gums • Examination of the oropharynx
Neck	• Examination of the neck • Examination of the thyroid
Respiratory	• Assessment of respiratory effort • Percussion of the chest • Palpation of the chest • Auscultation of the lungs
Cardiovascular	• Palpation of the heart • Auscultation of the heart • Examination of carotids, aorta, femoral arteries, pedal pulses, and extremities for edema/varicosities
Chest/breasts	• Inspection of the breasts • Palpation of the breasts and axillae
Gastrointestinal	• Examination of the abdomen • Examination of the liver and spleen • Presence or absence of hernia • Examination of the anus, perineum, and rectum (when indicated) • Stool sample for blood (when indicated)
Genitourinary (male)	• Examination of the scrotum • Examination of the penis • Digital rectal exam
Genitourinary (female)	• Pelvic exam • Examination of the uterus • Examination of the adnexa
Lymphatic	• Palpation in two or more areas: neck, axillae, groin, other
Musculoskeletal	• Examination of gait and station • Inspection/palpation of digits and nails • Examination of joints, bones, and muscles in one or more of the following: head and neck, spine, ribs and pelvis, right or left upper or lower extremities
Skin	• Inspection of skin and subcutaneous tissue • Palpation of skin and subcutaneous tissue
Neurologic	• Test cranial nerves • Examine deep tendon reflexes • Examination of sensation
Psychiatric	• Description of judgment and insight • Assessment of mental status: orientation, recent and remote memory, mood and affect

TABLE 147.2	Documentation Requirements Based Upon Extent of Service	
Extent of service	History	Physical examination
Problem focused	CC, brief HPI	Limited exam of affected part
Expanded	CC, brief HPI + Problem-pertinent system review	Limited exam of affected part plus other symptomatic or related organ system or body areas (6 elements total documented)
Detailed	Extended HPI + Extend review of systems + Pertinent past, family, and/or social history	Extended exam of the above (12 elements total documented)
Comprehensive	Extended HPI + Complete review of systems + Complete past, family, and social history	General multisystem exam or complete exam of a single organ system (must have at least 16 elements documented)

9 organ systems with every element in each system performed. Documentation of at least 2 defined elements from at least eight organ systems examined is expected (Table 147.2). Each organ system has specific exam requirements as well as exam elements from related organ systems.

MEDICAL DECISION MAKING (MDM)

There are four types of MDM: straightforward, low complexity, moderate complexity, and high complexity. This is measured by the number of possible diagnoses and/or management options; the amount and/or complexity of medical records, tests, and/or other information that must be obtained, reviewed, and analyzed; and the risk of significant complications, morbidity, and/or mortality, as well as comorbidities, associated with the patient's presenting problem, the diagnostic procedure, and/or possible management options.

Diagnoses

Listing diagnoses is an important part of the record. What is listed can support diagnostic testing as well as E/M coding level. List severe or traumatic diagnoses first. Listing the patient's chief complaint(s) is important in supporting the chart.

CRITICAL CARE

Current procedural terminology (CPT) currently defines a critical illness or injury as an illness or injury that "acutely impairs one or more vital organ systems such that there is a high probability of imminent or life threatening deterioration in the patient's condition." Critical care services are defined as care that "involves high complexity decision making to assess, manipulate, and support vital system functions(s) to treat single or multiple vital organ system failure and/or to prevent further life threatening deterioration of the patient's condition." Use of this code requires documentation of time directly managing the patient. This includes time spent documenting, reviewing labs and radiographs, discussing care with other health professionals, and discussion with family/HCPOA in patients who are unable to make medical decisions. Other services that can be included in critical care time are interpretation of cardiac output, chest plain radiographs, pulse oximetry, blood gases, gastric intubation, temporary transcutaneous pacing, ventilatory management, and peripheral vascular access procedures. These procedures should not be billed separately when counting toward critical care. Time spent on separately billable procedures and time spent teaching do not count toward critical care time. You must provide at least 30 minutes of services to bill. The "first hour" includes the first 74 minutes, and each additional 15–30 minutes time increment is billed separately. Time must be clearly documented and does not need to be continuous. Time spent on critical care services requires the full attention of the physician, and she/he, therefore, cannot provide services to other patients. If you were to work a 4-hour shift and provided two patients with a total of 4 hours of critical care, you are documenting that you only saw and billed for 2 patients that shift.

BEHAVIOR MODIFICATION COUNSELING

Tobacco cessation (intermediate) counseling must include face-to-face counseling and last 3–10 minutes. Documentation must include patient readiness for change, patient's barriers to change, advice in changing behavior, and specific suggested actions.

Substance abuse counseling (alcohol and/or drugs) can be billed but requires a documented evidence-based questionnaire followed by at least 15 minutes of face-to-face counseling with full documentation.

OBSERVATION

Nonsurgical extended duration therapeutic services, or observation as it is called, is a status, not a place. Observation care is a well-defined set of specific, clinically appropriate services. These services include ongoing short-term treatment, assessment, and reassessment to provide additional therapeutic treatment and avoid an inappropriate hospital admission or determine if the patient can be discharged from the hospital versus requirement of admission as an inpatient. Observation must last at least 8 hours, but no more than 48. The initial calendar day documentation must include 2 of the following: history, exam, and MDM. Observation services require an "admit to observation" order, periodic progress notes, and discharge summary.

SUGGESTED READING

CMS Manual System, Centers for Medicare & Medicaid Services (CMS), Department of Health & Human Services (DHHS). Pub 100-04 Medicare Claims Processing.

148 Social Media

Aldo Andino

GENERAL PRINCIPLES

- Social media is defined as internet-based resources that are used to share information, ideas, and other content (pictures and videos).
- Social media outlets include news/entertainment (Reddit), video (YouTube), social (Facebook, Instagram, Twitter), and professional networking (LinkedIn).

PROFESSIONALISM

- The American Medical Association has published a guideline for professionalism in the use of social media, summarized below:
  - Physicians should be aware of standards of patient privacy and confidentiality in all environments, including online.
  - Physicians on social networking sites should safeguard their privacy and content as much as possible but should understand that privacy settings are not absolute, and once content is on the internet, it is there permanently. Physicians should monitor their personal and professional information on their own sites, as well the content posted by others for accuracy and appropriateness.
  - The physician–patient relationship is held to the same ethical standards online as it is in any other context.
  - In order to maintain appropriate boundaries, physicians should consider separating personal and professional content online.
  - Physicians that observe unprofessional content online by a colleague are to bring it the attention of the individual and/or take other appropriate actions. If the behavior violates professional norms and the individual does not take appropriate action to resolve the situation, the physician should report the matter to the appropriate authorities.
  - Physicians must recognize that actions online and content posted may negatively affect their reputations, hinder their medical careers, and undermine public trust in the medical profession.

FREE OPEN-ACCESS MEDICAL EDUCATION (FOAM)

- Free Open-Access Medical Education (FOAM) is a dynamic collection of resources and tools for lifelong learning in medicine, as well as a community and an ethos.
- FOAM may be largely social media based but exists independent of a specific media or platform and includes blogs, podcasts, tweets, Google hangouts, web-based applications, online videos, text documents, photographs, and graphics.

SUGGESTED READINGS

Chretien KC, Greysen S, Chretien J, Kind T. Online posting of unprofessional content by medical students. *JAMA* 2009;302(12):1309–15. doi: 10.1001/jama.2009.1387.
Kavoussi SC, Huang JJ, Tsai JC, Kempton JE. HIPAA for physicians in the information age. *Conn Med* 2014;78(7):425–7.

Nickson CP, Cadogan MD. Free open access medical education (FOAM) for the emergency physician. *Emerg Med Australas* 2014;26:76–83. doi: 10.1111/1742-6723.12191.

Opinion 9.124—Professionalism in the Use of Social Media. From the AMA code of medical ethics. Available at: http://www.ama-assn.org/ama/pub/physician-resources/medical-ethics/code-medical-ethics/opinion9124.page?

Perrin A. Social Media Usage: 2005–2015. Available at: http://www.pewinternet.org/2015/10/08/social-networking-usage-2005-2015

Pillow MT, Hopson L, Bond M, et al. Social media guidelines and best practices: recommendations from the council of residency directors social media task force. *West J Emerg Med* 2014;15(1):26–30. doi: 10.5811/westjem.2013.7.14945. uciem_westjem_14945. Available at: http://escholarship.org/uc/item/8jh2p2mq

149 Violence in the Emergency Department

Vincent Boston and Robert Poirier

GENERAL PRINCIPLES

According to the Occupational Safety and Health Administration (OSHA), workplace violence is any act or threat of physical violence, harassment, intimidation, or other threatening disruptive behavior that occurs at the work site.[1] It is a growing safety concern for physicians, staff, and patients in the ED. The majority of reported incidents in the ED are verbal threats or abuse.[2,3]

Violence associated with patient care is the primary source of non-fatal injury in all health care organizations today. Hospital based medical workers currently have the highest rate of non-fatal assaults over all other sectors of employment.[4]

According to the Bureau of Labor Statistics' data, a nurse in the ED is three times more likely to be assaulted on the job than an average American worker, and health care workers are nearly four times as likely to require time away from work as a result of violence.[5]

The ED is the most common place in the hospital, regardless of hospital type, for violent incidents, and the majority of assaults on physicians are perpetrated by patients.[6]

Hospitals are especially high-risk areas for violence since they are open to the public 24 hours a day, every day of the year. The emergency department is particularly vulnerable since it is a high-traffic/high-stress area, making it difficult to secure.[7]

Factors that can lead to violence include unrestricted movement of individuals, the presence of gang members, drug or alcohol abusers, trauma patients, distraught family members, and long wait times.[8]

Methods of prevention can include posting uniformed officers in the ED, limiting the number of visitors, creating set visiting hours, screening the visitors for weapons, and conducting bag checks.

Profiling patients has been suggested as a preventative measure for preventing violence in the emergency department. Patients can be placed in a "high-risk" category for committing workplace violence that allows staff members to have the proper security and procedures in place to prevent incidents before they occur.

Patients who have previously been violent in emergency departments could have the potential to become violent again. A record of violence, if available to staff, may be helpful when assessing the patient's risk of behaving violently again.[9]

Workplace violence is often not reported to employers or law enforcement, particularly in the health care field. Incidents may be underreported because of the absence of institutional reporting policies, the perception that assaults are part of the job, employee beliefs that reporting will not benefit them, and employee concerns that assaults may be viewed as evidence of poor job performance or worker negligence.[10]

Recommendations for reducing violence include the following[8]:

- Training and education of health care employees in violence recognition and prevention methods
- Creating a code system, which alerts a specific violence response team
- Encouraging employees to report violent incidents without fear of repercussion
- Documenting violent encounters in patient's charts and flagging those charts to identify patients likely to become violent
- Restricting visiting access for persons with a history of violence
- Creating controlled access to waiting rooms and patient care areas of the emergency department
- Implementing the use of metal detectors and "bag checks" to screen patients for weapons

REFERENCES

1. Occupational Safety and Health Administration (OSHA). 2015. Guidelines for preventing workplace violence for healthcare and social service workers. No. 3148-04R. Available at: https://www.osha.gov/Publications/OSHA3826.pdf
2. Available at: https://www.osha.gov/OshDoc/data_General_Facts/factsheet-workplace-violence.pdf
3. Kowalenko T, Walters BL, Khare RK, Compton S. Workplace violence: a survey of emergency physicians in the state of Michigan. *Ann Emerg Med* 2005;46:142–7.
4. Rugala EA, Isaacs AR, eds. *Workplace Violence: Issues in Response.* Quantico, VA: Critical Incident Response Group, National Center for the Analysis of Violent Crime, FBI Academy, 2003. Available at: https://www.fbi.gov/stats-services/publications/workplace-violence
5. *Census of Fatal Occupational Injuries (CFOI)—Current and Revised Data.* Washington: Bureau of Labor Statistics, 2014. Available at: http://www.bls.gov/iif/oshcfoi1.htm
6. Stultz MS. Crime in hospitals 1995: the latest International Association for Healthcare Security and Safety Survey. *J Healthc Prot Manage* 1996–1997;13:1–45.
7. Preventing violence in the health care setting. *Sentinel Event Alert* 2010;45:1–3.
8. Rugala EA, Isaacs AR, eds. *Workplace Violence: Issues in Response.* Quantico, VA: Critical Incident Response Group, National Center for the Analysis of Violent Crime, FBI Academy, 2003. Available at: https://www.fbi.gov/stats-services/publications/workplace-violence
9. Kelen GD, Catlett CL, Kubit JG, Hsieh YH. Hospital-based shootings in the United States: 2000 to 2011. *Ann Emerg Med* 2012;60(6):790–8.e1.
10. Gacki-Smith J, Juarez AM, Boyett L, et al. Violence against nurses working in US emergency departments. *J Nurs Adm* 2009;39:340–9.

Index

Note: Page numbers in italics indicate figures; those followed by "t" indicates table.